Current Progress in Medicine and Health Science

Current Progress in Medicine and Health Science

Editor: Anna Garner

AMERICAN
MEDICAL PUBLISHERS
www.americanmedicalpublishers.com

AMERICAN
MEDICAL PUBLISHERS
www.americanmedicalpublishers.com

Cataloging-in-Publication Data

Current progress in medicine and health science / edited by Anna Garner.
p. cm.
Includes bibliographical references and index.
ISBN 978-1-63927-237-2
1. Medicine. 2. Health. 3. Medical sciences. 4. Public health. I. Garner, Anna.
R111 .C87 2022
610--dc23

American Medical Publishers,
41 Flatbush Avenue,
1st Floor, New York,
NY 11217, USA

ISBN 978-1-63927-237-2 (Hardback)

Contents

Preface

Medicine is a field of science that deals with the diagnosis, prognosis, treatment and prevention of diseases. Contemporary medicine or modern medicine uses biomedical sciences and research, genetics, surgeries, medical devices and technology for the diagnosis and treatment of different diseases. The branches of medicine are divided into three categories - basic sciences, medical specialties and interdisciplinary fields. Anatomy, biomechanics, genetics, immunology, physiology, etc. are a few branches that fall under basic sciences. Medical specialties include surgery, internal medicine, pathology, clinical neurophysiology, etc. Other interdisciplinary fields are aerospace medicine, evolutionary medicine, veterinary medicine, therapeutics, etc. Health science deals with the health of humans and animals. It has two divisions of study - the study and research of health, and its applications to promote health and functioning of the organisms. This book unravels the recent studies in the field of medicine and health science. It attempts to understand the multiple branches that fall under the discipline of medicine and health science and how such concepts have practical applications. The book will help the readers in keeping pace with the rapid changes in this field.

This book is the end result of constructive efforts and intensive research done by experts in this field. The aim of this book is to enlighten the readers with recent information in this area of research. The information provided in this profound book would serve as a valuable reference to students and researchers in this field.

At the end, I would like to thank all the authors for devoting their precious time and providing their valuable contribution to this book. I would also like to express my gratitude to my fellow colleagues who encouraged me throughout the process.

Editor

1

Efficacy and safety of methylene blue in the treatment of malaria

G. Lu[1,2], M. Nagbanshi[2], N. Goldau[2], M. Mendes Jorge[2], P. Meissner[3], A. Jahn[2], F. P. Mockenhaupt[4] and O. Müller[2*]

Abstract

Background: Methylene blue (MB) was the first synthetic antimalarial to be discovered and was used during the late 19th and early 20th centuries against all types of malaria. MB has been shown to be effective in inhibiting *Plasmodium falciparum* in culture, in the mouse model and in rhesus monkeys. MB was also shown to have a potent ex vivo activity against drug-resistant isolates of *P. falciparum* and *P. vivax*. In preclinical studies, MB acted synergistically with artemisinin derivates and demonstrated a strong effect on gametocyte reduction in *P. falciparum*. MB has, thus, been considered a potentially useful partner drug for artemisinin-based combination therapy (ACT), particularly when elimination is the final goal. The aim of this study was to review the scientific literature published until early 2017 to summarise existing knowledge on the efficacy and safety of MB in the treatment of malaria.

Methods: This systematic review followed PRISMA guidelines. Studies reporting on the efficacy and safety of MB were systematically searched for in relevant electronic databases according to a pre-designed search strategy. The search (without language restrictions) was limited to studies of humans published until February 2017.

Results: Out of 474 studies retrieved, a total of 22 articles reporting on 21 studies were eligible for analysis. The 21 included studies that reported data on 1504 malaria patients (2/3 were children). Older studies were case series and reports on MB monotherapy while recent studies were mainly controlled trials of combination regimens. MB was consistently shown to be highly effective in all endemic areas and demonstrated a strong effect on *P. falciparum* gametocyte reduction and synergy with ACT. MB treatment was associated with mild urogenital and gastrointestinal symptoms as well as blue coloration of urine. In G6PD-deficient African individuals, MB caused a slight but clinically non-significant haemoglobin reduction.

Conclusions: More studies are needed to define the effects of MB in *P. falciparum* malaria in areas outside Africa and against *P. vivax* malaria. Adding MB to ACT could be a valuable approach for the prevention of resistance development and for transmission reduction in control and elimination programs.

Systematic review registration: This study is registered at PROSPERO (registration number CRD42017062349).

Keywords: Malaria, Methylene blue, Efficacy and safety, Drug resistance, Elimination

* Correspondence: olaf.mueller@urz.uni-heidelberg.de
[2]Institute of Public Health, Medical School, Ruprecht-Karls-University Heidelberg, Heidelberg, Germany
Full list of author information is available at the end of the article

Background

Malaria remains the most important parasitic disease in humans [1]. Combination treatment of malaria has become the accepted paradigm in malaria control, with the particular aim of delaying and possibly reversing the development of drug resistance [2]. Artemisinin-based combination therapy (ACT) has become the standard treatment for falciparum malaria in virtually all endemic regions in the 21st century [3, 4]. However, artemisinin resistance is emerging in South-East Asia, and there is a clear need to develop strategies to protect the ACTs [5]. One potentially useful strategy could be to add a third drug with an independent anti-parasitic activity [6]. Moreover, the World Health Organization recommends the addition of a gametocytocidal drug such as primaquine (PQ) to current ACT regimens for malaria elimination programs [7].

Methylene blue (MB) is a water-soluble dye, which has been used for a long time in industry and medicine [8, 9]. The drug is rapidly and widely distributed throughout the body [10, 11]. The drug is well absorbed from the gastrointestinal tract and partly monodemethylated to azure B. Maximal plasma concentrations are reached 2 hours following oral administration, and the plasma half-life is about 20 h [12]. Renal excretion of MB and azure B (in oxidised blue or reduced uncoloured forms) is the main elimination pathway [13, 14].

MB is a registered drug in most countries for various indications, such as the treatment of both acquired and hereditary methaemoglobinaemia, the prevention of ifosfamide-induced encephalopathy in human cancer management, the prevention of urinary tract infections, the intraoperative visualisation of nerves and endocrine glands as well as of pathologic fistulae, and the sterilisation of transfusion blood [9, 15–23]. MB has also been considered to be effective in priapism, against septic shock (blocking the NO-dependant guanylate-cyclase) and in vasoplegic patients after cardiac surgery, and it is under investigation as an experimental drug against Alzheimer's disease [24–28]. MB was the first synthetic antimalarial to be used, which occurred in a German hospital some 120 years ago [29]. Its global use in malaria endemic areas is well documented for the late 19th and early 20th centuries [30, 31]. However, it stopped being used after new synthetic antimalarials were developed [9].

The interest in MB as an antimalarial drug was reactivated when *Plasmodium falciparum* glutathione reductase was identified as a new drug target [8, 32–34], although this concept has been questioned by other experimental evidence [35]. Like its major catabolite, azure B, MB is a subversive redox-cycling substrate, and like 4-aminoquinolines, it also interacts with the polymerisation of haem to hemozoin [34, 36–38]. Indeed, further but not yet fully understood mechanisms appear to be involved, which renders the development of resistance to MB with its multifactorial activity rather unlikely [9, 10]. The development of resistance to MB was proven to be difficult in vivo [39]. MB has been shown to be effective in inhibiting *P. falciparum* in culture, in the mouse model and in rhesus monkeys [40, 41]. MB was also shown to have a potent ex vivo activity against drug-resistant isolates of *P. falciparum* and *P. vivax* [42, 43]. In preclinical studies, MB acted synergistically with artemisinin derivates, but not with chloroquine (CQ), and was shown to have a strong effect on gametocyte reduction in *P. falciparum* [44–48]. MB has, thus, been considered a potentially useful partner drug for ACT, particularly when elimination is the final goal [49]. The aim of this study was to review the scientific literature published until early 2017 to summarise existing knowledge on the efficacy and safety of MB in the treatment of malaria.

Methods

This systematic review follows the PRISMA (Preferred Reporting Items for Systematic Reviews and Meta-Analyses) guidelines [50].

Study inclusion and exclusion criteria

All available and accessible data published until 28 February 2017 on the efficacy and/or safety of MB in the treatment of malaria were considered. Studies reporting data on MB given to humans of any age as monotherapy or in combination with other antimalarials and irrespective of drug formulations and sample size were included. In vitro and animal studies with MB, reports on the use of MB in humans for indications that were not malaria and review papers were excluded.

Search strategy and selection criteria

Standard electronic databases were searched for scientific papers on the subject, but also hand searches were done in scientific books of major libraries. The following databases were searched for studies published in any language: Medline, Embase, BIOSIS, Cochrane Central Register of Controlled Trials, Cochrane Library, Web of Science, and the China National Knowledge Infrastructure and the Chinese Biomedical databases. The search used combinations of the terms "malaria" and "methylene blue" as both medical subject headings and key or free text words and included a broad range of derivations to ensure as wide a search strategy as possible. A list of the detailed search strategy used is available online as Additional file 1. We also retrieved and manually searched articles with relevant titles but an unclear or no abstract. Bibliographies of reports were searched and additional relevant references identified and, where appropriate, included in the review.

Data extraction and analysis

The electronic reports identified were imported into the reference manager *Endnote* and duplicates removed. Each paper was assessed in two phases: first by screening title and abstract, and then by full-text review to ensure it met the inclusion criteria. The first assessment was done by two reviewers (MN and NG). The second assessment was done by GL and OM. An additional reviewer (AJ) settled any discordance between the reviewers.

Predetermined study characteristics were defined for extraction and documentation by two of the investigators (GL and OM), first independently and then in a consensus procedure. Reports selected were stratified according to study type. The primary outcome was the reported cure rate. Secondary outcomes were fever and parasite clearance rates, the effect on malaria gametocytes and adverse events (AEs).

Quality appraisal

Two of the investigators (GL and OM) evaluated the quality of included studies in a consensus procedure. The risk of bias of randomised controlled trials (RCTs) was evaluated by the tool described in the Cochrane Handbook for Systematic Reviews of Interventions [51]. The risk of bias in other controlled studies was evaluated by MINORS, for which 12 methodological items are reported [52]. Each domain was scored 0 (not reported), 1 (reported but inadequate) or 2 (reported and adequate). The maximum ideal score was 24.

Quality criteria for case series and case reports were developed from MINORS and the 2016 Critical Appraisal Checklist of the Joanna Briggs Institute for case reports and case series [52–54]. Seven methodological domains were evaluated (score 0 = not reported, score 1 = reported but inadequate or score 2 = reported and adequate). The maximum ideal score was 14. Where necessary, study authors have been contacted for clarification. Due to a lack of homogeneity among the studies, a meta-analysis was not possible.

Results

Study selection

Figure 1 summarises the selection process. After removing duplicates, the literature search identified 474 records of which 151 were selected for full text assessment (Additional file 2). Of these, 129 were excluded leaving 22 publications reporting on 21 studies for data extraction and further analysis [29, 55–75].

The most common reasons for exclusion were as follows: the manuscripts were reviews or comments or guidelines ($n = 47$), studies were not retrievable despite exhaustive efforts due to very old date ($n = 38$), manuscripts provided insufficient information ($n = 32$), preclinical studies ($n = 5$), MB was not used for treatment of malaria ($n = 4$), and patients were not treated with MB ($n = 3$).

General study characteristics

The 21 studies included are summarised in Table 1. They originated from Africa ($n = 7$), Asia ($n = 3$), the Americas ($n = 3$) and Europe ($n = 8$) and reported data on 1504 malaria patients (2/3 were children). The majority of reports were historical studies from around the year 1900 ($n = 15$), one was from the year 1949, and the remaining ($n = 5$) were published after the year 2000. The historical studies reported on malaria types diagnosed microscopically and/or clinically, which were not always well specified (of 368 cases, 30 were diagnosed as quartan malaria, 87 as tertian malaria, 183 as falciparum malaria, one as a double infection with tertian malaria and falciparum malaria, and the remaining were not specified). The more recently conducted controlled trials reported microscopically well determined outcomes on falciparum malaria ($n = 5$) and on vivax malaria ($n = 1$).

Study designs and MB regimens

Fifteen studies were historical case reports ($n = 5$) or case series ($n = 10$), while six studies were non-randomised controlled trials ($n = 3$) or RCTs ($n = 3$) from more recent years.

Summaries of treatment regimens are shown in Table 1. In the historical studies, MB was usually given in divided doses (e.g. five times per day) of 300–1000 mg per day in adults and 20–300 mg per day in children for 3–90 days as daily or interrupted (e.g. a 2-day pause after several days of treatment) oral monotherapy, with largely varying follow-up periods [29, 62, 64–67, 69]. In the controlled study on vivax malaria, MB was given to adults at a dose of 500 mg per day for 14 days in combination with isopentaquine (IQ) or in combination with IQ and quinine (Q) [61]. In the very recent RCTs on falciparum malaria, MB was given to children in various combination regimens [MB- CQ, MB-amodiaquine (AQ), MB-artesunate (AS) or MB-AQ-AS] in doses ranging from 4 mg/kg per day to 24 mg/kg per day, initially as 2–4 divided doses per day, and always for 3 days [56, 58, 60]. The latest dose regimen applied was 15 mg/kg per day in a single dose over 3 days [55]. In the only recently conducted MB monotherapy study, MB in adults was administrated at a fixed dose of 780 mg per day for 3, 5 or 7 days [59]. In the controlled studies, comparator regimens were CQ, AS-AQ, IQ and IQ-Q [56, 58, 60, 61].

Quality of included studies

Tables 2, 3 and 4 show the quality assessment of the studies included. The three RCTs had a low risk for bias and were consequently considered to be of high quality. Of the three non-RCTs, the two recently conducted

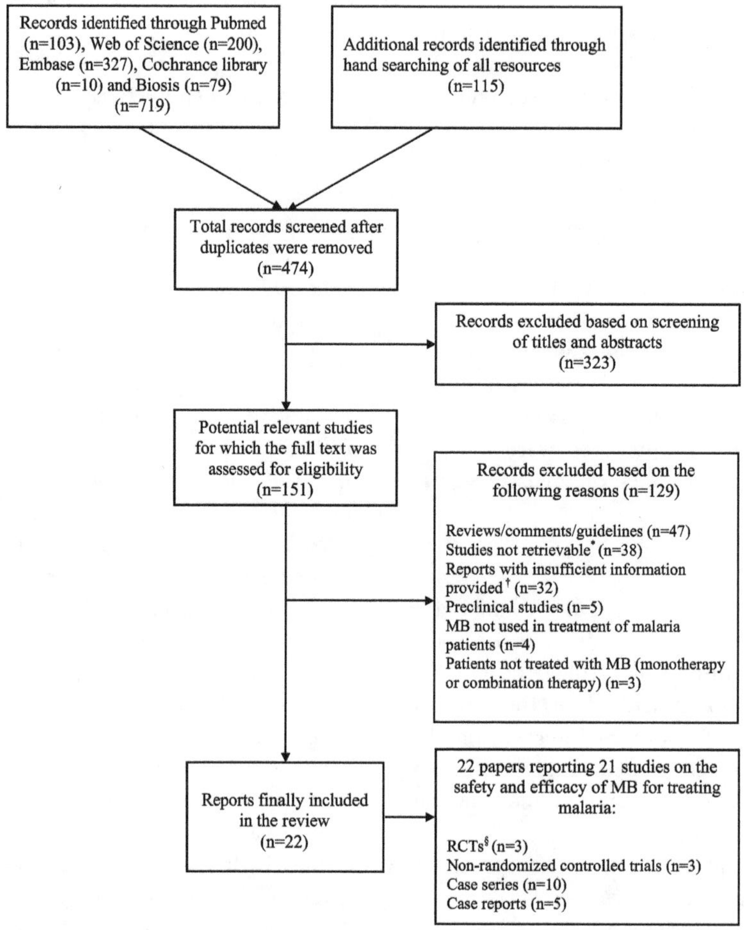

Fig. 1 Selection process of the review. * Original full article not available due to it being very old despite exhaustive searches of all possible resources including databases and libraries and making contact with journal archivists. † Information was missing on more than three parameters of the analysis and there was no possibility of getting this from other resources. MB methylene blue, RCT randomised controlled trial

studies scored rather high and were, thus, considered of high quality, while the study from 1949 had a relatively low quality score. The quality of the case series and case reports finally included in our review was overall high. The mean quality score was 10.53, and the majority of case series and case reports provided a clear description of malaria treatment and efficacy outcomes. The information most frequently missing from case series and reports was study participant characteristics (33.3%, 5/15) and safety outcomes (26.7%, 4/15).

Efficacy of MB against asexual parasites

In MB monotherapy studies conducted around the year 1900, 337/373 (90%) of malaria cases were reported to be cured. Reported potential reasons for treatment failure were: unsuccessful quinine pretreatment ($n = 8$), vomiting of treatment ($n = 3$), low dose of MB ($n = 6$) and unknown ($n = 19$). In a more recent trial, MB monotherapy in 60 West African adults with falciparum malaria (a fixed dose of 780 mg for 3 days) showed a 100% cure rate when MB was given for 7 days compared to a 85% cure rate when MB was given for a shorter time period; this difference was close to being statistically significant [59].

Like MB in the combination treatment, a controlled study on vivax malaria among US prisoners from 1949 reported a cure rate of 6/9 (67%) for MB plus IQ and of 3/3 (100%) for MB plus IQ plus quinine [61]. In the recent RCTs among West African children with falciparum malaria, MB-based regimens ($n = 391$) showed superior efficacy compared to control regimens ($n = 207$). In the first trial, the cure rate of MB (4 mg/kg per day) plus CQ (56%) was slightly but non-significantly higher compared to that of CQ alone (46%) [58]. A subsequent dose-finding study demonstrated an improved efficacy (77%) of MB-CQ when higher doses of MB (12–24 mg/kg per day) were used [60]. A third study compared the regimens MB-AQ, MB-AS (MB at 20 mg/kg per day) and

Table 1 Summary of included studies assessing methylene blue (MB) in the treatment of malaria

Study: First Author Place of study (Year)	Patient information	Malaria type	Malaria diagnosis	MB treatment	Follow-up	Efficacy outcome	Safety outcome	Other Information
Randomised controlled trials								
Coulibaly et al. Burkina Faso (2015) [55]	$n = 193$ (6–59-month-old children)	*P. falciparum*	By microscope	Arm 1: AS-AQ-MB ($n = 92$) (MB: 15 mg/kg per day for 3 days) Arm 2: AS-AQ ($n = 101$) Formulation: mini-tablets	28 days	ACPR was 80% in arm 1, and 85% in arm 2. Significant lower gametocyte prevalence on day 7 in arm 1 compared to arm 2 (both microscopically and molecular biologically) Clearance of *P. falciparum* asexual parasites in AS-AQ-MB took 1.82 days compared to 1.96 days in the AS-AQ group	MB regimen was associated with more vomiting. Haemoglobin values were significantly lower in arm 1 than in arm 2 at day 2 and day 7 (difference 0.5–1.0 mg/dl)	(1) There were no differences in parents and caregivers self-reported acceptance rate between groups (2) The MB mini-tablets were provided on a spoon with local food to improve the acceptability for children
Zoungrana et al. Burkina Faso (2008) [56, 57]	$n = 180$ (6–10-year-old children)	*P. falciparum*	By microscope	Arm 1: MB-AS ($n = 61$) Arm 2: MB-AQ ($n = 58$) (MB: 20 mg/kg per day for 3 days) Arm 3: AS-AQ ($n = 61$) Formulation: taste-masked tablets	28 days	ACPR was 62% in arm 1, 95% in arm 2 and 82% in arm 3 MB regimens were associated with a more rapid parasite clearance and significantly reduced gametocyte prevalence during follow-up	MB regimen was associated with vomiting and dysuria	Vomiting was shown to be much reduced by administering MB together with food
Meissner et al. Burkina Faso (2005) [58]	$n = 226$ (6–59-month-old children)	*P. falciparum*	By microscope	Arm 1: CQ-MB ($n = 181$) (MB: 4 mg/kg per day for 3 days) Arm 2: CQ ($n = 45$) Formulation: 0.5% MB solution	14 days	ACPR was 56% (93/166) in arm 1 compared to 46% (19/41) in arm 2	No differences in SAEs, and no cases of severe haemolysis No differences in haemoglobin over time in both the G6PD-deficient and G6PD-sufficient subgroups	Administration of the bitter-tasting MB solution was sometimes difficult, especially in younger children
Non-randomised control trials								
Bountogo et al. Burkina Faso (2010)[a] [59]	$n = 60$ (age range: 18–55 years, median 25)	*P. falciparum*	By microscope	Arm 1: MB for 7 days ($n = 20$) Arm 2: MB for 5 days ($n = 20$) Arm 3: MB for 3 days ($n = 20$) MB: 780 mg per day Formulation: taste-masked tablets	28 days	Arm 1: 0/20 recrudescence Arm 2: 4/19 recrudescence Arm 3: 2/20 recrudescence	Dysuria (47/60). Gastrointestinal symptoms (13/60). No significant differences in adverse events between groups	MB was given at a dose of 390 mg twice daily after breakfast and supper
Meissner et al. Burkina Faso (2006)[b] [60]	$n = 435$ (6–59-month-old children)	*P. falciparum*	By microscope	Arm 1: CQ-MB ($n = 156$) (MB: 12 mg/kg per day for 3 days) Arm 2: CQ-MB ($n = 155$) (MB: 18 mg/kg per day for 3 days) Arm 3: CQ-MB ($n = 123$) (MB: 24 mg/kg per day for 3 days) Formulation: 2.3% MB solution	14 days	Overall clinical and parasitological cure rate on day 14 was 90% (326/364) and 77% (278/364) respectively, without differences between groups	There were three SAEs, one probably associated with MB Haemoglobin development was not associated with G6PD deficiency	MB was given with fruit flavouring and honey supplement to mask the bitter taste

Table 1 Summary of included studies assessing methylene blue (MB) in the treatment of malaria *(Continued)*

Study: First Author Place of study (Year)	Patient information	Malaria type	Malaria diagnosis	MB treatment	Follow-up	Efficacy outcome	Safety outcome	Other Information
Alving (1949) Cited by Baird et al. USA (2012)[a] [61]	$n = 37$	*P. vivax*	Clinical	Arm 1: IQ ($n = 10$) Arm 2: IQ-quinine ($n = 15$) Arm 3: IQ-MB ($n = 9$) (MB: 500 mg per day) Arm 4: IQ-MB-quinine ($n = 3$) (MB: 500 mg per day) All treatments were for 14 days	14 days	Arm 1: 9/10 relapsed Arm 2: 5/15 relapsed Arm 3: 3/9 relapsed Arm 4: 0/3 relapsed	1/10 in arm 1 experienced severe haemolysis; after being treated again with IQ plus MB for 14 days, no haemolysis	–
Case series								
Mayer Russia (1919) [62]	$n = 3$	*P. malariae*	By microscope	1000 mg per day over 30 days (16 days MB and 14 days breaks); MB divided into five doses of 200 mg per day	52–72 days	2/3: cure 1/3: relapsed after 4 months	Mild urogenital symptoms despite daily nutmeg application	–
Panse Africa (1902) [63]	$n = 2$	*P. malariae*	By microscope	Case 1: 400–1000 mg per day for 14 days Case 2: 600–1000 mg per day for 32 days	14–32 days	Case 1: cure Case 2: failure	No safety information	Both patients were pretreated with quinine
Glogner Indonesia (1901) [64]	$n = 6$ (2 adults, 4 children)	*P. vivax/ovale*	By microscope	Adults: 1000 mg every 2 days; 1000 mg per day Children: 300 mg per day every 5 days; 300 mg per day every 2 days	2–7 months	6/6 relapsed	No safety information	All patients were pretreated with quinine
Ollwig (1899) Africa [65]	$n = 10$	*P. vivax/ovale* (3/10) *P. falciparum* (4/10) *P. malariae* (1/10) *P. vivax/ovale* and *P. falciparum* (1/10) Unspecified (1/10)	By microscope	300 mg per day to 1000 mg per day for 3 days to 14 days, followed by breaks of 5–8 days. The regimen was cycled up to 3 months	8 days to 3 months	7/10: cured 3/10: failure	Urogenital symptoms ($n = 2$) Vomiting after MB intake ($n = 3$) Diarrhoea ($n = 1$)	Frequent vomiting of MB reported in 2/3 failure cases 6/10 cases were pretreated with quinine Nutmeg was taken together with MB against urogenital symptoms
Cardamatis Greece (1898) [66]	$n = 275$ (157/118 male/female); 129 children, 91 youths, 55 adults	*P. vivax/ovale* (72/275) *P. falciparum* (178/275) *P. malariae* (21/275) Unspecified *(4/275)*	Clinical	In 245/275 MB monotherapy Adults: 400–500 mg per day Youth: 300 mg per day Children: 200 mg per day Infants: 20–40 mg per day Regimens given in four doses per day (every 2 hours) initially for 6–12 days and for a	Up to 1 year	257/275 cured 18/275 failure	Urogenital symptoms observed only with very high MB doses Colouring properties in particular in association with vomiting of children	Good efficacy in quinine non-responders Nutmeg was taken together with MB against urogenital symptoms

Table 1 Summary of included studies assessing methylene blue (MB) in the treatment of malaria *(Continued)*

Study: First Author Place of study (Year)	Patient information	Malaria type	Malaria diagnosis	MB treatment	Follow-up	Efficacy outcome	Safety outcome	Other Information
				total of 22–60 days (with variable pauses) In 30/275 MB in combination with quinine or arsenic				
Röttger Germany (1895) [67]	*n* = 7	No specific information	Clinical	600–800 mg per day for 8–33 days	8–33 days	6/7 cured 1/7 failure	1/7 vomiting after MB1/7 urogenital symptoms	Nutmeg helped to reduce the urogenital side effects
Ferreira Brazil (1893) [68]	*n* = 21 (2–180-month-old children, median 18 months)	No specific information	Clinical	200–600 mg per day, usually in divided doses, for 3–30 days	3–30 days (median 9 days)	21/21 cured	1/21 reported urogenital symptoms	5/21 initial treatment with quinine failed
Parenski and Blatteis Europe (1893) [69]	*n* = 35	No specific information	By microscope	800–1500 mg per day	7 days to 4 months	33/35 cases cured after 7 days 2/35 failure	Divided small doses (0.1–0.2 g) of MB rarely produced side effectsDivided higher doses (0.4–0.6 g) of MB produced more side effects, in particular vomiting and urogenital symptoms	Medicinale MB Merck free of chlorinated zinc, lead and arsenic was used
Thayer USA (1892) [70]	*n* = 7 (age range: 17–58 years, median 33)	*P. vivax/ovale* (3/7) *P. malariae* (1/7) Unspecified (3/7)	Clinical	400–1000 mg per day for 7–23 days	7–23 days	4/7 cured 3/7 failure	Urogenital symptoms (3/7) Dizziness (1/7)	Nutmeg was taken together with MB to reduce urogenital symptoms
Guttmann and Ehrlich Germany (1891) [29]	*n* = 2	*P. vivax/ovale*	By microscope	500 mg per day for 12–24 days	1–2 months	2/2 cured	Urogenital symptoms (*n* = 1)	Nutmeg was taken together with MB to reduce urogenital symptoms
Case reports								
Mühlens and Kirschbaum Germany (1921) [71]	*n* = 1	*P. vivax/ovale*	By microscope	1000 mg per day for 7 days followed by alternating 5-day breaks and 3-day treatments with 1000 mg per day for 3 months	3 months	Cured	No safety information	Nutmeg was taken together with MB to reduce urogenital symptoms
Atkinson China (1903) [72]	*n* = 1 (male child)	Unspecified	By microscope	300 mg per day	11 days	Cured	Gastrointestinal disorder	Initial treatment with quinine failed
Sivers Germany (1901) cited by Merck (1922) [73, 74]	*n* = 1 (15-year-old girl)	*P. vivax/ovale*	By microscope	500 mg per day	3 days	Cured	Vomiting	–

Table 1 Summary of included studies assessing methylene blue (MB) in the treatment of malaria *(Continued)*

Study: First Author Place of study (Year)	Patient information	Malaria type	Malaria diagnosis	MB treatment	Follow-up	Efficacy outcome	Safety outcome	Other Information
Anonymous Germany (1893) [75]	$n = 1$ (32-year-old man)	*P. vivax/ovale*	By microscope	1000 mg on day 1, 500 mg on day 2, then 300 mg for 14 days, then continued treatment for 6 weeks	2 months	Parasite-free on day 7, relapse on day 14, and cured without relapse on day 60	Urogenital symptoms	MB dose for treatment after relapse not specified Nutmeg helped to reduce urogenital side effects
Trintignan India (1882) cited by Röttger (1895) [67]	$n = 1$	*P. falciparum*	Clinical	2000 mg per day during acute attack, followed by 500 mg per day until day 20	20 days	Cured	None	–

ACPR **adequate clinical and parasitological response,** ***AQ*** **amodiaquine,** ***AS*** **artesunate,** ***CQ*** **chloroquine,** ***IQ*** **isopentaquine,** ***MB*** **methylene blue,** ***SAE*** **serious adverse event**
[a]Controlled phase II study
[b]Phase II dose-finding study

Table 2 Quality assessment of included randomised controlled trials

Study: First Author Place of study (Year)	Selection bias[a] (random sequence generation)	Allocation concealment bias[a]	Performance bias[a] (blinding of the participants and personnel)	Detection bias[a] (blinding of outcome assessment)	Attribution bias[a] (incomplete outcome data)	Reporting bias[a] (selective reporting)
Coulibaly et al. Burkina Faso (2015) [55]	Low	Low	Low	Low	Low	Low
Zoungrana et al. Burkina Faso (2008) [56, 57]	Low	Low	Low	Low	Low	Low
Meissner et al. Burkina Faso (2005) [58]	Low	Low	Low	Low	Low	Low

[a]Assessed as low, unclear or high risk of bias

AS-AQ. The cure rates were 95%, 62% and 82%, respectively, and these differences were statistically significant [56]. Finally, a trial that compared AS-AQ-MB (MB at 15 mg/kg per day) with AS-AQ produced similar cure rates in both regimens (80% vs 85%) [55].

Parasite clearance with MB appeared to be rather slow. In African adults treated with MB monotherapy, 9% were still parasitaemic on day 3 [59]. In children treated with MB-CQ or CQ, the median parasite clearance time did not differ (91.3 and 86.4 h) [58]. In children treated with MB-AS, only 2% were parasitaemic on day 3, i.e., a significantly lower proportion than following treatment with AS-AQ (5%) or MB-AQ (17%) [56]. The clearance time for the *P. falciparum* parasite was non-significantly shortened in children receiving AS-AQ-MB compared to the AS-AQ group (medians 43.7 vs 47.0 h) [55]. Fever was cleared rapidly in all of these studies without differences between MB and comparator regimens [55, 56, 58].

Table 3 Quality assessment of included non-randomised controlled trials

Methodological item	Score for studies[a] Bountogo et al. Burkina Faso (2010) [59]	Meissner et al. Burkina Faso (2006) [60]	Alving (1949) Cited by Baird et al. (2012) [61]
Clearly stated aim	2	2	1
Inclusion of consecutive patients	2	2	1
Prospective collection of data	2	2	0
End points appropriate to the aim of the study	1	2	1
Unbiased assessment of the study end point	2	2	0
Follow-up period appropriate to the aim of the study	2	2	1
Loss to follow-up less than 5%	2	2	0
Prospective calculation of the study size	2	2	0
Adequate control group	1	2	1
Contemporary groups	1	1	1
Baseline equivalence of groups	1	2	0
Adequate statistical analyses	2	2	0
Total score	20	23	6

[a]The items are scored 0 (not reported), 1 (reported but inadequate) or 2 (reported and adequate). The global ideal score was 24 for comparative studies

Efficacy of MB against gametocytes

Gametocyte clearance following MB-based treatment was investigated in two RCTs. The first study was a secondary analysis of data from an RCT in children. Compared to AS-AQ, both MB-containing regimens were associated with significantly reduced gametocyte carrier rates during follow-up days 3, 7 and 14 [57]. The second study, in which post-treatment gametocyte prevalence was the main outcome variable, demonstrated a significantly lower figure in children treated with MB-AS-AQ compared to AS-AQ on day 7 of follow-up (microscopically, 1% vs 9%; by QT-NASBA, 37% vs 63%) [55].

Safety and acceptability of MB

Treatment of malaria with MB was consistently associated with green-blue discoloration of urine. AEs concerning the urogenital system (urethritis) and the gastrointestinal system (vomiting) were reported to be associated with MB treatment. These AEs were more frequently reported with higher doses of MB [65, 66, 69, 75]. Vomiting in children was often associated with the bitter taste of MB, depending on the type of formulation. In two RCTs, vomiting in MB-containing regimens ranged from 24% to 68% [55, 56]. Urethritis was reported in 78% of adults and in 55% of older children treated with MB, but this symptom was not reported from RCTs in preschool children [56, 59]. In the controlled studies, severe adverse events (SAEs) were rarely reported and none were attributed to MB [60]. In particular, there were no cases of severe haemolysis associated with MB.

Despite some AEs being clearly associated with MB treatment, one study reported no differences between study groups in acceptance rates by parents and caregivers of children [55].

Discussion

This is the first review within the last 100 years to attempt systematically to collect and analyse all the data that have been published on the effects of MB in the treatment of human malaria. As MB was used for this indication globally in the late 19th and early 20th

Table 4 Quality assessment of included case series and case reports

Study: First Author Place of study (Year)	Score for studies[a]							Total score
	What is the overall degree of presentation of study details?	Detailed presentation of study participant characteristics?	Case definition clearly reported?	Clear description of malaria treatment reported?	Clear reporting on the follow-up period?	Appropriate reporting of efficacy outcomes?	Appropriate reporting of safety outcomes?	
Case series								
Mayer Russia (1919) [62]	2	0	2	2	2	2	2	12
Panse Africa (1902) [63]	2	0	2	2	1	1	0	8
Glogner Indonesia (1901) [64]	2	2	2	2	1	1	0	10
Ollwig Africa (1899) [65]	2	1	1	2	1	2	2	11
Cardamatis Greece (1898) [66]	1	0	1	2	1	1	1	7
Röttger Germany (1895) [67]	2	2	1	2	1	2	2	12
Ferreira Brazil (1893) [68]	2	2	1	2	2	2	2	13
Parenski and Blatteis Europe (1893) [69]	1	0	1	2	1	1	1	7
Thayer USA (1892) [70]	2	2	1	2	1	2	2	12
Guttmann and Ehrlich Germany (1891) [29]	2	2	2	2	1	2	2	13
Case reports								
Mühlens Germany (1921) [71]	1	0	2	2	2	2	0	9
Atkinson China (1903) [72]	1	1	1	2	2	2	1	10
Sivers Germany (1901) cited by Merck (1922) [73, 74]	1	2	2	2	1	1	2	11

Table 4 Quality assessment of included case series and case reports *(Continued)*

Study: First Author Place of study (Year)	Score for studies[a]							Total score
	What is the overall degree of presentation of study details?	Detailed presentation of study participant characteristics?	Case definition clearly reported?	Clear description of malaria treatment reported?	Clear reporting on the follow-up period?	Appropriate reporting of efficacy outcomes?	Appropriate reporting of safety outcomes?	
Anonymous Germany (1893) [75]	2	2	2	2	2	2	2	14
Trintignan India (1882) cited by Röttger (1895) [67]	1	1	1	2	2	2	0	9

[a]The items are scored 0 (not reported), 1 (reported but inadequate) or 2 (reported and adequate). The global ideal score was 14 for case series and case reports

centuries, some early reviews were published at that time. In 1904, a meta-analysis of 425 malaria cases from 11 publications concluded that MB was effective in 85% of patients [30].

In the early 20th century, MB was gradually replaced by new synthetic antimalarials with different characteristics and finally without colouring properties [9]. Scientists at Bayer used MB as the starting point for systematic antimalarial testing of synthetic compounds. Thus, the first synthetic drug designed as an antimalarial, pamaquine, was derived from MB [76].

The revival of MB as an antimalarial drug candidate began in 1995, at the height of the development of resistance against existing antimalarials, in three biochemical laboratories [32, 35, 38]. A key achievement was the detection that MB inhibits the glutathione reductase of *P. falciparum* [8]. Considerably elevated glutathione levels were found in CQ-resistant *P. falciparum* strains, triggering the hypothesis that combining MB and CQ might overcome resistance [8]. This was the rationale to start clinical trials with MB in the early 21st century.

Efficacy of MB against malaria

In our analysis of 15 case reports and case series, 339/373 (91%) of patients were cured, which provides evidence for the high efficacy of MB monotherapy in the treatment of malaria. Treatment failures were attributed to previously unsuccessful quinine treatment, vomiting and a low and/or short MB dosing regimen, which helps to explain early controversies on whether quinine or MB was more effective against malaria [63–65, 77]. Conducted in tropical as well as in non-tropical areas and including all types of human malaria, these early studies were of overall good external validity. Interestingly, the MB dosing schedules used in these early studies were rather similar to what has been found to be effective in a MB dose-finding study in African children as well as in a proof of principle MB monotherapy study in African adults [59, 60].

In the recent studies, MB was usually given in combination with other antimalarials and tested in RCTs. In an area of high CQ resistance, MB-CQ was more effective than CQ alone but not sufficiently so [58, 60]. Combining MB with AS, AQ or AS-AQ and increasing MB doses in these combinations did not lead to a substantial increase in efficacy [55, 56]. This indicates that the curative efficacy of MB in eliminating asexual parasitaemia appears to be limited in the study region of Burkina Faso compared to the cure rates observed roughly a hundred years ago in a variety of settings. There is no evidence for and—because of the lack of drug pressure—no reason to expect that MB resistance has emerged meanwhile. The actual causes of the comparatively lower efficacy of MB-containing regimens in the recent studies, thus, remains unclear. Total dosage and a generally longer treatment period in the older studies might be relevant, however.

Despite this limitation, other properties of MB are notable and promising. Adding MB to an ACT reinforced the particular beneficial effects of the artemisinins, i.e., it further accelerated the elimination of asexual *P. falciparum* parasites and reduced *P. falciparum* gametocytes [55–57]. The epidemiological relevance of the latter observation has recently been confirmed by a phase II study in Mali, which showed a 100% reduction of mosquito infectivity by day 7 both with PQ- and MB-containing drug regimens through membrane feeding assays [78]. This supports findings from preclinical studies on an existing synergy between MB and artemisinins as well as on the very strong effects of MB on *P. falciparum* gametocyte reduction [41, 44, 45, 79]. Interestingly, the efficacy of MB against gametocytes had been observed in historical studies [30]. However, further studies to identify the lowest effective dose for the gametocytocidal effect of MB in falciparum malaria should be conducted.

Safety of MB in malaria treatment

In the historical studies, MB was usually given orally and often in high doses and for prolonged periods of time, both in children and in adults, and without reports of major safety problems. During World War I for example, some European soldiers received more than 400 g of MB over several weeks without major side effects, apart from moderate urogenital symptoms [31]. Brazilian children were reported to tolerate 20–50 mg/kg per day of MB very well for long periods of time [68]. Also, in the recent RCTs conducted in West Africa, MB treatment was not associated with SAEs. However, while MB given orally seems to be largely well tolerated, MB given intravenously must be applied with caution. Intravenous MB is often routinely given as the first-line treatment for acute acquired methemoglobinemia in doses of 1–2 mg/kg, but a dose of 7 mg/kg can lead to severe gastrointestinal symptoms [9]. Moreover, a dose of 5 mg/kg has been reported to be associated with an altered mental status during parathyroidectomy [80]. For sheep, the LD50 of MB was found to be 42 mg/kg when applied intravenously [81].

AEs shown to be associated with MB treatment are mild gastrointestinal symptoms, which may manifest as vomiting, and mild urogenital symptoms, which usually manifest shortly after drug intake. This has consistently been reported, both in historical studies and in more recently conducted RCTs. Pure MB powder or MB dissolved in water has a very bitter and metallic taste. The gastrointestinal symptoms are clearly influenced by the formulation of MB, which suggests it is better to use taste-masked formulations. As the World Health

Organization is now also recommending solid formulations for small children, mini-tablets, which should also be taste-masked, will be preferred over liquid formulations [82]. MB given with food and with a small amount of grated nutmeg has consistently been described as being effective in suppressing the frequently reported gastrointestinal and urogenital AEs [30, 60, 66]. Finally, both MB and PQ were recently shown to be well tolerated in males in Mali [78].

MB is on the list of drugs potentially dangerous for patients with G6PD deficiency, but the clinical importance of this is still controversial [83, 84]. In this review, no association between MB and severe haemolysis has been detected. Nevertheless, in a pooled analysis of all recent studies conducted with MB against falciparum malaria in West African children (including one unpublished RCT), small effects were seen. In 844 MB-treated African children, two patients developed severe anaemia (Hb < 5 g/dL) during the first days of treatment and both were G6PD deficient. Minimal Hb concentrations following MB treatment did not significantly differ in children with and without G6PD deficiency. However, when modelling the Hb time course, an MB dose-dependent effect of lowering Hb concentrations was observed for children with a full G6PD defect (hemi- and homozygous deficiency; prevalence, 10%). The maximal difference compared to non-deficient peers was estimated as –0.9 g/dl on day 5 of the follow-up, which is, however, considered to be of limited clinical relevance [85]. In sub-Saharan Africa, the moderate A minus type of X-chromosomally inherited G6PD deficiency (15–25% enzyme activity) dominates and affects 10–25% of the population. G6PD-deficient red blood cells have increased sensitivity to oxidative stress originating from various triggers including antimalarial drugs [86]. Whether or not MB confers an increased risk in malaria patients with more severe variants of G6PD deficiency needs to be evaluated in future studies, e.g. in South-East Asia. There are, however, reports of MB being associated with severe haemolytic reactions in neonatal G6PD deficiency [87, 88]. Finally, MB at low concentration is a strong inhibitor of monoamine oxidase A and therefore, should not be given together with serotonin reuptake inhibitors [89].

Reassuringly and despite the characteristic AE profile, MB has been well accepted by patients and caregivers of children in West Africa, which was also supported by an anthropological study in Burkina Faso [90]. However, the acceptance of its colouring properties also needs to be studied in other populations and cultures.

Strengths and limitations

The strength of this review is that it includes all studies ever conducted with MB or MB-containing regimens in humans with malaria irrespective of study design and sample size and irrespective of the language of the report. Moreover, it can be considered as beneficial that a number of authors of this review have been the investigators of all recently conducted studies on this topic. Limitations of this review are the lower quality of the historical studies included compared to recent RCTs, the availability of three reports only in an abbreviated form from other sources [73, 91, 92] and the non-availability of a number of studies due to their old age despite extensive searches.

Conclusions

This review shows that MB has substantial antimalarial activity against all types of malaria in various endemic areas and, in combination with other antimalarials, against falciparum malaria in Africa. Although MB alone appears to act rather slowly against the asexual parasites of *P. falciparum*, it shows synergy with the artemisinin component in rapidly clearing the parasites and it is very effective in reducing the gametocytes and consequently mosquito transmission. MB is usually well tolerated and accepted with mild and regularly self-limiting gastrointestinal and urogenital symptoms, which are the main AEs. To avoid vomiting, the drug should be given in a taste-masked formulation and/or together with food. In historical studies, nutmeg has been shown to be effective in moderating the frequent occurrence of urethritis, which should be evaluated in future studies. Whether the small effect of MB on the haemoglobin development is of clinical significance needs to be monitored in future large-scale studies including regions with more severe forms of G6PD deficiency compared to African populations.

MB appears to be a potential alternative to PQ for reducing post-treatment infectivity in *P. falciparum* infections, a useful partner for triple combination therapy regimens with the goal of protecting the artemisinin component of the ACT and of reducing the spread of drug-resistant parasites, and a potentially valuable partner drug for mass drug administration in malaria elimination programs. Further studies should investigate the efficacy, safety and community acceptance of different ACT regimens in combination with MB against falciparum malaria in different areas inside and outside Africa, while well-designed pilot studies should investigate the effects of MB and MB-containing combination regimens as a treatment for vivax malaria.

Additional files

Additional file 1: Search strategy. (DOCX 12 kb)

Additional file 2: A list of all the records screened after duplicates were removed (*N* = 474). (PDF 329 kb)

Abbreviations

ACT: Artemisinin-based combination therapy; AE: Adverse event; AQ: Amodiaquine; AS: Artesunate; CQ: Chloroquine; IQ: Isopentaquine;

MB: Methylene blue; PQ: Primaquine; Q: Quinine; RCT: Randomised controlled trial; SAE: Severe adverse event

Acknowledgements
We thank Dr Olaf Horstick for his helpful comments on the draft paper.

Funding
The project was funded by BASF (Germany) to celebrate its 150th birthday and to acknowledge that MB was the first product patented by the firm. BASF was neither involved in the design and conduct of the study nor in data analysis and interpretation. The paper was written by the authors without any interference by BASF.

Authors' contributions
GL and OM designed the study. MN and NG did the initial literature searches. GL and OM, with support from MN and NG, analysed the data. All authors contributed to the interpretation of the data and to writing of the paper. All authors read and approved the final manuscript.

Competing interests
The authors declare that they have no competing interests.

Author details
[1]Medical College of Yangzhou University, Yangzhou University, Yangzhou 225001, China. [2]Institute of Public Health, Medical School, Ruprecht-Karls-University Heidelberg, Heidelberg, Germany. [3]Department of Paediatric and Adolescent Medicine, Ulm University, Ulm, Germany. [4]Institute of Tropical Medicine and International Health, Charité-Universitätsmedizin Berlin, Berlin, Germany.

References
1. White NJ, Pukrittayakamee S, Hien TT, Faiz MA, Mokuolu OA, Dondorp AM. Malaria. Lancet. 2014;383(9918):723–35.
2. Nosten F, Brasseur P. Combination therapy for malaria: the way forward? Drugs. 2002;62(9):1315–29.
3. Adjuik M, Babiker A, Garner P, Olliaro P, Taylor W, White N, International Artemisinin Study G. Artesunate combinations for treatment of malaria: meta-analysis. Lancet. 2004;363(9402):9–17.
4. WHO. World malaria report 2016. Geneva: World Health Organization; 2016
5. Noedl H, Se Y, Schaecher K, Smith BL, Socheat D, Fukuda MM, Artemisinin Resistance in Cambodia 1 Study C. Evidence of artemisinin-resistant malaria in western Cambodia. N Engl J Med. 2008;359(24):2619–20.
6. White NJ. Antimalarial drug resistance. J Clin Invest. 2004;113(8):1084–92.
7. WHO. Guidelines for the treatment of malaria-3rd edition. Geneva: World Health Organization; 2015.
8. Schirmer RH, Coulibaly B, Stich A, Scheiwein M, Merkle H, Eubel J, Becker K, Becher H, Muller O, Zich T, et al. Methylene blue as an antimalarial agent. Redox Rep. 2003;8(5):272–5.
9. Schirmer RH, Adler H, Pickhardt M, Mandelkow E. Lest we forget you–methylene blue. Neurobiol Aging. 2011;32(12):2325. e2327-2316
10. Wainwright M, Amaral L. The phenothiazinium chromophore and the evolution of antimalarial drugs. Tropical Med Int Health. 2005;10(6):501–11.
11. Warth A, Goeppert B, Bopp C, Schirmacher P, Flechtenmacher C, Burhenne J. Turquoise to dark green organs at autopsy. Virchows Arch. 2009;454(3):341–4.
12. Walter-Sack I, Rengelshausen J, Oberwittler H, Burhenne J, Mueller O, Meissner P, Mikus G. High absolute bioavailability of methylene blue given as an aqueous oral formulation. Eur J Clin Pharmacol. 2009;65(2):179–89.
13. DiSanto AR, Wagner JG. Pharmacokinetics of highly ionized drugs. II. Methylene blue–absorption, metabolism, and excretion in man and dog after oral administration. J Pharm Sci. 1972;61(7):1086–90.
14. Peter C, Hongwan D, Kupfer A, Lauterburg BH. Pharmacokinetics and organ distribution of intravenous and oral methylene blue. Eur J Clin Pharmacol. 2000;56(3):247–50.
15. Mansouri A, Lurie AA. Concise review: methemoglobinemia. Am J Hematol. 1993;42(1):7–12.
16. Coleman MD, Coleman NA. Drug-induced methaemoglobinaemia. Treatment issues. Drug Saf. 1996;14(6):394–405.
17. Cawein M, Behlen CH 2nd, Lappat EJ, Cohn JE. Hereditary Diaphorase Deficiency and Methemoglobinemia. Arch Intern Med. 1964;113:578–85.
18. Zulian GB, Tullen E, Maton B. Methylene blue for ifosfamide-associated encephalopathy. N Engl J Med. 1995;332(18):1239–40.
19. Kupfer A, Aeschlimann C, Wermuth B, Cerny T. Prophylaxis and reversal of ifosfamide encephalopathy with methylene-blue. Lancet. 1994;343(8900): 763–4.
20. Orth K, Ruck A, Stanescu A, Beger HG. Intraluminal treatment of inoperable oesophageal tumours by intralesional photodynamic therapy with methylene blue. Lancet. 1995;345(8948):519–20.
21. O'Leary JL, Petty J, Harris AB, Inukai J. Supravital staining of mammalian brain with intra-arterial methylene blue followed by pressurized oxygen. Stain Technol. 1968;43(4):197–201.
22. Williamson LM, Cardigan R, Prowse CV. Methylene blue-treated fresh-frozen plasma: what is its contribution to blood safety? Transfusion. 2003;43(9):1322–9.
23. Floyd RA, Schneider JE Jr, Dittmer DP. Methylene blue photoinactivation of RNA viruses. Antivir Res. 2004;61(3):141–51.
24. Van der Horst C, Stuebinger H, Seif C, Melchior D, Martinez-Portillo FJ, Juenemann KP. Priapism - etiology, pathophysiology and management. Int Braz J Urol. 2003;29(5):391–400.
25. Juffermans NP, Vervloet MG, Daemen-Gubbels CRG, Binnekade JM, de Jong M, Groeneveld ABJ. A dose-finding study of methylene blue to inhibit nitric oxide actions in the hemodynamics of human septic shock. Nitric Oxide-Biol Ch. 2010;22(4):275–80.
26. Levin RL, Degrange MA, Bruno GF, Del Mazo CD, Taborda DJ, Griotti JJ, Boullon FJ. Methylene blue reduces mortality and morbidity in vasoplegic patients after cardiac surgery. Ann Thorac Surg. 2004;77(2):496–9.
27. Oz M, Lorke DE, Petroianu GA. Methylene blue and Alzheimer's disease. Biochem Pharmacol. 2009;78(8):927–32.
28. Wischik CM, Edwards PC, Lai RY, Roth M, Harrington CR. Selective inhibition of Alzheimer disease-like tau aggregation by phenothiazines. Proc Natl Acad Sci U S A. 1996;93(20):11213–8.
29. Guttmann P, Ehrlich P. Über die wirkung des methylenblau bei malaria. Berliner Klin Wochenschr. 1891;28:935–56.
30. Wood HC. The use of methylene blue in malarial fevers. Proc Phila Co Med Soc. 1904;25:281–6.
31. Marshall DG. The "toxicity" of methylene-blue. Lancet. 1920;195(5051):1334.
32. Farber PM, Arscott LD, Williams CH Jr, Becker K, Schirmer RH. Recombinant Plasmodium falciparum glutathione reductase is inhibited by the antimalarial dye methylene blue. FEBS Lett. 1998;422(3):311–4.
33. Sarma GN, Savvides SN, Becker K, Schirmer M, Schirmer RH, Karplus PA. Glutathione reductase of the malarial parasite Plasmodium falciparum: crystal structure and inhibitor development. J Mol Biol. 2003;328(4):893–907.
34. Buchholz K, Schirmer RH, Eubel JK, Akoachere MB, Dandekar T, Becker K, Gromer S. Interactions of methylene blue with human disulfide reductases and their orthologues from Plasmodium falciparum. Antimicrob Agents Chemother. 2008;52(1):183–91.
35. Pastrana-Mena R, Dinglasan RR, Franke-Fayard B, Vega-Rodriguez J, Fuentes-Caraballo M, Baerga-Ortiz A, Coppens I, Jacobs-Lorena M, Janse CJ, Serrano AE. Glutathione reductase-null malaria parasites have normal blood stage growth but arrest during development in the mosquito. J Biol Chem. 2010; 285(35):27045–56.
36. Atamna H, Krugliak M, Shalmiev G, Deharo E, Pescarmona G, Ginsburg H. Mode of antimalarial effect of methylene blue and some of its analogues on Plasmodium falciparum in culture and their inhibition of P. vinckei petteri and P. yoelii nigeriensis in vivo. Biochem Pharmacol. 1996;51(5):693–700.
37. Kanzok SM, Schirmer RH, Turbachova I, Iozef R, Becker K. The thioredoxin system of the malaria parasite Plasmodium falciparum. Glutathione reduction revisited. J Biol Chem. 2000;275(51):40180–6.

38. Davioud-Charvet E, Delarue S, Biot C, Schwobel B, Boehme CC, Mussigbrodt A, Maes L, Sergheraert C, Grellier P, Schirmer RH, et al. A prodrug form of a Plasmodium falciparum glutathione reductase inhibitor conjugated with a 4-anilinoquinoline. J Med Chem. 2001;44(24):4268–76.
39. Thurston JP. The chemotherapy of Plasmodium berghei. I. Resistance to drugs. Parasitology. 1953;43(3–4):246–52.
40. Vennerstrom JL, Makler MT, Angerhofer CK, Williams JA. Antimalarial dyes revisited: xanthenes, azines, oxazines, and thiazines. Antimicrob Agents Chemother. 1995;39(12):2671–7.
41. Ohrt C, Li Q, Obaldia N, Im-Erbsin R, Xie L, Berman J. Efficacy of intravenous methylene blue, intravenous artesunate, and their combination in preclinical models of malaria. Malar J. 2014;13:415.
42. Pascual A, Henry M, Briolant S, Charras S, Baret E, Amalvict R, Huyghues d, Etages E, Feraud M, Rogier C, Pradines B. In vitro activity of Proveblue (methylene blue) on *Plasmodium falciparum* strains resistant to standard antimalarial drugs. Antimicrob Agents Chemother. 2011;55(5):2472–4.
43. Wirjanata G, Sebayang BF, Chalfein F, Prayoga, Handayuni I, Trianty L, Kenangalem E, Noviyanti R, Campo B, Poespoprodjo JR, et al. Potent Ex Vivo Activity of Naphthoquine and Methylene Blue against Drug-Resistant Clinical Isolates of Plasmodium falciparum and Plasmodium vivax. Antimicrob Agents Chemother. 2015;59(10):6117–24.
44. Akoachere M, Buchholz K, Fischer E, Burhenne J, Haefeli WE, Schirmer RH, Becker K. In vitro assessment of methylene blue on chloroquine-sensitive and -resistant Plasmodium falciparum strains reveals synergistic action with artemisinins. Antimicrob Agents Chemother. 2005;49(11):4592–7.
45. Adjalley SH, Johnston GL, Li T, Eastman RT, Ekland EH, Eappen AG, Richman A, Sim BK, Lee MC, Hoffman SL, et al. Quantitative assessment of Plasmodium falciparum sexual development reveals potent transmission-blocking activity by methylene blue. Proc Natl Acad Sci U S A. 2011;108(47):E1214–23.
46. Garavito G, Bertani S, Rincon J, Maurel S, Monje MC, Landau I, Valentin A, Deharo E. Blood schizontocidal activity of methylene blue in combination with antimalarials against Plasmodium falciparum. Parasite. 2007;14(2):135–40.
47. Haynes RK, Cheu KW, Li KY, Tang MM, Wong HN, Chen MJ, Guo ZF, Guo ZH, Coghi P, Monti D. A partial convergence in action of methylene blue and artemisinins: antagonism with chloroquine, a reversal with verapamil, and an insight into the antimalarial activity of chloroquine. ChemMedChem. 2011;6(9):1603–15.
48. Garavito G, Bertani S, Quiliano M, Valentin A, Aldana I, Deharo E. The in vivo antimalarial activity of methylene blue combined with pyrimethamine, chloroquine and quinine. Mem Inst Oswaldo Cruz. 2012;107(6):820–3.
49. Müller O, Sie A, Meissner P, Schirmer RH, Kouyate B. Artemisinin resistance on the Thai-Cambodian border. Lancet. 2009;374(9699):1419.
50. Liberati A, Altman DG, Tetzlaff J, Mulrow C, Gotzsche PC, Ioannidis JP, Clarke M, Devereaux PJ, Kleijnen J, Moher D. The PRISMA statement for reporting systematic reviews and meta-analyses of studies that evaluate health care interventions: explanation and elaboration. PLoS Med. 2009;6(7):e1000100.
51. Higgins JP, Altman DG, Gotzsche PC, Juni P, Moher D, Oxman AD, Savovic J, Schulz KF, Weeks L, Sterne JA, et al. The Cochrane Collaboration's tool for assessing risk of bias in randomised trials. BMJ. 2011;343:d5928.
52. Slim K, Nini E, Forestier D, Kwiatkowski F, Panis Y, Chipponi J. Methodological index for non-randomized studies (minors): development and validation of a new instrument. ANZ J Surg. 2003;73(9):712–6.
53. Critical appraisal tools-checklist for case reports. http://joannabriggs.org/assets/docs/critical-appraisal-tools/JBI_Critical_Appraisal-Checklist_for_Case_Reports2017.pdf.
54. Critical appraisal tools-checklist for case series. http://joannabriggs.org/assets/docs/critical-appraisal-tools/JBI_Critical_Appraisal-Checklist_for_Case_Series2017.pdf.
55. Coulibaly B, Pritsch M, Bountogo M, Meissner PE, Nebie E, Klose C, Kieser M, Berens-Riha N, Wieser A, Sirima SB, et al. Efficacy and safety of triple combination therapy with artesunate-amodiaquine-methylene blue for falciparum malaria in children: a randomized controlled trial in Burkina Faso. J Infect Dis. 2015;211(5):689–97.
56. Zoungrana A, Coulibaly B, Sie A, Walter-Sack I, Mockenhaupt FP, Kouyate B, Schirmer RH, Klose C, Mansmann U, Meissner P, et al. Safety and efficacy of methylene blue combined with artesunate or amodiaquine for uncomplicated falciparum malaria: a randomized controlled trial from Burkina Faso. PLoS One. 2008;3(2):e1630.
57. Coulibaly B, Zoungrana A, Mockenhaupt FP, Schirmer RH, Klose C, Mansmann U, Meissner PE, Muller O. Strong gametocytocidal effect of methylene blue-based combination therapy against falciparum malaria: a randomised controlled trial. PLoS One. 2009;4(5):e5318.
58. Meissner PE, Mandi G, Witte S, Coulibaly B, Mansmann U, Rengelshausen J, Schiek W, Jahn A, Sanon M, Tapsoba T, et al. Safety of the methylene blue plus chloroquine combination in the treatment of uncomplicated falciparum malaria in young children of Burkina Faso [ISRCTN27290841]. Malar J. 2005;4:45.
59. Bountogo M, Zoungrana A, Coulibaly B, Klose C, Mansmann U, Mockenhaupt FP, Burhenne J, Mikus G, Walter-Sack I, Schirmer RH, et al. Efficacy of methylene blue monotherapy in semi-immune adults with uncomplicated falciparum malaria: a controlled trial in Burkina Faso. Tropical Med Int Health. 2010;15(6):713–7.
60. Meissner PE, Mandi G, Coulibaly B, Witte S, Tapsoba T, Mansmann U, Rengelshausen J, Schiek W, Jahn A, Walter-Sack I, et al. Methylene blue for malaria in Africa: results from a dose-finding study in combination with chloroquine. Malar J. 2006;5:84.
61. Baird KJ, Maguire JD, Price RN. Diagnosis and treatment of Plasmodium vivax malaria. Adv Parasitol. 2012;80:203–70.
62. Mayer M. Über die Wirkung von Methylenblau bei Malaria quartana. Deutsch Med Wochenschrift. 1919;45:1052–3.
63. Panse O. Schwarzwasserfieber. Aus dem Gouvernementskrankenhaus Taga, Deutsch-Ostafrika. Veit & Comp: Leipzig; 1902.
64. Glogner M. Ein Beitrag zur Beurtheilung der Malaria Rezidive und ihrer Behandlung. Berlin: Springer; 1900.
65. Ollwig D. Ein Beitrag zur Behandlung der Malaria mit Methylenblau. Z Hyg. 1899;31(31):318–36.
66. Cardamatis JP. 275 klinische Beobachtungen über das Methylenblau. Deutsche Med Wochenschrift Ther Beilage. 1898;2(9):9–10.
67. Röttger W. Ein Beitrag zur Behandlung der Malaria mit Methylenblau. Kiel: University Kiel; 1895.
68. Ferreira MC. Sur l'emploi du bleu de méthylène dans la malaria infantile. Ther Medico-Chirugicale. 1893;124:488–525.
69. Parenski S, Blatteis S. Über das Methylenblau bei Malaria. Ther Monatshefte. 1893;7:16–9.
70. Thayer WS. On the Value of methylene blue in malarial fever. Bull Johns Hopkins Hosp. 1892;2(22):49–53.
71. Mühlens P, Kirschbaum W. Parasitologische und klinische Beobachtungen bei künstlichen Malaria und Recurrensübertragungen. Z Hyg Infekt. 1921;94:1–28.
72. Atkinson JM. Ocimum Viride and Malaria. Lancet. 1903;162(4169):265–6.
73. Sivers R. Finska Läkaresällskapets Handlingar. 1901;43:857.
74. Merck E. Merck's Wissenschaftliche Abhandlungen aus den Gebieten der Pharmakotherapie, Pharmazie und verwandter Disziplinen-Anilinfarben in der Therapie. Darmstadt: Darmstadt; 1922.
75. Anonymous. Über Methylenblau. Dtsch Med Wochenschr. 1893;19(1):23.
76. Krafts K, Hempelmann E, Skorska-Stania A. From methylene blue to chloroquine: a brief review of the development of an antimalarial therapy. Parasitol Res. 2012;111(1):1–6.
77. Kaufmann P. Ueber die Wirkung des Methylenblau bei Malaria. Dtsch Med Wochenschr. 1919;49:1365.
78. Dicko A, Roh ME, Diawara H, Mahamar A, Soumare HM, Lanke K, Bradley J, Sanogo K, Kone DT, Diarra K, et al. Efficacy and safety of primaquine and methylene blue for prevention of Plasmodium falciparum transmission in Mali: a phase 2, single-blind, randomised controlled trial. Lancet Infect Dis. 2018. https://doi.org/10.1016/S1473-3099(18)30044-6. Epub ahead of print.
79. Siciliano G, Santha Kumar TR, Bona R, Camarda G, Calabretta MM, Cevenini L, Davioud-Charvet E, Becker K, Cara A, Fidock DA, et al. A high susceptibility to redox imbalance of the transmissible stages of Plasmodium falciparum revealed with a luciferase-based mature gametocyte assay. Mol Microbiol. 2017;104(2):306–18.
80. Kahn M, North A, Chadwick D. Prolonged postoperative altered mental status after methylene blue infusion during parathyroidectomy: a case report and review of literature. Ann R Coll Surg Engl. 2007;89(2):W9–W11.
81. Burrows GE. Methylene blue: effects and disposition in sheep. J Vet Pharmacol Ther. 1984;7(3):225–31.
82. Orubu ES, Tuleu C. Medicines for children: flexible solid oral formulations. Bull World Health Organ. 2017;95(3):238–40.
83. Youngster I, Arcavi L, Schechmaster R, Akayzen Y, Popliski H, Shimonov J, Beig S, Berkovitch M. Medications and glucose-6-phosphate dehydrogenase deficiency: an evidence-based review. Drug Saf. 2010;33(9):713–26.

84. Müller O, Meissner P, Mansmann U. Glucose-6-phosphate dehydrogenase deficiency and safety of methylene blue. Drug Saf. 2012;35(1):85. author reply 85-86.
85. Müller O, Mockenhaupt FP, Marks B, Meissner P, Coulibaly B, Kuhnert R, Buchner H, Schirmer RH, Walter-Sack I, Sie A, et al. Haemolysis risk in methylene blue treatment of G6PD-sufficient and G6PD-deficient West-African children with uncomplicated falciparum malaria: a synopsis of four RCTs. Pharmacoepidem Dr S. 2013;22(4):376–85.
86. Cappellini MD, Fiorelli G. Glucose-6-phosphate dehydrogenase deficiency. Lancet. 2008;371(9606):64–74.
87. Gauthier TW. Methylene blue-induced hyperbilirubinemia in neonatal glucose-6-phosphate dehydrogenase (G6PD) deficiency. J Matern Fetal Med. 2000;9(4):252–4.
88. Kirsch I, Cohen H. Heinz body hemlytic anemia from the use of methylene blue in neonates. J Pediatr. 1980;96(2):276–8.
89. Ramsay RR, Dunford C, Gillman PK. Methylene blue and serotonin toxicity: inhibition of monoamine oxidase A (MAO A) confirms a theoretical prediction. Br J Pharmacol. 2007;152(6):946–51.
90. Sanon S, Ollivier E, Azas N, Mahiou V, Gasquet M, Ouattara CT, Nebie I, Traore AS, Esposito F, Balansard G, et al. Ethnobotanical survey and in vitro antiplasmodial activity of plants used in traditional medicine in Burkina Faso. J Ethnopharmacol. 2003;86(2–3):143–7.
91. Trintignan. Du bleu de methylene dans le paludisme et dans la blenhorragie. Bull Med Paris. 1892;46:943–4.
92. Alving AS, Eichelberger L, Arnold JJE. The clinical testing of antimalarial drugs at Stateville Penitentiary. Semi-Annual Report 1948–49 1949, NIH Malaria Report NO. 87. (USPHS Antimalarial Grant No.RG 198).

2

Validity of an online 24-h recall tool (myfood24) for dietary assessment in population studies: comparison with biomarkers and standard interviews

Petra A. Wark[1,2†], Laura J. Hardie[3†], Gary S. Frost[4†], Nisreen A. Alwan[5,10], Michelle Carter[6], Paul Elliott[7], Heather E. Ford[4], Neil Hancock[6], Michelle A. Morris[8], Umme Z. Mulla[1], Essra A. Noorwali[6,9], K. Petropoulou[4], David Murphy[3], Gregory D. M. Potter[3], Elio Riboli[7], Darren C. Greenwood[3,8†] and Janet E. Cade[6*†]

Abstract

Background: Online dietary assessment tools can reduce administrative costs and facilitate repeated dietary assessment during follow-up in large-scale studies. However, information on bias due to measurement error of such tools is limited. We developed an online 24-h recall (myfood24) and compared its performance with a traditional interviewer-administered multiple-pass 24-h recall, assessing both against biomarkers.

Methods: Metabolically stable adults were recruited and completed the new online dietary recall, an interviewer-based multiple pass recall and a suite of reference measures. Longer-term dietary intake was estimated from up to 3 × 24-h recalls taken 2 weeks apart. Estimated intakes of protein, potassium and sodium were compared with urinary biomarker concentrations. Estimated total sugar intake was compared with a predictive biomarker and estimated energy intake compared with energy expenditure measured by accelerometry and calorimetry. Nutrient intakes were also compared to those derived from an interviewer-administered multiple-pass 24-h recall.

Results: Biomarker samples were received from 212 participants on at least one occasion. Both self-reported dietary assessment tools led to attenuation compared to biomarkers. The online tools resulted in attenuation factors of around 0.2–0.3 and partial correlation coefficients, reflecting ranking intakes, of approximately 0.3–0.4. This was broadly similar to the more administratively burdensome interviewer-based tool. Other nutrient estimates derived from myfood24 were around 10–20% lower than those from the interviewer-based tool, with wide limits of agreement. Intraclass correlation coefficients were approximately 0.4–0.5, indicating consistent moderate agreement.

Conclusions: Our findings show that, whilst results from both measures of self-reported diet are attenuated compared to biomarker measures, the myfood24 online 24-h recall is comparable to the more time-consuming and costly interviewer-based 24-h recall across a range of measures.

Keywords: Nutrition assessment, Online, Biomarkers, Validation, Nutritional epidemiology, Nutrient intake, Food, Diet, Adult

* Correspondence: j.e.cade@leeds.ac.uk
†Petra A. Wark, Laura J. Hardie, Gary S. Frost, Darren C. Greenwood and Janet E. Cade contributed equally to this work.
[6]Nutritional Epidemiology Group, School of Food Science and Nutrition, University of Leeds, Leeds LS2 9JT, UK
Full list of author information is available at the end of the article

Background

Robust assessment of the association between diet and health in population-based studies requires accurate and often repeated measurements of diet [1]. Food frequency questionnaires (FFQs), often the method of choice in large population studies, provide a convenient assessment of usual, longer-term diet. Many assumptions are made with the use of FFQs, including lists of foods likely to be consumed, portion sizes and the frequency of consumption [2]. FFQs and food recall checklists are not easy to adapt for different population groups, including ethnic minorities, due to their reliance on previously defined lists of a limited number of foods. Only a minority allow for addition of foods not listed in the pre-set food lists. The use of 24-h dietary recalls can provide more accurate intake data, with reduced measurement error, for a given day [3–5]. Use of more detailed 24-h recalls traditionally administered by trained dietitians [6] are costly to implement, with large volumes of paper-based prompts, and if not automated, they are expensive and time-consuming to code. The 24-h recalls have been prohibitively expensive for large-scale studies, especially when repeat measures are required to estimate longer-term or usual intake [1]. The capability to collect an automated, self-administered 24-h recall makes it feasible to collect multiple days of recalls to characterise usual intake in large-scale observational studies and national dietary surveys. A single recall does not capture day-to-day variation and does not allow for examination of changes in dietary patterns over time or inclusion as time-dependent covariates [7, 8]. Repeated application would reduce bias from random measurement error and allow for changes in dietary patterns. Online dietary recall systems for research have been developed and tested in the USA and some European countries. The US National Cancer Institute's ASA24® (Automated Self-Administered 24-Hour Dietary Assessment Tool), for example, can be used to collect both 24-h dietary recalls and food records and as of August 2017 has been used by 3500 studies in the USA, Canada and Australia [9, 10]. DietDay is another online 24-h recall system being used in epidemiological research in the USA [11, 12], and a comprehensive 24-h online dietary assessment food record is being used in a large cohort study conducted in France [12, 13]. In the UK, INTAKE24 [14] and the Oxford WebQ [15] are new online tools measuring diet using a recall and questionnaire format respectively. Although most of these tools have been compared to other established dietary assessments, very few have been validated against independent dietary biomarkers [16, 17].

An automated 24-h dietary recall, such as the one we have developed and report here, has potential advantages over FFQs and interviewer-administered recalls with the opportunity for self-administration, reducing interviewer and possible coding costs. Whilst still retaining the detail of information acquired on food type and amount consumed, the number of prompts used in a paper-based system are minimised to avoid user fatigue and restricted to likely forgotten items and an overall check prior to submission. In addition, the automated system could also use a search engine of a much larger food database than, for example, the fixed food lists of FFQs or a generic food database which is commonly used in the UK for coding food diaries or recalls including 3500 foods [18]. An online searchable food database could include specific items more commonly consumed by minority groups, incorporate brand-level data and could be updated easily to reflect new products. Furthermore, such a tool could record time-varying intakes such as eating occasions, meal patterns, foods eaten in combination and portion size estimation not limited to standard portions and aided by the use of photographs. The tool we have developed is called myfood24 (Measure Your Food On One Day 24-h recall) [19], and this study aims to validate it against independent biomarkers and compare its performance with an interviewer-administered multiple-pass 24-h recall (MPR).

Methods

Ethics

All procedures and documents involving human subjects were reviewed and approved by the West London Research Ethics Committee (14/SC/1267) in advance of the study commencing. The study was conducted according to the guidelines of the Declaration of Helsinki, and full written informed consent was received from all participants.

Recruitment

Participants were intended to be broadly representative of the adult general population, and to be eligible for recruitment they had to be between 18 and 65 years old and metabolically stable. This was assessed at a screening visit by confirming their weight stability defined as weight stable (gained or lost ≥3 kg weight in the past 3 months?) and their willingness to maintain current dietary and physical activity habits for the duration of the study. To complete the dietary recalls and reference measures they had to have regular high-speed Internet access and a telephone, be able to speak and read English and be willing to visit the National Institute for Health Research (NIHR)/Wellcome Trust Clinical Research Facility (CRF) at Hammersmith Hospital (Imperial College Healthcare National Health Service (NHS) Trust, London, UK). Participants were recruited through a number of sources: the North West London Primary Care Research Network (WeLReN), a multidisciplinary network of primary care professionals and practices who have expressed prior interest in participating in research projects; lists of individuals known to CRF who had previously expressed an interest in participating in research projects; posters displayed in local general practices; and through a list of local addresses obtained from the post office, with potential participants receiving a postal invitation to take part. Approximately 2000 letters were sent out.

Respondents were invited to attend a screening visit to confirm eligibility, receive a detailed explanation of the study protocol, provide informed consent and undergo a health screen. This consisted of an electrocardiogram (ECG), blood pressure, height and weight measurement, a blood sample to check routine measures of liver and kidney function and cholesterol levels and a short questionnaire. Following the screening visit, participants were randomised into the different study arms as detailed in subsequent sections. Participants were provided with £100, as compensation for their time, upon completing the study.

Study design

Here we report on results from two different 24-h recalls (an interviewer-based dietary MPR and the myfood24 online dietary recall). This analysis compares the standard interviewer-based recall and the online myfood24 recall against the reference measures from biomarkers. At each clinic visit, the reference measures were followed 1 to 3 days later by the first 24-h recall, which was followed approximately 2 to 4 days later by the alternative 24-h recall method. Each 24-h recall and a suite of reference measures (i.e. biomarkers and total energy expenditure) were completed on three separate occasions separated by approximately 2 weeks to approximate longer-term intake (Fig. 1). The order of the different types of 24-h recalls was allocated by simple randomisation to reduce learning effects.

myfood24 online tool

The development of the myfood24 online 24-h dietary recall has been described in full elsewhere [19–21]. Briefly, myfood24 Version 1 was developed as an online self-administered 24-h dietary recall tool, targeting collection of automated dietary data in large-scale epidemiological studies. It was designed for speed and simplicity, requiring as few separate webpages, pop-ups and prompts as possible, but it includes an optional recipe builder, a detailed food search capability, an option to make an initial list for the first pass, prompts for commonly forgotten foods and foods often consumed together and a final review before submission. A large electronic food composition database (Version 1) was developed to reflect the variety of foods consumed in the UK. This was based on more than 3000 generic items from the UK Composition of Foods integrated dataset [18], nutrient content provided by fast food outlets and nutrient content as provided on the packaging of more than 50,000 branded food items [22] with remaining nutrients for branded items matched to the closest generic items on the basis of declared content

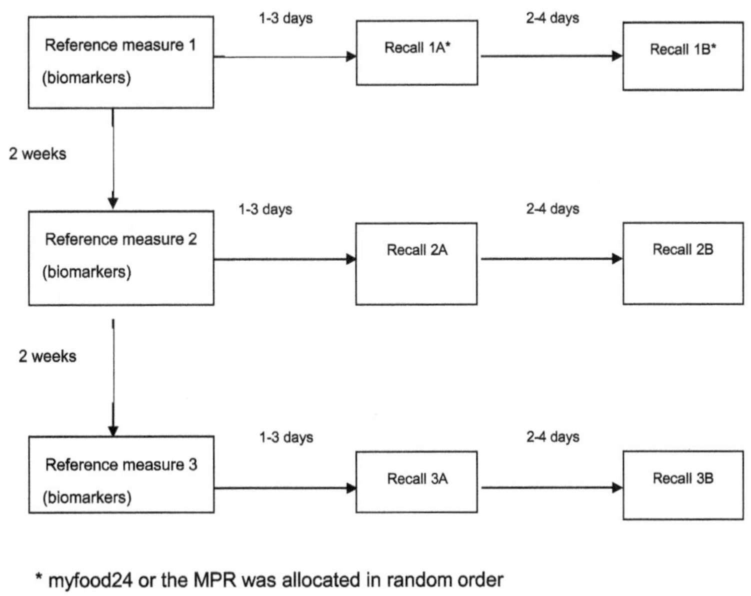

Fig. 1 myfood24 validation study design overview. Each 24-h recall (the interviewer-based multiple-pass 24-h recall and myfood24 online tool in random order) and a suite of reference measures (biomarkers and total energy expenditure) were completed on 3 separate occasions separated by approximately 2 weeks. At each occasion, the reference measure was followed 1–3 days later by the first 24-h recall method, which was followed 2–4 days later by the second 24-h recall method

[19]. Six thousand of the most common food items had photographic images to aid portion size recognition.

To test the online tool as an independent, stand-alone system, participants were not directly instructed in how to use myfood24 by the interviewers. However, all participants had access to a range of online help videos and frequently asked questions (https://www.youtube.com/watch?v=RI1C1AzvOBw; https://www.youtube.com/watch?v=CpLZ_NTH_O4).

Interviewer-administered 24-h recall

To standardise the telephone 24-h multiple-pass recall interviews, a standardised comprehensive prompt sheet based on the US Department of Agriculture (USDA) Automated Multiple-Pass Method was used by the interviewers [9]. This approach has also been applied in other myfood24 evaluation studies [20]. Nutritional intake was calculated using Dietplan 6.7 software (Forestfield Software, Horsham, UK), which is based on the McCance and Widdowson's 6th Edition Composition of Foods UK Nutritional Dataset (UKN). A team of trained coders matched the food and drink items recorded in the recalls to UKN database codes and portion sizes using a standard operating protocol provided in a detailed supplementary document attached to this reference [23]. This protocol was developed to reduce the number of subjective decisions made by coders by providing a series of flow diagrams to guide coders in the translation of food and drink records to database codes and portion sizes to weights (grams). This has been successfully used in other studies to reduce error code rates [23]. Composite dishes were broken down into their constituent parts with the use of retailer websites to check details of ingredients.

Urinary biomarkers

Participants were instructed to take one 80 mg 4-para-aminobenzoic acid (PABA) tablet with meals at approximately 8:00, 13:00 and 18:00 h in the 24 h preceding each study visit. They were requested to collect urine in dark containers for 24 h following the first void of the day including the first void of the next day. In addition, they recorded the timing of first and last collections, missed collections and supplement and medication use. Participants returned their 24-h urine samples to the CRF on the same day as collection ended. Urine volume was recorded before storage at − 20 °C and transportation to the Molecular Epidemiology Unit at the University of Leeds. Total urinary nitrogen was measured by the Kjeldahl method [24] with completeness of 24-h urine collection assessed by analysis of 4-para-aminobenzoic acid (PABA) concentration in the urine, using high performance liquid chromatography (HPLC) [25]. We assumed that 93% of PABA is excreted within 24 h [25] and that 81% of nitrogen is excreted within 24 h [26]. We used food-specific nitrogen-to-protein conversion ratios.

Urinary potassium and sodium concentrations were measured by the Clinical Biochemistry Department at the Leeds Teaching Hospitals NHS Trust using an ADVIA 2400 Clinical Chemistry System (Siemens AG, Munich, Germany) with ion selective electrode detection. We assumed that 80% of potassium [27] and 86% of sodium is excreted [28].

Urinary fructose and sucrose concentrations were quantified using a Sucrose/D-Glucose/D-Fructose Assay (Boehringer Mannheim/R-Biopharm AG, Darmstadt, Germany) scaled down to a microplate format. Multiplying by the total volume of urine collected over the 24 h allowed daily excretion of urinary sucrose and fructose to be estimated. This was then converted to a predicted intake of total sugars, based on a calibration equation derived from a controlled feeding study, which accounts for the age and sex of the individual [29]. As in the Observing Protein and Energy Nutrition (OPEN) study, we assumed that the relationship between urinary sucrose and fructose excretion and true intake of all sugars in our study was similar to that of an experimental sugar feeding study by Tasevska et al. [30].

Plasma biomarkers

During participant visits to the CRF, blood samples (40 ml) were collected in lithium heparin tubes before centrifugation at 2000×g for 10 min. Plasma was collected, aliquoted and frozen at − 80 °C. Plasma concentrations of total vitamin C (dehydroascorbic and ascorbic acid), vitamin E (α-tocopherol) and β-carotene were measured by HPLC as previously described [31] in the Molecular Epidemiology Unit at the University of Leeds with detection at 270 nm for ascorbic acid, 292 nm for α-tocopherol and 452 nm for β-carotene.

Total energy expenditure

Total energy expenditure (TEE) was estimated from combining measurements of resting energy expenditure (REE) and activity energy expenditure (AEE) and an assumed thermic effect of food. REE was measured by open-circuit indirect calorimetry (Gas Exchange Monitor; GEM Nutrition, Cheshire, UK). Following calorimeter calibration, volunteers were asked to lie in a semi-recumbent position under the canopy. Measurements were allowed to stabilise before oxygen consumption (VO_2) and carbon dioxide production (VCO_2) were recorded every minute for 15 min. The mean of the last 10 VO_2 and VCO_2 measurements was calculated and REE estimated from VO_2 and VCO_2 production in a given time using the equation by Weir [32]. AEE was estimated using a SenseWear three-plane accelerometer

(BodyMedia Inc., Pittsburgh, PA, USA) worn on the upper arm for a period of 24 h on one of the days preceding the patient's clinic visit. We assumed that the thermic effect of food was approximately 10% of TEE [33]. This method of estimating TEE has previously demonstrated close agreement to estimates using doubly labelled water [20, 34]. Estimated TEE served as a surrogate for total energy intake, assuming individuals were in energy balance.

Statistical analysis

Our a priori statistical analysis plan, approved by the study team and advisors, stated that our primary comparison was both long-term and short-term agreement between myfood24 and biomarkers, compared to the agreement between the interviewer-based multiple-pass method and biomarkers. Protein was the primary dietary component since it has a well-established recovery biomarker available. All participants were included in the main analyses unless they reported missing collection of two or more voids of urine during the 24-h collection period [35] or had a greater than 5% weight change from the first clinic appointment.

Our main analysis addressed longer-term intake. The attenuation factor (the parameter measuring the ability to detect diet-disease relationships using the dietary assessment tool) and the correlation coefficient between the dietary assessment tool and estimated true long-term intake (the parameter relating to the loss of power and to attenuation of log relative risks between categories of intake) were estimated from structural equation models using the method of maximum likelihood assuming multivariate normal distributions for the data after log transformation and also assuming that any missing observations were missing at random. We assumed a similar measurement error structure to that proposed in previous validation studies [36], with self-report dietary assessments having a person-specific systematic bias as well as a systematic bias related to level of intake. We also assumed that the person-specific biases for the interviewer-based 24-h recall and myfood24 were correlated. The structural equation models included linear associations between the longer-term usual intake and both the biomarkers and self-reported intakes, as suggested by Kipnis et al. [37]. Further details of the measurement error model are provided in Additional file 1: Table S1 and section Supplementary Materials and Methods.

For recovery biomarkers and equivalent reference instruments the attenuation factors are multipliers indicating the degree to which log relative risks are attenuated because of the measurement error in the dietary assessment tool. Attenuation factors are presented for a single administration of each self-report tool. From this model the bias in both of the self-report 24-h recalls compared to the biomarkers is also estimated, based on the mean self-reported intake over the replicates for each participant minus the mean over the replicates for the biomarker or equivalent reference tool, back-transformed and expressed as a percentage. This is the equivalent to the mean difference presented in the Bland-Altman approach [38].

A sensitivity analysis was conducted including only participants with complete PABA recovery (85–110%) and adjusting the urinary nitrogen, potassium and sodium to PABA recovery of 93% where the PABA recovery was 50–85% [39]. A sensitivity analysis was also conducted excluding participants who wore their SenseWear armbands for < 23 h or > 25 h, and the main analyses were also repeated excluding 24-h recalls that were collected within 24 h of a biomarker and therefore might give an optimistic estimate of agreement longer-term.

To reflect how myfood24 may be used in practice, the attenuation factors and correlations were re-estimated based on the average of a series of 2, 4 or 7 repeat administrations of the myfood24 tool, using the same approach as that of Schatzkin et al., 2003 [40]. To assess the robustness of results to participant characteristics, analyses were repeated stratified on sex, on age and on body mass index (BMI).

For nutrients with concentration biomarkers, β-carotene, vitamin C and vitamin E, intraclass correlation coefficients (ICCs) for absolute agreement between estimated intake and the reference tool were derived from two-way mixed effects models, with the dietary assessment method as the fixed effect. We included a subject-by-method interaction to allow for different responses for the two dietary assessment tools. We allowed the variance of random coefficients to vary and measurement error variances to vary between methods and focussed on individual 24-h periods rather than averages over the three time periods [4, 41, 42].

For nutrients with no adequate biomarkers, we also estimated the ICC between estimated intakes from the two different 24-h recalls. In addition, following the approach suggested by Altman and Bland, we also presented the mean difference in estimates between the two different 24-h recalls (an estimate of relative bias), alongside estimated limits of agreement (an estimate of precision for individual measures) [38].

We applied log transformations to all our analyses. All statistical analyses were performed in Stata SE version 14.2 [43].

Sample size

We aimed for a final sample size of 200 participants. Assuming similar parameters to those found in the OPEN study and EPIC Norfolk [37, 44], this sample size would allow the attenuation factor for protein intake to be estimated to approximately ± 0.08 and the correlation between myfood24 and true long-term intake to be estimated to approximately ± 0.1. This would also allow the mean difference between two tools to be estimated to within approximately ± 0.4 g nitrogen.

Results

Of the 289 respondents invited to the first clinic, 84% attended, provided consent and passed the health screen. Following random allocation of order of recalls, 31 participants (13%) withdrew during the course of the study. Completed myfood24 online 24-h recalls, interviewer-based 24-h recalls and samples for biomarker analysis were provided by 212 participants on at least one occasion. There were 12 24-h collection periods amongst 11 of these participants when more than one urine sample was missed. The biomarker measurements were excluded for those occasions. However, because samples were collected on up to three occasions, no participants were excluded entirely from the study as a result.

Table 1 shows the demographic characteristics of the participants on entry to the study. The mean age of participants was 43 years, 127 (60%) were female, 155 (73%) were white and 127 (60%) were educated past age 18 years. Only 25 (12%) reported being current smokers. Mean body weight was 81 kg for male and 67 kg for female participants at the first appointment. Participants' weights were generally stable over the course of the study, but 6 (3%) sets of energy expenditure results were excluded because of more than a 5% weight change in some participants.

Table 1 Demographic characteristics of participants by sex

	Men (*n* = 85)[a]	Women (*n* = 127)[a]
Mean age (years) (SD)	43 (15)	44(16)
Ethnicity		
White	63 (74%)	92 (72%)
Black	1 (1%)	9 (7%)
Asian	5 (6%)	8 (6%)
Mixed and other	15 (18%)	14 (11%)
Age left education		
16 or under	13 (15%)	11 (9%)
17 to 18	23 (27%)	36 (28%)
19+	49 (58%)	78 (61%)
Smoking status		
Non-smoker	65 (76%)	99 (78%)
Smoker	12 (14%)	13 (10%)
Mean weight (kg) (SD)	81 (13)	67 (13)
Mean body mass index (kg/m^2) (SD)	26 (4)	25 (5)

[a]Note, where numbers in each category do not sum to the totals for the column, it is due to incomplete data for that characteristic
SD standard deviation

Table 2 shows the geometric mean and 95% confidence interval (CI) for protein, potassium, sodium and total sugar intakes and associated nutrient densities as assessed by the myfood24 online recall, the interviewer-based 24-h recall and the biomarkers and reference tools relating to the first clinic visit. The myfood24 estimates of intake were similar to the biomarker measurements for protein, higher for potassium and sodium and lower for total sugars and estimated total energy intake compared to reference estimates. The two types of 24-h recall gave broadly similar results, but the online myfood24 typically provided slightly lower estimates compared to the interviewer-administered tool.

Table 3 lists the attenuation factors for the online myfood24 and interviewer-based 24-h recalls when used to estimate long-term intake and nutrient densities. The attenuation factors, the degree to which diet-disease relationships are attenuated, were low for both self-report tools, but both were higher than those seen with FFQs [37]. The attenuation factors for the online myfood24 tool were slightly lower than those for the interviewer-based tool. The partial correlation coefficients between the self-report tools and the estimated true longer-term intake, ranging between 0.2 to 0.4, indicating the attenuation of log relative risks between categorised levels of intake as well as the loss of power introduced by measurement error, were poor for both self-report tools. For this outcome both the online and interviewer-based tools performed similarly. The mean percentage difference between the self-report tools and the biomarker measures (Table 3) reflected the extent to which the self-report tools over-estimated potassium and sodium intakes and under-estimated total sugars and total energy intake. Results for total energy intake and nutrient densities were slightly worse than those for nutrient intakes. The estimated parameters from the full measurement models are provided in Additional file 1: Table S1.

Adjustment of urinary nitrogen, sodium and potassium for completeness of urine samples when PABA recovery was 50–85%, and exclusion of observations outside the range of 50–110%, led to increased derived protein (77 g vs 68 g), potassium (2.4 g vs 2.1 g) and sodium (2.1 g vs 1.8 g) intakes, which were closer to the self-reported intakes. This did not substantially influence the estimates of the attenuation factors (0.27 vs 0.30 for protein, 0.29 vs 0.31 for potassium and 0.19 vs 0.21 for sodium). However, the correlation between self-report intakes and true intake was somewhat improved, albeit with wider confidence intervals (0.50 vs 0.43 for protein, 0.48 vs 0.40 for potassium and 0.37 vs 0.30 for sodium).

Table 2 Geometric means and 95% confidence interval (CI) for protein, potassium, sodium and total sugar intake and density as assessed by myfood24, interviewer-based 24-h recall and biomarkers relating to the first clinic visit

	myfood24		Interviewer-based 24-h recall		Biomarker/reference tool	
	n	Geometric mean (95% CI)	*n*	Geometric mean (95% CI)	*n*	Geometric mean (95% CI)
Nutrient intake:						
Protein (g)	208	70.5 (66.1, 75.2)	197	81.7 (77.3, 86.4)	192	68.4 (64.1, 72.8)
Potassium (g)	208	2.7 (2.5, 2.9)	197	3.1 (3.0, 3.3)	192	2.1 (1.9, 2.3)
Sodium (g)	208	2.3 (2.1, 2.5)	197	2.4 (2.2, 2.6)	192	1.8 (1.7, 2.0)
Total sugars (g)	208	72.8 (66.4, 79.8)	197	91.0 (85.0, 97.5)	191	128.3 (115.9, 142.0)
Energy expenditure:						
Total energy expenditure (MJ)	208	7.5 (7.1, 7.9)	197	8.5 (8.1, 8.9)	185	11.0 (10.5, 11.6)
Nutrient density:[a]						
Protein (g/MJ)	208	9.5 (9.0, 9.9)	197	9.6 (9.2, 10.0)	180	6.2 (5.8, 6.7)
Potassium (g/MJ)	208	0.36 (0.35, 0.38)	197	0.37 (0.35, 0.39)	180	0.19 (0.18, 0.21)
Sodium (g/MJ)	208	0.31 (0.29, 0.33)	197	0.28 (0.27, 0.30)	180	0.16 (0.15, 0.18)
Total sugars (g/MJ)	208	9.8 (9.1, 10.5)	197	10.7 (10.1, 11.4)	179	11.6 (10.4, 12.9)

[a]Nutrient density for protein, potassium, sodium and total sugars was expressed in g/MJ of total energy intake
The n is the number of participants who had both the dietary assessment measure and the biomarker

Table 3 Attenuation factors, correlation between dietary assessment tool and true intake and mean difference between self-report tool and reference intake for protein, potassium, sodium and total sugar intake and density as assessed by myfood24 and interviewer-based 24-h recall

	Dietary assessment tool	Attenuation factor (95% CI)	Correlation with true intake (95% CI)	Mean % difference vs reference tool (95% CI)
Nutrient intake:				
Protein (g) (*n* = 192)	myfood24	0.30 (0.21, 0.38)	0.43 (0.32, 0.53)	+1% (−4%, + 7%)
	MPR[b]	0.38 (0.29, 0.47)	0.48 (0.39, 0.58)	+ 11% (+ 6%, + 17%)
Potassium (g) (*n* = 192)	myfood24	0.31 (0.21, 0.41)	0.40 (0.28, 0.52)	+ 26% (+ 19%, + 35%)
	MPR	0.35 (0.23, 0.46)	0.38 (0.27, 0.49)	+ 48% (+ 39%, + 57%)
Sodium (g) (*n* = 192)	myfood24	0.21 (0.12, 0.30)	0.30 (0.18, 0.41)	+ 22% (+ 13%, + 32%)
	MPR	0.22 (0.11, 0.32)	0.28 (0.15, 0.40)	+ 28% (+ 18%, + 38%)
Total sugars (g) (n = 191)	myfood24	0.15 (0.06, 0.24)	0.24 (0.09, 0.38)	−45% (− 39%, − 50%)
	MPR	0.25 (0.14, 0.36)	0.31 (0.18, 0.44)	−30% (−24%, − 35%)
Energy expenditure:				
Total energy expenditure (MJ) (*n* = 185)	myfood24	0.19 (0.10, 0.29)	0.29 (0.15, 0.42)	−31% (− 27%, − 35%)
	MPR	0.32 (0.21, 0.43)	0.37 (0.25, 0.49)	−23% (− 19%, − 27%)
Nutrient density:[a]				
Protein (g/MJ) (*n* = 180)	myfood24	0.16 (0.03, 0.29)	0.17 (0.03, 0.32)	+ 48% (+ 39%, + 58%)
	MPR	0.26 (0.11, 0.40)	0.24 (0.11, 0.37)	+ 46% (+ 38%, + 55%)
Potassium (g/MJ) (*n* = 180)	myfood24	0.25 (0.09, 0.41)	0.23 (0.09, 0.37)	+ 85% (+ 72%, + 99%)
	MPR	0.38 (0.23, 0.53)	0.34 (0.22, 0.47)	+ 93% (+ 81%, + 107%)
Sodium (g/MJ) (*n* = 180)	myfood24	0.08 (−0.03, 0.19)	0.09 (−0.04, 0.21)	+ 78% (+ 63%, + 94%)
	MPR	0.11 (−0.02, 0.24)	0.11 (− 0.02, 0.24)	+ 66% (+ 52%, + 80%)
Total sugars (g/MJ) (*n* = 179)	myfood24	0.16 (0.04, 0.28)	0.21 (0.06, 0.36)	−19% (− 11%, − 26%)
	MPR	0.23 (0.09, 0.37)	0.25 (0.10, 0.39)	−8% (+ 0%, − 15%)

All dietary measures and estimates were log-transformed
[a]Nutrient density for protein, potassium, sodium and total sugars was expressed in g/MJ of total energy intake
[b]Interviewer-based multiple-pass 24-h dietary recall

Attenuation factors were almost identical when participants who did not wear their armbands for 24 h were excluded (data not shown). When intakes estimated within 24 h of a biomarker collection were excluded, attenuation factors were marginally lower for protein, potassium and sodium, and essentially unchanged for total sugars and total energy intake, but all with wider confidence intervals (data not shown).

Using the average of a series of 2, 4 or 7 repeat administrations, attenuation was reduced and correlations improved with repeat administration of the myfood24 tool (Additional file 1: Table S2).

Attenuation factors from models stratified by BMI showed that BMI may modify attenuation factors and deviations from true values when using myfood24 and the traditional 24 h recall (Table 4), with somewhat lower attenuation for participants with BMI < 25 kg/m^2 for measures of protein and potassium. Other models stratifying by sex and age found attenuation of total energy intake and nutrient densities slightly better for males compared to females, and less attenuation for most nutrients with younger age (Additional file 1: Tables S3 and S4).

The intraclass correlation (95% CI) between plasma antioxidant concentrations and estimated intake from myfood24 were 0.56 (0.52, 0.60), 0.53 (0.50, 0.57) and 0.55 (0.50, 0.59) for β-carotene, vitamin C and vitamin E respectively (Table 5). These correlations were very similar to those obtained using the interviewer-based 24-h recall.

Table 6 shows the geometric mean intake and 95% CI for each nutrient estimated by the myfood24 online tool and the interviewer-administered tool at the time of first recall. It also presents the percent difference between the two methods with 95% CI, the Bland-Altman limits of agreement between the two methods and the intraclass correlation between the two methods, with 95% CI. The myfood24 estimates of nutrient intake were around 10–20% lower compared to the interviewer-based estimates. The ICCs comparing myfood24 and interviewer-based estimates were generally in the range 0.4–0.5, indicating moderate agreement between the two methods.

Table 4 Attenuation factors and correlation between dietary assessment tool and true intake for protein, potassium, sodium and total sugar intake and density as assessed by myfood24 and interviewer-based 24-h recall by body mass index

	Dietary assessment tool	Body mass index < 25 kg/m^2 (n = 99)		Body mass index 25+ kg/m^2 (n = 99)	
		Attenuation factor (95% CI)	Correlation with true intake (95% CI)	Attenuation factor (95% CI)	Correlation with true intake (95% CI)
Nutrient intake:					
Protein (g)	myfood24	0.32 (0.20, 0.45)	0.45 (0.30, 0.60)	0.28 (0.16, 0.40)	0.42 (0.26, 0.57)
	MPR[b]	0.37 (0.24, 0.50)	0.44 (0.32, 0.57)	0.33 (0.21, 0.45)	0.47 (0.33, 0.61)
Potassium (g)	myfood24	0.43 (0.28, 0.59)	0.51 (0.36, 0.66)	0.18 (0.04, 0.32)	0.40 (0.26, 0.54)
	MPR	0.40 (0.23, 0.57)	0.26 (0.06, 0.45)	0.27 (0.12, 0.41)	0.34 (0.18, 0.51)
Sodium (g)	myfood24	0.17 (0.04, 0.30)	0.24 (0.07, 0.42)	0.24 (0.12, 0.35)	0.34 (0.19, 0.49)
	MPR	0.17 (0.05, 0.29)	0.24 (0.08, 0.41)	0.15 (0.04, 0.26)	0.22 (0.07, 0.37)
Total sugars (g)	myfood24	0.14 (0.02, 0.26)	0.25 (0.04, 0.47)	0.14 (−0.01, 0.28)	0.19 (− 0.01, 0.39)
	MPR	0.14 (0.02, 0.26)	0.22 (0.05, 0.40)	0.24 (0.10, 0.37)	0.30 (0.14, 0.45)
Energy expenditure:					
Total energy expenditure (MJ)	myfood24	0.16 (0.04, 0.29)	0.28 (0.07, 0.48)	0.20 (0.06, 0.33)	0.27 (0.09, 0.45)
	MPR	0.27 (0.14, 0.39)	0.39 (0.23, 0.56)	0.23 (0.08, 0.39)	0.27 (0.11, 0.43)
Nutrient density:[a]					
Protein (g/MJ)	myfood24	0.29 (0.11, 0.48)	0.32 (0.14, 0.51)	−0.06 (− 0.25, 0.13)	−0.06 (− 0.27, 0.14)
	MPR	0.34 (0.17, 0.51)	0.34 (0.20, 0.49)	0.04 (−0.13, 0.20)	0.04 (−0.14, 0.23)
Potassium (g/MJ)	myfood24	0.35 (0.11, 0.59)	0.29 (0.10, 0.48)	0.15 (−0.07, 0.36)	0.15 (−0.07, 0.37)
	MPR	0.62 (0.37, 0.87)	0.47 (0.31, 0.62)	0.24 (0.01, 0.46)	0.24 (0.02, 0.46)
Sodium (g/MJ)	myfood24	0.05 (−0.13, 0.22)	0.05 (−0.13, 0.23)	0.14 (− 0.02, 0.29)	0.16 (− 0.01, 0.33)
	MPR	0.12 (−0.04, 0.28)	0.13 (− 0.04, 0.31)	0.07 (− 0.06, 0.21)	0.09 (− 0.07, 0.25)
Total sugars (g/MJ)	myfood24	0.07 (− 0.08, 0.22)	0.12 (− 0.15, 0.38)	0.24 (0.05, 0.43)	0.27 (0.07, 0.47)
	MPR	0.08 (−0.06, 0.22)	0.14 (−0.09, 0.37)	0.27 (0.09, 0.44)	0.28 (0.11, 0.44)

All dietary measures and estimates were log-transformed
[a]Nutrient density for protein, potassium, sodium and total sugars was expressed in g/MJ of total energy intake
[b]Interviewer-based multiple-pass 24-h dietary recall

Table 5 Geometric mean biomarker concentration, estimated intake at first dietary recall by myfood24 and interviewer-based tool and intraclass correlation coefficients between biomarker and each tool assessed over three time points

	Biomarker $n = 202$	myfood24 $n = 208$		Interviewer-based 24-h recall $n = 197$	
	Geometric mean (95% CI)	Geometric mean (95% CI)	Intraclass correlation with biomarker	Geometric mean (95% CI)	Intraclass correlation with biomarker
Nutrient intake:					
β-carotene	0.59 μM (0.52, 0.67)	0.65 mg (0.51, 0.83)	0.56 (0.52, 0.60)	1.53 mg (1.20, 1.95)	0.52 (0.48, 0.56)
Vitamin C	60 μM (57, 64)	59 mg (51, 69)	0.53 (0.50, 0.57)	75 mg (66, 85)	0.53 (0.49, 0.56)
Vitamin E	37 μM (35, 40)	1.6 mg (1.3, 1.9)	0.55 (0.50, 0.59)	2.3 mg (2.0, 2.8)	0.53 (0.49, 0.57)

Discussion

Our findings show that the myfood24 online 24-h recall is comparable to the more time-consuming and costly interviewer-based 24-h recall across a range of dietary measures. This is in line with previous reviews of online and computer-based dietary assessment tools [10, 45, 46]. Whilst both the online and interviewer-based 24 h recall tools suffer from the same problems of measurement error and correlated person-specific biases [47] to which all self-report tools are prone [39], they both perform broadly as well as other 24-h recalls in the USA, and most importantly, substantially better than widely used FFQs [3, 5, 37].

Our statistical approach to method validation was strong, although we did not set an a priori level of validity, which is not common practice in validation of dietary assessment tools, as shown by 78 validated tools included on the Nutritools website [48]. Rather than use Pearson's correlation, which tends to give a falsely optimistic view of a dietary assessment tool and does not provide a measure of agreement [38], we have used measures of agreement that estimate the extent to which the diet-disease association to be estimated in a large-scale study would be attenuated if the tool were being used, either to provide a continuous estimate of nutrient intake, or ranking intake in categories. The correlation coefficients reported in our paper are akin to intraclass correlations measuring agreement. In this way, we demonstrate the utility of the tool in practice and allow comparison with other tools assessed in the same way. As such, the myfood24 tool is better than FFQs and performs similarly to dietary MPRs assessed in the USA where similar approaches to validation have been used [37].

The mean percentage differences showed that both self-report tools under-estimated intakes of total sugars and energy and over-estimated intakes of potassium and sodium in comparison to the biomarkers. In this regard, use of the myfood24 tool is no better on a population level than an interviewer-based 24 h recall, which is prone to the same problems of under-reporting and over-reporting. This is also true of other self-report tools used in national surveys, such as the 4-day food diary currently used in the UK National Diet and Nutrition Survey (NDNS), where total energy intake is mis-reported by 46% in adults aged 16–64 years [49]. This could be as a result of systematic under-estimation or over-estimation using self-report measurement tools. Reporting error, daily variation in diet and limitations of food composition tables can all affect results. For example, although potassium intake may be captured accurately using self-report methods, the ability to assess sodium intake is more controversial as a result of addition of salt to foods in manufacture or at the table [5]. Biomarkers as a gold standard may also have limitations; for example, predictive biomarkers such as urinary sucrose and fructose may vary as a result of between-person differences in sucrose and fructose absorption, uptake by tissues or reabsorption in the kidneys [50].

The extent of under-reporting or over-reporting of self-reported dietary assessment tools compared to objective biomarkers is rarely reported as transparently as we have done here. Although the attenuation associated with using nutrient intakes derived from myfood24 is in the order of 0.2–0.3, and the attenuation associated with categorised intakes from myfood24 in the order of 0.3–0.4, the equivalent attenuation bias results from some FFQs have previously shown to be much worse, with attenuation factors almost half these figures. For example, the OPEN Study, including three different and well-used FFQs, showed attenuation factors for protein compared to a biomarker of 0.16 for men and 0.14 for women [37]. A more recently developed FFQ in the Netherlands fared somewhat better, with an adjusted attenuation factor of 0.28 for protein intake against the biomarker [51]. The favourable properties of the myfood24 tool do not simply reflect the close administration of the tool relative to biomarker sampling for a proportion of the recalls, as attenuation factors were similar when any intakes estimated within 24 h of a biomarker collection were excluded.

The agreement between plasma antioxidants and estimated intakes was good in our setting, as

Table 6 Geometric mean at first dietary recall, percent difference in means over all recalls, limits of agreement and intraclass correlation coefficients for nutrient intake estimated from myfood24 and interviewer-based 24-h recalls

	myfood24 $n = 208$	Interviewer-based 24-h recall $n = 197$			
	Geometric mean (95% CI)	Geometric mean (95% CI)	% Difference in means[a]	% Limits of agreement[a]	Intraclass correlation
Nutrient intake:					
Total energy intake (MJ)	7.5 (7.1, 7.9)	8.5 (8.1, 8.9)	−10% (− 14%, − 6%)	− 63% to + 118%	0.51 (0.48, 0.54)
Fat (g)	68 (64, 73)	82 (77, 88)	−14% (−18%, − 9%)	− 74% to + 182%	0.42 (0.40, 0.45)
Saturated fatty acids per 100 g food (g)	23 (21, 25)	28 (25, 30)	−13% (− 19%, − 8%)	− 79% to + 263%	0.40 (0.38, 0.43)
Monounsaturated fatty acids per 100 g food (g)	24 (22, 26)	28 (26, 30)	− 14% (− 19%, − 8%)	− 78% to + 238%	0.40 (0.38, 0.43)
Polyunsaturated fatty acids per 100 g food (g)	12 (11, 13)	14 (13, 15)	−11% (−17%, −5%)	− 80% to + 303%	0.39 (0.36, 0.41)
Protein (g)	72 (68, 78)	78 (73, 82)	−9% (− 14%, − 5%)	− 68% to + 158%	0.45 (0.42, 0.48)
Carbohydrate (g)	198 (186, 211)	224 (213, 236)	−12% (−17%, − 7%)	− 70% to + 162%	0.54 (0.51, 0.56)
Starch (g)	107 (99, 116)	117 (110, 126)	− 9% (− 15%, − 3%)	− 79% to + 263%	0.44 (0.41, 0.46)
Total sugars (g)	73 (67, 80)	92 (86, 98)	−20% (− 25%, − 15%)	−80% to + 216%	0.46 (0.43, 0.49)
Alcohol (g)	1.3 (1.0, 1.6)	1.5 (1.2, 2.0)	−9% (− 23%, + 7%)	− 98% to + 4177%	0.38 (0.35, 0.40)
Englyst fibre (g)	14 (13, 15)	15 (14, 16)	−14% (− 19%, − 9%)	−75% to + 199%	0.43 (0.41, 0.46)
Cholesterol (g)	0.17 (0.15, 0.20)	0.21 (0.18, 0.24)	−12% (− 20%, − 3%)	− 91% to + 793%	0.37 (0.35, 0.39)
Sodium (g)	2.3 (2.1, 2.5)	2.4 (2.2, 2.6)	−4% (− 10%, + 2%)	− 76% to + 283%	0.44 (0.41, 0.47)
Potassium (g)	2.7 (2.5, 2.9)	3.1 (3.0, 3.3)	− 14% (−18%, − 10%)	− 69% to + 137%	0.48 (0.45, 0.51)
Calcium (g)	0.68 (0.63, 0.74)	0.83 (0.77, 0.89)	−7% (− 22%, − 12%)	−79% to + 223%	0.46 (0.43, 0.49)
Phosphorous (g)	1.2 (1.1, 1.3)	1.4 (1.3, 1.4)	−12% (− 16%, −8%)	−68% to + 143%	0.51 (0.48, 0.53)
Iron (mg)	11.3 (10.6, 12.0)	12.3 (11.6, 13.0)	−10% (−14%, − 5%)	− 70% to + 170%	0.46 (0.43, 0.49)
Copper (mg)	1.8 (1.7, 1.9)	1.8 (1.7, 1.8)	−2% (−6%, + 2%)	− 63% to + 162%	0.42 (0.39, 0.45)
Zinc (mg)	8.6 (8.0, 9.2)	10.0 (9.4, 10.6)	−10% (−14%, −4%)	−72% to + 197%	0.46 (0.43, 0.48)
Selenium (μg)	38 (33, 42)	44 (40, 48)	−13% (−20%, −6%)	− 86% to + 445%	0.43 (0.40, 0.45)
Iodine (μg)	85 (75, 96)	128 (116, 140)	−27% (− 33%, −9%)	−91% to + 509%	0.44 (0.42, 0.47)
Retinol (μg)	143 (114, 179)	218 (181, 262)	−27% (− 36%, − 15%)	− 98% to + 2188%	0.37 (0.35, 0.40)
Vitamin D (μg)	2.1 (1.9, 2.4)	2.2 (1.9, 2.5)	−3% (− 13%, + 7%)	−91% to + 908%	0.37 (0.35, 0.39)
Vitamin E (mg)	7.7 (6.9, 8.5)	9.7 (8.9, 10.5)	−19% (− 25%, −12%)	−86% to + 381%	0.43 (0.40, 0.46)
Thiamin (mg)	1.9 (1.8, 2.0)	1.9 (1.9, 2.0)	−6% (−9%, −2%)	− 61% to + 129%	0.46 (0.43, 0.49)
Niacin (mg)	18.7 (17.4, 20.2)	20.0 (18.5, 21.5)	−5% (−10%, + 1%)	−75% to + 265%	0.41 (0.38, 0.43)
Vitamin B6 (mg)	2.2 (2.1, 2.3)	2.5 (2.4, 2.7)	−10% (−14%, −7%)	− 65% to 127%	0.42 (0.39, 0.45)
Vitamin B12 (μg)	3.4 (3.1, 3.9)	5.2 (4.8, 5.8)	−27% (− 33%, − 21%)	−90% to + 422%	0.40 (0.38, 0.43)
Folate (mg)	.22 (.20, .24)	.25 (.24, .27)	−14% (− 21%, −11%)	−78% to + 215%	0.45 (0.42, 0.48)
Pantothenic acid (mg)	4.6 (4.3, 4.9)	5.9 (5.5, 6.2)	−20% (− 24%, − 16%)	−74% to + 150%	0.43 (0.41, 0.46)
Biotin (μg)	30 (28, 33)	37 (35, 40)	−19% (−25%, −13%)	−81% to + 240%	0.45 (0.42, 0.48)
Vitamin C (mg)	59 (51, 69)	76 (66, 86)	−28% (− 36%, −20%)	−94% to + 765%	0.45 (0.42, 0.47)

[a]The difference in means and limits of agreement relate to the ratio of geometric means because of log transformation and are presented as % differences

indicated by ICCs between 0.5 and 0.6. Between interviewer-administered and Internet-administered 24-h recalls coefficients were generally in the range of 0.4–0.5, indicating moderate agreement, but there was a tendency for the online tool to be lower for most nutrients by around 10–20%. This relative bias may imply that myfood24 under-estimates, or the traditional interviewer-based multiple pass recall over-estimates, or that both tools are biased compared to the truth. For estimated intakes for individuals, this relative bias may be important, but it may be less important when diet is categorised and ranked, as is common in reporting large-scale epidemiological studies. As with all comparisons of dietary assessments conducted over different days, the limits of agreement were wide, reflecting the wide day-to-day variation in diets.

Sensitivity analyses found potentially lower attenuation for participants with BMI < 25 kg/m^2 for measures of protein and potassium, highlighting the need to take account of participant characteristics when measuring diet.

Some previous comparisons between interviewer-administered 24-h recalls over the telephone and self-administered 24-h recalls over the Internet compared dietary intake on the same day using the same computerised interface for data entry [12, 13]. Both the same 24-h period and the same data entry interface lead to much closer agreement between the self-administered and interviewer-administered approaches, but either could lead to potentially substantial learning effects, as participants may simply repeat what was recalled using the previous tool. The same data entry interface also eliminates differences in estimated portion size options between the two approaches, exaggerating the apparent agreement. Finally, using the same 24-h period means that the validation relates to short-term use, rather than longer-term average intake, where agreement would be expected to be lower anyway. By contrast, our methodology directly assesses agreement between the two dietary assessment tools, rather than correlation which would exaggerate similarities between the tools [28], and it does not use the same day for each tool. Our focus is on agreement in estimated longer-term intake, by spreading different dietary assessments over a number of weeks, each recorded at different time points [52].

For large-scale prospective studies and health surveys, FFQs are the common choice due to interviewer-based 24-h recalls being prohibitively expensive to administer in person or over the telephone by trained researchers, and time-consuming to identify food items and analyse for nutrient content, despite the 24-h recall capturing intake with less bias in validation studies [3]. The myfood24 tool has a substantially better measurement error profile than many FFQs and would lead to less attenuation of diet-disease association estimates and greater power to detect associations as statistically significant, particularly given the lower attenuation following repeat administrations. Moreover, for the online myfood24 tool there would be negligible additional financial and staff costs associated with increasing the number of 24-h recalls that each individual provides, contrasting with costly interviewer-based 24-h recalls. This allows greater precision of estimated longer-term intake, for intake to be assessed across different seasons, for estimated intake to be updated frequently throughout follow-up, improved capture of episodically consumed items and for intra-person variability to be estimated as well as inter-person variability [1]. We believe that these strengths make online 24-h recall such as myfood24 the tool of choice for future large-scale studies, either alone or in combination with FFQs, potentially addressing some of the current criticism of self-reported dietary data.

We have compared the myfood24 tool with objective biomarker measures that are not prone to person-specific bias that might be correlated with the self-report tool being assessed. This provides a better evaluation of the tool than a comparison with another self-report 24-h recall alone, which would be prone to similar measurement errors and might be equally poor. The use of objective reference measures such as biomarkers of intake and energy expenditure is therefore a major strength of our validation study.

One weakness of our study was not being able to use the gold standard measure for energy of doubly labelled water because of the prohibitive expense [3]. However, the activity monitor equipment we used provides an alternative measure of TEE that is also objective and therefore meets the same purpose. However, this might explain why agreement between biomarker measures for nutrient densities was not as high as that for the absolute nutrients. Another weakness common to all validation studies using biomarkers is that most nutrients do not have adequate recovery biomarkers with which to validate estimated intake [53]. Whilst other objective measures exist that could be used for such nutrients, such as larder inventories and itemised till receipts, these have their own weaknesses such as being measured at a household level and not allowing for food waste [54].

One further potential challenge of this online approach is that Internet-based tools may be more acceptable to younger than to older people, and may be more accessible to individuals who are more educated or have greater income. However, our study covered a wide age range, including anyone between 18 and 65 years old, with a mean age in the middle of this range. Our participants were motivated and reimbursed for participation. Use of an Internet tool is no substitute for good study design and consideration of approaches to maximise participation rates. In developing the tool we assessed the acceptability of the tool in different age groups [19–21] and in pregnancy [55], with system usability scores being 'good'. When we stratified our results by age group, by sex and by BMI, the myfood24 tool appeared to offer less attenuation with younger participants who were not obese. However, the same was seen for the interviewer-based tool as well. Furthermore, the unique use of brand-specific nutrient information [19, 22] means that in principle the tool is more able to match the different diets found across different demographic groups around the country.

These encouraging results provide a platform to develop country-specific versions of the tool, incorporating local foods, with estimated nutrient intakes based on food composition tables local to that country.

Conclusions

To conclude, whilst all self-report tools are prone to substantial measurement error and associated bias, the attenuation and bias from the online myfood24 tool are substantially better than those of many alternative FFQs. The estimated attenuation factors for the myfood24 tool are similar to those of the more resource-consuming expert interviewer-administered MPR. It is therefore more likely to be of use in large-scale population surveys, prospective cohorts and trials to give more valid estimates of diet-disease associations than an FFQ and may be able to better measure the effect of dietary exposures on health and disease outcomes.

Additional file

Additional file 1: Table S1. Measurement error structure for protein, potassium, sodium and total sugar intake and density as assessed by myfood24 and interviewer-based 24-h recall. **Table S2.** Attenuation factors and correlation between dietary assessment tool and true intake for protein, potassium, sodium and total sugar intake as assessed by myfood24 for different numbers of repeat administrations of the tool. **Table S3.** Attenuation factors and correlation between dietary assessment tool and true intake for protein, potassium, sodium and total sugar intake and density as assessed by myfood24 and interviewer-based 24-h recall by sex. **Table S4.** Attenuation factors and correlation between dietary assessment tool and true intake for protein, potassium, sodium and total sugar intake and density as assessed by myfood24 and interviewer-based 24-h recall by age group. (DOCX 27 kb)

Abbreviations

BMI: Body mass index; FFQ: Food frequency questionnaire; ICC: Intraclass correlation coefficient

Acknowledgements

Salwa A Albar contributed to the development of the myfood24 tool, Sarah Beer contributed to myfood24 data, Charlotte Evans contributed to the study proposal and development of the myfood24 tool, Laurence S Freedman advised on statistical methods, Jozef Hooson contributed to myfood24 data, Simon Futers contributed to concentration biomarker analysis, Claire McLoughlin contributed to project administration, Amy F Subar is external scientific advisor, contributed to study design and advised on statistical methods, Kay L White contributed to laboratory methods development and conducted PABA analysis, Cybele P Wong contributed to database design, Kamal Wahab contributed to data entry. Thanks go to the student and administration team who supported the data entry and development phases of myfood24.

We acknowledge the support of the NIHR Imperial Centre for Translational and Experimental Medicine for hosting the study. Gary Frost is an NIHR Senior Investigator. The opinions expressed in this study are those of the authors and do not necessarily reflect those of the NHS nor the NIHR.

Funding

The project was funded by the Medical Research Council (GB) grant MRC G1100235.

Authors' contributions

PAW is Co-Investigator (Co-I), jointly conceived the project, oversaw the project in London, co-drafted the participant protocol and associated study material, contributed to the study design and is joint guarantor for the project. LJH is Co-I, contributed to the study design, developed biomarker methods and takes responsibility for laboratory analyses. GSF is Co-I, contributed to the study design, oversaw the practical conduct of the participant study and is Director of the Clinical Research Facility at Hammersmith Hospital, London (Imperial College Healthcare NHS Trust). NAA is Co-I and contributed to the study design. MC managed the project in Leeds for 2 years and contributed to development of myfood24. PE is Co-I and contributed to the study design. HEF led participant recruitment and biological sample collection. NH is Co-I, contributed to the study design, contributed to development of myfood24 and is responsible for the myfood24 database and data linkage. MAM managed the project in Leeds for 1 year and contributed to development of myfood24. UZM co-drafted the participant protocol and associated study material, managed the project in London for 2 years and led participant recruitment and biological sample collection. KP managed the project in London for 1 year and led participant recruitment and biomarker collection. GDMP conducted the urinary nitrogen and sugars analyses. DM conducted the plasma β-carotene, α-tocopherol and vitamin C analyses. EN conducted plasma vitamin C analysis. ER is Co-I and contributed to the study design. DCG is Co-I, contributed to the study design, developed the statistical methods, takes responsibility for statistical analysis and wrote the manuscript. JEC is Principal Investigator, conceived the project, had overall oversight of the project, contributed to the study design, contributed to development of myfood24 and is joint guarantor for the project. All authors contributed to interpretation of data and revising the manuscript critically for important intellectual content. All authors read and approved the final manuscript.

Competing interests

Janet Cade is a director of a University of Leeds spin out private company, Dietary Assessment Ltd., supporting the development of myfood24. Michelle Morris and Michelle Carter are shareholders in Dietary Assessment Ltd. The company has been running for 1 year and has not made a profit (or loss). Janet Cade acknowledges additional support from the Medical Research Council (MR/L02019X/1). Paul Elliott is Director of the MRC-PHE Centre for Environment and Health and acknowledges support from the Medical Research Council and Public Health England (MR/L01341X/1). He also acknowledges support from the NIHR Biomedical Research Centre at Imperial College Healthcare NHS Trust and Imperial College London; the NIHR Health Protection Research Unit in Health Impact of Environmental Hazards (HPRU-2012-10,141). Gary Frost has worked as a consultant for a number of food companies including Nestle, Unilever, Quorn, New Food Innovations and Malaysian Palm Oil.

Author details

[1]Centre for Innovative Research Across the Life Course (CIRAL), Faculty of Health and Life Sciences, Coventry University, Coventry CV1 5FB, UK. [2]Global eHealth Unit, Department of Primary Care and Public Health, Imperial College, Imperial College, London SW7 2AZ, UK. [3]Division of Epidemiology and Biostatistics, Leeds Institute for Cardiovascular and Metabolic Medicine, School of Medicine, University of Leeds, Leeds LS2 9JT, UK. [4]Nutrition and Dietetic Research Group, Division of Diabetes, Endocrinology and Metabolism, Faculty of Medicine, Imperial College London, London W12 0NN, UK. [5]Academic Unit of Primary Care and Population Sciences, Faculty of Medicine, University of Southampton, Southampton SO16 6YD, UK. [6]Nutritional Epidemiology Group, School of Food Science and Nutrition, University of Leeds, Leeds LS2 9JT, UK. [7]MRC-PHE Centre for Environment and Health, Department of Epidemiology and Biostatistics, School of Public Health, Faculty of Medicine, Imperial College London, London W2 1PG, UK. [8]Leeds Institute of Data Analytics, University of Leeds, Leeds LS2 9JT, UK. [9]Department of Clinical Nutrition, Faculty of Applied Medical Sciences, Umm Al-Qura University, P.O. Box 715, Makkah 21955, Saudi Arabia. [10]NIHR Southampton Biomedical Research Centre, University of Southampton and University Hospital Southampton NHS Foundation Trust, Southampton SO16 6YD, UK.

References

1. Schatzkin A, Subar AF, Moore S, Park Y, Potischman N, Thompson FE, Leitzmann M, Hollenbeck A, Morrissey KG, Kipnis V. Observational

epidemiologic studies of nutrition and cancer: the next generation (with better observation). Cancer Epidemiol Biomark Prev. 2009;18(4):1026–32.
2. Cade JE, Warthon-Medina M, Albar S, Alwan NA, Ness A, Roe M, Wark PA, Greathead K, Burley VJ, Finglas P, et al. DIET@NET: best practice guidelines for dietary assessment in health research. BMC Med. 2017;15(1):202.
3. Freedman LS, Commins JM, Moler JE, Arab L, Baer DJ, Kipnis V, Midthune D, Moshfegh AJ, Neuhouser ML, Prentice RL, et al. Pooled results from 5 validation studies of dietary self-report instruments using recovery biomarkers for energy and protein intake. Am J Epidemiol. 2014;180(2):172–88.
4. Bland JM, Altman DG. Agreement between methods of measurement with multiple observations per individual. J Biopharm Stat. 2007;17(4):571–82.
5. Freedman LS, Commins JM, Moler JE, Willett W, Tinker LF, Subar AF, Spiegelman D, Rhodes D, Potischman N, Neuhouser ML, et al. Pooled results from 5 validation studies of dietary self-report instruments using recovery biomarkers for potassium and sodium intake. Am J Epidemiol. 2015;181(7):473–87.
6. Thompson FE, Subar AF, Loria CM, Reedy JL, Baranowski T. Need for technological innovation in dietary assessment. J Am Diet Assoc. 2010; 110(1):48–51.
7. Moreno-Betancur M, Carlin JB, Brilleman SL, Tanamas SK, Peeters A, Wolfe R: Survival analysis with time-dependent covariates subject to missing data or measurement error: multiple imputation for joint modeling (MIJM). Biostatistics 2017. https://doi.org/10.1093/biostatistics/kxx046.
8. Freedman LS, Midthune D, Dodd KW, Carroll RJ, Kipnis V. A statistical model for measurement error that incorporates variation over time in the target measure, with application to nutritional epidemiology. Stat Med. 2015; 34(27):3590–605.
9. Raper N, Perloff B, Ingwersen L, Steinfeldt L, Anand J. An overview of USDA's dietary intake data system. J Food Compos Anal. 2004;17(3–4):545–55.
10. Timon CM, van den Barg R, Blain RJ, Kehoe L, Evans K, Walton J, Flynn A, Gibney ER. A review of the design and validation of web- and computer-based 24-h dietary recall tools. Nutr Res Rev. 2016;29(2):268–80.
11. Arab L, Hahn H, Henry J, Chacko S, Winter A, Cambou MC. Using the web for recruitment, screen, tracking, data management, and quality control in a dietary assessment clinical validation trial. Contemporary Clinical Trials. 2010; 31(2):138–46.
12. Touvier M, Kesse-Guyot E, Mejean C, Pollet C, Malon A, Castetbon K, Hercberg S. Comparison between an interactive web-based self-administered 24 h dietary record and an interview by a dietitian for large-scale epidemiological studies. Br J Nutr. 2011;105(7):1055–64.
13. Andreeva VA, Deschamps V, Salanave B, Castetbon K, Verdot C, Kesse-Guyot E, Hercberg S. Comparison of dietary intakes between a large online cohort study (Etude NutriNet-Sant,) and a nationally representative cross-sectional study (Etude Nationale Nutrition Sant,) in France: addressing the issue of generalizability in E-epidemiology. Am J Epidemiol. 2016;184(9):660–9.
14. Bradley J, Simpson E, Poliakov I, Matthews JNS, Olivier P, Adamson AJ, Foster E. Comparison of INTAKE24 (an online 24-h dietary recall tool) with interviewer-led 24-h recall in 11–24 year-old. Nutrients. 2016;8(6):358.
15. Liu B, Young H, Crowe FL, Benson VS, Spencer EA, Key TJ, Appleby PN, Beral V. Development and evaluation of the Oxford WebQ, a low-cost, web-based method for assessment of previous 24 h dietary intakes in large-scale prospective studies. Public Health Nutr. 2011;14(11):1998–2005.
16. Yuan C, Spiegelman D, Rimm EB, Rosner BA, Stampfer MJ, Barnett JB, Chavarro JE, Rood JC, Harnack LJ, Sampson LK, et al. Relative validity of nutrient intakes assessed by questionnaire, 24-hour recalls, and diet records compared with urinary recovery and plasma concentration biomarkers: findings for women. Am J Epidemiol. 2018;187(5):1051–63.
17. Lassale C, Castetbon K, Laporte F, Camilleri GM, Deschamps V, Vernay M, Faure P, Hercberg S, Galan P, Kesse-Guyot E. Validation of a web-based, self-administered, non-consecutive-day dietary record tool against urinary biomarkers. Br J Nutr. 2015;113(6):953–62.
18. Food Standards Agency. McCance and Widdowson's the composition of foods. London: Royal Society of Chemistry; 2014.
19. Carter MC, Albar SA, Morris MA, Mulla UZ, Hancock N, Evans CE, Alwan NA, Greenwood DC, Hardie LJ, Frost GS, et al. Development of a UK online 24-h dietary assessment tool: myfood24. Nutrients. 2015;7(6): 4016–32.
20. Albar SA, Alwan NA, Evans CEL, Greenwood DC, Cade JE, Myfood24 Consortium Group. Agreement between an online dietary assessment tool (myfood24) and an interviewer-administered 24-h dietary recall in British adolescents aged 11-18 years. Br J Nutr. 2016;115(9):1678–86.
21. Albar SA, Carter MC, Alwan NA, Evans CEL, Cade JE, On behalf of the myfood24 Consortium Group. Formative evaluation of the usability and acceptability of myfood24 among adolecents: a UK online dietary assessment tool. BMC Nutrition. 2015;1(29).
22. Brandbank Ltd. Brandbank. 2016. http://www.brandbank.com. Accessed 18 July 2017.
23. Gibson R, Eriksen R, Lamb K, McMeel Y, Vergnaud A-C, Spear J, Aresu M, Chan Q, Elliott P, Frost G. Dietary assessment of British police force employees: a description of diet record coding procedures and cross-sectional evaluation of dietary energy intake reporting (the Airwave Health Monitoring Study). BMJ Open. 2017;7(4):e012927.
24. Bingham SA. Urine nitrogen as a biomarker for the validation of dietary protein intake. J Nutr. 2003;133(3):921S–4S.
25. Bingham S, Cummings JH. The use of 4-aminobenzoic acid as a marker to validate the completeness of 24 h urine collections in man. Clin Sci. 1983; 64(6):629–35.
26. Bingham SA, Cummings JH. Urine nitrogen as an independent validatory measure of dietary intake: a study of nitrogen-balance in individuals consuming their normal diet. Am J Clin Nutr. 1985;42(6): 1276–89.
27. Freedman LS, Midthune D, Carroll RJ, Krebs-Smith S, Subar AF, Troiano RP, Dodd K, Schatzkin A, Ferrari P, Kipnis V. Adjustments to improve the estimation of usual dietary intake distributions in the population. J Nutr. 2004;134(7):1836–43.
28. Holbrook JT, Patterson KY, Bodner JE, Douglas LW, Veillon C, Kelsay JL, Mertz W, Smith JC. Sodium and potassium intake and balance in adults consuming self-selected diets. Am J Clin Nutr. 1984;40(4):786–93.
29. Tasevska N, Midthune D, Potischman N, Subar AF, Cross AJ, Bingham SA. Use of the predictive sugars biomarker to evaluate self-reported total sugars intake in the Observing Protein and Energy Nutrition (OPEN) study. Cancer Epidemiol Biomark Prev. 2011;20(3):490–500.
30. Tasevska N, Runswick SA, McTaggart A, Bingham SA. Urinary sucrose and fructose as biomarkers for sugar consumption. Cancer Epidemiol Biomark Prev. 2005;14(5):1287–94.
31. White KLM, Chalmers DM, Martin IG, Everett SM, Neville PM, Naylor G, Sutcliffe AE, Dixon MF, Turner PC, Schorah CJ. Dietary antioxidants and DNA damage in patients on long-term acid-suppression therapy: a randomized controlled study. Br J Nutr. 2002;88(3):265–71.
32. Weir JBD. New methods for calculating metabolic rate with special reference to protein metabolism. J Physiol London. 1949;109(1–2):1–9.
33. Tataranni PA, Larson DE, Snitker S, Ravussin E. Thermal effect of food in humans: methods and results from use of a respiratory chamber. Am J Clin Nutr. 1995;61(5):1013–9.
34. Johannsen DL, Calabro MA, Stewart J, Franke W, Rood JC, Welk GJ. Accuracy of armband monitors for measuring daily energy expenditure in healthy adults. Med Sci Sports Exerc. 2010;42(11):2134–40.
35. Subar AF, Midthune D, Tasevska N, Kipnis V, Freedman LS. Checking for completeness of 24-h urine collection using para-amino benzoic acid not necessary in the Observing Protein and Energy Nutrition study. Eur J Clin Nutr. 2013;67(8):863–7.
36. Kipnis V, Carroll RJ, Freedman LS, Li L. Implications of a new dietary measurement error model for estimation of relative risk: application to four calibration studies. Am J Epidemiol. 1999;150(6):642–51.
37. Kipnis V, Subar AF, Midthune D, Freedman LS, Ballard-Barbash R, Troiano RP, Bingham S, Schoeller DA, Schatzkin A, Carroll RJ. Structure of dietary measurement error: results of the OPEN biomarker study. Am J Epidemiol. 2003;158(1):14–21.
38. Altman DG, Bland JM. Measurement in medicine: the analysis of method comparison studies. Statistician. 1983;32(3):307–17.
39. Johansson G, Bingham S, Vahter M. A method to compensate for incomplete 24-hour urine collections in nutritional epidemiology studies. Public Health Nutr. 1999;2(4):587–91.
40. Schatzkin A, Kipnis V, Carroll RJ, Midthune D, Subar AF, Bingham S, Schoeller DA, Troiano RP, Freedman LS. A comparison of a food frequency questionnaire with a 24-hour recall for use in an epidemiological cohort study: results from the biomarker-based Observing Protein and Energy Nutrition (OPEN) study. Int J Epidemiol. 2003;32(6):1054–62.
41. Bland JM, Altman DG. Measuring agreement in method comparison studies. Stat Methods Med Res. 1999;8(2):135–60.
42. Rabe-Hesketh S, Skrondal A. Multilevel and longitudinal modeling using Stata. 3rd edition. College Station: Stata Press; 2012.

43. StataCorp. Stata statistical software: Release 14.2. College Station, TX: Stata Corporation, 2015.
44. Bingham S, Luben R, Welch A, Tasevska N, Wareham N, Khaw KT. Epidemiologic assessment of sugars consumption using biomarkers: comparisons of obese and nonobese individuals in the European Prospective Investigation of Cancer Norfolk. Cancer Epidemiol Biomark Prev. 2007;16(8):1651–4.
45. Thompson FE, Dixit-Joshi S, Potischman N, Dodd KW, Kirkpatrick SI, Kushi LH, Alexander GL, Coleman LA, Zimmerman TP, Sundaram ME, et al. Comparison of interviewer-administered and automated self-administered 24-hour dietary recalls in 3 diverse integrated health systems. Am J Epidemiol. 2015;181(12):970–8.
46. Kirkpatrick SI, Subar AF, Douglass D, Zimmerman TP, Thompson FE, Kahle LL, George SM, Dodd KW, Potischtnan N. Performance of the automated self-administered 24-hour recall relative to a measure of true intakes and to an interviewer-administered 24-h recall. Am J Clin Nutr. 2014;100(1):233–40.
47. Kipnis V, Midthune D, Freedman LS, Bingham S, Schatzkin A, Subar A, Carroll RJ. Empirical evidence of correlated biases in dietary assessment instruments and its implications. Am J Epidemiol. 2001;153(4):394–403.
48. DIET@NET (DIETary Assessment Tools NETwork): Nutritools. 2018. https://www.nutritools.org/. Accessed 15 Mar 2018.
49. Murakami K, Livingstone MBE. Greenhouse gas emissions of self-selected diets in the UK and their association with diet quality: is energy under-reporting a problem? Nutr J. 2018;17(1):27.
50. Tasevska N. Urinary sugars—a biomarker of total sugars intake. Nutrients. 2015;7(7):5816–33.
51. Sluik D, Geelen A, de Vries JH, Eussen SJ, Brants HA, Meijboom S, van Dongen MC, Bueno-de-Mesquita HB, Wijckmans-Duysens NE, van 't Veer P, et al. A national FFQ for the Netherlands (the FFQ-NL 1.0): validation of a comprehensive FFQ for adults. Br J Nutr. 2016;116(5):913–23.
52. Tucker KL, Smith CE, Lai C-Q, Ordovas JM. Quantifying diet for nutrigenomic studies. Ann Rev Nutr. 2013;33:349–71.
53. Bingham SA. Biomarkers in nutritional epidemiology. Public Health Nutr. 2002;5(6A):821–7.
54. Greenwood DC, Ransley JK, Gilthorpe MS, Cade JE. Use of itemized till receipts to adjust for correlated dietary measurement error. Am J Epidemiol. 2006;164(10):1012–8.
55. Morris MA, Carter MC, Brown H, Hancock N, Scott E, Endersby D, Alwan N, Cade JE. Is blood glucose control in women with gestational diabetes associated with fruit and veg intake? Eur J Pub Health. 2016;26:108.

3

Abortion-related emergency department visits in the United States: An analysis of a national emergency department sample

Ushma D. Upadhyay[1*], Nicole E. Johns[1], Rebecca Barron[2], Alice F. Cartwright[1], Chantal Tapé[2], Alyssa Mierjeski[2] and Alyson J. McGregor[2]

Abstract

Background: Media depictions and laws passed in state legislatures regulating abortion suggest abortion-related medical emergencies are common. An accurate understanding of abortion-related emergencies is important for informing policy and practice. We assessed the incidence of abortion-related emergency department (ED) visits in the United States (U.S.).

Methods: We used a retrospective observational study design using 2009–2013 data from the Nationwide Emergency Department Sample, a nationally representative sample of U.S. ED visits from 947 to 964 hospitals across the U.S. per year. All ED visits among women of reproductive age (15–49) were included. We categorized ED visits by abortion relatedness and treatments received, and assessed whether the visit was for a major incident (defined as requiring blood transfusion, surgery, or overnight inpatient stay). We estimated the proportion of visits that were abortion-related and described the characteristics of patients making these visits, the diagnoses and subsequent treatments received by these patients, the sociodemographic and hospital characteristics associated with the incidents and observation care only (defined as receiving no treatments), and the rate of major incidents for all abortion patients in the U.S.

Results: Among all ED visits by women aged 15–49 (189,480,685), 0.01% ($n = 27,941$) were abortion-related. Of these visits, 51% (95% confidence interval, 95% CI 49.3–51.9%) of the women received observation care only. A total of 20% (95% CI 19.3–21.3%) of abortion-related ED visits were for major incidents. One-fifth (22%, 95% CI 20.9–23.0%) of abortion-related visits resulted in admission to the same hospital for abortion-related reasons. Of the visits, 1.4% ($n = 390$, 95% CI 1. 1–1.7%) were potentially due to attempts at self-induced abortion. In multivariable models, women using Medicaid (adjusted odds ratio, AOR 1.28, 95% CI 1.08–1.52) and women with a comorbid condition (AORs 2.47–4.63) had higher odds of having a major incident than women using private insurance and those without comorbid conditions. During the study period, 0.11% of all abortions in the U.S. resulted in major incidents as seen in EDs.

Conclusions: Abortion-related ED visits comprise a small proportion of women's ED visits. Many abortion-related ED visits may not be indicated or could have been managed at a less costly level of care. Given the low rate of major incidents, perceptions that abortion is unsafe are not based on evidence.

Keywords: Abortion, Emergency department, Emergencies, Hospital admission, Complications, Health policies

* Correspondence: ushma.upadhyay@ucsf.edu
[1]Department of Obstetrics, Gynecology & Reproductive Sciences, University of California, San Francisco, 1330 Broadway, Suite 1100, Oakland, California 94612, USA
Full list of author information is available at the end of the article

Background

Emergency departments (EDs) are key sites of health-care delivery in the United States (U.S.), with 141.4 million visits in 2014 alone [1], and 55% of these visits are made by women. Although abortion-related complications are rare [2], the surge in legislation aimed at regulating abortion access [3] suggests that complications are common and that abortion is generally unsafe.

Since 2011, state legislatures across the U.S. have passed numerous laws that regulate abortion provision, many requiring abortion providers to obtain local hospital admitting privileges and have transfer agreements with nearby hospitals [3]. These laws are passed under a presumption that they are needed to protect women's health and safety [4, 5] and that hospitalization as a result of abortion is an occurrence frequent enough to necessitate legislation formalizing the relationship between hospitals, abortion providers, and clinics.

National-level estimates of abortion-related ED visits do not exist. However, data from one state suggests that abortion-related ED visits are rare. In a study using data from California's Medicaid program, Upadhyay et al. found that 0.03% of abortions were followed by an immediate ambulance transfer to an ED and 2.6% of abortions were followed by an abortion-related ED visit within 6 weeks of the abortion [2]. Another study that examined all medication abortions done by Planned Parenthood in 2009 and 2010 found an ED treatment rate of 0.10%, although medication abortions represented only about 23% of abortions at the time, and this study included only those ED visits that involved treatment [6]. In a study of outcomes of abortion procedures by family physicians in New York and Philadelphia, 0.3% of first-trimester medication and aspiration abortion patients were referred or went to an ED for assessment [7].

There is a paucity of published national data on the incidence and outcomes of ED visits after abortion. In this study, we examine the frequency of abortion-related ED visits, the frequency of major abortion-related incidents, and the characteristics of abortion-related ED visits in the U.S. using a nationally representative sample of ED visits.

Methods

Study design and data source

We conducted a retrospective observational study of abortion-related ED visits using data from the Nationwide Emergency Department Sample (NEDS), a nationally representative sample of ED visits. NEDS is a database of ED visits from 947 to 964 hospitals across the U.S. per year. Annually it includes more than 30 million unweighted visits, which represent more than 135 million weighted visits. NEDS was developed for the Healthcare Cost and Utilization Project (HCUP) and is maintained by the Agency for Healthcare Research and Quality. Data are available from 2006 onward. For this study, we utilized the five most recent years of data available (2009–2013). The study was certified exempt by the institutional review board of the University of California, San Francisco.

Unweighted visits are data collected on actual visits, which are then weighted proportionately to the total number of ED visits in the country based on the sampling strategy. The NEDS is a stratified single-stage cluster sample of state-level ED data reported to HCUP. Using the American Hospital Association Annual Survey of Hospitals as the target universe, the available data are selected to approximate a 20% stratified sample of all U.S. hospital-based EDs. More details of the sampling of hospitals can be found on the HCUP website [8, 9]. The characteristics used for sample stratification in the NEDS are U.S. region, urban or rural location, teaching status, ownership, and trauma level (see Fig. 1 for region definitions and states contributing data).

The NEDS includes patient-level and hospital-level information. Each ED visit has patient-level demographic characteristics including age, sex, primary and secondary payment source, and zip code-based urbanicity and income quartile. Each ED visit also has clinical characteristics, including up to 15 diagnoses (International Classification of Diseases, 9th Revision [ICD-9] codes), up to 15 procedures or treatments (Healthcare Common Procedure Coding System [HCPCS] and Current Procedural Terminology [CPT] codes), injury codes, admission and discharge status, diagnosis and treatment codes for inpatient care if admitted to the same hospital, and total charges. Each visit also has the corresponding hospital code, and hospital characteristics such as region, trauma level, urban-rural location, and teaching status. In this dataset, 5 of 13 states in the West, 11 of 12 states in the Midwest, 8 of 16 states in the South, and 8 of 9 states in the Northeast were represented in the data. Midwest hospitals were represented the most. The trauma level of a hospital refers to how well equipped it is to provide care to patients with traumatic injuries. Trauma level influences patient composition and was key to sample stratification in the dataset. Hospital ownership was categorized by the data distributor according to information reported in the American Hospital Association Annual Survey Database. Ownership could be governmental, private non-profit, or private for-profit. Hospitals with religious affiliations, including Catholic hospitals, are included, but are not distinguished as such and may fall into private for-profit or private non-profit categories. Federal hospitals (Veterans Affairs and Department of Defense) were not included in the sample. Patient-level and hospital-level weights were also provided to generate nationally representative estimates. HCUP provided weights for the NEDS data and these

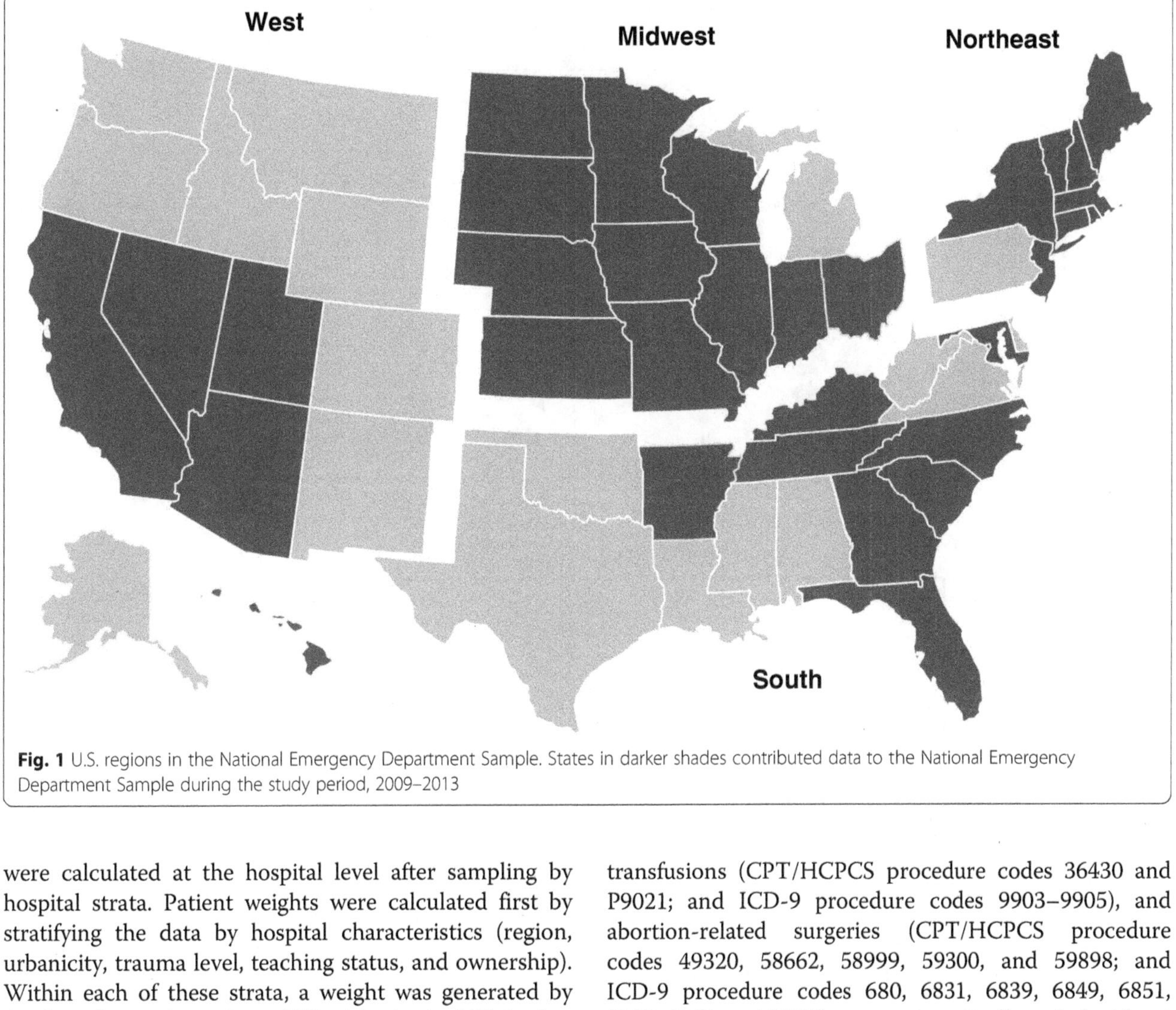

Fig. 1 U.S. regions in the National Emergency Department Sample. States in darker shades contributed data to the National Emergency Department Sample during the study period, 2009–2013

were calculated at the hospital level after sampling by hospital strata. Patient weights were calculated first by stratifying the data by hospital characteristics (region, urbanicity, trauma level, teaching status, and ownership). Within each of these strata, a weight was generated by dividing the total number of ED visits in the U.S. in that year for that stratum (from American Hospital Association data) by the number of ED visits for that stratum in the NEDS data. Weighted data thus represent all ED visits in the U.S. for a year.

Data preparation

We identified all ED visits that had an ICD-9 diagnosis code for abortion (ICD-9 diagnosis codes 635, 636, 637, and 638). We categorized ED visits by abortion relatedness and treatments received, and assessed whether the visit was for a major or minor incident. Visit categorization was based on the previously developed Procedural Abortion Incident Reporting and Surveillance (PAIRS) Framework [10]. Based on procedure codes, visits that were for observation care, repeat procedures (codes present in the dataset were CPT/HCPCS procedure codes 59812, 59820, 59821, 59840, 59841, 59851, 59855, and 59856; and ICD-9 procedure codes 6901, 6902, 6909, 6951, 6952, 6959, 734, and 750), blood transfusions (CPT/HCPCS procedure codes 36430 and P9021; and ICD-9 procedure codes 9903–9905), and abortion-related surgeries (CPT/HCPCS procedure codes 49320, 58662, 58999, 59300, and 59898; and ICD-9 procedure codes 680, 6831, 6839, 6849, 6851, 6859, 6869, and 7491) were systematically coded without individual visit review. Where procedure and diagnosis codes for a visit did not fall into one of these categories, several authors who are emergency medicine physicians or students with physician supervision provided an individual review of each visit following a modified version of the PAIRS framework (see Fig. 2). After a joint review of 100 visits with refinement of the decision rules, the physicians reviewed the remaining uncategorized visits, resulting in 1642 reviewed ED visits in total.

For each reviewed visit, the emergency medicine physicians assigned the reason for the patient's ED visit to one of five categories: abortion-related, concurrent condition, pre-existing condition, not abortion-related, or cannot determine. They classified an ED visit as abortion-related based on the constellation of diagnosis and procedure codes for that visit. Abortion-related visits included adverse events, such as hemorrhage or infection, and symptoms directly related to the procedure, such as abdominal pain and vomiting. Concurrent conditions were defined as

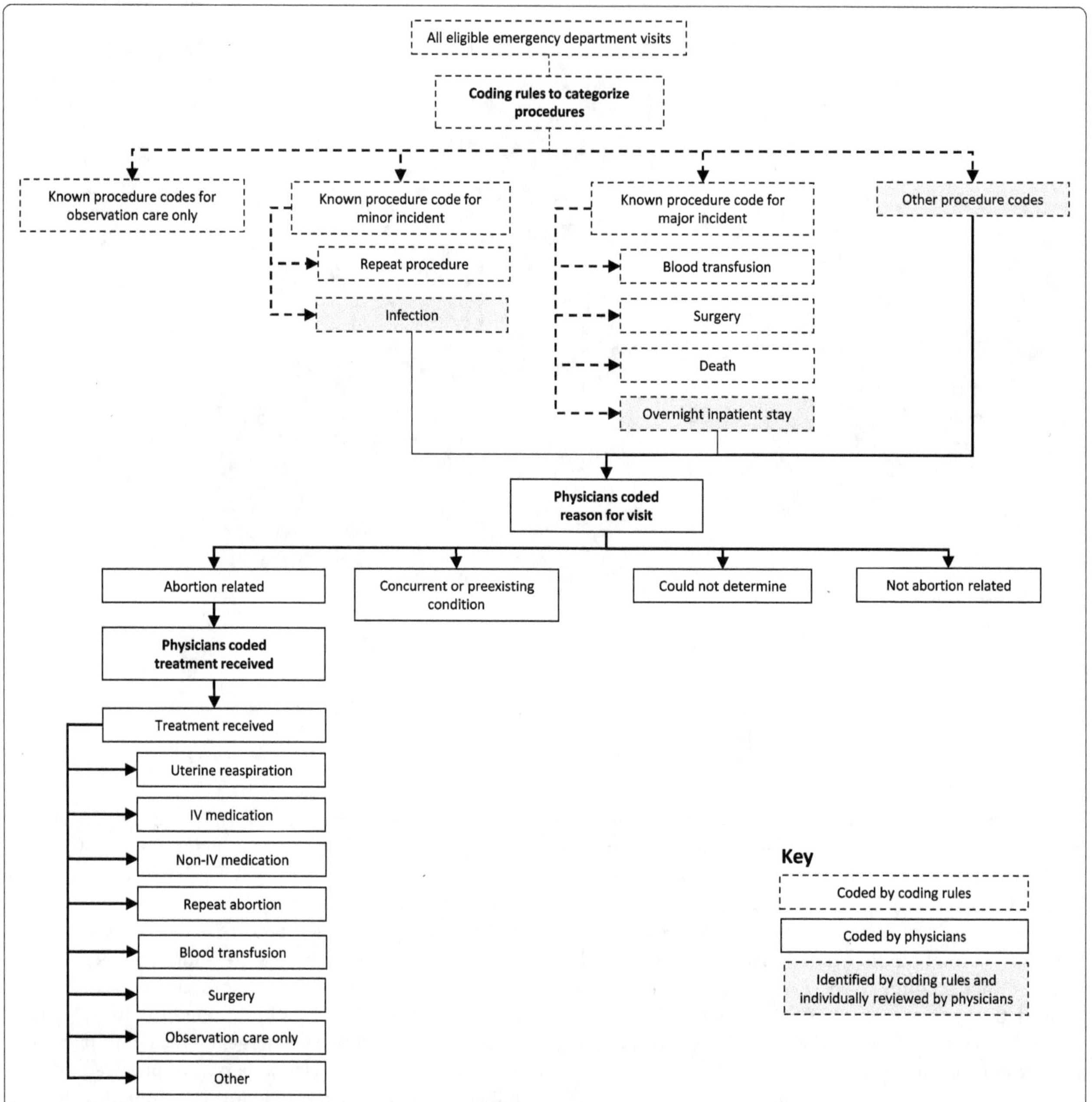

Fig. 2 Flow chart for coding of abortion-related emergency department visits. IV intravenous

conditions that may have been noticed during or exacerbated by abortion, but were not directly caused by the abortion, such as ovarian cysts, vaginitis, urinary tract infection, or anxiety/depression. Pre-existing conditions were defined as chronic conditions such as hypertension or diabetes. The data were also categorized with regards to treatments received for abortion-related complaints. Categories of treatment included uterine reaspiration (which involves suction, not an incision, and does not meet the criteria for surgery), intravenous (IV) and non-IV medication, repeat abortion, blood transfusion, surgery, observation care, or other. The medication category excluded codes for injections or infusion of a therapeutic substance if no accompanying medication was listed. The observation care category included women who had routine testing for their symptoms but did not receive any medications or other treatments. This included women who had IV fluids, blood work, testing for sexually transmitted infections, and diagnostic imaging studies, but no treatments. The NEDS dataset also included information on whether patients were admitted as an inpatient to the same hospital, discharged home, transferred to another facility, or left against medical advice. Among women who were admitted, the reason for visit and treatment information in their chart was used to determine if the admission was likely abortion-related.

Major and minor incidents were systematically coded, with major incidents defined as those requiring an overnight inpatient stay, blood transfusion, or surgery. Minor incidents were defined as all other incidents that involved an abortion-related diagnosis or treatment. All overnight stays were further reviewed by physicians, and a group of treatments for an abortion-related diagnosis that together required the patient to stay overnight qualified as a major incident. Visits that involved concurrent conditions, pre-existing conditions, or visits that were not abortion-related were categorized as no incident. We identified the prevalence of comorbid conditions based on diagnosis codes. These included three key conditions hypothesized to be associated with abortion-related adverse events: diabetes, hypertension, and having an overweight/obese body mass index (BMI) [11–14].

ED visits were additionally categorized as being potentially indicative of a self-induced abortion. The physician team individually reviewed all abortion-related visits that had diagnosis codes of illegal abortion, failed attempted abortion, and certain injury codes (including poisonings and indications of self-harm). They looked at all of the diagnosis codes for that case and made a clinical judgement based on the group of codes together and their ED experience. Visits that were coded as illegal abortions, particularly those that included injury codes, were more often considered potentially self-induced. In addition, visits that included injury codes consistent with self-induction were categorized as such. Cases which were unlikely to have been abortion-related were removed.

Statistical analysis

We estimated the number of abortion-related ED visits annually in the U.S. and the proportion of ED visits among women of reproductive age (15–49) that were for abortion-related care. We examined the characteristics of the sample and compared these to published estimates of the characteristics of abortion patients [15]. We also described outcomes including treatments received and discharge status. Based on treatments received, ED visits were categorized as being for a major incident, a minor incident, no incident, or that the incident type could not be determined. We then built multivariable logistic regression models to examine the factors associated with major incidents and observation care, controlling for sociodemographic characteristics, comorbidities, and hospital characteristics with the ED visit as the unit of analysis. Per the recommendation of the HCUP, the organization which oversees the NEDS database, sample weights were not used in the multivariable models [16]. We also estimated the proportion of ED visits that were potentially due to attempted self-induced abortion. Because the weighted estimates are nationally representative, we were also able to use published national estimates of abortion incidence [17] to estimate the major incident rate for abortion in the U.S. during the study period. This assumes that the vast majority of major incidents go through an ED evaluation (although we acknowledge that a small percentage do not). For all analyses, we report weighted results unless otherwise specified. Where data were missing, a missing category was retained for all analyses. Statistical significance was set at $P < 0.05$ for all chi-squared tests and adjusted odds ratios (AORs). We used STATA 14 for all analyses.

Results

Among 42,493,214 unweighted visits among women of reproductive age (15–49) during the study period, 6342 visits had an abortion diagnosis. Among these, 70 visits were determined to be unrelated to abortion based on clinician review and 33 visits were duplicates (all variables were identical other than ID number); these 103 visits were excluded, leaving an analytical sample of 6239 unweighted abortion-related ED visits. We did not include an additional 101 visits with abortion diagnoses for women outside the age range of interest (younger than 15 or older than 49).

The final analytical sample corresponded to 27,941 weighted ED visits for abortion-related reasons among 189,480,685 weighted ED visits among women of reproductive age. Thus abortion-related ED visits represented 0.01% of all ED visits among women of reproductive age during the study period. All subsequent results are weighted.

The average age of the population seeking abortion-related ED care was 26, and 12.9% of visits were by women under 20 (Table 1). Women using Medicaid were most common (45.2% of visits), followed by those using private insurance (31.4%), and those who self-paid (17.1%). The population seeking abortion-related ED care was overwhelmingly of urban residence (91.0%). Low-income zip code residences were overrepresented in the sample; 27.5% of women lived in a zip code with the lowest national income quartile, while 20.5% lived in the highest income quartile. Comorbid conditions including diabetes (1.5%), hypertension (3.2%), and overweight/obese BMI (1.8%) were noted in abortion-related ED visits. Hospitals in the South (35.5%) and West (31.7%) had the largest number of abortion-related ED visits. Most visits were to non-trauma or trauma level III hospitals (62.8%) and most were to hospitals in urban locations (92.3%). Visit numbers remained approximately constant throughout the study period. Average ED costs were $4719, with 8.6% of ED visits costing $10,000 or more.

Table 1 Characteristics of abortion-related emergency department visits, 2009–2013 weighted $n = 27{,}941$

	Weighted N	Weighted %	Abortion patients in the U.S., 2014% [15]
Total	27,941	100	100
Patient characteristics			
Age			
15–19	3605	12.9	11.7
20–24	9686	34.7	33.6
25–29	6952	24.9	26.5
30–39	6809	24.4	25.0
40–49	888	0.3	3.1
Primary payer			
Private insurance	8787	31.4	31.3
Medicaid	12,624	45.2	34.6
Medicare	410	1.5	–
Self-pay	4764	17.1	27.6[A]
No charge	188	0.7	–
Other	1049	3.8	6.5[B]
Missing	118	0.4	–
Urban/rural residence			
Urban	25,435	91.0	
Rural	2401	8.6	
Missing	104	0.4	
Zip code-based national income quartile			
First quartile (low)	7686	27.5	65.3[C]
Second quartile	7014	25.1	
Third quartile	7082	25.3	21.7
Fourth quartile (high)	5721	20.5	
Missing	437	1.6	13.0
Comorbidities			
Diabetes	415	1.5	
Hypertension	879	3.1	
Overweight/obese BMI	507	1.8	
Hospital characteristics			
Region			
Northeast	4539	16.2	
Midwest	4627	16.6	
South	9912	35.5	
West	8862	31.7	
Trauma level of hospital			
Level I or II	9429	33.7	
Nontrauma or level III	17,537	62.8	
Not specified	974	3.5	
Urban/rural location of hospital			
Urban	25,796	92.3	
Rural	2145	7.7	
Visit characteristics			
ED visit day			
Weekday	20,640	73.9	
Weekend	7301	26.1	
ED visit season			
Fall	5628	20.1	
Winter	5989	21.4	
Spring	6343	22.7	
Summer	6174	22.1	
Missing	3808	13.6	
Year			
2009	5350	19.1	
2010	5899	21.1	
2011	5448	19.5	
2012	5627	20.1	
2013	5617	20.1	
Total ED charges			
<$1000	2643	9.5	
$1000–$1999	4290	15.4	
$2000–$4999	7188	25.7	
$5000–$9999	3083	11.0	
$10,000+	2407	8.6	
Missing	8330	29.8	

BMI body mass index, *ED* Emergency department
[A]Defined as no coverage
[B]Defined as had either insurance through Healthcare.gov or a different type of insurance
[C]Defined as poor (<100% federal poverty level) or low income (<200% federal poverty level). At the time of the study, the national income median was approximately equal to 200% federal poverty level

Half of abortion-related visits received observation care only (50.6%, 95% confidence interval, 95% CI 49.3–51.9%) (Table 2). Nearly a third of visits resulted in a uterine reaspiration or repeat abortion procedure (32.2%, 95% CI 31.0–33.4%). Medications were used in 16.1% of ED visits (95% CI 15.2–17.1%): IV-medications in 13.7% of visits and non-IV medications in 7.4% of visits. The most commonly administered medication was pain medication (10.4%, 95% CI 9.7–11.2%), followed by anti-nausea medication (7.4%, 95% CI 6.8–8.1%) and antibiotics (3.2%, 95% CI 2.8–3.7%). A minority of ED visits involved blood transfusion (5.0%, 95% CI 4.5–

Table 2 Diagnoses and treatments received, weighted $n = 27,941$

	Weighted N	Weighted percentage	Weighted percentage 95% confidence interval
Incident type			
Minor incident[A]	10,089	36.1	34.9–37.4
Major incident[B]	5673	20.3	19.3–21.3
No incident	16,087	57.6	56.3–58.8
Could not be determined	426	1.5	1.2–1.9
Treatment received			
Repeat abortion or uterine reaspiration	8994	32.2	31.0–33.4
IV medications	3838	13.7	12.9–14.6
Non-IV medications	2072	7.4	6.8–8.1
Unspecified type medication	232	0.8	0.6–1.1
Type of medication			
Pain	2912	10.4	9.7–11.2
Nausea	2080	7.4	6.8–8.1
Antibiotics	895	3.2	2.8–3.7
Other	1361	4.9	4.3–5.5
Blood transfusion	1397	5.0	4.5–5.6
Surgery	267	1.0	0.7–1.2
Observation care only	14,126	50.6	49.3–51.9
Other treatment[C]	81	0.3	0.1–0.5
Discharge status			
Routine discharge from ED	20,992	75.1	74.0–76.2
Admission to hospital	6136	22.0	20.9–23.0
Transferred to other medical facility	464	1.7	1.4–2.0
Left against medical advice	277	1.0	0.8–1.3
Other or unknown	57	0.2	0.1–0.4
Death	15	0.05	0.02–0.2

ED emergency department, *IV* intravenous
[A]Minor incident includes all other incidents that involved an abortion-related diagnosis or treatment, such as those requiring medication or repeat procedure
[B]Major incident includes those requiring overnight inpatient stay, blood transfusion, or surgery
[C]Other treatments include suture of laceration to the cervix, laminaria insertion, and abscess drainage

5.6%), abortion-related surgery (1.0%, 95% CI 0.7–1.2%), or other treatments (0.3%, 95% CI 0.2–0.5%), and 19.4% (95% CI 18.5–20.5%) of all abortion-related visits resulted in an overnight inpatient stay at the same hospital. Major incidents, treated with blood transfusion, surgery, or overnight inpatient stay, accounted for 20.3% (95% CI 19.3–21.3%) of all visits. Minor incidents accounted for 36.1% (95% CI 34.9–37.4%) of visits.

Three-quarters (75.1%) of abortion-related ED visits resulted in discharge from the ED. Another 21.2% were admitted to the same hospital for abortion-related reasons and 0.8% were admitted for non-abortion-related reasons. For the remaining 3%, the disposition was unknown or they were transferred to another medical facility or left against medical advice. Among all abortion-related ED visits over the 5 years of data ($n = 27,941$), 15 ended in the patient's death.

Several demographic and hospital factors were significantly associated with major incidents in a multivariable model (Table 3). Women over 30 were more likely than women aged 20–24 to have major incidents ($P < 0.001$), and women using Medicaid ($P = 0.004$) were more likely than women with private insurance to have a major incident. Women who paid out of pocket for the ED visit were less likely to have a major incident than women with private insurance ($P = 0.001$). The presence of any of the three examined comorbid conditions was associated with more than double the odds of a major incident compared to women without those comorbid conditions ($P < 0.01$). ED visits at trauma hospitals were more likely to be for major incidents than those at non-trauma hospitals ($P < 0.001$). ED visits in all regions were significantly more likely to be for a major incident than those in the Midwest ($P < 0.001$). There was a decreasing trend in major incidents over time. Similar significant relationships were found for factors associated with receipt of observation care only, but factors associated with increased likelihood of major incidents were associated with a lower likelihood of requiring observation care only. Two notable exceptions are a significantly higher likelihood of observation care only in the West compared to the Midwest ($P < 0.001$) and the absence of a trend over time for receipt of observation care only.

We used published rates of the total number of abortions to calculate the percentage of all abortions seen in an ED that resulted in a major incident. During the 5-year study period, there were an estimated 5,282,500 total abortions in the U.S. [17]. Using this number as the denominator, we estimate the rate of major incidents seen in EDs for abortion in the U.S. is 0.11%, or 108 per 100,000 abortions.

We identified 390 ED visits that represented potential self-induced abortion and accounted for 1.4% of abortion-related ED visits during the study period (95% CI 1.1–1.7%). There were slightly higher rates of potential self-induced abortion in the South (2.0%) than in the Midwest (1.0%), West (1.1%), and Northeast (1.3%) ($P = 0.05$) (Table 4). There were no time trends or other factors associated with self-induced abortion.

Discussion

We found that abortion-related ED visits comprised 0.01% of ED visits among women aged 15–49. In other

Table 3 Factors associated with major incidents and observation care only, weighted $n = 27,941$

	Major incident	Observation care
	Adjusted odds ratio (95% confidence interval)	Adjusted odds ratio (95% confidence interval)
Age		
15–19	0.94 (0.74–1.21)	1.18 (0.97–1.42)
20–24	Reference	Reference
25–29	1.08 (0.91–1.28)	0.81** (0.71–0.94)
30–39	1.49*** (1.24–1.79)	0.72*** (0.62–0.83)
40–49	1.75** (1.21–2.53)	0.55*** (0.39–0.77)
Primary payer		
Private insurance	Reference	Reference
Medicaid	1.28** (1.08–1.52)	0.83* (0.72–0.96)
Medicare	1.30 (0.79–2.15)	0.94 (0.55–1.62)
Self-pay	0.66** (0.52–0.85)	1.33** (1.12–1.57)
No charge	1.20 (0.39–3.69)	0.73 (0.34–1.59)
Other	1.35 (0.93–1.97)	0.95 (0.68–1.31)
Missing	0.32 (0.06–1.70)	0.85 (0.36–2.00)
Urban/rural residence		
Urban	Reference	Reference
Rural	1.02 (0.59–1.75)	0.86 (0.58–1.28)
Missing	1.67 (0.58–4.75)	0.43 (0.14–1.28)
Zip code-based income quartile		
First quartile	Reference	Reference
Second quartile	1.11 (0.90–1.36)	0.95 (0.82–1.10)
Third quartile	0.93 (0.75–1.15)	0.89 (0.76–1.04)
Fourth quartile	1.04 (0.82–1.32)	0.92 (0.77–1.11)
Missing	0.90 (0.46–1.75)	0.96 (0.54–1.70)
Diabetes indicated		
No	Reference	Reference
Yes	2.47** (1.42–4.31)	0.28*** (0.14–0.54)
Hypertension indicated		
No	Reference	Reference
Yes	3.79*** (2.46–5.83)	0.52** (0.34–0.80)
Overweight/obese BMI indicated		
No	Reference	Reference
Yes	4.63*** (2.65–8.10)	0.18*** (0.10–0.33)
Hospital characteristics		
Region		
Northeast	1.89*** (1.32–2.71)	0.65** (0.48–0.88)
Midwest	Reference	Reference
South	2.11*** (1.53–2.90)	0.69** (0.54–0.86)
West	1.80*** (1.30–2.49)	2.19*** (1.71–2.80)
Trauma level of hospital		
Level I or II	1.52*** (1.23–1.88)	0.81* (0.68–0.98)

Table 3 Factors associated with major incidents and observation care only, weighted $n = 27,941$ *(Continued)*

	Major incident	Observation care
	Adjusted odds ratio (95% confidence interval)	Adjusted odds ratio (95% confidence interval)
Nontrauma or level III	Reference	Reference
Not specified	1.40 (0.88–2.23)	0.86 (0.55–1.35)
Urban or rural location of hospital		
Urban	Reference	Reference
Rural	0.65 (0.36–1.17)	1.20 (0.77–1.86)
Year		
2009	Reference	Reference
2010	0.85 (0.68–1.07)	1.04 (0.85–1.28)
2011	0.77* (0.61–0.98)	1.09 (0.88–1.36)
2012	0.73** (0.57–0.92)	0.95 (0.76–1.19)
2013	0.71** (0.56–0.90)	0.87 (0.70–1.08)

* $P < 0.05$, ** $P < 0.01$, *** $P < 0.001$
BMI body mass index

words, 14 of every 100,000 ED visits among women aged 15–49 were for abortion-related reasons. The majority (51%) of these were visits involving observation care only.

These data also allowed us to estimate the national major incident rate after an abortion. The rate of 0.11% (108 per 100,000) abortion patients is slightly higher than the rate of 0.05% found in a study of first trimester abortion patients in California [18], and slightly lower than the rate of 0.23% found in a study of all abortions covered by California's Medicaid program [2]. While not all abortion-related incidents lead to an ED visit and thus, are not reflected in this estimate, we believe that the vast majority of major incidents (those involving a blood transfusion, surgery, or hospital admission) are reflected here. Those that would be missed from this analysis are cases that skip the ED and are directly admitted to a hospital or an outpatient surgicenter (usually for scheduled hospitalization) and complications arising from the small proportion (4%) of abortions done in hospitals [17] and are then directly admitted. Thus, the major incident rate may be slightly underestimated.

The major incident rate for abortion (0.1%) is lower than the published rates for pregnancy (1.4%) [19], as well as other common procedures such as colonoscopy (0.2%) [20], wisdom tooth removal (1.0%) [21], and tonsillectomy (1.4%) [22]. Abortion care is, thus, safer than many other unregulated outpatient procedures. Additionally, we found 15 deaths between 2009 and 2013, which is slightly lower than the total number of abortion-related deaths reported in 2009–2012, the most recent years available ($n = 24$) [23].

Notably, the majority of visits involved observation care only, which is consistent with a previous study [2].

Table 4 Potential self-induced abortion, by region

	Weighted N	Weighted percentage of all abortion-related emergency department visits	Weighted percentage 95% confidence interval	Chi-squared test P value
Overall	390	1.4	1.1–1.7	
Region				0.048
Northeast	58	1.3	0.7–2.2	
Midwest	44	1.0	0.5–1.9	
South	195	2.0	1.5–2.6	
West	94	1.1	0.7–1.6	

Patients experience a range of post-abortion symptoms, including ongoing uterine cramping and bleeding for up to 3 weeks after the abortion. Patients may not realize that this is normal. Some women do not start to bleed until several days after the abortion, while some stop bleeding and then start again. Increased cramping and bleeding could start several days after the abortion. Patients may not be given ample information about what to expect or they may have trouble differentiating normal post-abortion symptoms from signs of a complication. Patient visits to EDs for non-urgent care have the potential to be costly to the health system. Such visits could be due to several reasons and little research has been done on factors that contribute to patients' decisions to visit an ED after abortion. EDs offer 24-h access to care compared to abortion facilities, which have relatively limited hours and may require an appointment [24]. The long distances that many women across the U.S. must travel to reach an abortion provider may make return visits for follow-up too arduous [25, 26]. Indeed, research found that patients who travel longer distances to reach an abortion provider are more likely to visit an ED for follow-up care or to manage subsequent symptoms and less likely to return to the original abortion provider [27]. We note that patients presenting to the ED were disproportionately of urban residence (91% in the sample compared to 81% of the U.S. population) [28]. This is likely explained in that 91% of abortion patients live in urban areas [29] and 92% of EDs in the sample were in urban areas, attracting mainly local residents who may find them convenient geographically.

Post-abortion visits to the ED may also be driven by stigma, worry, or distrust of abortion providers. A perception that abortion is unsafe [30–32] may lead women to worry about mild symptoms, such as cramping and bleeding, even though they are an expected result of abortion. Such perceptions may stem from abortion portrayals in the media and popular culture. A study of abortion-related storylines in fictional American television shows found a major incident rate of 34% [33], over 34,000% greater than the real-life major incident rate of 0.1% found here. The long-term consequences of these fictional abortions were much more likely to be severe, including frequent depictions of negative mental health sequelae, infertility, and even death.

Women using Medicaid had higher odds of major incidents than those not using Medicaid and lower odds of observation care. In this context, insurance type may be a proxy for socioeconomic status, as women requiring Medicaid are low income and as a result, face a multitude of barriers to accessing health care and are known to have poorer health status, including multiple chronic conditions, than women with private insurance. Women who were self-pay were less likely to have major incidents and more likely to receive observation care only, suggesting that patients without healthcare coverage may not have been given treatments to reduce patient costs.

We found that the pre-existing chronic conditions that have previously been suspected to be associated with major abortion-related incidents were indeed associated with a significantly higher rate of those incidents in this sample. While there is limited previous research on the impact of chronic health conditions on the risk of abortion complications, it is well established that women with chronic conditions are more likely to have pregnancy-related complications [34]. Our findings are consistent with provider guidance that suggests women with multiple chronic medical conditions may be at increased risk [35], but conflicting with previous studies that find that obesity and chronic health conditions confer no increased risk among women having abortions [11–14]. This increased risk might be explained in that women who had overnight inpatient stays (one of the categories of a major incident) were more likely to have their obesity or other chronic diseases documented in their charts than those who did not have an overnight stay.

We found some cases of potential self-induced abortions using such means as poisoning or other methods of self-harm. While self-induced abortions are safe when appropriate dosages of mifepristone and misoprostol or misoprostol alone are used, other methods are hazardous, as evidenced by ED visits. Rates were highest in the South, which is known to have the most barriers to abortion access, including the fewest providers [17, 26], and the most state-level restrictions. States that are hostile to abortion may see more ED visits due to self-induced abortion than non-hostile states, potentially due to stigma, protesters, and other barriers to in-clinic abortion.

This study included a large, nationally representative sample of ED visits, allowing us to draw national- and regional-level conclusions about abortion safety. However, using billing codes to understand the nature of the ED visit can be imprecise and incomplete. The estimates produced here may be conservative if patients did not report having had an abortion due to fear of stigmatization or if relevant diagnosis and procedure codes were not reported or were systematically misreported. The lack of full clinical data to determine abortion relatedness could cause errors. For example, the visits in this study could include cases of miscarriage. Likewise, this study may miss abortion-related incidents that were inaccurately coded as a miscarriage.

Conclusions

These new findings can inform policy debates regarding abortion regulation in the U.S. Regulations on abortion provider or facility relationships to hospitals or EDs should be considered in light of their relative impact on improving women's health. Because abortion-related ED visits comprise a very small proportion of women's ED visits, and the rate of major incidents is very low, regulations on abortion are unlikely to have any impact on women's health outcomes. Many abortion-related ED visits are for observation only and may not be indicated or could be managed at a less costly level of care. Perceptions that abortion is unsafe are not based on evidence.

Abbreviations

AOR: Adjusted odds ratio; BMI: Body mass index; CI: Confidence interval; CPT: Current Procedural Terminology; ED: Emergency department; HCPCS: Healthcare Common Procedure Coding System; HCUP: Healthcare Cost and Utilization Project; ICD-9: International Classification of Diseases, 9th Revision; IV: Intravenous; NEDS: Nationwide Emergency Department Sample; PAIRS: Procedural Abortion Incident Reporting and Surveillance; U.S.: United States

Funding

This work was supported by a research grant to UDU from the Society of Family Planning (grant SFPRF10). The funder had no role in study design, data collection and analysis, decision to publish, or preparation of the manuscript.

Authors' contributions

UDU, NEJ, and AFC conceived and designed the study. NEJ acquired the data and led the data analysis. RB, CT, AM, and AJM conducted the review and analysis of records. NEJ and UDU drafted the manuscript. All authors contributed to interpretation of the data, revised the draft manuscript for important intellectual content, and approved the final version.

Competing interests

The authors declare that they have no competing interests.

Author details

[1]Department of Obstetrics, Gynecology & Reproductive Sciences, University of California, San Francisco, 1330 Broadway, Suite 1100, Oakland, California 94612, USA. [2]Department of Emergency Medicine, Warren Alpert Medical School of Brown University, 593 Eddy Street, Providence, RI 02903, USA.

References

1. Rui P, Kang K: National Hospital Ambulatory Medical Care Survey: 2014 Emergency Department Summary Tables; 2014.
2. Upadhyay UD, Desai S, Zlidar V, Weitz TA, Grossman D, Anderson P, Taylor D. Incidence of emergency department visits and complications after abortion. Obstet Gynecol. 2015;125(1):175–83.
3. Guttmacher Institute. State Policies in Brief: Targeted Regulation of Abortion Providers. Guttmacher Institute: New York; 2017. https://www.guttmacher.org/state-policy/explore/targeted-regulation-abortion-providers. Accessed 23 May 2018.
4. U.S. Court of Appeals for the Fifth Circuit. Planned Parenthood of Greater Tex. Surgical Health Servs. v. Abbot. 769 F.3d 330, 335; 2014.
5. Fernandez M, Eckholm E. Court Upholds Texas Limits on Abortion. In: The New York Times; 2015.
6. Cleland K, Creinin MD, Nucatola D, Nshom M, Trussell J. Significant adverse events and outcomes after medical abortion. Obstet Gynecol. 2013;121(1): 166–71.
7. Bennett IM, Baylson M, Kalkstein K, Gillespie G, Bellamy SL, Fleischman J. Early abortion in family medicine: clinical outcomes. Ann Fam Med. 2009; 7(6):527–33.
8. NEDS Database Documentation. https://www.hcup-us.ahrq.gov/db/nation/neds/nedsdbdocumentation.jsp. Accessed 23 May 2017.
9. Healthcare Cost and Utilization Project: Introduction to the HCUP Nationwide Emergency Department Sample (NEDS) 2015; 2017.
10. Taylor D, Upadhyay UD, Fjerstad M, Battistelli MF, Weitz TA, Paul ME. Standardizing the classification of abortion incidents: the Procedural Abortion Incident Reporting and Surveillance (PAIRS) Framework. Contraception. 2017;96(1):1–13.
11. Guiahi M, Schiller G, Sheeder J, Teal S. Safety of first-trimester uterine evacuation in the outpatient setting for women with common chronic conditions. Contraception. 2015;92(5):453–7.
12. Benson LS, Micks EA, Ingalls C, Prager SW. Safety of outpatient surgical abortion for obese patients in the first and second trimesters. Obstet Gynecol. 2016;128(5):1065–70.
13. Ingalls C, Benson L, Micks E, Prager S. Obesity in Surgical Abortion: A Risk Factor for Complications?[13N]. Obstet Gynecol. 2016;127:117S–8S.
14. Lederle L, Steinauer JE, Montgomery A, Aksel S, Drey EA, Kerns JL. Obesity as a Risk Factor for Complications After Second-Trimester Abortion by Dilation and Evacuation. Obstet Gynecol. 2015;126(3):585–92.
15. Jerman J, Jones RK, Onda T. Characteristics of U.S. Abortion Patients in 2014 and Changes Since 2008. New York: Guttmacher Institute; 2016.
16. Houchens R, Chu B, Steiner C. Hierarchal Modeling using HCUP Data. In: HCUP Methods Series Report #2007-01 Online. Rockville: U.S. Agency for Healthcare Research and Quality; 2007.
17. Jones RK, Jerman J. Abortion Incidence and Service Availability In the United States, 2014. Perspect Sex Reprod Health. 2017;49(1):17–27.
18. Weitz TA, Taylor D, Desai S, Upadhyay UD, Waldman J, Battistelli MF, Drey EA. Safety of aspiration abortion performed by nurse practitioners, certified nurse midwives, and physician assistants under a California legal waiver. Am J Public Health. 2013;103(3):454–61.
19. Division of Reproductive Health, National Center for Chronic Disease Prevention and Promotion: Severe Maternal Morbidity in the United States; 2017.
20. Castro G, Azrak MF, Seeff LC, Royalty J. Outpatient colonoscopy complications in the CDC's Colorectal Cancer Screening Demonstration Program: a prospective analysis. Cancer. 2013;119(Suppl 15):2849–54.

21. Bui CH, Seldin EB, Dodson TB. Types, frequencies, and risk factors for complications after third molar extraction. J Oral Maxillofac Surg. 2003; 61(12):1379–89.
22. Gallagher TQ, Wilcox L, McGuire E, Derkay CS. Analyzing factors associated with major complications after adenotonsillectomy in 4776 patients: comparing three tonsillectomy techniques. Otolaryngol Head Neck Surg. 2010;142(6):886–92.
23. Jatlaoui TC, Ewing A, Mandel MG, Simmons KB, Suchdev DB, Jamieson DJ, Pazol K. Abortion Surveillance - United States, 2013. MMWR Surveill Summ. 2016;65(12):1–44.
24. Uscher-Pines L, Pines J, Kellermann A, Gillen E, Mehrotra A. Emergency department visits for nonurgent conditions: systematic literature review. Am J Manag Care. 2013;19(1):47–59.
25. Johns NE, Foster DG, Upadhyay UD. Distance traveled for Medicaid-covered abortion care in California. BMC Health Serv Res. 2017;17(1):287.
26. Cartwright AF, Karunaratne M, Barr-Walker J, Johns NE, Upadhyay UD. Identifying National Availability of Abortion Care and Distance From Major US Cities: Systematic Online Search. J Med Internet Res. 2018;20(5):e186.
27. Upadhyay UD, Johns NE, Meckstroth KR, Kerns JL. Distance Traveled for an Abortion and Source of Care After Abortion. Obstet Gynecol. 2017;130(3): 616–24.
28. United States Census Bureau: New Census Data Show Differences Between Urban and Rural Populations; 2016.
29. Jones RK, Jerman J. How far did U.S. women travel for abortion services in 2008? J Womens Health (Larchmt). 2013;22(8):706–13.
30. Gelman A, Rosenfeld EA, Nikolajski C, Freedman LR, Steinberg JR, Borrero S. Abortion Stigma Among Low-Income Women Obtaining Abortions in Western Pennsylvania: A Qualitative Assessment. Perspect Sex Reprod Health. 2017;49(1):29–36.
31. Littman LL, Jacobs A, Negron R, Shochet T, Gold M, Cremer M. Beliefs about abortion risks in women returning to the clinic after their abortions: a pilot study. Contraception. 2014;90(1):19–22.
32. Bessett D, Gerdts C, Littman LL, Kavanaugh ML, Norris A. Does state-level context matter for individuals' knowledge about abortion, legality and health? Challenging the 'red states v. blue states' hypothesis. Cult Health Sex. 2015;17(6):733–46.
33. Sisson G, Rowland B. "I was close to death!": abortion and medical risk on American television, 2005–2016. Contraception. 2017;96(1):25–9.
34. Berg CJ, Mackay AP, Qin C, Callaghan WM. Overview of maternal morbidity during hospitalization for labor and delivery in the United States: 1993–1997 and 2001–2005. Obstet Gynecol. 2009;113(5):1075–81.
35. Davis A, Easterling T. Medical Evaluation and Management. In: Management of Unintended and Abnormal Pregnancy. Chichester: Blackwell Publishing Ltd; 2009. p. 78–89.

4

Can community health worker home visiting improve care-seeking and maternal and newborn care practices in fragile states such as Afghanistan?

Karen M. Edmond[1*], Khaksar Yousufi[1], Zelaikha Anwari[2], Sayed Masoud Sadat[3], Shah Mansoor Staniczai[4], Ariel Higgins-Steele[1], Alexandra L. Bellows[5] and Emily R. Smith[5]

Abstract

Background: The effects of community health worker (CHW) home visiting during the antenatal and postnatal periods in fragile- and conflicted-affected countries such as Afghanistan are not known.

Methods: We conducted a non-randomised population-based intervention study from March 2015 to February 2016. Two intervention and two control districts were selected.
All female CHWs in the intervention districts were trained to provide eight home visits and behaviour change communication messages from pregnancy to 28 days postpartum. The primary outcome was the proportion of women who reported delivering in a health facility. Secondary outcomes were the proportion of women who reported attending a health facility for at least one antenatal and one postnatal visit. Outcomes were analysed at 12 months using multivariable difference-in-difference linear regression models adjusted for clustering.

Results: Overall, 289 female CHWs in the intervention districts performed home visits and 1407 eligible women (less than 12 months postpartum) at baseline and 1320 endline women provided outcome data (94% response rate). Facility delivery increased in intervention villages by 8.2% and decreased in the control villages by 6.3% (adjusted mean difference (AMD) 11.0%, 95% confidence interval (CI) 4.0–18.0%, $p = 0.002$). Attendance for at least one antenatal care visit (AMD 10.5%, 95% CI 4.2–16.9%, $p = 0.001$) and postnatal care visit (AMD 7.2%, 95% CI 0.2–14.2%, $p = 0.040$) increased in the intervention compared to the control districts.

Conclusions: CHW home visiting during the antenatal and postnatal periods can improve health service use in fragile- and conflict-affected countries. Commitment to scale-up from Ministries and donors is now needed.

Trial registration: This trial was retrospectively registered at the Australian and New Zealand Clinical Trial Registry (ACTRN12618000609257).

Keywords: Community, maternal, newborn

* Correspondence: kedmond@unicef.org
[1]UNICEF Afghanistan, UNOCA, Jalalabad Road, Kabul, Afghanistan
Full list of author information is available at the end of the article

Background

There have been substantial improvements in the provision of maternal and newborn health (MCH) services in Afghanistan in recent years [1]. However, key indicators, such as receipt of any antenatal care (ANC) (59%) or postnatal care (PNC) for newborns (9%), remain low [2]. Afghanistan continues to have a fragile and challenging environment for women wishing to obtain healthcare, with maternal and newborn mortality rates remaining among the highest globally [2–4]. Reasons for this include persistent levels of violence and conflict, which limit the ability of many mothers and families to leave the home to receive health and social care [5–7]. Other important barriers are poverty, the mountainous terrain and lack of decision-making 'power' of women within the family [2].

Studies over the last 5 years in poor communities in south Asia and Africa have conclusively shown that community health worker (CHW) home visiting during the antenatal and postnatal periods can improve both the demand for and use of ANC, delivery and PNC services, and reduce maternal and newborn mortality by at least 15–20% [8–11]. CHWs are increasingly being 'institutionalised' in the workforce in south Asia and Africa through enhanced training and incentive packages [12–14].

Home visiting from female CHWs during the antenatal and postnatal periods is likely to be an important way to improve the demand for and use of MCH services in fragile and conflict-affected countries such as Afghanistan [7, 12, 15, 16]. Many CHW studies have been conducted in Africa and South Asia [8, 10]. However, to our knowledge, there have been no published studies of the effectiveness of home visiting by CHWs in conflict-affected districts or provinces.

Volunteer CHWs have been part of the health system in Afghanistan since 2001, but have not been routinely used for home visiting during the antenatal and postnatal periods [17]. In 2015, the Ministry of Public Health in Afghanistan, together with UNICEF and Save the Children, implemented a study to understand if home visiting by CHW for MCH could be effective in conflict-affected districts. The overall aim was to assess whether a CHW home visiting programme could improve care-seeking and newborn care practices in mothers living in the challenging environment of rural Afghanistan.

The primary objective was to assess the effects of the Afghanistan CHW home visiting programme on the proportion of women delivering in a health facility. Secondary outcomes were to assess the effects on the proportion of women who attended a health facility for at least one ANC and one PNC visit. In addition, we assessed effects on birth preparedness and newborn care practices, especially early initiation of exclusive breastfeeding. Effects on the knowledge of mothers about their own and their infant's health were also assessed.

Methods

Study setting

This study was based in Bamyan and Kandahar provinces of Afghanistan. Bamyan is located in the central, mountainous, highland region of Afghanistan and Kandahar is in the southern, sub-desert region bordering eastern Pakistan.

The primary healthcare system includes accredited nurses and doctors who work in sub-centres, basic health centres, comprehensive health centres, and national, regional, provincial and district hospitals [17, 18]. The doctors and midwives provide all medical tests, medical examinations, and ANC, PNC and birthing services in the health facilities. The primary healthcare system also includes volunteer CHWs who work in 'health posts' (usually their own home in their own villages) [17]. New CHWs receive 3 months of initial training followed by annual refresher training. CHWs perform annual censuses through house-to-house visiting, which are recorded on pictorial tally sheets. Women of reproductive age are visited quarterly, new pregnancies are recorded and household listings are updated. CHWs are also trained to act as 'civil registration vital statistics' key informants in the villages. Village members are asked to report all pregnancies, births and deaths to the CHWs. The CHWs report the civil registration vital statistics data to their supervisors monthly. CHWs are also trained to provide family planning, maternal and child health promotion education, basic medicines (e.g. oral contraceptives, iron and folic acid, antibiotics, oral rehydration solution), and to refer mothers and children with significant illness and danger signs. CHWs are not accredited to provide medical or birthing services, these must be provided by accredited doctors and midwives. The CHWs are supervised by paid community health supervisors who provide monthly village-based supportive supervision.

Design

This was a non-randomised, population-based intervention study conducted over a 12-month period from September 2015 to August 2016 in Bamyan and Kandahar provinces. For the evaluation, the baseline survey was conducted over a 1-month period in August 2015 and the endline survey was conducted in July 2016.

We used World Bank and Central Statistics Organization definitions to categorise all districts in Bamyan and Kandahar provinces into 'conflict-affected', 'remote', 'mountainous' and 'poor quintile' categories and to quantify their health services [2, 19–21]. The project team purposively selected two intervention districts per province (Arghandab, Dand, Bamyan, Yakawalang) to ensure 'conflict-affected' areas, 'remote' and 'mountainous' regions were represented. Two control districts per province (Speenboldak, Daman, Panjab and Waras) were then purposively chosen with similar sociodemographics, access and conflict status. Figure 1 displays the map of the study area. Tables 1 and 2 display district profile data and definitions. Intervention and control districts were similar in terms of population size, conflict risk, remoteness, mountainous terrain, wealth quintile and number of health centres. All districts had poor road infrastructure (over 50% of roads unsealed).

Intervention

The intervention was a standardised training and supportive supervision package aimed at improving existing CHW capacity to provide maternal and neonatal home visits and behaviour change communication (BCC) messages from as early as possible in the antenatal period to 28 days postpartum. It was specifically targeted to female CHWs in the study area. All (100%) 289 female CHWs in the study area received the training package.

The intervention had five components. (1) Structured home visiting schedule. Each CHW was trained to provide eight home visits (four during the antenatal period and four in the postnatal period (days 1, 3, 7 and 28) and to provide health promotion and BCC messages at each visit. (2) Structured and simplified MCH BCC training 'curriculum'. This was based on the standardised World Health Organization/UNICEF CHW training package [22]. It included key messages that the CHW should provide to mothers about birth preparedness, care-seeking for ANC, delivery care and newborn care. As most of the CHWs in Afghanistan cannot read or write, locally appropriate tools were developed and pre-tested, including pictorial counselling flip cards for birth preparedness, ANC, facility delivery, newborn greetings, PNC of mother and newborn, and maternal and newborn danger signs. Each training session lasted for 5 days and was followed by three 4-hour 'on the job' refresher sessions over a 12-month intervention period. (3) Structured 'Training of Trainers' programme. Two female government reproductive health provincial officers, one per district, were trained over a 5-day period using locally developed tools and training curriculum. The supervisors then provided training to the female CHWs as described above. (4) Supportive supervision programme. The female CHWs were visited once per month by their supervisors, who provided advice and monitoring, over a period of 12 months. These visits included both scheduled and random unscheduled visits. (5) Performance-based incentive programme. CHWs were provided with a family kit (consisting of cooking and eating utensils including pots, plates, spoons, towels and soap) (total cost approximately $21 USD per kit) for their own use at the beginning of the project if they mapped and registered pregnant women in their catchment areas. They were provided with an additional kit if the woman delivered at a health facility. Programmatic data about the number of CHWs and the intensity of their work and monitoring in the intervention districts are provided in Table 3. These data were collected by the study supervisors during their monthly supervision visits.

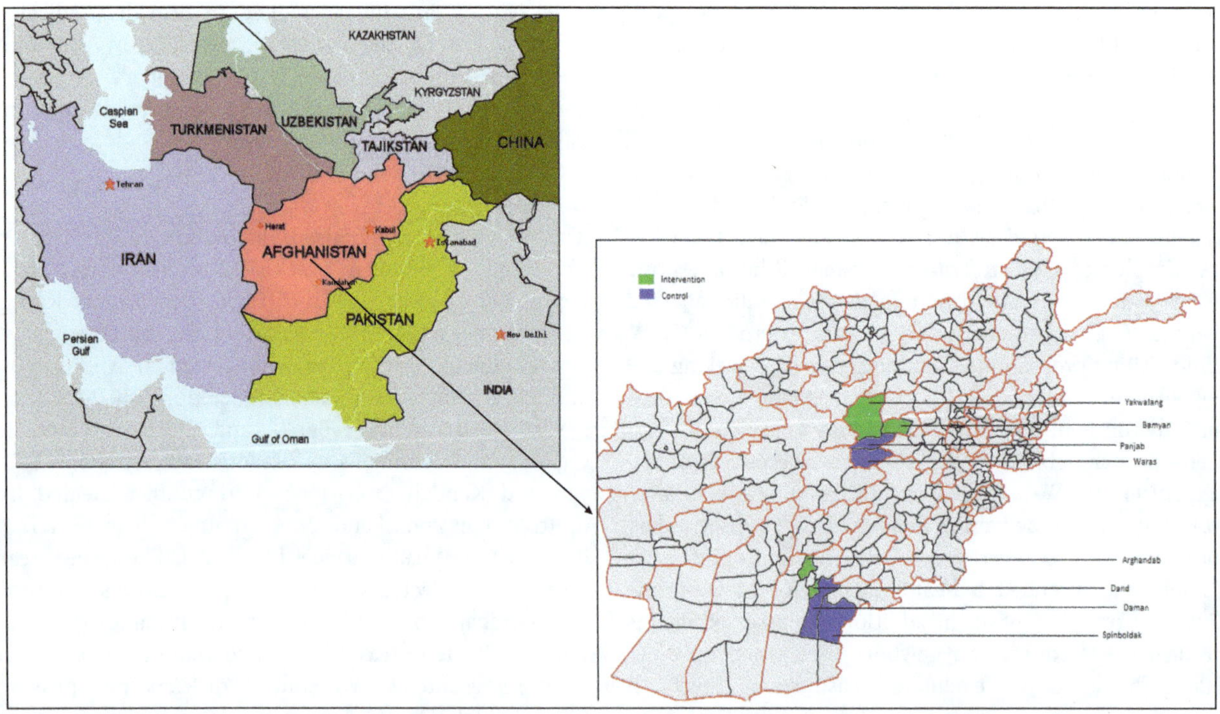

Fig. 1 Map of Afghanistan and intervention and control districts

Table 1 Sociodemographic characteristics of women included in the study compared between intervention and control villages

	Number (%) of mothers in intervention villages		Number (%) of mothers in control villages	
	Baseline	Endline	Baseline	Endline
	(*n* = 709)	(*n* = 689)	(*n* = 699)	(*n* = 689)
Mother's age (mean, SD)	27.9 (6.4)	27.8 (6.6)	28.8 (6.3)	28.4 (6.7)
Mother's education level				
None	459 (64.7%)	460 (66.9%)	408 (58.4%)	448 (66.2%)
Primary (grade 6)	94 (13.3%)	48 (7.0%)	213 (30.5%)	53 (7.8%)
Secondary (grade 9)	27 (3.8%)	27 (3.9%)	21 (3.0%)	34 (5.0%)
High school (grade 12)	23 (3.2%)	21 (3.1%)	24 (3.4%)	28 (4.1%)
University	20 (2.8%)	10 (1.5%)	11 (1.6%)	10 (1.5%)
Madrassa	86 (12.1%)	116 (16.9%)	22 (3.2%)	92 (13.6%)
Ethnic language group				
Dari	356 (50.2%)	331 (49.8%)	353 (50.6%)	358 (52.1%)
Pashtun	353 (49.8%)	334 (50.2%)	345 (49.4%)	329 (47.9%)
Husband/partner's education				
None	335 (47.3%)	278 (40.7%)	286 (41.1%)	360 (53.4%)
Primary (grade 6)	96 (13.5%)	80 (11.7%)	214 (30.6%)	51 (7.6%)
Secondary (grade 9)	62 (8.7%)	60 (8.8%)	57 (8.2%)	31 (4.6%)
High school (grade 12)	52 (7.3%)	56 (8.2%)	37 (5.3%)	37 (5.5%)
University	45 (6.4%)	48 (7.0%)	32 (4.6%)	37 (5.5%)
Madrassa	119 (16.8%)	165 (24.2%)	72 (10.3%)	156 (23.2%)
Husband/partner's occupation				
Does not work	29 (4.2%)	25 (3.7%)	34 (5.0%)	19 (2.8%)
Servant/household worker	6 (0.9%)	5 (0.7%)	17 (2.5%)	10 (1.5%)
Farmer	259 (37.4%)	266 (39.2%)	229 (33.8%)	199 (20.8%)
Livestock herder	15 (2.2%)	10 (1.5%)	17 (2.5%)	18 (2.7%)
Labourer	116 (16.7%)	142 (20.9%)	144 (21.2%)	202 (30.2%)
Street seller/vendor	12 (1.7%)	22 (3.1%)	14 (2.1%)	19 (2.8%)
Shopkeeper	156 (22.5%)	103 (15.2%)	137 (20.2%)	126 (18.9%)
Businessman	18 (2.6%)	10 (1.5%)	8 (1.2%)	11 (1.7%)

Control areas

The control districts received standard care by CHWs who did not receive specific training in home visiting, MCH and BCC. All health facilities in the intervention and control areas received a health system strengthening package over the 12 months prior to the intervention delivery and throughout the intervention period. This included (1) the standard World Health Organization/UNICEF training package to midwives and neonatal nurses in essential newborn care (ENC) and Emergency Obstetric and Newborn Care and (2) training to local community health action groups on the importance of essential antenatal and newborn care.

Data collection

Baseline and endline data were collected from women who were less than 12 months postpartum using a standardised structured survey questionnaire based on the Centers for Disease Control KPC 2000 tool [23]. Survey domains included self-reported baseline socioeconomic status, service use for ANC, delivery and PNC, birth preparedness (including seeking care for maternal postnatal complications, saving money for transportation for emergency obstetric care, pre-planning for a skilled birth attendant (SBA), arranging for a blood donor and newborn care practices (initiating breastfeeding within 1 hour of birth)), and knowledge about ANC, delivery, PNC and birth preparedness.

A separate independent team of female data collectors were trained over a 5-day period and were supervised by two independent data supervisors. The data supervisors performed spot (unscheduled) checks of approximately 10% of the surveys together with a member of the study team. An additional 10% of surveys were selected for re-survey. The data supervisors reviewed each survey

Table 2 Sociodemographic characteristics of the intervention and control districts

Intervention or control area	Intervention	Intervention	Intervention	Intervention	Control	Control	Control	Control
Design								
Province	Bamyan	Bamyan	Kandahar	Kandahar	Bamyan	Bamyan	Kandahar	Kandahar
District	Bamyan	Yakawlang	Arghandaab	Dand	Panjab	Waras	Damaan	Speen Boldak
District population data								
Total population	55,123	57,559	69,094	83,392	53,501	84,826	15,815	88,622
Women of child-bearing age	11,198	11,870	14,356	15,678	11,456	16,743	3678	18,765
Distance in km from provincial capital	110	130	110	155	140	160	100	120
Health system characteristics								
Sub-centres	4	3	4	5	4	5	2	4
Basic health centres	3	3	3	3	3	4	2	3
Comprehensive health centres	3	2	3	4	3	4	2	3
District hospitals	1	1	1	1	1	1	1	1
Mobile health teams	1	2	0	0	2	3	0	1
Demographic characteristics								
Conflict risk[a]	Low	Medium	High	High	Low	Medium	High	High
Remote[b]	Yes	Yes	Yes	Yes	Yes	Yes	Yes	Yes
Mountainous[c]	Yes	Yes	No	No	Yes	Yes	No	No
Lowest wealth quintile[d]	81%	39%	74%	32%	65%	35%	71%	40%

[a]Conflict affected = use of armed force between warring parties in a conflict dyad, be it state based or non-state, resulting in deaths); 25 deaths or less in the previous 12 months is categorised as low intensity, 25–100 is categorised as moderate intensity and 100+ is categorised as high intensity [20, 21]
[b]Remote = District centre more than 2 h away by any form of transport from provincial capital [20, 21]
[c]Mountainous = more than 1800 km elevation at highest point of district [20, 21, 41]
[d]Lowest wealth quintile = As per the Afghanistan Living Standards Survey 2015 using Principal Components Analysis [41]

form and they were not submitted for data entry until they were considered complete and without error. An additional random subsample of 10% of survey forms were also reviewed in the first month of data collection.

Data analysis

For the outcome evaluation, we assessed mean differences in key variables from baseline (data collection immediately prior to the intervention) to endline (data collection 12 months after the intervention commenced) and compared the effects in the intervention areas compared to control areas. We randomly selected households to be visited in each district using a standard two-stage sampling method with probability of selection proportional to size (i.e. random selection of villages followed by random selection of households) [24–26]. The sampling frame was obtained from the Central Statistics Organization, which listed the names of the districts, their villages and their population size. Use of the same cooking hearth was used to define a household.

The primary outcome measure was the proportion of women who reported delivering in a health facility in the study area. Secondary outcome measures were the proportion of women who received at least one ANC visit, proportion of women who received at least one PNC visit, and the proportion of women who initiated breastfeeding within 1 h postpartum. Information on improvements in mothers' knowledge about their own and their infant's health was also analysed.

We calculated that we required a sample size of 1400 women to provide 80% power at a 5% significance level for the primary outcome. These calculations were based on recent data at the provincial level, which indicated that there would be a baseline level of facility delivery of 61% [2], and previous studies that indicated that there would be at least a 20% change in service use due to the intervention [8]. We also assumed that there would be one eligible woman per household. We calculated that this sample size would also provide adequate power for the secondary outcomes.

We used a multivariable 'difference-in-differences' approach to estimate the mean effect of the intervention on each outcome [27]. The difference-in-differences approach is based on comparing mean differences in the intervention group (before and after the intervention) to mean differences in the control group and assumes that trends in both groups are the same in the absence of the intervention [24]. Multivariable linear regression models were constructed to adjust for clustering by district and potential confounders decided a priori and to calculate adjusted mean differences (AMD), 95% confidence intervals (95% CI) and corresponding p values.

Table 3 Community health worker home visiting in intervention districts

	Bamyan	Kandahar	Total[a]
Population	112,682	152,486	265,168
Number of villages	150	131	281
Number of female CHWs	154	135	289
Population size per CHW	732	1130	918
Number of pregnant women in study area	2050	3730	5780
Number of pregnant women per CHW	13	28	20
Number (%) of women who received:			
First CHW antenatal visit	1242 (60.6%)	3436 (92.1%)	4125 (71.4%)
Second CHW antenatal visit	575 (28.0%)	393 (10.5%)	968 (16.7%)
Third CHW antenatal visit	598 (29.2%)	382 (10.2%)	980 (17.0%)
Fourth CHW antenatal visit	458 (22.3%)	272 (7.3%)	730 (12.6%)
First CHW postnatal visit day 1–2[b]	1421 (69.3%)	3029 (81.2%)	4129 (71.7%)
Second CHW postnatal visit day 3	368 (18.0%)	113 (3.0%)	481 (8.3%)
Third CHW postnatal visit day 7	330 (16.1%)	113 (3.0%)	443 (7.7%)
Fourth CHW postnatal visit day 28	198 (9.7%)	82 (2.2%)	280 (4.8%)
Total number of CHW visits in 12-month period	5180	7706	12,886
Number of visits per CHW in 12-month period	33.6	57.1	44.6
Number of visits per CHW per month	2.8	4.8	3.7
Number of visits per woman	2.5	2.1	2.2
Monitoring			
Number (%) of CHWs who received at least one supportive supervision visit	154 (100%)	135 (100%)	289 (100%)
Number (%) of CHWs who received two or more supportive supervision visits	150 (97.4%)	129 (95.6%)	279 (96.5%)

CHW community health worker
[a]Kandahar intervention districts: Arghandab, Dand; Bamyan intervention districts: Bamyan, Yakawalang
[b]This is a visit within the first 48 h after birth. We had exact timing data for 4393 of the 5780 mothers (76%); 966 (22%) were visited at 0–23 h and 3427 (88%) were visited at 24–47 h post birth

In the endline sample, we also assessed whether attending ANC, knowledge about birth preparedness, or sociodemographic factors were associated with facility or SBA-attended birth. Log Binomial and Poisson models with robust variances were used to estimate adjusted relative risks (adjRR), 95% CIs and corresponding p values [28]. SAS version 9.4 was used for all analyses.

Results

All 289 female CHWs in the intervention districts were trained (135 in Kandahar Province (Arghandab and Dand districts) and 154 in Bamyan Province (Yakawalang and Bamyan) districts) (Table 3); 94% (2780 out of 2947) of the women in the study area agreed to participate (1408 women at baseline and 1372 women at endline). The CHWs performed 12,886 home visits to pregnant or postpartum women over the 12-month intervention period (3.7 visits per CHW per month) (Table 3). In total, 5780 pregnant or postpartum women were estimated to receive the intervention. Each CHW visited approximately 20 women and each woman received an average of 2.2 home visits throughout the antenatal and postpartum periods (mean 2.5 Bamyan, mean 2.1 Kandahar) (Table 3). Overall, 4125 (71.4%) women received a first ANC visit and 4127 (71.5%) received a visit within 48 h of birth, but only 730 (12.6%) received a fourth ANC visit and 280 (4.8%) received a fourth PNC visit on approximately day 28 postpartum.

Evaluation survey data were collected from 2780 women. Demographic characteristics were similar between intervention and control districts (Table 1). Overall, 66% of women had no education and 80% of their partners worked as farmers or labourers or were unemployed (Tables 1 and 2). Only maternal primary school education was statistically significantly different between the intervention and control groups ($p = 0.02$).

Service use

Facility delivery increased in intervention villages by 8.2% and decreased in the control villages by 6.3% (AMD 11.0%, 95% CI 4.0–18.0%, p = 0.002). There were similar significant increases in the proportion of women whose delivery was attended by a SBA in the intervention areas as compared to the control areas (AMD 14.2%, 95% CI 7.3–21.2%, $p < 0.0001$) (Table 4). Attendance for at least one ANC visit improved 3.4% in intervention villages (from 71.5% to 74.9%), while ANC attendance declined in control villages (from 80.8% to 70.9%) (AMD 10.5%, 95% CI 4.2%–16.9%, $p = 0.040$). Attendance for at least one PNC visit (AMD 7.2%, 95% CI 0.2–14.2%, $p = 0.040$) increased in the intervention compared to the control districts (Table 4). The proportion of women who sought care for maternal postnatal complications increased by 14.0% in the intervention compared to the control villages (AMD 14.0%, 95% CI 4.1–23.9%, $p = 0.006$). The proportion of women who sought care for maternal antenatal complications also increased in the intervention compared to the control villages (AMD 2.8%, 95% CI −6.2 to −11.8%, $p = 0.540$), though this change was not statistically significant (Table 4).

Birth preparedness

The intervention appeared to have little effect on birth preparedness. The proportion of women who reported that they saved money for transportation for emergency obstetric care, pre-planned for a SBA and arranged for a blood donor was similar between intervention and control districts (Table 5).

Table 4 Service use and care seeking in women included in the study compared between intervention and control villages

	Number (%) of mothers in intervention villages	Number (%) of mothers in control villages	Crude mean difference (95% CI)	*p* value	Adjusted mean difference[a] (95% CI)	*p* value
Antenatal care						
Attended at least one antenatal care visit with a skilled healthcare provider in the previous 6 months						
Baseline (*n* = 1400)	507 (71.5%)	558 (80.8%)				
Endline (*n* = 1366)	513 (74.9%)	483 (70.9%)				
Difference	3.38%	−9.82%	13.21% (6.7 to 19.7)	< 0.0001	10.54% (4.2 to 16.9)	0.001
Care seeking for antenatal or delivery complications						
Baseline (*n* = 866)	329 (75.8%)	352 (81.5%)				
Endline (*n* = 576)	229 (77.9%)	215 (76.2%)				
Difference	2.10%	−5.30%	7.33% (−1.4 to 16.0)	0.10	2.81% (−6.2 to 11.8)	0.54
Delivery care						
Facility delivery						
Baseline (*n* = 1407)	448 (63.2%)	488 (69.9%)				
Endline (*n* = 1300)	446 (71.4%)	429 (63.6%)				
Difference	8.20%	−6.30%	14.53% (7.5 to 21.6)	< 0.0001	10.97% (4.0 to 18.0)	0.002
Delivery attended by a skilled birth attendant						
Baseline (*n* = 1407)	454 (64.0%)	499 (71.5%)				
Endline (*n* = 1320)	479 (74.2%)	428 (63.5%)				
Difference	9.8%	−8.0%	18.1% (11.1 to 25.1)	< 0.0001	14.22% (7.3 to 21.2)	< 0.0001
Sought care for complications during delivery or postpartum						
Baseline (*n* = 655)	268 (82.5%)	292 (85.9%)				
Endline (*n* = 377)	170 (87.6%)	164 (89.6%)				
Difference	5.10%	3.70%	1.43% (−7.3 to 10.2)	0.75	2.36% (−6.8 to 11.5)	0.61
Postnatal care						
Attended at least one postnatal care visit with a skilled healthcare provider in the previous 6 months						
Baseline (*n* = 1392)	337 (47.9%)	369 (53.6%)				
Endline (*n* = 1309)	319 (49.6%)	300 (45.1%)				
Difference	1.7%	−8.5%	10.33% (2.8 to 17.9)	0.0072	7.20% (0.2 to 14.2)	0.04
Sought care for maternal postnatal complications						
Baseline (*n* = 739)	210 (61.4%)	302 (76.1%)				
Endline (*n* = 486)	165 (73.3%)	189 (72.4%)				
Difference	11.90%	−3.70%	15.59% (5.2 to 26.0)	0.0032	14.0% (4.05 to 23.9)	0.006

[a]Adjusted for clustering by district, maternal age, maternal education and paternal education

Newborn care practices

The proportion of women who initiated breastfeeding within 1 h of birth decreased in the intervention villages from 77.9% to 67.4%; however, the proportion increased in the control villages (from 55.8% to 73.7%) (AMD −28.22%, 95% CI −35.7 to −20.8%, $p < 0.0001$) (Table 5). Immediate breastfeeding rates appeared higher in home (260, 76.9%) than facility deliveries (472, 67.5%). Over 94% of women reported that they were providing breast milk to their babies in the intervention and control villages at a mean of 4 months (SD 2.5 months) postnatal in both baseline and endline samples (Table 5).

Knowledge

In general, knowledge related to birth preparedness increased in the intervention compared to the control villages (Table 6). In particular, the proportion of women who could list at least one reason for arranging for travel around the time of birth increased by almost 9% (AMD 8.7%, 95% CI 2.9–14.0%, $p = 0.003$) (Table 6).

Predictors of service use

Maternal and paternal educational level did not appear to influence delivery at a facility or use of a SBA (Table 7). However, young mothers (< 20 years) were almost 20% more likely to give birth in a facility or with a SBA as compared to women aged 25–30 years (adjRR 1.19, 95% CI 1.05–1.34, $p = 0.007$) (Table 7). Women who attended at least one ANC visit with a skilled care provider during their pregnancy were 41% more likely to deliver at a facility or with a SBA (adjRR 1.41, 95% CI 1.27–1.58, $p < 0.001$) than women who did not (Table 7). Birth preparedness was also associated with facility or SBA-attended delivery. In particular, women who could list at least one reason why saving money was important before childbirth were 32% more likely to deliver in a facility or use a SBA (adjRR 1.32, 95% CI 1.18–1.47, $p < 0.001$) than women who could not list these reasons.

Discussion

Training of CHWs in home visiting and BCC skills during the antenatal and postnatal periods was associated with significantly improved care-seeking and service utilisation for facility delivery and ANC in the rural districts of Afghanistan included in our study. Facility delivery increased by 11%, delivery by a SBA increased by 14%, ANC attendance increased by 10% and care-seeking for

Table 5 Birth preparedness and newborn care practices in women included in the study compared between intervention and control villages

	Number (%) of mothers in intervention villages	Number (%) of mothers in control villages	Crude mean difference (95% CI)	*p* value	Adjusted mean difference[a] (95% CI)	*p* value
Birth preparedness						
Saved money for transportation for emergency obstetric care						
Baseline ($n = 1377$)	475 (67.6%)	405 (60.1%)				
Endline ($n = 1226$)	373 (60.7%)	286 (46.8%)				
Difference	−6.90%	−13.30%	6.36% (−1.1 to 13.8)	0.10	2.31% (−4.8 to 9.4)	0.53
Arranged blood donors						
Baseline ($n = 1365$)	172 (24.9%)	84 (12.4%)				
Endline ($n = 1192$)	123 (20.9%)	98 (16.3%)				
Difference	−4.00%	3.90%	−7.91% (−13.9 to −1.9)	0.0098	−9.59% (−15.4 to −3.8)	0.0013
Pre-planned for a skilled birth attendant						
Baseline ($n = 1345$)	467 (68.2%)	396 (55.9%)				
Endline ($n = 1226$)	339 (55.7%)	238 (38.6%)				
Difference	−12.50%	−17.30%	4.83% (−2.7 to 12.4)	0.21	5.32% (−2.0 to 12.7)	0.16
Breastfeeding						
Initiated breastfeeding within the first hour after birth						
Baseline ($n = 1216$)	471 (77.9%)	341 (55.8%)				
Endline ($n = 1037$)	345 (67.4%)	387 (73.7%)				
Difference	−10.50%	17.90%	−28.4% (−35.9 to −20.8)	< 0.0001	−28.22% (−35.7 to −20.8)	< 0.0001
Currently breastfeeding						
Baseline ($n = 1385$)	659 (93.2%)	640 (94.4%)				
Endline ($n = 1366$)	603 (93.8%)	631 (94.5%)				
Difference	0.6%	0.1%	0.50% (−3.1 to 4.1)	0.78	1.13% (−2.4 to 4.7)	0.39

[a]Adjusted for clustering by district, maternal age, maternal education and paternal education

Table 6 Knowledge about birth preparedness in women included in the study compared between intervention and control villages

	Number (%) of mothers in intervention villages	Number (%) of mothers in control villages	Crude mean difference (95% CI)	*p* value	Adjusted mean difference[a] (95% CI)	*p* value
Knowledge of importance of saving money during pregnancy						
Baseline ($n = 1398$)	605 (85.4%)	517 (74.9%)				
Endline ($n = 1291$)	509 (82.6%)	441 (65.3%)				
Difference	−2.8%	−9.6%	6.77% (0.5 to 13.0)	0.04	4.13% (−2.0 to 10.3)	0.19
Knowledge of importance of preplanning travel for birth						
Baseline ($n = 1392$)	623 (88.4%)	575 (83.7%)				
Endline ($n = 1289$)	540 (87.7%)	490 (72.8%)				
Difference	−0.7%	−10.9%	10.18% (4.6 to 15.8)	0.0004	8.46% (2.9 to 14.0)	0.003
Knowledge of importance of arranging a skilled birth attendant						
Baseline ($n = 1390$)	625 (88.7%)	572 (83.5%)				
Endline ($n = 1285$)	513 (83.7%)	502 (74.7%)				
Difference	−5.0%	−8.8%	3.84% (−1.9 to 9.5)	0.19	2.13% (−3.5 to 7.7)	0.45

[a]Adjusted for clustering by district, maternal age, maternal education and paternal education

Table 7 Predictors of facility delivery or skilled birth attendant among women participating in the endline survey ($n = 1376$)

	Univariable model[a]		Multivariable model[a,b]	
	RR (95% CI)	*p* value	RR (95% CI)	*p* value
Maternal educational level				
No education	Reference			
Primary school	1.22 (1.09–1.36)	0.0005	1.07 (0.96–1.19)	0.21
Secondary school or higher	1.21 (1.09–1.33)	0.0003	0.99 (0.89–1.11)	0.91
Madrassa	1.10 (1.01–1.22)	0.04	1.07 (0.97–1.18)	0.20
Paternal educational level				
No education	Reference			
Primary school	1.15 (1.02–1.29)	0.02	1.08 (0.96–1.22)	0.19
Secondary school or higher	1.22 (1.12–1.33)	< 0.0001	1.07 (0.98–1.17)	0.12
Madrassa	1.01 (0.91–1.11)	0.89	0.96 (0.88–1.06)	0.46
Maternal age (years)				
15–19	1.27 (1.12–1.43)	0.0001	1.19 (1.05–1.34)	0.007
20–24	1.05 (0.96–1.16)	0.29	1.01 (0.92–1.11)	0.85
25–29	Reference			
30–34	1.09 (0.98–1.21)	0.10	1.08 (0.99–1.19)	0.10
35–40	0.98 (0.86–1.11)	0.74	1.02 (0.9–1.14)	0.80
> 40	0.97 (0.82–1.16)	0.75	1.02 (0.87–1.2)	0.76
Attended at least one antenatal care visit	1.60 (1.43–1.79)	< 0.0001	1.41 (1.27–1.58)	< 0.0001
Mothers reported having knowledge about the importance of:				
Skilled birth attendance	1.41 (1.26–1.59)	< 0.0001	1.12 (0.99–1.25)	0.06
Preplanning for travel	1.47 (1.30–1.67)	< 0.0001	1.14 (1.01–1.3)	0.04
Saving money in preparation for delivery	1.53 (1.37–1.71)	< 0.0001	1.32 (1.18–1.47)	< 0.0001

[a]Relative risk estimated by log binomial regression models
[b]Adjusted for maternal education, paternal education, maternal age, antenatal care attendance, maternal knowledge, clustering by district

antenatal and postnatal complications improved by 14% in the intervention compared to the control districts. PNC attendance was maintained in the intervention districts but declined in the control districts. Mothers' knowledge also appeared to improve but there was little change in birth preparedness or newborn care practices.

Overall, our findings are encouraging, as the dose of our programmatic intervention was low. Each woman in our study received only two home visits from the onset of pregnancy to 28 days postpartum. Each CHW performed an average of 45 home visits over the 12-month intervention period (almost four per month); 70% of women received a first ANC visit, but only 13% of women received a fourth antenatal visit. Further, 70% of women received a visit from a CHW on the first 2 days after birth but only 8% received a PNC visit on day 7 postpartum and only 5% received a PNC on day 28 postpartum. Over the study period, the levels of conflict and insecurity in both Kandahar and Bamyan provinces increased and restricted movement of some CHWs. Some CHWs were also not allowed by other family members to visit the mothers. A particular barrier was entry to the indoor area of the home, though some CHWs were able to interact with the women in the seating area in front of their home. Competing workload priorities and other employment also restricted the time the CHWs could devote to the home visiting programme. Other challenges included the winter season limiting movement of CHWs and project staff and the dynamic nature of the conflict with new restrictions occurring on a weekly basis.

'Dropout' after initial engagement is a well-known part of 'real world' MCH service delivery [29–31]. Analyses of Demographic and Health Surveys (DHS) conducted in Pakistan, Uganda and Ethiopia describe coverage of 70–80% at the first ANC visit declining to 10–20% by the fourth visit [29, 32, 33]. Coverage of CHW home visits (50–70%) in 'real world' programmatic settings is also substantially lower than experimental research sites (95–100%) [8, 34, 35].

Encouragingly, our study shows that a dose as low as two home visits per pregnant woman can have an important effect on care seeking for service delivery. Increasing the dose of home visits per woman is likely to result in an even greater effect on service use and neonatal morbidity and mortality in our setting in rural Afghanistan. A clear dose response of increasing ANC and PNC service use with increasing intensity of CHW home visiting has been shown in analyses of observational data from Asia and Africa [8, 36, 37]. Clinical trial data also indicate that neonatal mortality can be reduced by up to 45% if a coverage of 90–100% of CHW home visits can be achieved [8, 35–38]. Of note, the Ministry is considering implementation of a 'focused' package of home visits limited to one ANC and one PNC visit, which may be more feasible to implement in our study area.

Mechanisms to increase MCH coverage must include demand generation. A recent Cochrane systematic review reported that CHW packages that included community mobilisation strategies had a 20% greater impact on coverage and health outcomes compared to CHW home visits alone [8, 10]. In our study, the Ministry of Public Health village level community health action groups were trained in intervention and control districts as part of the health system strengthening strategy. However, their activities were limited throughout the study period due to difficulties in implementing supportive supervision for them.

The intervention was made up of five components (home visits, training curriculum, training programme, supervision, incentives). Supportive supervision and in-kind payments are important for the operationalisation of home visits by volunteer CHWs [8–10, 39, 40]. Many studies have shown that cash and in-kind incentives are highly valued by a volunteer CHW workforce [8–10], yet the training stipend is also an important incentive and must be considered part of the essential intervention package [17]. Support to the CHWs through careful monthly supervision was also essential in this fragile context. However, the difficulties with monthly supervision should not be underestimated and are well described in other studies (e.g. ensuring that the most remote area CHWs are supervised, maintaining transport links and ensuring that the correct travel and accommodation per diem is paid) [8–10]. In Afghanistan, community health supervisors are paid staff members and have been embedded within the health system for the last 10 years [17, 22]. Their role is much needed and we are working with the Ministry to ensure sustainability of community health supervisor funding, training and supervision.

Overall, our baseline ANC, facility delivery, PNC and other service utilisation rates were similar to Afghanistan DHS 2015 provincial data [2], indicating that our data collection procedures worked well. The 2015 Afghanistan DHS reported slightly lower national level rates than those provided herein (national level ANC (59%), facility delivery (48%), PNC to mother (40%), PNC to infant (9%)) [2]. However, the Afghanistan DHS also reported a wide variation in coverage including rates as low as 10–20% in very poor provinces such as Nuristan and Urzugan, where attendance at community health facilities requires a longer than 4-hour walk and where the ability to leave the home is markedly restricted [2]. The modest increases reported in our study will mean much for the mothers and infants who live in similar poor and deprived districts across Afghanistan.

Mothers' knowledge about birth preparedness (saving money for transportation, preplanning travel for facility delivery, preplanning for a SBA) appeared to be maintained in the intervention villages compared to the control villages, and also appeared to be significantly predictive of later service use. However, there appeared to be little difference between the intervention and control groups in mothers' actual actions in saving money for transportation, preplanning travel for facility delivery or preplanning for a SBA. These findings may reflect the limited resources and financial decision-making power of the women in the deprived villages that participated in our study. Increasing the intensity and quality of CHW home visiting is needed to change the complex behaviours required for birth preparedness. This includes CHW interaction with other family members, such as fathers and grandfathers, who are the traditional decision-makers in the family setting. Other initiatives, such as cash transfers, demand side financing and provision of local transport options, are also needed [10, 39, 40].

Little improvement in neonatal care practices was observed. In particular, the proportion of women who initiated breastfeeding within 1 hour of birth declined in the intervention villages by 10%. Other studies have indicated difficulties in changing breastfeeding behaviour at both community and facility level [37, 40]. Our health system strengthening included facility-based ENC training and the importance of early initiation of breastfeeding. However, we had few resources available for ongoing supportive supervision and we were aware that quality of ENC may have been poor in both the intervention and control facilities. We also reported that breastfeeding rates appeared higher after home (260, 76.9%) than facility deliveries; thus, we feel that more facility-based work is needed in our study area. Increasing rates of referral and care seeking will not be effective in improving morbidity and mortality if health facilities cannot deal with the work load or have poor quality of care [31–33]. Interestingly, our levels of breastfeeding (94%) were maintained at high levels postpartum in both intervention and control villages at baseline and endline. These data require more investigation as to their accuracy.

Our study had some limitations. It was non-randomised and we purposively chose the intervention and control districts to ensure that both fragile and conflict-affected areas were included. However, we used adjusted difference-in-difference analyses to account for baseline differences and any potentially differing trends in the intervention and control areas [27]. Our intervention dose was low, as described above, due to implementation in difficult conflict-affected areas but we were still able to show an important difference on key outcomes. Our data collectors were allowed to spend only a short period of time in the locations to collect data due to concerns about security. Thus, our evaluation questionnaire, especially the newborn and knowledge sections, was more restricted than previously planned. Our outcome data were also all self-reported and we were not able to verify even a subsample due to project restrictions. Additionally, there was some deterioration in facility delivery, SBA and ANC coverage in the study area, likely due to increasing levels of conflict restricting access; however, longer term surveillance is needed to understand the ongoing trends.

Strengths of our study included our ability to adhere to our data quality and supportive supervision plan, which included random re-visits and verification. Other strengths included our population- and community-based implementation and evaluation. We also had a large sample size and a high response rate. Finally, definitions of 'fragile' and 'conflict affected' also vary; herein, we used clear World Bank and Organisation for Economic Co-operation and Development (OEDC) categories ('fragile' districts requiring external assistance for peacekeeping, governance and financial assistance, and 'conflict affected' districts requiring armed force resulting in battle-related deaths) [19–21], which do not include 'natural disasters' such as earthquakes, floods or fire.

Conclusion

Overall, our CHW home visiting intervention appeared to improve care seeking and knowledge but not birth preparedness and newborn care practices. Our results indicate that home visiting from CHWs during the antenatal and postnatal periods is likely to be a valuable part of the health system in rural Afghanistan, but that improved training packages are also needed for more complex behaviours such as birth preparedness and newborn care. More work is also needed in strengthening of knowledge and quality of care, especially in specific essential care components including the promotion of early initiation of breastfeeding and other newborn care practices. Further system changes are also required to ensure the sustainability of the CHW programme in Afghanistan, including performance-based payments for completion of home visits and outcomes such as facility delivery. Increasing the intensity and engagement of CHW with families of pregnant and postpartum women and increasing demand generation is also important. Encouraging new findings have arisen from studies focused on cash transfers to CHWs and mothers for facility delivery and 'mini motorcycle ambulances' for transport of unwell pregnant mothers and their young children in Afghanistan, which will be presented in subsequent papers. Our results also indicate that CHW home visiting will be highly effective in other conflict-affected countries where women have little power to seek care for themselves or their young children. However, more studies are urgently needed especially from African states and other cultural contexts.

Appendix

Table 8 Sociodemographic characteristics of women included in the study in Kandahar and Bamyan villages at baseline

	Number (%) of mothers in Bamyan intervention and control villages at baseline ($n = 709$)	Number (%) of mothers in Kandahar intervention and control villages at baseline ($n = 699$)
Mother's age (mean, SD) ($n = 1397$)	27.8 (5.9)	28.8 (6.7)
Mother's education level ($n = 1408$)		
None	502 (70.8%)	365 (52.2%)
Primary (grade 6)	70 (9.9%)	237 (33.9%)
Secondary (grade 9)	24 (3.4%)	24 (3.4%)
High School (grade 12)	41 (5.8%)	6 (0.9%)
University	26 (3.7%)	5 (0.7%)
Madrassa	46 (6.5%)	62 (8.9%)
Ethnic language group ($n = 1407$)		
Dari	709 (100%)	0 (0%)
Pashto	0 (0%)	699 (100%)
Husband/Partner's education ($n = 1408$)		
None	272 (38.4%)	350 (50.1%)
Primary (grade 6)	98 (13.8%)	212 (30.3%)
Secondary (grade 9)	68 (9.6%)	51 (7.3%)
High school (grade 12)	64 (9.0%)	25 (3.6%)
University	70 (9.9%)	7 (1.0%)
Madrassa	137 (19.3%)	54 (7.7%)
Husband/Partner's occupation ($n = 1370$)		
Does not work	30 (4.4%)	33 (4.9%)
Servant/household worker	4 (0.6%)	19 (2.8%)
Farmer	345 (50.1%)	143 (21.0%)
Livestock herder	4 (0.6%)	28 (4.1%)
Labourer	118 (17.1%)	142 (20.9%)
Street seller/vendor	2 (0.3%)	24 (3.5%)
Shopkeeper	55 (8.0%)	238 (35.0%)
Businessman	11 (1.6%)	15 (2.2%)

Acknowledgements
The authors would like to acknowledge the dedicated work of the other members of the study implementation team: Mohammad Attai, Emal Mujadidi, Ahmad Wahidi, Akmal Samsor, Malalai Naziri and Sherin Varkey. The authors would also like to thank colleagues and collaborations from the Ministry of Public Health, UNICEF and other UN agencies.

Funding
UNICEF Afghanistan Country Office.

Authors' contributions
KME conceptualised and wrote the first draft of the paper and analyses. The other authors all supervised or conducted the data collection or analyses. All authors reviewed and approved the final manuscript.

Competing interests
The authors declare that they have no competing interests.

Author details
[1]UNICEF Afghanistan, UNOCA, Jalalabad Road, Kabul, Afghanistan. [2]Ministry of Public Health, Reproductive, Maternal, Newborn, Child and Adolescent Directorate, Kabul, Afghanistan. [3]Ministry of Public Health, Community Based Health Care Department, Kabul, Afghanistan. [4]Save The Children, Kabul, Afghanistan. [5]Department of Global Health and Population, Harvard TH Chan School of Public Health, Boston, USA.

References

1. Akseer N, Bhatti Z, Rizvi A, Salehi AS, Mashal T, Bhutta ZA. Coverage and inequalities in maternal and child health interventions in Afghanistan. BMC Public Health. 2016;16(Suppl 2):797.
2. Central Statistics Organisation. Ministry Public Health (MoPH) and ICF 2017. Demographic and Health Survey. Kabul Afghanistan: Central Statistics Organization; 2015.
3. Akseer N, Kamali M, Husain S, Mirza M, Bakhache N, Bhutta ZA. Strategies to avert preventable mortality among mothers and children in the eastern Mediterranean region: new initiatives, new hope. East Mediterr Health J. 2015;21(5):361–73.

4. Akseer N, Salehi AS, Hossain SM, et al. Achieving maternal and child health gains in Afghanistan: a Countdown to 2015 country case study. Lancet Glob Health. 2016;4(6):e395–413.
5. Hirose A, Borchert M, Cox J, Alkozai AS, Filippi V. Determinants of delays in travelling to an emergency obstetric care facility in Herat, Afghanistan: an analysis of cross-sectional survey data and spatial modelling. BMC Pregnancy Childbirth. 2015;15:14.
6. Hirose A, Borchert M, Niksear H, et al. Difficulties leaving home: a cross-sectional study of delays in seeking emergency obstetric care in Herat, Afghanistan. Soc Sci Med. 2011;73(7):1003–13.
7. Burki T. Conflict in Afghanistan takes an increasing toll on civilians. Lancet. 2016;388(10040):117–8.
8. Lassi ZS, Bhutta ZA. Community-based intervention packages for reducing maternal and neonatal morbidity and mortality and improving neonatal outcomes. Cochrane Database Syst Rev. 2015;3:CD007754.
9. Colvin CJ, de Heer J, Winterton L, et al. A systematic review of qualitative evidence on barriers and facilitators to the implementation of task-shifting in midwifery services. Midwifery. 2013;29(10):1211–21.
10. Glenton C, Colvin CJ, Carlsen B, et al. Barriers and facilitators to the implementation of lay health worker programmes to improve access to maternal and child health: qualitative evidence synthesis. Cochrane Database Syst Rev. 2013;10:CD010414.
11. Yonemoto N, Dowswell T, Nagai S, Mori R. Schedules for home visits in the early postpartum period. Cochrane Database Syst Rev. 2017;8:CD009326.
12. Pfaffmann Zambruni J, Rasanathan K, Hipgrave D, et al. Community health systems: allowing community health workers to emerge from the shadows. Lancet Glob Health. 2017;5(9):e866–e7.
13. The Lancet Global Health. Community health workers: emerging from the shadows? Lancet Glob Health. 2017;5(5):e467.
14. USAID Unicef Institutionalizing Community Health Conference, Johannesberg 2017. http://www.ichc2017.org/sites/default/files/images/Plenary%205/Plenary%205%20-%20Jerome%20Pfaffmann.pdf. Accessed 24 Apr 2018.
15. Black RE, Taylor CE, Arole S, Bang A, Bhutta ZA, Chowdhury AMR, Kirkwood BR, Kureshy N, Lanata CF, Phillips JF, Taylor M, Victora CG, Zhu Z, Perry HB. Comprehensive review of the evidence regarding the effectiveness of community-based primary health care in improving maternal, neonatal and child health: 8. Summary and recommendations of the expert panel. J Glob Health. 2017;7(1):010908.
16. Gopalan SS, Das A, Howard N. Maternal and neonatal service usage and determinants in fragile and conflict-affected situations: a systematic review of Asia and the middle-east. BMC Womens Health. 2017;17(1):20.
17. Newbrander W, Paul I, Feroz F, Stanekzai H. Afghanistan's Basic Package of Health Services: Its Development and Effects on Rebuilding the Health System. 25, 2014. http://moph.gov.af/en/article/afghanistans-basic-package-of-health-services-its-development-and-effects-on-rebuilding-the-health-system. Accessed 24 Apr 2018.
18. Frost A, Wilkinson M, Boyle P, Patel P, Sullivan R. An assessment of the barriers to accessing the basic package of health services (BPHS) in Afghanistan: was the BPHS a success? Glob Health. 2016;12(1):71.
19. World Bank. The World Bank Group's harmonized list of fragile situations. 2016. http://pubdocs.worldbank.org/en/586581437416356109/FCS-List-FY16-Information-Note.pdf. Accessed 24 Apr 2018.
20. The World Bank Data. Fragile and conflict affected situations. 2018. https://data.worldbank.org/region/fragile-and-conflict-affected-situations. Accessed 24 Apr 2018.
21. OECD. States of Fragility 2016: Understanding Violence. Paris: OECD Publishing; 2016. https://doi.org/10.1787/9789264267213-en. Accessed 24 Apr 2018
22. Caring for the Newborn at Home. A Training Course for Community Health Workers. http://www.who.int/maternal_child_adolescent/news/events/2012/CHW_Manual.pdf. Accessed 8 Dec 2017.
23. Centers for Disease Control KPC 2000+ Survey tool. https://www.spring-nutrition.org/sites/default/files/publications/tools/spring_context_assessment_tools_all.pdf Accessed 8 Dec 2017.
24. Bierrenbach AL. World Health Organization. Geneva http://www.who.int/tb/advisory_bodies/impact_measurement_taskforce/meetings/prevalence_survey/psws_probability_prop_size_bierrenbach.pdf. Accessed 25 Nov 2017.
25. Bierrenbach B. Steps in Applying Probability Proportional to Size and Calculating Basic Probability Weights. Geneva: World Health Organization 2012.
26. Bennett S. A Simplified General Method for Cluster Sample Surveys of Health in Developing Countries. http://apps.who.int/iris/bitstream/10665/47585/1/WHSQ_1991_44(3)_98-106_eng.pdf. Accessed 8 Dec 2017.
27. Dimick JB, Ryan AM. Methods for evaluating changes in health care policy: the difference-in-differences approach. JAMA. 2014;312(22):2401–2.
28. Spiegelman D, Hertzmark E. Easy SAS calculations for risk or prevalence ratios and differences. Am J Epidemiol. 2005;162(3):199–200.
29. Anastasi E, Borchert M, Campbell OM, et al. Losing women along the path to safe motherhood: why is there such a gap between women's use of antenatal care and skilled birth attendance? A mixed methods study in northern Uganda. BMC Pregnancy Childbirth. 2015;15:287.
30. Mohan D, LeFevre AE, George A, et al. Analysis of dropout across the continuum of maternal health care in Tanzania: findings from a cross-sectional household survey. Health Policy Plan. 2017;32(6):791–9.
31. Singh K, Story WT, Moran AC. Assessing the continuum of care pathway for maternal health in South Asia and sub-Saharan Africa. Matern Child Health J. 2016;20(2):281–9.
32. Iqbal S, Maqsood S, Zakar R, Zakar MZ, Fischer F. Continuum of care in maternal, newborn and child health in Pakistan: analysis of trends and determinants from 2006 to 2012. BMC Health Serv Res. 2017;17(1):189.
33. Yaya S, Bishwajit G, Ekholuenetale M, Shah V, Kadio B, Udenigwe O. Timing and adequate attendance of antenatal care visits among women in Ethiopia. PLoS One. 2017;12(9):e0184934.
34. Mbuagbaw L, Medley N, Darzi AJ, Richardson M, Habiba Garga K, Ongolo-Zogo P. Health system and community level interventions for improving antenatal care coverage and health outcomes. Cochrane Database Syst Rev. 2015;12:CD010994.
35. Kirkwood BR, Manu A, ten Asbroek AH, et al. Effect of the Newhints home-visits intervention on neonatal mortality rate and care practices in Ghana: a cluster randomised controlled trial. Lancet. 2013;381(9884):2184–92.
36. Friberg IK, Bhutta ZA, Darmstadt GL, et al. Comparing modelled predictions of neonatal mortality impacts using LiST with observed results of community-based intervention trials in South Asia. Int J Epidemiol. 2010; 39(Suppl 1):i11–20.
37. Karim AM, Admassu K, Schellenberg J. Effect of Ethiopia's health extension program on maternal and newborn health care practices in 101 rural districts: a dose-response study. PLoS One. 2013;8(6):e65160.
38. Johnson AD, Thiero O, Whidden C, Poudiougou B, Diakité D, Traoré F, Samaké S, Koné D, Cissé I, Kayentao K. Proactive community case management and child survival in periurban Mali. BMJ Glob Health. 2018; 3(2):e000634.
39. Wiysonge CS, Paulsen E, Lewin S, Ciapponi A, Herrera CA, Opiyo N, Pantoja T, Rada G, Oxman AD. Financial arrangements for health systems in low-income countries: an overview of systematic reviews. Cochrane Database Syst Rev. 2017;9:CD011084.
40. Mian NU, Alvi MA, Malik MZ, Iqbal S, Zakar R, Zakar MZ, Awan SH, Shahid F, Chaudhry MA, Fischer F. Approaches towards improving the quality of maternal and newborn health services in South Asia: challenges and opportunities for healthcare systems. Glob Health. 2018;14(1):17.
41. Islamic Republic of Afghanistan, Central Statistics Organization Afghanistan Living Standards Survey 2013–2014. http://cso.gov.af/Content/files/ALCS/ALCS%20ENGLISH%20REPORT%202014.pdf. Accessed 22 April 2018.

5

Translating evidence to patient care through caregivers: a systematic review of caregiver-mediated interventions

Kirsten M. Fiest[1*], Christiane Job McIntosh[2], Danielle Demiantschuk[2], Jeanna Parsons Leigh[3] and Henry T. Stelfox[4]

Abstract

Background: Caregivers may promote the uptake of science into patient care and the practice of evidence-informed medicine. The purpose of this study was to determine whether caregiver-mediated (non-clinical caregiver-delivered) interventions are effective in improving patient, caregiver, provider, or health system outcomes.

Methods: We searched the MEDLINE, Embase, PsycINFO, Cumulative Index of Nursing and Allied Health, and Scopus databases from inception to February 27, 2017. Interventions (with a comparison group) reporting on a quality improvement intervention mediated by a caregiver and directed to a patient, in all ages and patient-care settings, were selected for inclusion. A three-category framework was developed to characterize caregiver-mediated interventions: inform (e.g., provide knowledge), activate (e.g., prompt action), and collaborate (e.g., lead to interaction between caregivers and other groups [e.g., care providers]).

Results: Fifty-six studies met the inclusion criteria, and 64% were randomized controlled trials (RCTs). The most commonly assessed outcomes were patient- ($n = 40$) and caregiver-oriented ($n = 33$); few health system- ($n = 10$) and provider-oriented ($n = 2$) outcomes were reported. Patient outcomes (e.g., satisfaction) were most improved by caregiver-mediated interventions that provided condition and treatment education (e.g., symptom management information) and practical condition-management support (e.g., practicing medication protocol). Caregiver outcomes (e.g., stress-related/psychiatric outcomes) were most improved by interventions that activated caregiver roles (e.g., monitoring blood glucose) and provided information related to that action (e.g., why and how to monitor). The risk of bias was generally high, and the overall quality of the evidence was low-moderate, based on Grading of Recommendations Assessment Development and Evaluation ratings.

Conclusions: There is a large body of research, including many RCTs, to support the use of caregiver-mediated interventions that inform and activate caregivers to improve patient and caregiver outcomes. Select caregiver-mediated interventions improve patient (*inform-activate*) and caregiver (*inform-activate-collaborate*) outcomes and should be considered by all researchers implementing patient- and family-oriented research.

Systematic review: PROSPERO, CRD42016052509.

Keywords: Systematic review, Caregiver-mediated, Quality improvement, Knowledge translation, Implementation science, Intervention, Review, Translational medical research

* Correspondence: kmfiest@ucalgary.ca
[1]Departments of Critical Care Medicine and Community Health Sciences, O'Brien Institute for Public Health and Hotchkiss Brain Institute, Cumming School of Medicine, University of Calgary, 2500 University Drive NW, Calgary, AB T2N 1N4, Canada
Full list of author information is available at the end of the article

Background

Patient- and family-centered care (PFCC) research, where patients and families partner with providers in the planning and delivery of healthcare, represents a shift from solely studying provider-identified priorities [1, 2]. PFCC represents a cultural change in healthcare that acknowledges that patients and their caregivers are central figures in decision-making and the delivery of care [1, 2]. Perceptions of PFCC and its benefits are high among patients and family members, though there are barriers to its implementation, including a purported lack of provider knowledge of PFCC, system barriers (e.g., lack of personnel, visiting hours), and a perceived increase in provider burden [3–5]. The uptake of PFCC interventions is limited by these barriers, and the science of PFCC is lagging behind scientific, clinical, operational, and public interest and desire.

PFCC may provide a mechanism for quality improvement initiatives designed to implement evidence-informed practices into patient care. Patients and caregivers can act as agents of change, making evidence more accessible and providing a method for implementing science into patient care, regardless of the clinical setting [2]. Due to the nature of their illness and the use of invasive therapies, some patients may not be able to act as active agents of change [6]; children, and a growing number of adults with complex care needs, represent populations who require a caregiver. This presents a unique role for caregivers to be engaged in PFCC, though the evidence supporting the delivery and effectiveness of caregiver-mediated interventions is limited. Because of the growing role of patients and caregivers in care, there is an opportunity to engage and empower them to promote the uptake of science into patient care and the practice of evidence-informed medicine.

In order to effectively carry out PFCC, we must create, implement, and measure the effect of PFCC interventions. A recent systematic review of patient-mediated interventions suggested benefit [7]. There is a large and diverse literature on caregiver-mediated interventions, though no systematic review has been conducted. We therefore asked the question: Are caregiver-mediated interventions (interventions delivered in some part by the caregiver) effective in improving patient, caregiver, provider, or health system outcomes?

Methods

This systematic review was conducted and reported per the Preferred Reporting Items for Systematic Reviews and Meta-Analyses (PRISMA) criteria [8] (see Additional file 1 for the checklist). An a priori protocol was published online through PROSPERO (registration number CRD42016052509; Additional file 2). Ethical approval was not required, as previously published data were used.

Patient and stakeholder involvement

Our methods were informed by our stakeholders: a 2-day stakeholder (patients, families, researchers, care providers) engagement meeting was held (November 17–18, 2016, Calgary, Canada) to determine relevant, patient-oriented priorities. Attendees included three former intensive care unit (ICU) patients, four family members of former ICU patients, 19 researchers, and 10 care providers. Patients and family members were asked to identify relevant and important patient-oriented priorities in critical care medicine; the discussion was open and guided by an experienced facilitator. Study findings will be presented to these patients and family members at the next stakeholder engagement meeting planned for the Fall of 2018.

Outcome measures

Based on feedback from stakeholders, the primary research question was: Are caregiver-mediated interventions effective in improving patient, caregiver, provider, or health system outcomes? Secondary research questions were the following: (1) What types of interventions have been deemed effective? (2) Does effectiveness vary according to the intervention type, patient population, caregiver group, contextual factors, or implementation strategy? (3) How have these interventions been evaluated?

Populations, interventions, comparators, settings, and study designs

Inclusion criteria for studies were as follows: (1) interventional study design with a comparison group; (2) reporting on an intervention *mediated* by caregivers and directed to a patient; (3) conducted in a patient-care setting of any age group; and (4) in any language, and published at any time. Studies were excluded if they were not interventional in design, reported on interventions *directed* at the caregiver, or were not conducted in the context of patient care (e.g., took place at home). For the purposes of this review, we established definitions for key concepts and defined: (1) a caregiver as any non-clinical person who regularly provides support to the patient and is in some way directly implicated in the patient's care or directly affected by the patient's health problem; (2) caregiver-mediated as the caregiver being directly involved in delivering the intervention; (3) a patient as someone who has a health condition, is at risk for developing a health condition, or is attending a patient-care setting to receive care; and (4) a patient-care setting as any setting where a patient may receive care for an existing health condition or preventative care from a healthcare professional. We distinguish caregiver-*mediated* interventions from caregiver-*directed* interventions—where the caregiver is the target of the intervention and is not involved in delivering the intervention him/herself. Quality improvement (or implementation science or knowledge translation) was defined as the synthesis, dissemination, exchange, and application of health-related knowledge and research [9]. Studies were excluded if they were only abstracts or were not primary research.

Data sources and searches

The search strategy (Additional file 3) was developed with the assistance of a medical librarian (H.G.) and in consultation with experts in quality improvement in healthcare (H.T.S., J.P.L.). The MEDLINE (OVID), Embase (OVID), PsycINFO (OVID), Cumulative Index of Nursing and Allied Health (CINAHL [EBSCO]), and Scopus (Elsevier) bibliographic databases were searched from inception to February 27, 2017. Using subject headings, keywords, and synonyms, we searched the following domains: (1) caregivers; (2) intervention; (3) mediated; (4) quality improvement/knowledge translation; (5) clinical care. The reference lists of included papers were reviewed to identify potential studies missed in the search.

Study selection

All titles and abstracts were reviewed independently in duplicate by two reviewers (K.M.F., C.J.M.); any study selected by either reviewer at this stage was selected to move on to the next stage. The full text of all articles was reviewed independently in duplicate by two of three reviewers (K.M.F., C.J.M., D.D.); all articles selected by both reviewers at this stage were included in the final review. Disagreements were resolved by discussion or the involvement of a third reviewer when necessary. References were managed in EndNote X7 (Clarivate Analytics, Philadelphia, PA, USA).

Data extraction and quality assessment

Two reviewers (C.J.M., D.D.) abstracted data independently, in duplicate, using a data collection sheet developed and piloted by the study team. Information on study design, study characteristics (e.g., age, setting), patient population (e.g., infants, older adults; as defined by the individual papers), caregiver group (e.g., spouses, parents, family caregivers [which may include parents when undefined]), intervention, and control group was abstracted, and risk of bias and strength of the evidence (see below) assessed. Translation was sought for all non-English articles ($n = 7$; 2 French, 2 Cantonese, 1 Spanish, 1 Turkish, 1 Serbo-Croatian).

The Cochrane Collaboration's risk of bias tool was used to evaluate the internal validity of all included studies [10]. To be assigned an overall low risk of bias, all domains needed to be rated as low. The presence of a single high or unclear item resulted in the overall risk of bias being rated as high or unclear, respectively. The strength of the evidence was described as low, moderate, or high according to the Grading of Recommendations Assessment Development and Evaluation (GRADE) working group approach [11].

Data synthesis and analysis

Findings were summarized using descriptive statistics (median, frequencies) and their accompanying measures of variability (interquartile range [IQR]) where appropriate using STATA 14.1. Meta-analysis was not possible due to heterogeneity in study design, type of intervention, and outcomes reported. Using a framework of engagement described in previous research on patient-mediated interventions [7] and adapted from a previous meta-review [12], we categorized interventions into three engagement strategies: *inform* (interventions that provide knowledge), *activate* (interventions that prompt action), and *collaborate* (interventions that lead to interaction between the caregiver and other groups such as providers or other caregivers) (Additional file 1). Within these three strategies were 13 types of engagement support, including lifestyle advice, psychological strategies, and information on available resources (examples in Additional file 1). Interventions were further classified as single-component (involving a single component/engagement support) or complex interventions (involving more than one component/engagement support) [13]. Study outcomes were classified as patient-oriented, caregiver-oriented, provider-oriented, or health system-oriented.

Role of the funding source

The study funder had no role in the study design; in the collection, analysis, or interpretation of data; in the writing of the report; or in the decision to submit the article for publication. The researchers are independent from the study funders.

Results

Results of the search

We screened 4273 unique abstracts and reviewed 231 full-text articles; 175 full-text articles were excluded, the most common reasons being that the intervention was not mediated by a caregiver 110/175) or that the study did not include an intervention (37/175) (Fig. 1). Hand searching resulted in the inclusion of 18 additional studies. Characteristics of the 56 studies meeting all inclusion criteria are described in Additional file 2.

Description of included studies

The 56 intervention studies [1, 2, 14–67] were published between 1984 and 2017 and conducted in the USA ($n = 32$, 57.1%), Canada ($n = 3$, 5.4%), and 14 other countries ($n = 1$ or 2 studies each) (Additional file 2). Most

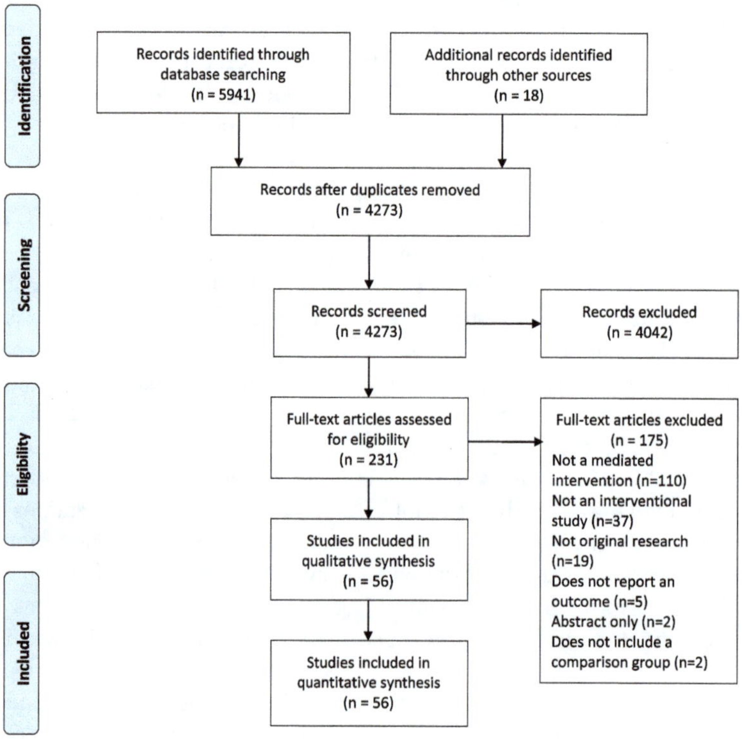

Fig. 1 Study flow diagram

studies ($n = 36$, 64.3%) were randomized controlled trials [14, 15, 18, 20, 24, 26–31, 33–36, 38, 39, 41–47, 50, 51, 54–59, 62, 64–66] and conducted in outpatient settings (including primary care and the community) ($n = 33$). Caregivers were most commonly parents ($n = 25$, 44.6%) [14–18, 20, 25, 28, 30, 34, 36, 37, 39–41, 46–48, 49, 53, 58, 60, 64–66] and family caregivers more broadly—family caregivers could include parents, but the term was broadly defined—($n = 17$, 30.4%) [1, 2, 22, 23, 31–33, 35, 42, 44, 45, 54, 56, 59, 61, 63, 67], with the most common populations receiving care being premature/low birth weight infants ($n = 8$, 14.3%) [14, 17, 18, 40, 47, 49, 65, 66], children with asthma ($n = 6$, 10.7%) [26, 27, 34, 41, 46, 56], and stroke survivors ($n = 4$, 7.0%) [33, 45, 51, 55]. More than half of the interventions ($n = 30$, 53.6%) were directed towards children, with the interventions mediated by parents or family caregivers [14–18, 20, 22, 24–28, 30, 34, 36, 37, 39–41, 46–49, 53, 56, 58, 60, 64–66].

Interventions and assessments

Caregiver-mediated interventions were categorized by the type of engagement strategy and support provided (Additional file 1). Figure 2 provides a conceptual framework of the engagement strategy and supports, caregiver-mediated interventions employed, and reported outcomes. All interventions were considered complex, with a median of 4 (IQR 2–6) engagement supports. The most common type of engagement strategy was *inform* ($n = 55$, 98.2%), followed by *activate* ($n = 54$, 96.4%), and *collaborate* ($n = 27$, 48.2%). The most common engagement support used as part of the *inform* strategies was condition/treatment education ($n = 47$, 83.9%), for the *activate* strategies the most common engagement support was practical management activities ($n = 40$, 71.4%), and for the *collaborate* strategies the most common engagement support was providing a safety net to caregivers ($n = 11$, 19.6%). All *inform* engagement strategies were accompanied by either *activate* and/or *collaborate* strategies. The most common pairing of engagement strategies was *inform-activate* ($n = 28$, 50.0%), and among those, educational engagement supports combined with practical management strategies ($n = 8$). For example, one *inform-activate* engagement strategy included family caregiver education and involvement in the basic care of patients admitted to the ICU; specifically, caregivers were provided with information on the advantages of their involvement in the basic care of the patient and details on the activities they could carry out, including general hygiene, mouth hygiene, mobilization, and feeding [42]. Similarly, two *inform-collaborate* engagement strategies included an education program aimed to improve knowledge about stroke and stroke prevention (*inform*), described services available in hospital and the community (*collaborate*), and provided an opportunity to ask questions and receive group support (*collaborate*) [51].

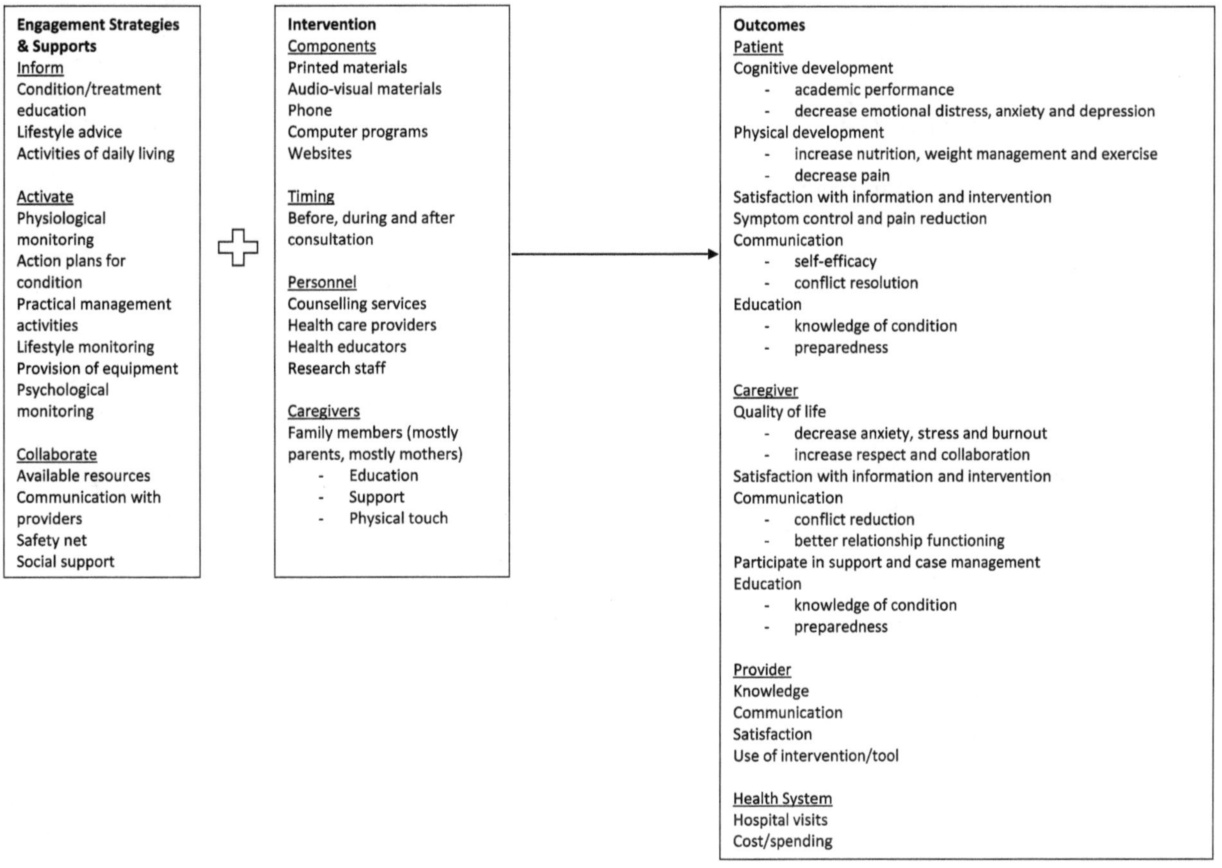

Fig. 2 Conceptual framework derived from synthesis of data

Outcomes

Patient- and caregiver-oriented outcomes were most commonly reported ($n = 40$ and $n = 33$, respectively) (Table 1). Health system-oriented outcomes were reported in 10 studies and provider-oriented outcomes in two studies. Patient-oriented outcomes included cognitive development, symptom control, and communication. Caregiver-oriented outcomes included anxiety, depression, and satisfaction. Provider-oriented outcomes included improved communication with caregivers and satisfaction with the intervention. Health system-oriented outcomes included length of hospital stay, number of hospital visits, and costs. Interventions with condition and treatment education (*inform*) and practical management (*activate*) engagement supports were generally effective in improving patient-reported outcomes. For caregiver-reported outcomes, engagement supports that included action plans (*activate*), practical management (*activate*), or lifestyle monitoring (*activate*), and condition and treatment education (*inform*) or lifestyle advice (*inform*) engagement supports were generally effective in improving outcomes. Provider outcomes were improved by providing caregivers engagement supports related to activities of daily living (*inform*) and notice of available resources (*collaborate*). Interventions with social support and safety net engagement supports (*collaborate*) tended to improve health system outcomes. No studies reported whether harmful effects were associated with the interventions.

Table 1 Type and effectiveness of interventions for primary study outcomes

Type of engagement	Patient outcomes	Caregiver outcomes	Provider outcomes	Health system outcomes
Inform-activate-collaborate	5⇑ 9⇔	11⇑ 4⇔	–	5⇑ 3⇔
Inform-activate	18⇑ 5⇔	9⇑ 5⇔	1⇑	1⇑ 1⇔
Inform-collaborate	1⇔	2⇑	1⇑	–
Activate-collaborate	1⇑ 1⇔	2⇔	–	–

Numbers represent the number of studies reporting on each outcome
⇑ statistically significant positive effect of intervention, ⇔ no statistically significant effect of intervention or mixed effect of intervention, ⇓ statistically significant harmful effect of intervention

Location of patient care

Interventions conducted in inpatient (or combined inpatient and outpatient) settings ($n = 34$) had more statistically significant positive effects on patient and caregiver outcomes than no/mixed effects (Table 2). In outpatient settings (including primary care and the community) ($n = 39$), interventions examining caregiver outcomes had more statistically significant positive effects than no/mixed effects. The same trend was observed for patient outcomes. Most inpatient interventions ($n = 15$, 44.1%) were *inform-activate*, while most outpatient interventions ($n = 18$, 46.2%) were *inform-activate-collaborate*.

Patient population

The majority of interventions were directed towards children (newborn–18 years) ($n = 30$, 53.6%), followed by adults (greater than 18 years) ($n = 11$, 19.6%) and older adults (greater than 55 years) ($n = 15$, 26.8%). Ten pediatric studies focused on newborn, low birth weight, or premature infants, while the remainder ($n = 20$) reported on children overall. In studies of infants, mothers ($n = 6$) delivered the intervention more frequently than both parents ($n = 4$), while in studies of children, both parents ($n = 15$) or a caregiver ($n = 5$) delivered the intervention. In studies of adults, the most commonly studied populations were persons with stroke ($n = 3$), persons with comorbid substance misuse, and persons in the ICU ($n = 2$). Among adult populations, the persons providing care were caregivers broadly (not specifically defined) ($n = 10$) or spouses ($n = 1$). Engagement strategies for adults were either *inform-activate* ($n = 6$) or *inform-activate-collaborate* ($n = 5$). Interventions directed at older adults were most commonly conducted in persons with dementia or Alzheimer's disease ($n = 8$) and utilized an *inform-activate-collaborate* engagement strategy ($n = 11$). Caregiver outcomes were reported in more studies of older adults ($n = 13$) than patient ($n = 8$), health system ($n = 4$), and provider ($n = 1$) outcomes. For both patient and caregiver outcomes in infants, children, or adolescents, there was a similar number of positive effects and mixed effects (Table 2). In adults, there were considerably more positive effects observed for both patient and caregiver outcomes. In older adults, caregiver outcomes were more frequently improved, though this was not observed for patient outcomes.

Table 2 Type and effectiveness of interventions for select subgroup analyses

Study population	Patient outcomes	Caregiver outcomes
All	24⇑ 16⇔	22⇑ 11⇔
Location of care		
Inpatient	11⇑ 7⇔	10⇑ 6⇔
Outpatient	13⇑ 9⇔	12⇑ 5⇔
Patient population		
Infants/children/adolescents	14⇑12⇔	7⇑7⇔
Adults	7⇑1⇔	6⇑1⇔
Older adults	3⇑3⇔	9⇑3⇔
GRADE criteria		
Very low-low	8⇑ 9⇔	7⇑ 6⇔
Moderate-high	16⇑7⇔	15⇑ 5⇔

Numbers represent the number of studies reporting on each outcome
⇑ statistically significant positive effect of intervention, ⇔ no statistically significant effect of intervention or mixed effect of intervention, ⇓: statistically significant harmful effect of intervention

Acceptability and feasibility

The acceptability and feasibility of caregiver-mediated interventions were inconsistently reported in the included studies, with less than half ($n = 26$, 46.4%) reporting response rates or process evaluations.

Risk of bias assessment and strength of evidence

None of the 56 included studies had a low overall risk of bias; risk of bias was high in 47 studies (83.9%) and unclear in nine studies (16.1%) (Additional file 4). The overall strength of the evidence based on GRADE criteria was low-moderate (Additional file 5). A lack of blinding of participants (i.e., caregivers and patients) and outcome assessors (i.e., patients not blinded to patient reported outcomes) was the main factor that limited the strength of the evidence.

When the analyses were restricted to studies with moderate or greater strength of evidence ($n = 33$, 58.9%), the results were similar, with most statistically significant effects observed for *inform-activate* engagement strategies for patient outcomes (Additional file 6).

Discussion

We utilized systematic review methodology to synthesize the literature on the effectiveness of caregiver-mediated interventions. There is a large and recent body of literature (including many randomized controlled trials [RCTs]) suggesting that complex interventions comprised of *inform-activate* and *inform-activate-collaborate* engagement strategies are associated with improved patient and caregiver outcomes. In contrast, there is very little literature regarding provider and health system outcomes, though all interventions involved care providers and/or the health system in some way. The potential for unintended consequences or harm from caregiver-mediated interventions was not explored in the included studies, and much of the literature focused on the parent-child relationship.

That interventions with an *inform* engagement strategy always included parts of *activate* and/or *collaborate* engagement strategies is noteworthy, as research suggests that education-only interventions (*inform* in this language) in various settings and populations are some of the weakest [68–71]. Education with prompts for action or education with active collaboration may circumvent the limitations of education alone [68–71]. Most interventions were mediated by parents or family caregivers (any family member, though not defined specifically), though there was heterogeneity in both the type of caregiver included and in how caregiver was defined. It is important to recognize that one caregiver is not the same as another; they may differ in their commitment, readiness, and capacity to fulfill the role. Validated tools to assess caregiver readiness (Willingness to Care Scale [72], Caregiver Self Expectations Inventory [73]) should be employed alongside caregiver-mediated interventions in this context [74]. Interventions to support caregivers once they are already in a caregiving role dominate the literature [75–77], with little or no information supporting the use of interventions to prepare the caregiver prior to entering the caregiving role. Nearly all studies of adults found improvement in both patient and caregiver outcomes, though in pediatric studies only half found improvement in patient and caregiver outcomes. Improved outcomes may be dependent on whether the caregiver-patient relationship is parent-child (i.e., parents providing support to children) versus child-parent (i.e., children providing support to parents).

All included interventions were complex (including multiple components). Thus, we are uncertain of the "active ingredients" of the interventions and how these components affect outcomes. The knowledge translation literature suggests that complex interventions may be no better than single-component interventions [68, 69]. If this holds true for caregiver-mediated interventions, then single-component interventions may represent a resource-efficient means of improving patient, caregiver, provider, and health system outcomes. We observed variation in reported outcomes according to the types of engagement pairings, suggesting that different combinations of interventions might have differing effects: the previously observed effect of simple-component versus complex interventions may not hold true for caregiver-mediated interventions. *Inform-activate* engagement strategies provide the strongest evidence for improving patient outcomes through caregiver-mediated interventions. Based on the results of the current study, we recommend interventions that provide both condition-specific information and prompts or tools to support action for managing a condition to the caregiver. For example, an intervention to encourage early mobilization of patients recovering from a serious illness might include both information about how the illness affects the patient's conditioning (*inform*) paired with instructions and prompts for caregiver-directed bedside physical therapy (*activate*). It is unclear how these interventions will apply in other contexts, though they appear to work in children and adults with any family caregiver in an inpatient setting. There was a trend towards more positive than equivocal effects for improved caregiver outcomes in an outpatient setting. *Inform-activate-collaborate* engagement strategies are supported by the strongest evidence to improve caregiver outcomes. We recommend utilizing this type of strategy for infants or children in outpatient or community settings with any family caregiver. For example, there could be a three-component (*inform-activate-collaborate*) telephone coaching intervention for parents of children with asthma (*activate*) combined with lifestyle advice on how to avoid asthma triggers (*inform*) and the provision of contact information for extra information or clinical supports (*collaborate*). These interventions have the potential to improve caregiver outcomes. At this time, there have been few evaluations of interventions using *inform-collaborate* (e.g., providing information to support activities of daily living and a list of available resources) or *activate-collaborate* (e.g., creating action plans specific to a medical condition and the provision of contact information for extra support) engagement strategies. For interventions conducted in the community (either partially or fully), it appears that *collaborate* engagement supports are necessary to improve outcomes.

Despite the large body of literature, there are a number of key gaps that must be addressed: provider and health system outcomes, the role of caregiver, the potential harms of caregiver-mediated interventions; and the economic impact of these interventions. Only two studies explored provider outcomes of caregiver-mediated interventions. Providers represent an important mechanism for implementing PFCC research [4, 78, 79]; it is essential to measure the impact that caregiver-mediated interventions have on this population. Ten studies reported on health system outcomes, which included hospital and emergency room visits and associated costs. As all caregiver-mediated interventions engage with the healthcare system, it is important to measure the impact they have on these limited resources. Within our aging population, investigations should explore whether the inverse effect of the parent-child dyad applies to caregiver-mediated interventions—that is, when children become the caregiver, are the same outcomes observed? The evidence from parent-child relationships may not inform the child-parent caregiver relationship in this context. No included studies reported on potential harms of caregiver-mediated interventions (e.g., falls among patients being mobilized by caregivers, caregiver feelings of guilt related to intervention adherence, conflict with providers); unintended effects of these interventions are an important area that requires further study. Caregiver-mediated interventions represent an opportunity for healthcare cost savings by transferring select care responsibilities from the clinical team to the caregiver. Future studies should assess the financial impact of employing caregiver-mediated interventions.

This study has a number of strengths, including the use of rigorous methodology defined by an a priori published protocol and adherence to recommended reporting criteria. We utilized previously validated tools to assess both the quality and strength of the evidence presented. The search was executed in five bibliographic databases, it was not restricted by language, and it was intentionally broad to ensure that caregiver-mediated interventions across all areas of healthcare were included. By focusing on healthcare settings, home-based interventions were excluded, including many studies of caregiver-mediated interventions in persons with dementia. In spite of these strengths, there are limitations to note. Our findings are limited by the methodological quality of the included studies; the risk of bias was generally high, and the overall quality of the evidence was low-moderate. When restricted to studies of at least moderate quality, there was a trend towards observing more positive effects. Risk of bias tends to be high in studies where blinding does not occur, as is the case in many of these interventions, and does not necessarily mean they are methodologically poor [80]. The literature is rich with RCTs, the quality of which is limited by methodological factors inherent in this type of research (e.g., lack of blinding) that are unlikely to be overcome in the future. We did not search the gray literature and could have missed studies, though our comprehensive search strategy included databases indexing both North American and European journals and full-text hand-searching was completed. We noted a lack of scientific abstracts, limited use of applicable keywords, and variable terminology to describe caregiver-mediated interventions in the included studies. This highlights the importance of full-text hand-searching, as these papers may not be found through standard database searching. All included papers reported on complex interventions, and thus it is not possible to determine which parts of the interventions were effective. The lack of effect in some studies may be a failure of implementation (few process evaluations conducted to inform) or a failure of measurement (i.e., use of the wrong measure) and not the intervention itself.

Conclusions

There is a large body of research, including many RCTs, to support the use of caregiver-mediated interventions that inform and activate caregivers to improve patient and caregiver outcomes. Additional study is needed to evaluate provider and health system outcomes, interventions for relationships outside of the parent-child role, potential harms, and economic implications. We recommend consideration of *inform-activate* and *inform-activate-collaborate* interventions when implementing patient and family-oriented research.

Additional files

Additional file 1: Characteristics of Caregiver-Mediated Interventions. Description of the engagement strategies and engagement supports and examples of each utilized in the study. (DOCX 17 kb)

Additional file 2: Characteristics of Included Studies. Table of the studies included in the systematic review with information including setting, participant population, intervention, and outcomes. (DOCX 120 kb)

Additional file 3: PRISMA Checklist. A completed PRISMA checklist for study transparency. (DOCX 24 kb)

Additional file 4: Risk of Bias Assessment. Risk of bias ratings for each included study. (DOCX 20 kb)

Additional file 5: GRADE Ratings. GRADE ratings for each included study. (DOCX 19 kb)

Additional file 6: Type and Effectiveness of Interventions for Primary Study Outcomes in Studies with Moderate or High Strength Evidence According to the GRADE Criteria. Main results restricted to those studies with a moderate or high strength of evidence according to the GRADE criteria. (DOCX 13 kb)

Abbreviations

GRADE: Grading of Recommendations Assessment Development and Evaluation; IQR: Interquartile range; PFCC: Patient and family-centered care; PRISMA: Preferred Reporting Items for Systematic Reviews and Meta-Analyses; RCT: Randomized controlled trial

Acknowledgements

The authors would like to acknowledge Ms. Heather Ganshorn (University of Calgary) for the development of the search strategies and the patients and family members who participated in the stakeholder engagement meeting. We would also like to acknowledge Dr. Khara Sauro (University of Calgary) and Dr. Daniel Niven (University of Calgary) for providing valuable feedback on the manuscript.

Funding

Canadian Institutes of Health Research. The funding body had no role in the design of the study or in the collection, analysis, or interpretation of data, or in writing the manuscript.

Authors' contributions

KMF, JPL, and HTS conceived the study. KMF, CJM, and DD analyzed the data. All authors interpreted the data, and KMF wrote the manuscript. All authors read and approved the final manuscript.

Competing interests

The authors declare that they have no competing interests.

Author details

[1]Departments of Critical Care Medicine and Community Health Sciences, O'Brien Institute for Public Health and Hotchkiss Brain Institute, Cumming School of Medicine, University of Calgary, 2500 University Drive NW, Calgary, AB T2N 1N4, Canada. [2]Department of Critical Care Medicine, Cumming School of Medicine, University of Calgary, 2500 University Drive NW, Calgary, AB T2N 1N4, Canada. [3]Department of Critical Care Medicine, O'Brien Institute for Public Health, Cumming School of Medicine, University of Calgary, 2500

University Drive NW, Calgary, AB T2N 1N4, Canada. [4]Departments of Critical Care Medicine, Medicine and Community Health Sciences, O'Brien Institute for Public Health, Cumming School of Medicine, University of Calgary, 2500 University Drive NW, Calgary, AB T2N 1N4, Canada.

References

1. Li H, Melnyk BM, McCann R, Chatcheydang J, Koulouglioti C, Nichols LW, Lee MD, Ghassemi A. Creating avenues for relative empowerment (CARE): a pilot test of an intervention to improve outcomes of hospitalized elders and family caregivers. Res Nurs Health. 2003;26(4):284–99.
2. Mitchell M, Chaboyer W, Burmeister E, Foster M. Positive effects of a nursing intervention on family-centered care in adult critical care. Am J Crit Care. 2009;18(6):543–52.
3. Gasparini R, Champagne M, Stephany A, Hudson J, Fuchs MA. Policy to practice: increased family presence and the impact on patient- and family-centered care adoption. J Nurs Adm. 2015;45(1):28–34.
4. Bauman G, Watling CJ, Hahn K. Oncologists' attitudes towards patient and family-centered care. J Clin Oncol. 2015;33(29_suppl):111.
5. Baird J, Davies B, Hinds PS, Baggott C, Rehm RS. What impact do hospital and unit-based rules have upon patient and family-centered care in the pediatric intensive care unit? J Pediatr Nurs. 2015;30(1):133–42.
6. Tonelli MR, Misak CJ. Compromised autonomy and the seriously ill patient. Chest. 2010;137(4):926–31.
7. Gagliardi AR, Legare F, Brouwers MC, Webster F, Badley E, Straus S. Patient-mediated knowledge translation (PKT) interventions for clinical encounters: a systematic review. Implement Sci. 2016;11:26.
8. Moher D, Liberati A, Tetzlaff J, Altman DG, Group P. Preferred reporting items for systematic reviews and meta-analyses: the PRISMA statement. BMJ. 2009;339:b2535.
9. Knowledge Translation. http://www.cihr-irsc.gc.ca/e/29418.html. Accessed 2 Feb 2018.
10. Higgins JP, Altman DG, Gotzsche PC, Juni P, Moher D, Oxman AD, Savovic J, Schulz KF, Weeks L, Sterne JA, et al. The Cochrane Collaboration's tool for assessing risk of bias in randomised trials. BMJ. 2011;343:d5928.
11. Guyatt GH, Oxman AD, Vist GE, Kunz R, Falck-Ytter Y, Alonso-Coello P, Schunemann HJ, GRADE Working Group. GRADE: an emerging consensus on rating quality of evidence and strength of recommendations. BMJ. 2008;336(7650):924–6.
12. Taylor SJC, Pinnock H, Epiphaniou E, Pearce G, Parke HL, Schwappach A, Purushotham N, Jacob S, Griffiths CJ, Greenhalgh T, et al. A rapid synthesis of the evidence on interventions supporting self-management for people with long-term conditions: PRISMS - Practical systematic Review of Self-Management Support for long-term conditions. Southampton: University of Southampton; 2014.
13. Craig P, Dieppe P, Macintyre S, Michie S, Nazareth I, Petticrew M, Medical Research Council G. Developing and evaluating complex interventions: the new Medical Research Council guidance. BMJ. 2008;337:a1655.
14. Achenbach TMH, T C, Aoki MF, Rauh VA. Nine-year outcome of the Vermont intervention program for low birth weight infants. Pediatrics. 1993;91(1):45–55.
15. Anderson BJ, Brackett J, Ho J, Laffel LM. An office-based intervention to maintain parent-adolescent teamwork in diabetes management: impact on parent involvement, family conflict, and subsequent glycemic control. Diabetes Care. 1999;22(5):713–21.
16. Bagner DM. Father's role in parent training for children with developmental delay. J Fam Psychol. 2013;27(4):650–7.
17. Bao XL, National Cooperative Research Group for Lowering Incidence of Cerebral Palsy of Premature Infants through Early Intervention. Lowering incidence of cerebral palsy of premature infants through early intervention. Zhonghua Er Ke Za Zhi. 2005;43(4):244–7.
18. Barrera ME, Rosenbaum PL, Cunningham CE. Early home intervention with low-birth-weight infants and their parents. Child Dev. 1986;57(1):20–33.
19. Bass DM, Judge KS, Snow AL, Wilson NL, Morgan R, Looman WJ, McCarthy CA, Maslow K, Moye JA, Randazzo R, Garcia-Maldonado M, Elbein R, Odenheimer G, Kunik ME. Caregiver outcomes of partners in dementia care: effect of a care coordination program for veterans with dementia and their family members and friends. J Am Geriatr Soc. 2013;61(8):1377–86.
20. Beeghly MB, Brazelton TB, Flannery KA, Nugent JK, Barrett DE, Tronick EZ. Specificity of preventative pediatric intervention effects in early infancy. J Dev Behav Pediatr. 1995;16(3):158–66.
21. Berthelsen CB, Kristensson J. The SICAM-trial: evaluating the effect of spouses' involvement through case management in older patients' fast-track programmes during and after total hip replacement. J Adv Nurs. 2016;4:4.
22. Blauw-Hospers CH, Dirks T, Hulshof LJ, Bos AF, Hadders-Algra M. Pediatric physical therapy in infancy: from nightmare to dream? A two-arm randomized trial. Phys Ther. 2011;91(9):1323–38.
23. Boltz M, Resnick B, Chippendale T, Galvin J. Testing a family-centered intervention to promote functional and cognitive recovery in hospitalized older adults. J Am Geriatr Soc. 2014;62(12):2398–407.
24. Arauz Boudreau AD, Kurowski DS, Gonzalez WI, Dimond MA, Oreskovic NM. Latino families, primary care, and childhood obesity: a randomized controlled trial. Am J Prev Med. 2013;44(3 SUPPL. 3):S247–57.
25. Brown JAW, Juliann J. Effects of a triadic parent-implemented home-based communication intervention for toddlers. J Early Interv. 2015;37(1):44–68.
26. Butz A, Kub J, Donithan M, James NT, Thompson RE, Bellin M, Tsoukleris M, Bollinger ME. Influence of caregiver and provider communication on symptom days and medication use for inner-city children with asthma. J Asthma. 2010;47(4):478–85.
27. Chen SH,H, L J, Yeh KW, Tsai YF. Interactive support interventions for caregivers of asthmatic children. J Asthma. 2013;50(6):649–57.
28. Dawson AM, Brown DA, Cox A, Williams SM, Treacy L, Haszard J, Meredith-Jones K, Hargreaves E, Taylor BJ, Ross J, Taylor RW. Using motivational interviewing for weight feedback to parents of young children. J Paediatr Child Health. 2014;50(6):461–70.
29. Eloniemi-Sulkava U, Saarenheimo M, Laakkonen ML, Pietila M, Savikko N, Kautiainen H, Tilvis RS, Pitkala KH. Family care as collaboration: effectiveness of a multicomponent support program for elderly couples with dementia. Randomized controlled intervention study. J Am Geriatr Soc. 2009;57(12):2200–8.
30. Fiks AG,M, L S, Karavite DJ, Suh A, O'Hara R, Localio AR, Ross M, Grundmeier RW. Parent-reported outcomes of a shared decision-making portal in asthma: a practice-based RCT. Pediatrics. 2015;135(4):e965–73.
31. Fortinsky RH, Kulldorf M, Kleppinger A, Kenyon-Pesce L. Dementia care consultation for family caregivers: collaborative model linking an Alzheimer's association chapter with primary care physicians. Aging Ment Health. 2009;13(2):162–70.
32. Fortinsky RHU, Christine G, Garcia RI. Helping family caregivers by linking primary care physicians with community-based dementia care services: the Alzheimer's Service Coordination Program. Dementia. 2002;1(2):227–40.
33. Galvin R, Cusack T, O'Grady E, Murphy B, Stokes E. Family mediated exercise intervention [fame]: evaluation of a novel form of exercise delivery after stroke. Physiotherapy (United Kingdom). 2011;97:eS387–8.
34. Garbutt JM, Banister C, Highstein G, Sterkel R, Epstein J, Bruns J, Swerczek L, Wells S, Waterman B, Strunk RC, et al. Telephone coaching for parents of children with asthma: impact and lessons learned. Arch Pediatr Adolesc Med. 2010;164(7):625–30.
35. Garcia-Huidobro D, Bittner M, Brahm P, Puschel K. Family intervention to control type 2 diabetes: a controlled clinical trial. Fam Pract. 2011;28(1):4–11.
36. Golley RK, Magarey AM, Baur LA, Steinbeck KS, Daniels LA. Twelve-month effectiveness of a parent-led, family-focused weight-management program for prepubertal children: a randomized, controlled trial. Pediatrics. 2007;119(3):517–25.
37. Gomez DB, Ana J, Andrews AR III, Cavell TA, Pastrana FA, Gregus SJ, Ojeda CA. Delivering parent management training in an integrated primary care setting: description and preliminary outcome data. Cogn Behav Pract. 2014;21(3):296–309.
38. Grover M, Naumann U, Mohammad-Dar L, Glennon D, Ringwood S, Eisler I, Williams C, Treasure J, Schmidt U. A randomized controlled trial of an internet-based cognitive-behavioural skills package for carers of people with anorexia nervosa. Psychol Med. 2011;41(12):2581–91.
39. Helgadottir HL, Wilson ME. A randomized controlled trial of the effectiveness of educating parents about distraction to decrease postoperative pain in children at home after tonsillectomy. Pain Manag Nurs. 2014;15(3):632–40.
40. Holditch-Davis D, White-Traut RC, Levy JA, O'Shea TM, Geraldo V, David RJ. Maternally administered interventions for preterm infants in the NICU: Effects on maternal psychological distress and mother-infant relationship. Infant Behav Dev. 2014;37(4):695–710.
41. Horn IB, Mitchell SJ, Gillespie CW, Burke KM, Godoy L, Teach SJ. Randomized trial of a health communication intervention for parents of children with asthma. J Asthma. 2014;51(9):989–95.
42. Martínez RM del C, Morilla FR, del Pino AR, Almenara MIM, Bannik JT, Caballero LJF, Macías GC, Bernet LA, González CA. Family involvement in

the critically ill patient basic care. Enfermería Intensiva. 2003;14(3):96–108.
43. Mittelman MS, Ferris SH, Shulman E, Steinberg G, Levin B. A family intervention to delay nursing home placement of patients with Alzheimer disease. A randomized controlled trial. JAMA. 1996;276(21):1725–31.
44. Mueser KT, Glynn SM, Cather C, Xie H, Zarate R, Smith LF, Clark RE, Gottlieb JD, Wolfe R, Feldman J. A randomized controlled trial of family intervention for co-occurring substance use and severe psychiatric disorders. Schizophr Bull. 2013;39(3):658–72.
45. Nayeri ND, Mohammadi S, Razi SP, Kazemnejad A. Investigating the effects of a family-centered care program on stroke patients' adherence to their therapeutic regimens. Contemporary Nurse. 2014;47(1/2):88–96.
46. Nelson KA, Highstein GR, Garbutt J, Trinkaus K, Fisher EB, Smith SR, Strunk RC. A randomized controlled trial of parental asthma coaching to improve outcomes among urban minority children. Arch Pediatr Adolesc Med. 2011; 165(6):520–6.
47. Nurcombe B, Howell DC, Rauh VA, Teti DM, Ruoff P, Brennan J. An intervention program for mothers of low-birthweight infants: preliminary results. J Am Acad Child Psychiatry. 1984;23(3):319–25.
48. Ozonoff S, Cathcart K. Effectiveness of a home program intervention for young children with autism. J Autism Dev Disord. 1998;28(1):25–32.
49. Pridham KA, Krolikowski MM, Limbo RK, Paradowski J, Rudd N, Meurer JR, Uttech A, Henriques JB. Guiding mothers' management of health problems of very low birth-weight infants. Public Health Nurs. 2006;23(3):205–15.
50. Robinson JK, Turrisi R, Stapleton J. Examination of mediating variables in a partner assistance intervention designed to increase performance of skin self-examination. J Am Acad Dermatol. 2007;56(3):391–7.
51. Rodgers H, Atkinson C, Bond S, Suddes M, Dobson R, Curless R. Randomized controlled trial of a comprehensive stroke education program for patients and caregivers. Stroke. 1999;30(12):2585–91.
52. Rodríguez-Gonzalo A, García-Martí C, Ocaña-Colorado A, Baquera-De Micheo MJ, Morel-Fernández S. Efficiency of an intensive educational program for informal caregivers of hospitalized, dependent patients: cluster randomized trial. BMC Nurs. 2015;14(1):1–12.
53. Sénéchal C, Larivée S, Thermidor G. Parents as co-therapists: a winning solution for treating autistic children. Annales Medico-Psychologiques. 2013; 171(9):603–9.
54. Tantirangsee N, Assanangkornchai S, Marsden J. Effects of a brief intervention for substance use on tobacco smoking and family relationship functioning in schizophrenia and related psychoses: a randomised controlled trial. J Subst Abus Treat. 2015;51:30–7.
55. Wang T-C, Tsai AC, Wang J-Y, Lin Y-T, Lin K-L, Chen JJ, Lin BY, Lin TC. Caregiver-mediated intervention can improve physical functional recovery of patients with chronic stroke: a randomized controlled trial. Neurorehabil Neural Repair. 2015;29(1):3–12.
56. Watson WT, Gillespie C, Thomas N, Filuk SE, McColm J, Piwniuk MP, Becker AB. Small-group, interactive education and the effect on asthma control by children and their families. CMAJ. 2009;181(5):257–63.
57. Mavandadi S, Wright EM, Graydon MM, Oslin DW, Wray LO. A randomized pilot trial of a telephone-based collaborative care management program for caregivers of individuals with dementia. Psychol Serv. 2017;14(1):102–11.
58. Sun G-C, Hsu M-C. Effects of nurse-led child- and parent-focused violence intervention on mentally ill adult patients and victimized parents: a randomized controlled trial. Int J Nurs Stud. 2016;60:79–90.
59. Toye C, Parsons R, Slatyer S, Aoun SM, Moorin R, Osseiran-Moisson R, Hill KD. Outcomes for family carers of a nurse-delivered hospital discharge intervention for older people (the Further Enabling Care at Home Program): single blind randomised controlled trial. Int J Nurs Stud. 2016;64:32–41.
60. Tyler DO, Horner SD. A primary care intervention to improve weight in obese children: a feasibility study. J Am Assoc Nurse Pract. 2016;28(2):98–106.
61. Souaibi L, Choueifati D, Kerbage H, Richa S. Therapeutic education of families of patients with schizophrenia: the Lebanese Hôtel-Dieu de France model. Annales Medico-Psychologiques. 2016;174(8):677–82.
62. Callahan CM, Boustani MA, Unverzagt FW, Austrom MG, Damush TM, Perkins AJ, Fultz BA, Hui SL, Counsell SR, Hendrie HC. Effectiveness of collaborative care for older adults with Alzheimer disease in primary care: a randomized controlled trial. JAMA. 2006;295(18):2148–57.
63. Gitlin LN, Reever K, Dennis MP, Mathieu E, Hauck WW. Enhancing quality of life of families who use adult day services: short- and long-term effects of the adult day services plus program. Gerontologist. 2006;46(5):630–9.
64. Melnyk BM, Alpert-Gillis L, Feinstein NF, Crean HF, Johnson J, Fairbanks E, Small L, Rubenstein J, Slota M, Corbo-Richert B. Creating opportunities for parent empowerment: program effects on the mental health/coping outcomes of critically ill young children and their mothers. Pediatrics. 2004; 113(6):e597–607.
65. Melnyk BM, Alpert-Gillis L, Feinstein NF, Fairbanks E, Schultz-Czarniak J, Hust D, Sherman L, LeMoine C, Moldenhauer Z, Small L, et al. Improving cognitive development of low-birth-weight premature infants with the COPE program: a pilot study of the benefit of early NICU intervention with mothers. Res Nurs Health. 2001;24(5):373–89.
66. Melnyk BM, Feinstein NF, Alpert-Gillis L, Fairbanks E, Crean HF, Sinkin RA, Stone PW, Small L, Tu X, Gross SJ. Reducing premature infants' length of stay and improving parents' mental health outcomes with the Creating Opportunities for Parent Empowerment (COPE) neonatal intensive care unit program: a randomized, controlled trial. Pediatrics. 2006;118(5):e1414–27.
67. Skoog M, Milner KA, Gatti-Petito J, Dintyala K. The impact of family engagement on anxiety levels in a cardiothoracic intensive care unit. Crit Care Nurse. 2016;36(2):84–9.
68. Oxman AD, Thomson MA, Davis DA, Haynes RB. No magic bullets: a systematic review of 102 trials of interventions to improve professional practice. CMAJ. 1995;153(10):1423–31.
69. Wensing M, van der Weijden T, Grol R. Implementing guidelines and innovations in general practice: which interventions are effective? Br J Gen Pract. 1998;48(427):991–7.
70. Grimshaw JM, Russell IT. Effect of clinical guidelines on medical practice: a systematic review of rigorous evaluations. Lancet. 1993;342(8883):1317–22.
71. Grol R, Grimshaw J. From best evidence to best practice: effective implementation of change in patients' care. Lancet. 2003;362(9391):1225–30.
72. Abell N. Assessing willingness to care for persons with AIDS: validation of a new measure. Res Soc Work Pract. 2001;11:118–30.
73. Y-IL S. Development and testing of the Family Caregiving Factors Inventory for home health assessment in Taiwan. J Adv Nurs. 2000;32:226–34.
74. Alliance FC. Selected caregiver assessment measures: a resource inventory for practitioners. 2nd ed; 2012.
75. Stockle HS, Haarmann-Doetkotte S, Bausewein C, Fegg MJ. The feasibility and acceptability of short-term, individual existential behavioural therapy for informal caregivers of patients recruited in a specialist palliative care unit. BMC Palliat Care. 2016;15(1):88.
76. Rexhaj S, Leclerc C, Bonsack C, Golay P, Favrod J. Feasibility and accessibility of a tailored intervention for informal caregivers of people with severe psychiatric disorders: a pilot study. Frontiers of Psychiatry. 2017;8:178.
77. Dam AEH, van Boxtel MPJ, Rozendaal N, Verhey FRJ, de Vugt ME. Development and feasibility of Inlife: a pilot study of an online social support intervention for informal caregivers of people with dementia. PLoS One. 2017;12(9):e0183386.
78. Philibert I, Patow C, Cichon J. Incorporating patient- and family-centered care into resident education: approaches, benefits, and challenges. J Grad Med Educ. 2011;3(2):272–8.
79. Ayub EM, Sampayo EM, Shah MI, Doughty CB. Prehospital Providers' perceptions on providing patient and family centered care. Prehosp Emerg Care. 2017;21(2):233–41.
80. Boutron I, Guittet L, Estellat C, Moher D, Hrobjartsson A, Ravaud P. Reporting methods of blinding in randomized trials assessing nonpharmacological treatments. PLoS Med. 2007;4(2):e61.

6

Effective coverage of essential inpatient care for small and sick newborns in a high mortality urban setting: a cross-sectional study in Nairobi City County, Kenya

Georgina A. V. Murphy[1,2*], David Gathara[2], Jacintah Mwachiro[2], Nancy Abuya[2,3], Jalemba Aluvaala[2], Mike English[2,1] and on behalf of the Health Services that Deliver for Newborns Expert Group

Abstract

Background: Effective coverage requires that those in need can access skilled care supported by adequate resources. There are, however, few studies of effective coverage of facility-based neonatal care in low-income settings, despite the recognition that improving newborn survival is a global priority.

Methods: We used a detailed retrospective review of medical records for neonatal admissions to public, private not-for-profit (mission) and private-for-profit (private) sector facilities providing 24×7 inpatient neonatal care in Nairobi City County to estimate the proportion of small and sick newborns receiving nationally recommended care across six process domains. We used our findings to explore the relationship between facility measures of structure and process and estimate effective coverage.

Results: Of 33 eligible facilities, 28 (four public, six mission and 18 private), providing an estimated 98.7% of inpatient neonatal care in the county, agreed to partake. Data from 1184 admission episodes were collected. Overall performance was lowest (weighted mean score 0.35 [95% confidence interval or CI: 0.22–0.48] out of 1) for correct prescription of fluid and feed volumes and best (0.86 [95% CI: 0.80–0.93]) for documentation of demographic characteristics. Doses of gentamicin, when prescribed, were at least 20% higher than recommended in 11.7% cases. Larger (often public) facilities tended to have higher process and structural quality scores compared with smaller, predominantly private, facilities. We estimate effective coverage to be 25% (estimate range: 21–31%). These newborns received high-quality inpatient care, while almost half (44.5%) of newborns needed care but did not receive it and a further 30.4% of newborns received an inadequate service.

Conclusions: Failure to receive services and gaps in quality of care both contribute to a shortfall in effective coverage in Nairobi City County. Three-quarters of small and sick newborns do not have access to high-quality facility-based care. Substantial improvements in effective coverage will be required to tackle high neonatal mortality in this urban setting with high levels of poverty.

Keywords: Newborn health, Neonatal care, Effective coverage, Inpatient newborn services, Quality of care, Paediatrics, Health services research, Kenya, Africa

* Correspondence: murphygina@gmail.com
[1]Centre for Tropical Medicine and Global Health, Nuffield Department of Medicine, University of Oxford, Oxford, UK
[2]Kenya Medical Research Institute - Wellcome Trust Research Programme, Nairobi, Kenya
Full list of author information is available at the end of the article

Background

The provision of good quality inpatient care for small and sick newborns is crucial if efforts to achieve the sustainable development goal 3 target to reduce neonatal mortality to 12 per 1000 live births or lower is to be achieved [1]. To date, progress in addressing neonatal mortality has been slow and insufficient emphasis has been placed on the importance of quality health care for small and sick newborns [2–5].

The main causes of neonatal mortality are intrapartum-related neonatal encephalopathy, prematurity and neonatal sepsis [3], which together accounted for more than 75% of the observed mortality in Kenya in 2014 [6]. Much of the mortality and long-term morbidity associated with these conditions is preventable with cost-effective interventions and the provision of universal access to basic but high-quality health services [7, 8], including interventions provided to inpatients, such as intravenous antibiotics for sepsis, assisted feeding for premature newborns and oxygen for respiratory distress syndrome [9, 10]. Yet, many sick and small (preterm and small for gestational age) newborns are not receiving appropriate inpatient neonatal services, and those who are may be treated in suboptimal conditions [4, 11–13]. Failures in the delivery of best care may reduce the effectiveness of available services or even cause harm [14].

Despite having a high density of health facilities and 89% of women delivering in a health facility, Nairobi City County has the highest neonatal mortality of all regions in Kenya [15, 16]. Gaps in provision and access to effective services for neonatal care in Kenya have previously been highlighted in the public sector [11–13], yet little has been described about the non-public sector.

To address this, the Nairobi Newborn Study aimed to examine the provision, access and quality of inpatient neonatal care in Nairobi City County—a population of approximately four million, 60–70% of whom are slum dwellers [17]. Previous reports deal with the need for health services [18] and characterise structural aspects of quality of care [19]. Here we report on the quality of the process of care delivered to small and sick inpatient newborns across diverse facility settings in Nairobi with a view to understanding effective coverage.

Methods

We conducted a structural assessment and medical record review of neonatal patients admitted between 1 July 2014 and 30 June 2015 to health facilities providing inpatient neonatal care for 24 h a day, seven days a week (24×7) (hereafter referred to as INC facilities), in Nairobi City County, Kenya. All INC facilities were eligible to partake in the study; we explain how facilities were identified in a separate report [19]. Full details of the study protocol have been published elsewhere and all study tools are publicly available [20, 21].

Study population and sampling

We aimed to provide summary measures of performance for specific indicators of the clinical processes of care across Nairobi City County. To do this, we use proportional sampling (with weighting where this was not achieved) and calculate summary estimates so that each health facility contributes in proportion to its contribution to the total number of annual neonatal admissions across all sites. We estimated that an examination of at least 800 records across the 28 participating sites would be required to meet our aims [19]. The sample of records at each facility was obtained beginning with admissions on 30 June 2015 and moving backwards through admission dates until the desired proportional sample size for that facility was achieved. This strategy was revised for low-volume facilities, for which proportional sampling would lead to <1 record being sampled. For facilities (11 of 28) with 20 or fewer admissions between 1 July 2014 and 30 June 2015, all records of admissions for the entire year were captured. This full record review was also conducted for an additional six facilities that did not have neonatal registers, so we could ascertain the total annual admission numbers for Nairobi.

Medical record review

Data from neonatal medical records were entered onsite in facilities by trained clerks, following strict standard operating procedures (SOPs), into a purpose-designed standardised data capture tool created in REDCap with inbuilt range and validity checks. Prior to data collection, a mock survey was conducted to pilot the tool, finalise SOPs and train data clerks. During data collection, a 10% random sample of records was independently abstracted by a team supervisor and the two entries were compared. Agreement rates were consistently greater than 95%. Predesigned error-checking scripts were run daily and weekly on collected data and corrections made where possible by referring to source documents.

Data analysis

Data analysis was conducted using Stata version 13 (Stata Corporation, TX, USA). Correct approaches to care were defined a priori in line with national guidelines that are based on World Health Organization guidelines [22]. Weights were applied during analysis to account for oversampling of records in some facilities. The weighting ensured that each facility contributed to the results as a proportion of their contribution to the total admissions (or sector or size group) across all 28 participating facilities, after exclusion of admissions for supportive care only (e.g. observation after caesarean).

Facilities are presented grouped by sector and size. Three sectors were considered: public, not-for-profit private (mission) and for-profit private (private). Small, medium and large facilities were defined as facilities with <100, 100–900 and >900 admissions between 1 July 2014 and 30 June 2015, respectively. Results by sector and size are presented as pooled patient-level weighted means. Estimates and 95% confidence intervals (CIs) were derived using the svy command in Stata to apply survey weights. MS Excel 2013 was used to produce radar plots, scatter plots and pie charts to present findings on process score domains, heterogeneity of scores across facilities and effective coverage, respectively.

Process scores

We assessed six domains of process quality against prespecified indicators: (I) documentation of newborn characteristics (nine items), (II) documentation of signs and symptoms (16 items), (III) evidence of monitoring (three items), (IV) correct antibiotic dose, (V) correct oxygen treatment and (VI) correct fluids and feeds prescribed (Box 1). For domain IV and domain VI, an overdose and underdose of antibiotics or fluids and feeds were defined as 20% more or less, respectively, than the recommended dose per kilogram body weight per day in the national guidelines [22, 23]. Unrecorded details of a prescription (e.g. oxygen route) were considered as incorrect prescriptions and included in the denominator when calculating correct prescriptions for domains IV–VI.

Domain scores were calculated at a patient level, as a proportion of the number of correct items within each of the domains I, II and III. In addition, patient-level domain scores (0 = incorrect and 1 = correct) were created for domains IV, V and VI for patients prescribed antibiotics, oxygen or fluids and feeds, respectively. An overall patient-level process score was calculated for each patient by taking the mean of their domain scores. Summary process scores were calculated per facility by taking the mean of all patient process scores within a facility.

Box 1: Process score domains

Domain I: Documentation of newborn characteristics

- **Characteristics:** Age, sex, mode of delivery, weight, gestational age, Apgar score at 5 min, HIV status, diagnosis, outcome
- Score of 0–1 as a proportion of 0–9 characteristics among all patients

Domain II: Documentation of signs and symptoms (documentation of absence or presence)

- **Signs** (evaluation on admission): Temperature, bulging fontanelle, can suck or breastfeed, reduced mobility or floppy, respiratory rate, indrawing, grunting, central cyanosis
- **Symptoms** (history): Prolonged rupture of membranes (ROM) (>18 h), fever, difficulty breathing, severe vomiting, difficulty feeding or breastfeeding, convulsions, partial or focal fits, apnoea
- Score of 0–1 as a proportion of 0–16 signs and symptoms among all patients

Domain III: Evidence of monitoring

- **Evidence:** Treatment sheet available and filled, vital signs chart available and filled, evidence of weight monitoring
- Score of 0–1 as a proportion of 0–3 monitoring evidences among all patients

Domain IV: Appropriate antibiotic prescription

- **Dose** of gentamicin and/or penicillin as per national guidelines, allowing for ±20% margin of error
- Score of 1 for correct dose and 0 for incorrect dose among patients with prescription for gentamicin or penicillin

Domain V: Correct oxygen prescription

- **Correct oxygen prescription:** Correct route and prescribed to patients requiring oxygen treatment as per recorded signs and symptoms
- Score of 1 for both components correct, 0.5 for one component correct and 0 for neither correct among patients prescribed oxygen treatment

Domain VI: Correct fluids and feeds volume

- **Volume** as per national guidelines, allowing for ±20% margin of error
- Score 1 for correct volume and 0 for incorrect volume among patients with fluid or feed prescription

Structural score

Direct estimation of the overall structural score and the approach taken to data collection have been described elsewhere [19]. Briefly, a structural assessment was conducted in study facilities by clinically trained research team members to examine eight domains in the maternity and neonatal units: (i) infrastructure (three items), (ii) laboratory services (10 items), (iii) hygiene equipment (14 items), (iv) safe delivery equipment and drugs for mothers (37 items), (v) resuscitation equipment for newborns on the delivery ward (20 items), (vi) essential equipment in the newborn unit (NBU) (18 items), (vii) intravenous fluids and feeds in the NBU (eight items) and (viii) NBU drugs (17 items) (listed in Additional file 1: Table S2). An overall structure score was calculated as a percentage from the sum of scores for the eight domains for a facility and divided by the total possible score.

Effective coverage

We defined effective coverage as newborns attending a facility providing high-quality care, taking the number of newborns requiring care as the denominator. The gap in receiving INC services and the gaps in quality are calculated as follows.

The gap in receiving INC services was calculated by comparing the number of newborns requiring care to the total number of neonatal admissions to INC facilities recorded in NBU registers during the study period, as previously described [19]. The former was calculated by estimating the number of live births for the 12 months from mid-2014 to mid-2015 in Nairobi City County (120,032) and then we applied a rate of 183 (estimate range 148–221) per 1000 live births requiring inpatient services to this total birth cohort, as also previously described [18]. Thus, the number of newborns requiring care that was used as a denominator when estimating effective coverage was 21,966 (estimate range 17,765–26,527).

Facilities were stratified into high, medium and low quality based on their structural score and summary process score. Facilities with both a summary process score >0.6 and structure score ≥0.8 were considered to be high quality. Newborns attending these facilities were regarded to be receiving effective care. The remaining facilities were stratified as medium quality (summary process score 0.5–0.6 and structure score ≥0.8) or low quality (summary process score ≤0.5 or structure score <0.8). We considered that all newborns admitted to a facility were receiving care equivalent to the level of the facility.

Ethics and permission

Ethical approval has been granted by the Scientific and Ethics Review Unit of the Kenya Medical Research Institute (KEMRI) (SSC protocol 2999). The study was conducted in collaboration with the Nairobi City County government. Written informed consent to conduct this study was obtained from the medical supervisor or equivalent authority in charge of each facility.

Results

Of the 34 eligible INC facilities, one was a military hospital with a restrictive access policy and was excluded. Two private facilities (estimated 250–350 maternal deliveries [24] and <50 neonatal admissions each per year) declined to partake in the study and three private facilities (accounting for a combined total of 59 annual neonatal admissions) agreed to the collection of structure data but not to an examination of medical records. We, therefore, report findings from 28 INC facilities: four public hospitals (one medium and three large), six mission hospitals (one small, four medium and one large) and 18 private hospitals (15 small and three large).

After removing admissions for supportive care only (n = 98), 1184 admissions of small and sick newborns across the 28 facilities (490 from public, 221 from mission and 473 from private facilities) between 1 July 2014 and 30 June 2015 were sampled from a total of 12,143 admissions.

Newborn characteristics and outcomes

Newborns were mostly admitted on the first day of life (Table 1). A substantial proportion of newborns weighed <2.5 kg (29.3%). Similarly, a large proportion were preterm (23.2%, <37 weeks gestational age); however, information on gestational age was missing for 39.8% of newborns (Table 1). Admission diagnosis was documented for most (87.0%, 1029/1183) newborns. The most common admission diagnoses were respiratory distress (35.2%), birth asphyxia (32.4%), preterm birth (24.6%), severe infection (18.9%) and jaundice (12.9%). Congenital malformations (3.1%), large for gestational age (3.0%) and dehydration (2.6%) were less common. More than one diagnosis was recorded for 43.8% of newborns.

Outcome was missing for 3.0% of newborns. Where recorded (n = 1104), 90.6% were discharged alive, 7.2% died, 1.7% were referred and 0.5% absconded. Crude mortality, without adjustment for case-mix or acuity, was higher in public facilities (8.8% [95% CI: 6.5–11.7%]) compared with mission facilities (2.1% [95% CI: 0.3–12.3%]) and private-sector facilities (3.8% [95% CI: 2.2–6.5%]).

Quality of process of care

Figure 1 presents radar plots summarising domain scores for Nairobi City County as a whole (Fig. 1a), by sector (Fig. 1b, c and d) and facility size (Fig. 1e, f and g). Mean (95% CI) scores are presented in Additional file 1: Table S3. Overall, performance was lowest for domain VI, correct fluid and feed volume (weighted mean score 0.35 [95% CI: 0.22–0.48]); whereas, performance was best for domain I, documentation of newborn characteristics (0.86 [95% CI: 0.80–0.93]).

When stratifying by sector and size, different patterns emerge, with generally lower domain scores for the process of care in the private (summary process score = 0.49 [95% CI: 0.44–0.54]) and mission sectors (0.48 [95% CI: 0.43–0.53]) compared with public-sector facilities (0.61 [95% CI: 0.56–0.67]), which account for 71% of admissions. Large facilities (three public, one mission and three private facilities) tended to have higher domain scores (summary process score = 0.59 [95% CI: 0.52–0.66]), while medium and small facilities scored less well (0.54 [95% CI: 0.48–0.60] and 0.45 [95% CI: 0.42–0.48], respectively), with suggestions of a trend of improving scores from small to larger facilities (Fig. 2).

Table 1 Newborn patient characteristics, weighted proportions (%)

	Total (*n* = 1184)	Public (*n* = 490)	Mission (*n* = 221)	Private (*n* = 473)
Age at admission				
<24 h	50.7	48.0	55.2	62.0
1 day	20.0	23.0	15.5	6.3
2–7 days	16.3	17.3	12.3	15.3
>1 week	5.5	5.3	1.7	13.1
Not recorded	7.5	6.4	15.2	3.3
Length of stay				
<7 days	63.8	64.3	81.4	55.0
7–13 days	14.9	18.0	6.3	15.6
14–28 days	7.5	8.4	0.9	9.7
>28 days	4.7	3.9	3.2	6.3
Not recorded	9.1	5.5	8.1	13.3
Sex				
Male	51.2	51.1	50.6	52.8
Female	42.9	42.3	45.4	42.9
Not recorded	5.9	6.6	3.9	4.3
Delivery mode				
Spontaneous	52.4	57.9	44.9	26.1
Caesarean section	40.4	36.7	48.9	52.5
Assisted or breech	1.3	0.7	1.9	4.4
Not recorded	6.0	4.8	4.3	17.0
Birthweight				
<1 kg	1.2	0.8	0.6	4.8
1–1.4 kg	6.2	6.5	2.1	10.9
1.5–2.4 kg	21.9	23.4	13.7	24.3
2.5–4 kg	58.8	59.7	67.5	39.2
>4 kg	5.4	4.6	8.9	5.4
Not recorded	6.4	4.9	7.2	15.3
Gestational age				
Very preterm (<32 wk)	7.0	7.0	2.2	14.6
Moderate or late preterm (32–36 wk)	16.2	15.5	13.3	25.4
Term (37–42 wk)	37.0	44.3	13.2	24.5
Not recorded	39.8	33.1	71.3	35.5
Apgar at 5 min				
0–3	2.2	2.9	0.6	0.2
4–6	14.6	15.9	12.9	8.2
7–10	69.3	69.6	74.9	58.9
Not recorded	13.8	11.6	11.5	32.8
HIV exposure status				
Exposed	4.4	5.0	3.2	2.6
Not exposed	58.2	66.5	41.6	27.1
Not recorded	37.3	28.5	55.2	70.4

Weighted proportions ensure that each facility contributed to the results as a proportion of their contribution to the total admissions across facilities and within their sector. The total refers to weighted results across all 28 facilities

Domain-specific indicators

Specific and additional details of domain indicators are presented in Table 2. Of note for domains I and II, documentation in the public sector was slightly better than in the private and mission sectors, particularly for documentation of key signs and symptoms.

Most newborns had evidence of a further clinical review after admission and vital signs monitoring within the first 48 h after admission. However, vital signs were predominantly recorded only in nursing notes (to which clinicians rarely have access). Only 39.4% of newborns had a vital signs chart available and completed in the medical record (Table 2). Similar proportions of newborns had feeding charts and fluids charts available and filled. The level of evidence for weight monitoring was particularly low (21.3%).

Almost two-thirds (63.4%) of the population were prescribed antibiotics, of whom the majority (92.6%) were prescribed both gentamicin and penicillin, suggesting good adherence to recommended first-line treatment across sectors. A large proportion (62.5%) of newborns who had no admission diagnosis of severe infection (n = 821) were nonetheless prescribed antibiotics. Incorrect doses were prescribed to 19.4% of newborns. An overdose of gentamicin was the most common error (11.7%) (Table 2).

Of those prescribed oxygen, 36.4% were prescribed oxygen via the correct route (nasal prongs or catheter); 32.5% had no route prescribed and 23.5% were prescribed oxygen via a mask. Recorded signs and symptoms suggested 39.7% (n = 894) might have required oxygen; 60.8% (n = 316) of these newborns had an oxygen prescription documented, of whom 40.7% (n = 191) were also prescribed the correct route.

Feeds were prescribed to 33.6% of newborns and 51.1% were prescribed fluids. Of those prescribed either feed or fluid (n = 721), 17.8% were prescribed both. Only 34.9% of newborns were found to be prescribed the correct volume of feed or fluid based on their admission age and weight (Table 2).

Structural and process quality

The weighted mean overall process of care score was 0.58 (95% CI: 0.52–0.64) across newborn records (Additional file 1: Table S3). The score was higher

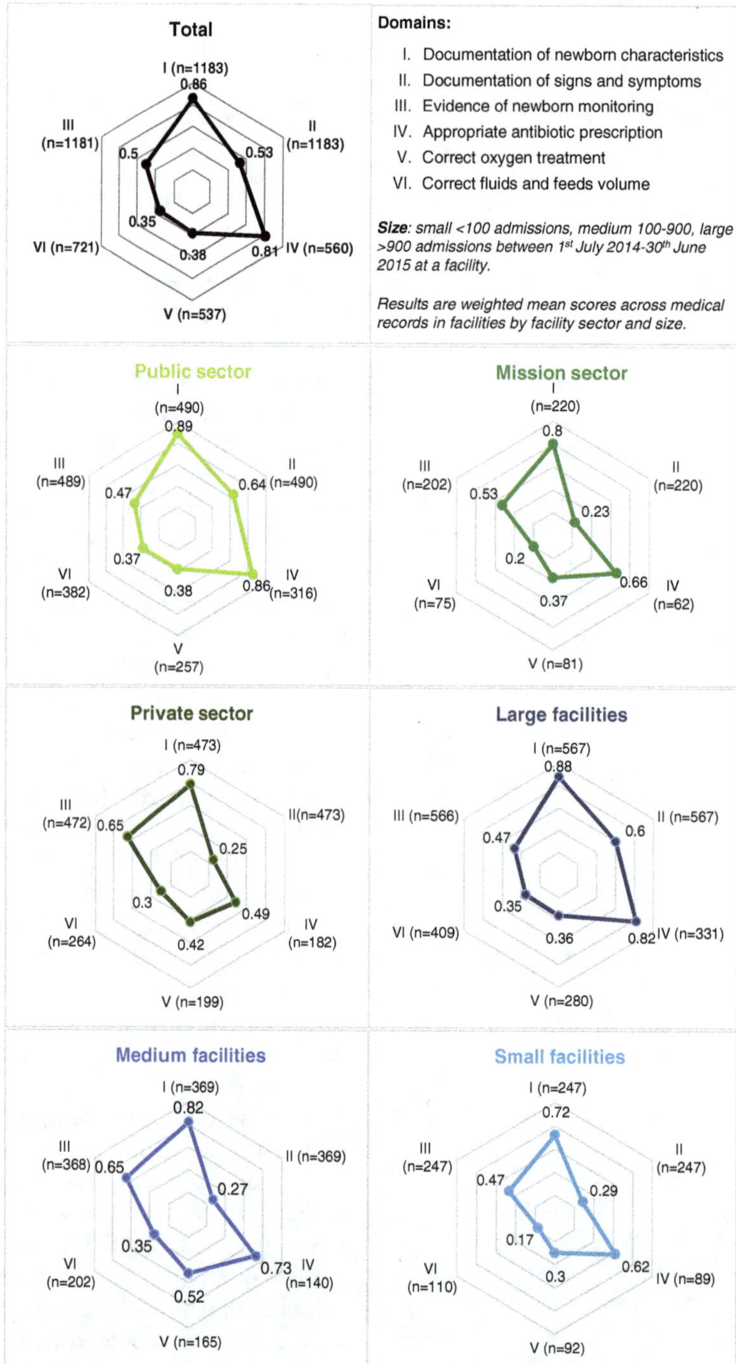

Fig. 1 Quality of care domain scores by sector and size of facilities

among public (0.61, 95% CI: 0.56–0.67), compared with mission (0.48, 95% CI: 0.43–0.53) and private (0.49, 95% CI: 0.44–0.54) facilities.

Visual assessment of Fig. 2 suggests a possible relationship between facility size and summary process and structural capacity scores, with larger facilities tending towards higher scores and smaller facilities tending towards lower scores for both process and structure. Large heterogeneity in process scores exists among facilities with high structural capacity scores.

Facilities with an absence of dedicated nursing staff on the NBU (associated with small facility size) had a lower mean process score than where facilities had nurses specifically assigned to NBUs (mean scores 0.47 [95%

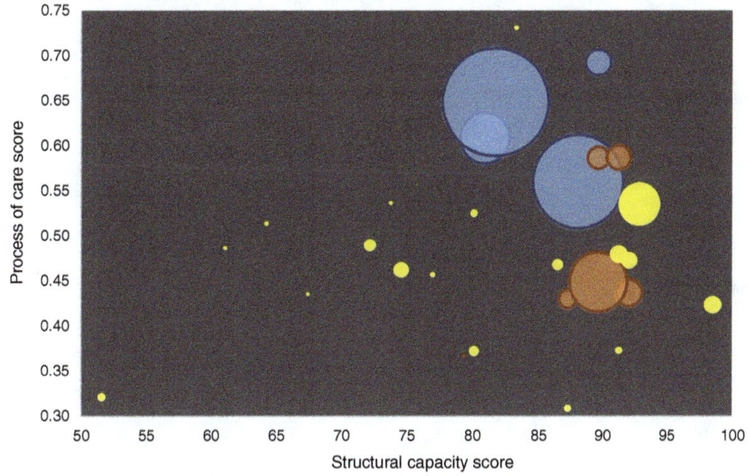

Fig. 2 Relationship between summary process of care score and structural capacity score for each facility, by patient volume and sector. Each bubble represents a facility. Bubble sizes are proportional to the number of admissions received by the facility between 1 July 2014 and 30 June 2015. Sectors are represented by bubble colours: blue = public, mission = orange and private = yellow. Scores are summary scores for patient records within each facility. Note that the *x*- and *y*-axes do not begin at zero

CI: 0.43–0.51], $n = 410$ and 0.60 [95% CI: 0.54–0.65], $n = 774$, respectively).

Effective coverage

Of newborns receiving services at one of the 28 study facilities, we estimate that 45.0% (5459/12,143) are receiving care associated with high to medium summary process scores (>0.6), while 35.4% (4300/12,143) and 19.6% (2384/12,143) are receiving care associated with medium to low (0.5–0.6) and low summary process quality scores (≤0.5), respectively.

We estimate that 24.9% [5459/21,966; estimate range 20.6% (5459/17,765) to 30.7% (5459/26,527)] of newborns needing care are admitted to a facility that provides high-quality care (process score >0.6 and structure score ≥80%), and are, hence, receiving effective coverage (Fig. 3). A further 30.4% of newborns needing care are receiving services either in a medium-quality care environment (19.5%, process score 0.5–0.6 and structure score ≥ 80%) or a low-quality care environment (10.9%, process score ≤ 0.5 or structural score <80%). Previous reports [18] estimated that 44.5% [9764/21,966; estimated range 37% (9764/17,765) to 55% (9764/26,527)] of newborns requiring care do not attend an INC facility in Nairobi City County and we regard these newborns as not receiving care. A further 0.3% (59/21,966) receive services at the remaining INC facilities not included in this process of care assessment.

Discussion

Our study examines the quality of neonatal care across an entire population, capturing information across sectors, and working towards defining effective coverage [25]. Our results provide insight into key actionable quality gaps and unearthed large heterogeneity in care contexts and quality for neonatal patients in this high-mortality setting. Deficits were most commonly identified in small, often private facilities, although severe workforce deficits and overcrowding undermine the quality of care in the public sector. Taken together with results of linked studies, we estimate that effective service provision is unavailable for 75% of sick newborns in Nairobi City County, this gap being made up of failures in access (44.5%) and receipt of lower quality services (30.4%).

Documentation of basic newborn characteristics, diagnoses and outcomes are important sources of data for local statistics to inform public health and health-care planning. As others have also found, improvement in the documentation of patient characteristics and care is needed, especially in mission and private-sector facilities [11, 13]. Standard admission forms that are aligned with national guidelines, used more often in public-sector facilities, may help to improve documentation [26, 27]. Structured vital signs charts were found to be commonly available but only completed in a third of records. Instead, newborn monitoring was often documented in the unstructured nursing Kardex (nursing-specific notes), to which clinicians do not have access. Combined medical and nursing records (a suggestion made over 60 years ago [28]) might, therefore, be a useful intervention to improve documentation and clinical communication.

Documented clinical care that does not align with national guidelines was common. Of particular concern is the possible harm caused by the inappropriate prescription of antibiotics, one of five indicators of quality neonatal care recommended by international and national

Table 2 Documented newborn assessment, monitoring and clinical care in newborn medical records, weighted proportions (%, 95% CI)

	Total	Public	Mission	Private
Documentation of newborn characteristics	$n = 1182$	$n = 490$	$n = 220$	$n = 472$
Characteristics documented (of nine), mean (95% CI)	7.8 (7.2–8.3)	8.0 (7.3–8.7)	7.2 (6.9–7.5)	7.1 (6.4–7.7)
Documentation of signs and symptoms	$n = 1182$	$n = 490$	$n = 220$	$n = 472$
Signs documented (of eight), mean (95% CI)	4.3 (2.7–5.9)	5.2 (4.0–6.5)	1.7 (0.8–2.5)	2.1 (1.7–2.5)
Symptoms documented (of eight), mean (95% CI)	4.2 (2.2–6.2)	5.0 (2.9–7.2)	2.0 (1.5–2.6)	1.9 (1.3–2.6)
Evidence of patient monitoring	$n = 1182$	$n = 490$	$n = 220$	$n = 472$
Evidence of further clinical review	89.6 (85.5–92.6)	90.7 (87.2–93.3)	83.6 (77.9–88.0)	91.6 (72.2–97.9)
Frequency of temperature recorded in first 48 h, mean (95% CI)	6.6 (5.0–8.2)	5.2 (4.5–5.8)	6.9 (5.6–8.2)	9.6 (8.2–10.9)
Treatment sheet available and filled	88.7 (79.9–93.9)	91.0 (81.7–95.9)	80.0 (54.2–93.1)	86.3 (76.8–92.2)
Vital signs chart available and filled	39.4 (13.3–73.4)	26.6 (4.7–72.8)	72.9 (48.8–88.3)	75.2 (39.0–93.5)
Feeding chart available and filled*	35.7 (23.3–50.3)	31.7 (20.7–45.1)	30.4 (9.6–64.3)	81.5 (48.3–95.4)
Fluid chart available and filled**	41.4 (17.7–70.0)	35.1 (9.8–72.8)	42.2 (23.9–62.9)	79.8 (40.9–95.8)
Weight monitored and filled	21.3 (7.8–46.3)	22.9 (6.2–57.1)	5.9 (3.0–11.2)	34.8 (14.6–62.6)
Appropriate antibiotic prescription				
Antibiotic dose	$n = 556$	$n = 316$	$n = 62$	$n = 178$
Incorrect dose	19.4 (11.8–30.2)	14.4 (8.6–23.1)	34.2 (15.9–58.7)	51.0 (38.6–63.4)
Gentamicin dose‡	$n = 539$	$n = 315$	$n = 62$	$n = 162$
Overdose	11.7 (7.1–18.5)	9.4 (5.5–15.5)	11.6 (7.4–17.8)	36.0 (26.0–47.3)
Under-dose	4.6 (2.3–9.1)	2.9 (1.6–5.5)	15.4 (7.0–30.8)	8.5 (6.0–11.8)
Penicillin dose‡	$n = 512$	$n = 302$	$n = 43$	$n = 167$
Overdose	2.8 (1.4–5.3)	2.7 (1.2–5.8)	0.0 (0.0–0.0)	5.8 (4.0–8.5)
Under-dose	3.6 (1.2–10.6)	1.3 (0.8–2.2)	21.6 (2.5–74.8)	11.1 (8.1–14.9)
Correct oxygen treatment				
Those requiring and prescribed	60.8 (54.8–66.5) ($n = 316$)	59.2 (53.6–64.6) ($n = 187$)	70.8 (42.0–89.0) ($n = 26$)	69.0 (53.9–80.9) ($n = 103$)
Correct route (nasal prongs or catheter)	36.4 (24.6–50.0) ($n = 412$)	36.5 (21.5–54.7) ($n = 181$)	35.4 (16.9–59.5) ($n = 73$)	37.0 (27.5–47.6) ($n = 158$)
Correctly prescribed (required and correct route)	40.7 (23.7–60.4) ($n = 191$)	39.4 (19.7–63.2) ($n = 111$)	57.1 (39.8–72.8) ($n = 18$)	39.1 (26.6–53.3) ($n = 62$)
Correct fluids and feeds	$n = 721$	$n = 382$	$n = 75$	$n = 264$
Correct fluid and feed volumes	34.9 (23.2–48.7)	37.4 (23.6–53.6)	19.9 (5.5–51.6)	30.1 (20.0–42.6)

Overdose and under-dose was defined as 20% more and less, respectively, than the recommended dose per kilogram body weight per day as per national guidelines. Correct fluid and feed volume allow for 20% margin of error from national guidelines
*Of those patients who received a prescription for feeding (n: total = 307, public = 199, mission = 16 and private = 92)
**Of those patients who received a prescription for fluids (n: total = 529, public = 252, mission = 66 and private = 211)
‡ Of those patients who received antibiotics ($n = 640$) and had their weight, prescription frequency and dose recorded
CI confidence interval

experts [23]. In our study, antibiotics were prescribed to the majority (63.4%) of newborns, regardless of a diagnosis of sepsis. Encouragingly though, first-line antibiotic regimens were used in over 90% of cases. Despite this, consistent with previous findings [13], antibiotic doses that were 20% too high or too low were prescribed for more than a fifth of newborns. Overdosing of gentamicin, which may cause toxicity in newborns, was of most concern. Mitigating this risk, however, the length of stay of newborns was often short (median = 4 days, interquartile range = 2–7.6, *unpublished data*). Nonetheless, inaccurate prescribing of a potentially toxic drug is an important

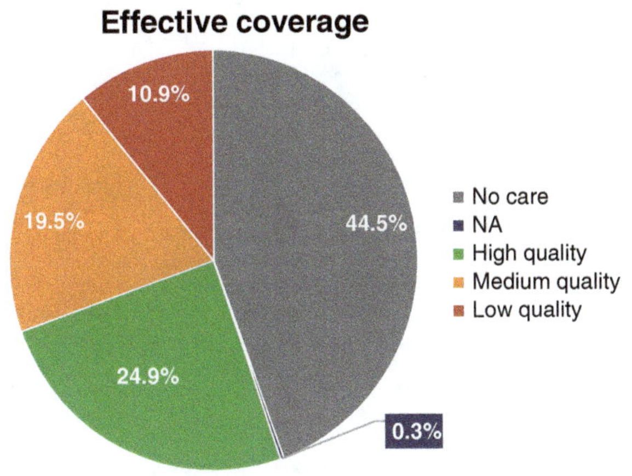

Fig. 3 Levels of care environment for newborns requiring inpatient services (n = 21,966) in Nairobi City County. No care: Not attending one of the 31 INC facilities. NA: Attended one of the 31 inpatient neonatal care facilities but did not partake in process assessment. High quality: Facility process score >0.6 and structure score ≥0.8. Medium quality: Facility process score 0.5–0.6 and structure score ≥0.8. Low quality: Facility process score ≤0.5 or structure score <0.8

patient safety issue. Also of concern are the prescribing inaccuracies in 65% of newborns receiving feeds or fluids. As with inaccurate drug prescription, this was more common in smaller facilities.

A distinct group of small facilities were found to have very low structural and process quality. This clustering of deficits was found primarily among private facilities, specifically smaller private facilities. Though highly heterogeneous as a sector, private facilities are least likely to be involved in training and quality improvement activities initiated by the government or partners. Minimum standards should be ensured across all settings and sectors, perhaps through benchmarking, accreditation and external audits. In some settings, this has been achieved through voluntary networks across public and private facilities [29].

Until recently, neonatal health care was not prominent on the global or national agendas, limiting investment in services for this patient group. Although providing good quality neonatal care poses specific challenges, many of the health system's weaknesses experienced in low-resource settings are also evident in Nairobi, impacting on neonatal survival. These weaknesses included health worker shortages in the public sector, poor staff motivation and inadequate health-care financing more broadly (as evidenced by the recent doctors' and nurses' strikes over pay and working conditions). The specific reasons behind gaps in quality of care for neonates and the challenges faced by nurses working in NBUs are being examined through ongoing qualitative research in Nairobi.

There are strengths and limitations to our study. Our use of routine medical records for the evaluation of quality of care is a pragmatic approach that can be integrated into routine on-site quality assessment in facilities [26, 30]. However, it also limits assessment to indicators that are routinely documented. Furthermore, medical records are not standardised across facilities, which may have contributed to the lower performance in non-public-sector facilities. We defined correct care a priori based on national standards of care, which have been widely disseminated in Kenya [22]. However, such guidelines may have less penetration in the private sector and, in particular, large private hospitals may have their own standards of care drawn from high-income practice settings. This may slightly disadvantage large private facilities in our scoring approach. Due to the lack of adequate data on acuity and case mix, we were unable to evaluate links between the quality scores and mortality meaningfully. We took a non-randomised approach to sampling records where this was needed (11/28), focusing on the most recent admissions. We do not anticipate that this should bias our findings unless seasonality differences in quality of care exist. Our aim was to provide insight into the entire population of neonatal patients receiving 24×7 inpatient care in Nairobi City County. Four of the 32 eligible facilities declined to partake. However, it is estimated that their contribution to annual admissions was a maximum of 1.3% (159/12,302) and, hence, we do not anticipate that our overall results would change upon their inclusion. Our denominator for effective coverage relies on estimating the number of live births in Nairobi City County during the study period and the proportion of those live births requiring admission. Although we have provided uncertainty estimates for the latter, we are unable to quantify uncertainty around the former estimate. The true range of uncertainty around our estimate for effective coverage is, therefore, higher than presented, which should be taken into consideration when interpreting these results. A detailed description of the methods and limitations of calculating the coverage denominator are presented in a separate publication [19].

Conclusions

Effective coverage of interventions delivered at facility level will become increasingly important for reducing neonatal mortality. Our multi-sector landscape evaluation of almost all facilities providing INC services to small and sick newborns in Nairobi City County demonstrates the value of estimating effective coverage and identifying gaps in access and quality. To improve these estimates continuously and ensure progress in addressing gaps can be tracked, it is important to develop the capacity to monitor access and quality across all sectors routinely. Efforts to improve care would be facilitated by the development and implementation of common minimum standards for facilities and processes of care, including the standardisation of medical and nursing records. Strategies to improve facility-based care for newborns will need to consider substantial deficits in access, resources and processes of care as part of long-term planning to improve service delivery equitably.

Abbreviations

CI: Confidence interval; INC: Inpatient neonatal care; KEMRI: Kenya Medical Research Institute; NBU: Newborn unit; SOP: Standard operating procedure

Acknowledgements

We would like to thank Hannah Leslie, Anna Gage and Margaret Kruk for their helpful comments on this manuscript. Ann Mwaniki, Grace Nabea, Beatrice Amboko, Wycliffe Nyachiro and Mercy Chepkirui contributed enormously to data collection and data entry for this study. We are grateful for the ongoing support and intellectual contributions to this project from Nairobi City County government, the Ministry of Health Kenya and the Kenya Paediatric Association. We would like also to thank all the facilities, including their management and staff, for participating in this study and their dedication to improving the care for sick newborns in Kenya.

Health Services that Deliver for Newborns Expert Group: Dr Sam Ochola (Nairobi City County Government), Dr Robert Ayisi (Nairobi City County Government), Prof Aggrey Wasunna (University of Nairobi), Prof Fred Were (University of Nairobi), Dr Catherine Mutinda and Dr Beth Maina (Pumwani Maternity Hospital), Dr Cecilia Mutiso (Mama Lucy Kibaki Hospital), Dr David Githanga (Kenya Paediatric Association), Dr David Kimutai (Mbagathi District Hospital), Prof Rachel Musoke (University of Nairobi), Dr Roseline Ochieng (Aga Khan University), Prof William Macharia (Aga Khan University) and Dr Rachel Nyamai (Ministry of Health).

Funding

This work was supported by a Health Systems Research Initiative joint grant provided by the Department for International Development, UK, the Economic and Social Research Council, the Medical Research Council and Wellcome Trust, grant MR/M015386/1. ME is supported by a Wellcome Trust Senior Fellowship (097170).

Authors' contributions

GM, JA and ME designed the study, with input from the expert group. GM, JM, NA and DG led the data collection and study coordination. GM analysed the data and wrote the manuscript, with support from ME and DG. All authors reviewed and provided input into the final version of the manuscript. All authors read and approved the final manuscript.

Competing interests

The authors declare that they have no competing interests.

Author details

[1]Centre for Tropical Medicine and Global Health, Nuffield Department of Medicine, University of Oxford, Oxford, UK. [2]Kenya Medical Research Institute - Wellcome Trust Research Programme, Nairobi, Kenya. [3]Nairobi City County Government, Nairobi, Kenya.

References

1. United Nations. Sustainable Development Goals: Goal 3. https://sustainabledevelopment.un.org/sdg3. (Accessed 26 May 2017).
2. Countdown to 2015. A Decade of Tracking Progress for Maternal, Newborn and Child Survival: The 2015 Report. Geneva: UNICEF and World Health Organisation. 2015.
3. Lawn JE, Blencowe H, Oza S, et al. Every Newborn: progress, priorities, and potential beyond survival. Lancet. 2014;384(9938):189–205.
4. Moxon SG, Lawn JE, Dickson KE, et al. Inpatient care of small and sick newborns: a multi-country analysis of health system bottlenecks and potential solutions. BMC Pregnancy Childbirth. 2015;15(Suppl 2):S7.
5. Dickson KE, Simen-Kapeu A, Kinney MV, et al. Every Newborn: Health-systems bottlenecks and strategies to accelerate scale-up in countries. Lancet. 2014;384:438–54.
6. Keats EC, Ngugi A, Macharia W, et al. Progress and priorities for reproductive, maternal, newborn, and child health in Kenya: a Countdown to 2015 country case study. Lancet Glob Health. 2017;5(8):e782–e95.
7. Bhutta ZA, Das JK, Bahl R, et al. Can available interventions end preventable deaths in mothers, newborn babies, and stillbirths, and at what cost? Lancet. 2014;384:347–70.
8. Wang W, Alva S, Wang S, Fort A. Levels and Trends in the Use of Maternal Health Services in Developing Countries. DHS Comparative Reports No. 26. Calverton: USAID; 2011.
9. Gabrysch S, Civitelli G, Edmond KM, et al. New signal functions to measure the ability of health facilities to provide routine and emergency newborn care. PLoS Med. 2012;9(11):e1001340.
10. The Partnership for Maternal Newborn & Child Health. A Global Review of the Key Interventions Related to Reproductive, Maternal, Newborn and Child Health (RMNCH). Geneva: Partnership for Maternal Newborn & Child Health; 2011.
11. Gathara D, Opiyo N, Wagai J, et al. Quality of hospital care for sick newborns and severely malnourished children in Kenya: a two-year descriptive study in 8 hospitals. BMC Health Serv Res. 2011;11:307.
12. Opondo C, Ntoburi S, Wagai J, et al. Are hospitals prepared to support newborn survival? - An evaluation of eight first-referral level hospitals in Kenya. Tropical Med Int Health. 2009;14(10):1165–72.
13. Aluvaala J, Nyamai R, Were F, et al. Assessment of neonatal care in clinical training facilities in Kenya. Arch Dis Child. 2015;100:42–7.
14. Glasziou P, Straus S, Brownlee S, et al. Evidence for underuse of effective medical services around the world. Lancet. 2017;390(10090): 169–77.
15. O'Neill K, Takane M, Sheffel A, Abou-Zahr C, Boerma T. Monitoring service delivery for universal health coverage: the Service Availability and Readiness Assessment. Bull World Health Organ. 2013;91(12):923–31.
16. Kenya National Bureau of Statistics. 2014 Kenya Demographic and Health Survey (2014 KDHS). Nairobi: Kenya National Bureau of Statistics; 2015.
17. African Population and Health Research Center (APHRC). Population and Health Dynamics in Nairobi's Informal Settlements: Report of the Nairobi Cross-sectional Slums Survey (NCSS) 2012. Nairobi: APHRC; 2014.
18. Murphy GAV, Waters D, Ouma PO, et al. Estimating the need for inpatient neonatal services: an iterative approach employing evidence and expert consensus to guide local policy in Kenya. BMJ Glob Health. 2017;2(4): e000472.
19. Murphy GAV, Gathara D, Abuya N, Mwachiro J, Ochola S, et al. What capacity exists to provide essential inpatient care to small and sick newborns in a high mortality urban setting? - A cross-sectional study in Nairobi City County, Kenya. PLOS ONE 2018;13(4):e0196585. https://doi.org/10.1371/journal.pone.0196585.
20. Murphy GA, Gathara D, Aluvaala J, et al. Nairobi Newborn Study: a protocol for an observational study to estimate the gaps in provision and quality of inpatient newborn care in Nairobi City County, Kenya. BMJ Open. 2016; 6(12):e012448.
21. The Global Health Network. Estimating the gaps in provision and quality of inpatient newborn care. https://globalresearchmethods.tghn.org/methodology-projects/estimating-gaps-provision-and-quality-inpatient-newborn-care/. Accessed 20 Apr 2018.
22. Ministry of Health Republic of Kenya. Basic Paediatric Protocols: for ages up to 5 years. 3rd ed; 2013.
23. Ntoburi S, Hutchings A, Sanderson C, et al. Development of paediatric quality of inpatient care indicators for low-income countries - A Delphi study. BMC Pediatr. 2010;10:90.
24. District health information software 2 (DHIS2). hiskenya.org. Accessed 9 Dec 2015.
25. Kinney MV, Cocoman O, Dickson KE, et al. Implementation of the Every Newborn Action Plan: Progress and lessons learned. Semin Perinatol. 2015; 39(5):326–37.
26. Tuti T, Bitok M, Malla L, et al. Improving documentation of clinical care within a clinical information network: an essential initial step in efforts to understand and improve care in Kenyan hospitals. BMJ Glob Health. 2016; 1(1):e000028.

27. Ayieko P, Ntoburi S, Wagai J, et al. A multifaceted intervention to implement guidelines and improve admission paediatric care in Kenyan district hospitals: a cluster randomised trial. PLoS Med. 2011;8(4):e1001018.
28. Dickerson LA. Coordinating medical and nursing records. Public Health Rep. 1953;68(12):1205–9.
29. Suresh G, Horbar JD, Plsek P, et al. Voluntary anonymous reporting of medical errors for neonatal intensive care. Pediatrics. 2004;113(6):1609–18.
30. Rubin HR, Pronovost P, Diette GB. The advantages and disadvantages of process-based measures of health care quality. Int J Qual Health Care. 2001; 13(6):469–74.

7

Stratified survival of resected and overall pancreatic cancer patients in Europe and the USA in the early twenty-first century: a large, international population-based study

Lei Huang[1,2], Lina Jansen[1,3], Yesilda Balavarca[4], Masoud Babaei[1], Lydia van der Geest[5], Valery Lemmens[5], Liesbet Van Eycken[6], Harlinde De Schutter[6], Tom B. Johannesen[7], Maja Primic-Žakelj[8], Vesna Zadnik[8], Marc G. Besselink[9], Petra Schrotz-King[4] and Hermann Brenner[1,3,4*]

Abstract

Background: The prognosis of pancreatic cancer (PaC) strongly varies across different stages and age groups, which has unfortunately not been well recorded in the literature. This international population-based study aimed to provide tumor-node-metastasis (TNM) stage- and age-specific survival estimates and trends in resected and overall (resected and unresected) PaC in the early twenty-first century.

Methods: Using data from the US Surveillance, Epidemiology, and End Results-18 Program and the national cancer registries of the Netherlands, Belgium, Norway, and Slovenia, short-term and long-term overall survival results stratified by TNM stage and age in resected and overall primary PaC, *irrespective of being microscopically confirmed or not*, in 2003–2014 were computed using the Kaplan-Meier method. The temporal survival trends over three predefined periods (2003–2005, 2006–2008, and 2009–2011) were further examined using the log-rank test.

Results: In total, data for 125,183 patients were analyzed. Overall, age-stratified 3-year survival was 20–34% (< 60 years), 14–25% (60–69 years), and 9–13% (≥ 70 years) in stages I–II PaC; and 2–5% (< 60 years), 1–2% (60–69 years), and < 1–1% (≥ 70 years) in stages III–IV cancer. Patients who underwent operation had higher 3-year survival in each stage and age group (stages I–II: 23–39% (< 60 years), 16–31% (60–69 years), and 17–30% (≥ 70 years); stages III–IV: 5–19% (< 70 years) and 2–14% (≥ 70 years)). Perioperative survival also decreased with advancing stage and older age (stages I–II: 98–100% (< 60 years), 97–99% (60–69 years), and 94–99% (≥ 70 years); stages III–IV: 94–99% (< 70 years) and 81–96% (≥ 70 years)). Between 2003 and 2005 and 2009–2011, for overall PaC, both short-term and long-term survival improvements were observed in all countries except Belgium; for resected disease, short-term improvements were present only in the USA and Slovenia, but long-term improvements were observed in all countries except Slovenia, with stage-specific variations.

(Continued on next page)

* Correspondence: h.brenner@dkfz-heidelberg.de
[1]Division of Clinical Epidemiology and Aging Research, German Cancer Research Center (DKFZ), Im Neuenheimer Feld 581, 69120 Heidelberg, Germany
[3]German Cancer Consortium (DKTK), German Cancer Research Center (DKFZ), Heidelberg, Germany
Full list of author information is available at the end of the article

(Continued from previous page)

Conclusions: Our large international study provides TNM stage- and age-specific population-based survival in overall and resected PaC that will facilitate clinical counseling. While the survival expectations for patients with resected PaC are substantially higher than the widely available and known dismal survival predictions for overall patients, conclusions on the benefits of resection cannot be made from this observational study. Patients with advanced-stage disease and/or older age should undergo careful risk assessment before treatment. Limited but inspiring improvement in survival is observed.

Keywords: Pancreatic cancer, Resection, Survival, TNM stage, Age, Population-based, Early twenty-first century

Background

Pancreatic cancer (PaC) is one of the deadliest malignancies worldwide; > 340,000 individuals receive this diagnosis annually with similar incidence and mortality rates [1]. PaC incidence is especially high in developed countries, being the fourth leading cause of cancer-related deaths in Western societies [2]. In the EU, PaC incidence has been stable or moderately increasing over the past decades, and it was estimated to have caused 91,500 deaths in 2017 and to cause 111,500 deaths in 2025, potentially becoming the third leading cause of cancer death [3].

The prognosis for PaC is poor, with 5-year survival of only ~ 5% [4]. Due to lack of effective early screening methods, more than half of PaCs are detected at advanced stages and are treated largely palliatively [5, 6]. According to the current guidelines [7–11], only tumor-node-metastasis (TNM) stages I–II PaCs are usually resectable, although the resectability criteria are differentially and arguably defined [12]. While resection could markedly improve the long-term survival in selected patients, less than one-fifth of diagnosed cases are considered eligible for resection [5, 10]. Patients with resectable PaC who undergo resection have much better survival rates than those who cannot undergo resection [8, 10].

We previously described the low and varying resection rates for PaC in Europe and the USA [13]. When counseling PaC patients who are considering surgery or who have already undergone resection, it is important to provide survival estimates for the resected subgroup. However, at this time, population-based survival estimates are only available for overall patients without differentiation by resection or TNM stage [4], according to which, however, survival might vary greatly. Survival odds in resected PaC data from institutional reports would be accompanied with relatively high patient selection, making the generalizability questionable. Based on multiple national databases, this large investigation aimed to comprehensively and robustly provide 1-month to 5-year overall survival estimates at the population level for overall (resected and unresected) and resected PaC patients diagnosed in the early twenty-first century in Europe and the USA stratified by TNM stage and age. Furthermore, survival trends over time in each country were explored.

Methods

Study design

A list of all contacted cancer registries together with reasons for exclusion are provided in Additional file 1: Table S1. Population-based PaC data from the US Surveillance, Epidemiology, and End Results (SEER)-18 Program, the Netherlands Cancer Registry, the Belgian Cancer Registry, the Cancer Registry of Norway, and the Cancer Registry of Slovenia were investigated in this large real-world observational study (Additional file 1: Table S2). The data quality of each registry was described in a previous publication [13], focusing on resection rates only. Among the previous participants [13], the Danish registry withdrew its participation due to some legislation issues, and the small population size for resected patients in Estonia did not allow for reasonable survival analyses. Institution-based data were not included due to the relatively high risk of patient selection bias. The participating European national registries, located in western, northern, and southern Europe, respectively, were those able to provide data of relatively high quality, according to a uniform data-request sheet, to ensure the robustness of the results. All variables were uniformly (re)coded across registries. National population-based registries were not included if they were not able to provide eligible treatment, TNM staging, or survival data. This study was approved by the Ethics Committee of Medical Faculty Heidelberg and reported following the Strengthening the Reporting of Observational Studies in Epidemiology (STROBE) guidelines.

Patients

Only patients with pathologic and/or clinical diagnoses of invasive primary malignant tumors of the exocrine pancreas were included. Patients were included irrespective of being microscopically diagnosed or not in this real-world study on survival for resected and overall PaC following the EUROCARE studies [4, 14], since consensus has been reached by the International Study Group of Pancreatic Surgery (ISGPS) that, in the presence of a solid mass suspicious for malignancy, biopsy proof has not been and is not required before proceeding with resection [15]. Those with benign/premalignant tumors, non-pancreatic neoplasms involving the pancreas, neuroendocrine tumors, carcinoids, sarcomas/stromal tumors, germ cell neoplasms, lymphomas, or periampullar tumors (Additional file 1: Table S3), with diagnosis based on autopsy or death certificate only, or with unknown diagnosis/follow-up date or survival status were excluded. Patients without TNM staging were also excluded. As the fifth edition of the TNM staging system was incompatible with the later versions in effect during 2003–2017 [8], only patients with PaC diagnosed after 2002 were included.

Collected information

Information on patient (year of diagnosis, sex, and age) and tumor characteristics (microscopic confirmation, TNM stage, location, and differentiation), treatment (resection, (neo) adjuvant chemotherapy, and radiotherapy), follow-up, and survival status was obtained. Tumor morphology and topography were coded according to the International Classification of Diseases for Oncology, Third Edition. Tumor stage was based on the TNM staging system, sixth/seventh edition [8]. In stage classification, pathologic (pTNM) stages were prioritized over clinical (cTNM) ones. Resection was defined as surgical removal of the primary tumor, regardless of being curative or palliative. Survival status was obtained from official population registers and/or national death registrations.

Outcome measures

Short-term (1-month to 6-month) and relatively long-term (1-year to 5-year) survival data in overall and resected PaC stratified by TNM stage (I–II and III–IV) and age group (< 60, 60–69, and ≥ 70 years) were presented. Cancer stage was divided into stages I–II and III–IV, considering the former to be clearly resectable and the latter mostly unresectable, and to ensure an adequate number for assessment in each subgroup. When describing survival for resected stages III–IV PaC, the subgroups < 60 and 60–69 years were combined considering the small size of either. Survival trends over 3 calendar years (2003–2005, 2006–2008, and 2009–2011) in each country were further reported. All these categories were predefined.

Statistical analyses

Complete-case analysis was performed for patients with known TNM stages. Results were described for each country separately without pooling, considering the potential heterogeneity across countries. Overall survival was defined as the months between diagnosis and death from any cause/last follow-up, and was estimated for overall and resected PaC patients by TNM stage and age group using the Kaplan-Meier method, with the 1-, 3-, 6-, 12-, 24-, 36-, and 60-month survival rates calculated. Sensitivity analyses were conducted by limiting the overall patients to those with microscopic confirmation. Changes in survival rates of overall and operated patients diagnosed between 2003 and 2005 and 2009–2011 were examined using the log-rank test. Statistical significance was defined by two-sided $P < 0.05$. The SAS software (version 9.4, Cary, NC, USA) was used.

Results

Patient characteristics

In total, data for 125,183 patients (stages I–II, 42,955 (34%); stages III–IV, 82,228 (66%)) were analyzed. Patients were diagnosed in comparable periods in all countries (2003/2004 until 2013/2014). Demographic and clinical characteristics for overall and operated patients with stages I–II and III–IV PaCs are shown in Table 1 and described in Additional file 1. In overall PaCs, 66% (Norway) to 91% (Belgium) of stages I–II cancers and 53% (Slovenia) to 86% (Belgium) of stages III–IV cancers were microscopically confirmed. Nearly all resected PaCs were microscopically confirmed (stages I–II, 99– ≥ 99%; stages III–IV, 92–100%).

Survival in overall and resected stages I–II PaCs

Survival in overall and resected stages I–II tumors is shown in Fig. 1, and the corresponding 1-month to 5-year survival rates are detailed in Table 2. For total patients, survival was lower in older patients and decreased strongly after diagnosis, with 3-year rates of 20–34% (< 60 years), 14–25% (60–69 years), and 9–13% (≥ 70 years), respectively. The subgroup of resected patients of all age groups in all countries had higher survival estimates, with 1-month (perioperative) rates of 98–100% (< 60 years), 97–99% (60–69 years), and 94–99% (≥ 70 years); and 3-year rates of 23–39% (< 60 years), 16–31% (60–69 years), and 17–30% (≥ 70 years), respectively. Again, younger patients had a better prognosis than older ones. However, age-specific differences were smaller, especially between those aged 60–69 and ≥ 70 years.

Survival in overall and resected stages III–IV PaCs

Considering the potentially varying proportions of underreporting of advanced-stage disease, survival results for stages III–IV PaCs should be interpreted with caution. Survival in overall and resected stages III–IV cancers is shown in Additional file 1: Figure S1, and the corresponding 1-month to 5-year survival rates are detailed in Additional file 1: Table S4. Generally, patients with stages III–IV PaCs had much lower survival results than those with stages I–II tumors, and already had high mortality shortly after diagnosis. In the total group, survival decreased with increasing age, with 3-year rates of 2–5% (< 60 years), 1–2% (60–69 years), and 1–1% (≥ 70 years), respectively. The resected subgroups showed higher survival estimates than the

Table 1 Demographic and clinical characteristics of patients with stages I–II and III–IV pancreatic cancer

Parameter	USA (2004–2013)		The Netherlands (2003–2014)		Belgium (2004–2013)		Norway (2003–2014)		Slovenia (2003–2013)	
Group	Overall	Resected	Overall	Resected	Overall	Resected	Overall	Resected	Overall	Resected
Stages I–II										
Number (n)	31,313	13,303 (43)	5710	2675 (47)	3437	2155 (63)	1545	526 (34)	667	406 (61)
Microscopically confirmed	27,290 (87)	13,290 (> 99)	4046 (71)	2673 (> 99)	3127 (91)	2148 (> 99)	1017 (66)	520 (99)	475 (71)	401 (99)
Gender, female	16,193 (52)	6604 (50)	2951 (52)	1268 (47)	1684 (49)	993 (46)	853 (55)	261 (50)	361 (54)	209 (52)
Age, years	70 ± 12	66 ± 11	71 ± 11	65 ± 10	69 ± 11	66 ± 10	72 ± 12	65 ± 11	69 ± 11	65 ± 10
Age group										
< 60 years	6100 (20)	3574 (27)	981 (17)	693 (26)	686 (20)	546 (25)	234 (15)	134 (26)	144 (22)	122 (30)
60–69 years	7817 (25)	4272 (32)	1477 (26)	978 (37)	937 (27)	698 (32)	375 (24)	195 (37)	166 (25)	131 (32)
≥ 70 years	17,396 (56)	5457 (41)	3252 (57)	1004 (38)	1814 (53)	911 (42)	936 (61)	197 (37)	357 (54)	153 (38)
Tumor location[a]										
Pancreas head	22,412 (83)	9573 (80)	4666 (89)	2187 (89)	1807 (81)	1207 (82)	851 (85)	394 (84)	471 (88)	321 (87)
Pancreas body	2502 (9)	890 (8)	255 (5)	91 (4)	179 (8)	100 (7)	87 (9)	33 (7)	35 (7)	26 (7)
Pancreas tail	2196 (8)	1448 (12)	296 (6)	191 (8)	244 (11)	169 (11)	62 (6)	41 (9)	32 (6)	21 (6)
Other	4203 (13)	1392 (11)	493 (9)	206 (8)	1207 (35)	679 (32)	545 (35)	58 (11)	129 (19)	38 (9)
Differentiation[b]										
Well	2145 (13)	1428 (12)	283 (12)	244 (11)	389 (18)	302 (17)	61 (10)	27 (6)	41 (10)	37 (10)
Intermediate	7574 (47)	6026 (51)	1225 (51)	1138 (52)	1072 (48)	901 (50)	352 (55)	259 (61)	153 (37)	142 (38)
Poor/undifferentiated	6264 (39)	4464 (38)	920 (38)	802 (37)	762 (34)	608 (34)	223 (35)	135 (32)	221 (53)	192 (52)
Neoadjuvant chemotherapy	–	NA	–	50 (2)	–	53 (3)	–	NA	–	2 (1)
Neoadjuvant radiotherapy	–	522 (4)	–	34 (1)	–	20 (1)	–	0 (0)	–	1 (< 1)
Resection type										
Pancreatoduodenectomy	–	9479 (71)	–	2269 (85)	–	NA	–	NA	–	NA
Distal pancreatectomy	–	1878 (14)	–	256 (10)	–	NA	–	NA	–	NA
Total pancreatectomy	–	1629 (12)	–	42 (2)	–	NA	–	NA	–	NA
Other[c]	–	314 (2)	–	108 (4)	–	NA	–	NA	–	NA
Adjuvant/palliative chemotherapy	NA	NA	1392 (24)	1078 (40)	1796 (52)	1200 (56)	265 (17)	127 (24)	131 (20)	120 (30)
Adjuvant/palliative radiotherapy	4460 (14)	4193 (32)	120 (2)	33 (1)	326 (10)	190 (9)	64 (4)	17 (3)	9 (1)	8 (2)
Stages III–IV										
Number (n)	55,153	1998 (4)	13,974	237 (2)	5632	298 (5)	4633	108 (2)	1997	135 (7)
Microscopically confirmed	46,973 (85)	1994 (> 99)	10,375 (74)	237 (100)	4837 (86)	297 (> 99)	3224 (70)	105 (97)	1056 (53)	124 (92)
Gender, female	26,427 (48)	969 (49)	6755 (48)	106 (45)	2700 (48)	154 (52)	2332 (50)	47 (44)	967 (48)	56 (42)
Age, years	69 ± 12	65 ± 12	68 ± 11	64 ± 10	69 ± 11	64 ± 10	71 ± 12	64 ± 10	69 ± 11	65 ± 10

Table 1 Demographic and clinical characteristics of patients with stages I–II and III–IV pancreatic cancer *(Continued)*

Parameter	USA (2004–2013)		The Netherlands (2003–2014)		Belgium (2004–2013)		Norway (2003–2014)		Slovenia (2003–2013)	
Group	Overall	Resected	Overall	Resected	Overall	Resected	Overall	Resected	Overall	Resected
Age group										
< 60 years	12,582 (23)	636 (32)	2938 (21)	69 (29)	1043 (19)	92 (31)	759 (16)	32 (30)	393 (20)	40 (30)
60–69 years	15,081 (27)	622 (31)	4412 (32)	96 (41)	1608 (29)	103 (35)	1268 (27)	43 (40)	513 (26)	45 (33)
≥ 70 years	27,490 (50)	740 (37)	6624 (47)	72 (30)	2981 (53)	103 (35)	2606 (56)	26 (24)	1091 (55)	43 (32)
Tumor location[a]										
Pancreas head	21,244 (56)	1069 (66)	7202 (62)	166 (79)	1585 (58)	126 (69)	1245 (63)	57 (66)	653 (64)	80 (78)
Pancreas body	7893 (21)	168 (10)	1844 (16)	11 (5)	508 (19)	19 (10)	340 (17)	8 (9)	160 (16)	12 (12)
Pancreas tail	9003 (24)	381 (24)	2666 (23)	34 (16)	649 (24)	37 (20)	382 (19)	21 (24)	215 (21)	10 (10)
Other	17,013 (31)	380 (19)	2262 (16)	26 (11)	2890 (51)	116 (39)	2666 (58)	22 (20)	969 (49)	33 (24)
Differentiation[d]										
Well	1213 (10)	173 (11)	222 (9)	20 (11)	425 (17)	42 (17)	122 (8)	6 (7)	33 (8)	6 (7)
Intermediate	4518 (35)	680 (45)	833 (35)	98 (51)	962 (39)	113 (47)	596 (40)	50 (61)	112 (25)	30 (34)
Poor/undifferentiated	6795 (56)	670 (44)	1340 (56)	73 (38)	1082 (44)	88 (36)	765 (52)	26 (32)	297 (67)	52 (59)
Neoadjuvant chemotherapy	–	NA	–	15 (6)	–	24 (8)	–	NA	–	0 (0)
Neoadjuvant radiotherapy	–	139 (7)	–	5 (2)	–	9 (3)	–	0 (0)	–	0 (0)
Resection type										
Pancreatoduodenectomy	–	1140 (57)	–	178 (75)	–	NA	–	NA	–	NA
Distal pancreatectomy	–	295 (15)	–	39 (17)	–	NA	–	NA	–	NA
Total pancreatectomy	–	211 (11)	–	5 (2)	–	NA	–	NA	–	NA
Other[c]	–	352 (18)	–	15 (6)	–	NA	–	NA	–	NA
Adjuvant/palliative chemotherapy	NA	NA	3475 (25)	81 (34)	3661 (65)	195 (65)	1159 (25)	25 (23)	368 (18)	39 (29)
Adjuvant/palliative radiotherapy	770 (1)	383 (19)	328 (2)	7 (3)	358 (6)	35 (12)	198 (4)	4 (4)	46 (2)	5 (4)

NOS not otherwise specified, *NA* not available; –, not applicable

Enumeration data are shown as count (percentage [%]), and measurement data as mean ± standard deviation. Records are complete, otherwise specified below

[a]The percentages of pancreas head, body, and tail are the proportions compared to the total tumor cases of the 3 locations; "other" includes pancreas duct, overlapping lesion, NOS, and other specified parts, and its proportion is relative to the whole cases

[b]Unknown differentiation in stages I–II cancer: USA, overall 15,330 (49%), resected 1385 (10%); the Netherlands, overall 3282 (58%), resected 491 (18%); Belgium, overall 1214 (35%), resected 344 (16%); Norway, overall 909 (59%), resected 100 (19%); Slovenia, overall 252 (38%), resected 35 (9%); Estonia, overall 134 (47%), resected 32 (20%)

[c]Pancreatectomy (NOS) and local resection

[d]Unknown differentiation in stages III–IV cancer: USA, overall 42,627 (77%), resected 475 (24%); the Netherlands, overall 11,579 (83%), resected 46 (19%); Belgium, overall 3163 (56%), resected 55 (19%); Norway, overall 3150 (68%), resected 26 (24%); Slovenia, overall 1555 (78%), resected 47 (35%); Estonia, overall 718 (86%), resected 5 (28%)

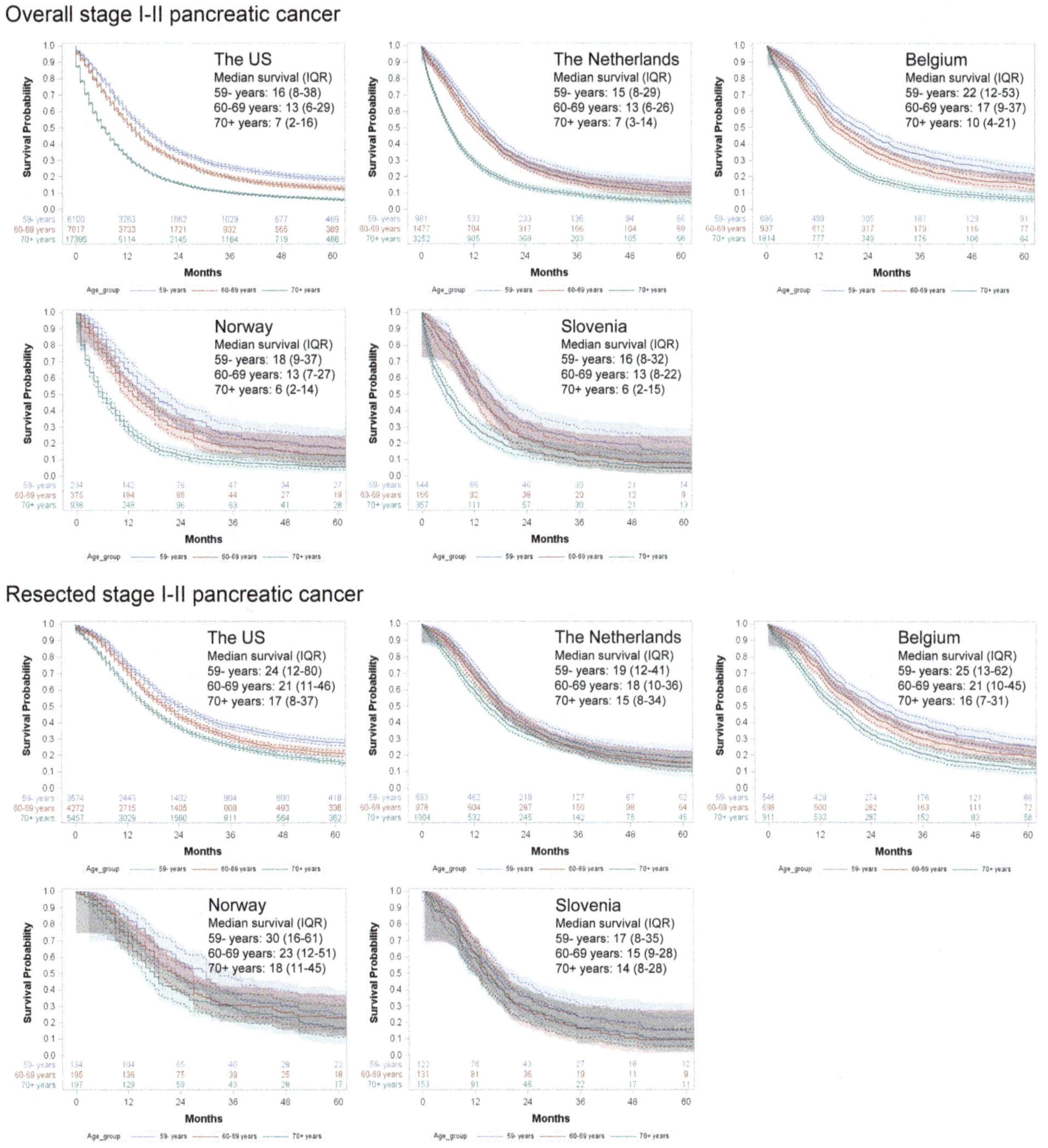

Fig. 1 Kaplan-Meier curves (*solid lines*) of age group-specific survival in overall (*upper panel*) and resected patients (*lower panel*) with TNM stages I-II pancreatic cancers. The *dashed lines* indicate the 95% confidence limits, and the *shadows* represent the Hall-Wellner confidence bands. Numbers of patients at risk are also reported. Median survival is in months. *IQR* interquartile range

overall population in all countries and all age groups (perioperative rates: < 70 years, 94–99%; ≥ 70 years, 81–96%; 3-year rates: < 70 years, 5–19%; ≥ 70 years, 2–14%). Differences between age groups were smaller in the resected subgroups than the overall patient population.

Survival in overall stages I-II and III-IV PaCs with microscopic confirmation

Considering the relatively high proportions of non-microscopically confirmed overall PaC patients, we conducted sensitivity analyses by limiting the patients with

Table 2 Unadjusted survival proportions in patients with overall and resected stages I–II pancreatic cancer

Time	USA		The Netherlands		Belgium		Norway		Slovenia	
	Overall	Resected	Overall	Resected	Overall	Resected	Overall	Resected	Overall	Resected
	OS (95% CI)[a]	OS (95% CI)	OS (95% CI)	OS (95% CI)	OS (95% CI)	OS (95% CI)	OS (95% CI)	OS (95% CI)	OS (95% CI)	OS (95% CI)
1 month										
< 60 years	95 (94–95)	98 (98–99)	97 (96–98)	98 (97–99)	98 (97–99)	99 (97–99)	98 (96–99)	100 (100–100)	97 (93–99)	98 (93–99)
60–69 years	92 (91–93)	97 (96–97)	95 (94–96)	97 (96–98)	97 (96–98)	98 (97–99)	97 (94–98)	99 (95–100)	96 (92–98)	99 (94–100)
≥ 70 years	79 (78–79)	94 (93–94)	88 (87–89)	96 (95–97)	93 (92–94)	96 (94–97)	89 (86–90)	99 (95–100)	85 (81–89)	99 (95–100)
3 months										
< 60 years	89 (88–90)	96 (95–97)	92 (90–94)	97 (95–98)	95 (93–96)	96 (94–98)	95 (92–97)	99 (95–100)	92 (86–95)	94 (88–97)
60–69 years	84 (84–85)	94 (93–95)	87 (85–89)	94 (93–96)	93 (91–94)	94 (92–96)	90 (86–93)	97 (93–99)	90 (84–94)	96 (91–98)
≥ 70 years	65 (64–66)	89 (88–90)	72 (70–73)	91 (89–92)	83 (81–84)	90 (88–92)	68 (65–71)	95 (91–98)	66 (61–71)	88 (82–92)
6 months										
< 60 years	80 (79–81)	91 (90–92)	81 (78–83)	92 (90–94)	90 (87–92)	93 (90–95)	86 (81–90)	96 (90–98)	88 (81–92)	89 (82–94)
60–69 years	73 (72–74)	88 (86–89)	76 (74–78)	89 (86–91)	86 (83–88)	89 (87–91)	77 (72–81)	91 (86–95)	78 (71–84)	85 (77–90)
≥ 70 years	51 (50–51)	80 (79–81)	53 (51–55)	81 (78–83)	67 (65–69)	80 (77–83)	50 (47–53)	88 (83–92)	50 (45–55)	82 (75–88)
12 months										
< 60 years	59 (57–60)	75 (73–76)	60 (56–63)	74 (70–77)	73 (70–76)	78 (75–82)	64 (57–70)	82 (75–88)	60 (52–68)	63 (54–71)
60–69 years	52 (51–53)	71 (69–72)	53 (50–55)	68 (65–71)	65 (62–68)	72 (68–75)	52 (47–57)	73 (66–79)	55 (48–63)	62 (53–70)
≥ 70 years	31 (31–32)	61 (59–62)	30 (29–32)	61 (57–64)	43 (40–45)	58 (55–62)	28 (25–31)	70 (63–76)	31 (26–36)	60 (51–67)
24 months										
< 60 years	35 (34–37)	50 (48–52)	30 (27–33)	40 (36–44)	47 (43–51)	53 (49–57)	38 (32–45)	58 (48–66)	33 (25–41)	36 (27–44)
60–69 years	29 (28–30)	44 (42–45)	28 (25–30)	38 (35–42)	38 (35–41)	45 (41–48)	29 (24–34)	48 (40–55)	23 (17–30)	28 (20–35)
≥ 70 years	16 (15–16)	37 (35–38)	14 (13–15)	33 (30–37)	21 (19–23)	33 (30–36)	13 (10–15)	38 (31–45)	16 (12–20)	30 (23–37)
36 months										
< 60 years	26 (24–27)	37 (36–39)	20 (18–23)	27 (24–31)	34 (30–37)	39 (35–43)	26 (20–32)	39 (30–48)	22 (16–29)	23 (16–31)
60–69 years	20 (19–21)	31 (29–32)	18 (16–20)	25 (22–28)	25 (22–28)	30 (27–34)	18 (14–23)	31 (24–38)	14 (9–19)	16 (11–23)
≥ 70 years	10 (10–11)	26 (24–27)	9 (8–11)	24 (21–27)	13 (11–14)	21 (19–24)	9 (7–11)	30 (23–37)	9 (7–13)	17 (11–23)
60 months										
< 60 years	19 (18–20)	28 (26–30)	14 (12–17)	19 (16–23)	23 (19–26)	26 (22–30)	17 (12–23)	25 (17–34)	15 (9–21)	15 (9–23)
60–69 years	13 (12–14)	21 (20–23)	11 (9–13)	16 (13–19)	16 (14–19)	20 (17–23)	13 (9–17)	23 (16–30)	8 (5–13)	10 (5–16)
≥ 70 years	6 (6–7)	16 (15–17)	5 (4–6)	13 (10–16)	7 (6–8)	12 (10–15)	6 (4–7)	17 (11–24)	5 (3–8)	10 (6–16)

OS overall survival, *CI* confidence interval

[a]Data are shown as survival proportion (95% confidence interval) [%]

overall stages I–II and III–IV cancer to those with microscopic confirmation (Table 3 and Additional file 1: Figure S2). Microscopically confirmed patients with stages I–II and III–IV cancer generally had higher survival especially in those ≥ 70 years old and within 24 months after diagnosis, in all participating countries except Belgium, where microscopic confirmation rates were high and where survival remained very similar. The 3-year survival rates remained mostly similar to those of the main analyses, and were 21–34% (< 60 years), 14–25% (60–69 years), and 12–14% (≥ 70 years) in stages I–II PaC, and 2–5% (< 60 years), 1–2% (60–69 years), and 1%–1% (≥ 70 years) in stages III–IV cancer.

Temporal survival trends in overall and resected PaCs by stage

Trends in 1-month to 5-year survival of patients diagnosed in 2003–2005, 2006–2008, and 2009–2011 are shown in Table 4 and Additional file 1: Figures S3–S7. Significant survival changes between 2003 and 2005 and 2009–2011 are detailed below.

Short-term survival

Significant increases in 1-month survival for overall PaC patients were observed in the USA and the Netherlands, with 3 and 3% units increase (UI) for stage I–II and 2 and 3 UI for stages III–IV tumors. In Slovenia, an increment by 6 UI in 1-month survival was observed among total stages III–IV cancer patients. For the subgroup of resected patients, a significant survival increase was only observed for stages I–II cancer patients in the USA (2 UI). Improvements in 3-month survival were generally larger and also significant among total patients in the USA and the Netherlands, with 4 and 6 UI in stages I–II and 3 and 3 UI in stages III–IV cancers, respectively. In Norway, an increment by 6 UI was observed in patients with stages I–II cancer. In Slovenia, a significant increasing trend by 8 UI persisted in stages III–IV cancers. Within the resected subgroup, significant increasing trends were observed in both stages I–II (2 UI) and III–IV cancer patients (7 UI) in the USA, and in patients with stages III–IV cancer (10 UI) in Slovenia.

Longer-term survival

While in all countries 1-year survival increased for patients with stages I–II PaC, increases were only significant in the USA (6 UI), the Netherlands (12 UI), and Norway (10 UI). For the subgroup of resected patients, again 1-year survival increased in all countries, but changes were only significant in the USA (5 UI) and Norway (11 UI). For overall stages III–IV patients, 1-year survival increased significantly in the USA (3 UI), the Netherlands (1 UI), Norway (2 UI), and Slovenia (6 UI). For resected stages III–IV PaC patients, significant increases were only observed in the USA (13 UI). Improvements in 3-year survival for total stages I–II PaC patients were generally smaller and significant in the USA (4 UI), the Netherlands (8 UI), and Norway (2 UI). For the subgroup of resected stages I–II patients, significant increases were observed in the USA (5 UI), the Netherlands (11 UI), and Belgium (5 UI). Changes in 3-year survival for stages III–IV PaC were minor and significant only in the USA (< 1 UI) and the Netherlands (< 1 UI). Significant changes for the subgroup of resected stages III–IV PaC patients were observed only in the USA (5 UI). Regarding 5-year survival, significant increases were observed only in patients with stages I–II cancers. Survival rates increased by 6 and 1 UI in the Netherlands and Norway, respectively, for overall patients, and by 8 UI in the Netherlands for the resected patients.

Discussion

This comprehensive, multinational, large-scale, population-based investigation provided overall survival estimates for overall patients and those with resected PaC by TNM stage and age. Furthermore, temporal trends for overall and resected cancer patients with clearly resectable (stages I–II) nd mostly unresectable (stages III–IV) PaCs in four European countries and the USA were shown respectively. In both stages I–II and III–IV tumors, survival rates decreased obviously with increasing age. Limited but encouraging progress in survival over time was detected.

According to EUROCARE-5 [4, 14], overall, the 1-, 3-, and 5-year survival rates of patients with PaC diagnosed during 1999–2007 in Europe were only 26%, 9%, and 7%, respectively. For the European countries investigated in this study, the 1-year survival was 19–34% and 5-year survival was 4–11%. In the USA, 5-year survival was 7–10% [16, 17]. Stage- and treatment-specific survival was not provided by the previous reports [4, 14]. Our study provided more up-to-date estimates by including patients diagnosed during 2003–2014 and further showed survival by TNM stage and age. Survival decreased with advancing stage and age. It is important to provide stratified survival for clinical counseling.

Guidelines [7–11] state that localized PaCs (stages I–II) are mostly resectable, while T4/stage III and M1/stage IV diseases are largely unresectable. Our results showed that resected patients with stages I–II PaCs had higher survival estimates in all age groups compared to the commonly reported and widely available overall ones. For example, resected patients < 60 years had 3–19%, 1–13%, and 1–9% units higher 1-, 3-, and 5-year survival than overall across countries, respectively. These differences may reflect effects of both resection and selection of fitter patients for resection. Given that most patients would perceive a general PaC prognosis as dismal and thus feel extremely

Table 3 Unadjusted survival proportions in overall microscopically confirmed stages I–II and III–IV pancreatic cancer patients

Time	USA		The Netherlands		Belgium		Norway		Slovenia	
	Stages I–II OS (95% CI)[a]	Stages III–IV OS (95% CI)	Stages I–II OS (95% CI)	Stages III–IV OS (95% CI)	Stages I–II OS (95% CI)	Stages III–IV OS (95% CI)	Stages I–II OS (95% CI)	Stages III–IV OS (95% CI)	Stages I–II OS (95% CI)	Stages III–IV OS (95% CI)
1 month										
≤ 60 years	96 (95–96)	77 (76–78)	98 (97–99)	87 (86–89)	98 (97–99)	93 (91–95)	99 (96–100)	92 (90–94)	98 (93–99)	87 (82–90)
60–69 years	93 (92–93)	72 (71–72)	96 (95–97)	83 (82–84)	97 (96–98)	89 (87–91)	97 (94–98)	87 (85–89)	97 (92–99)	82 (77–86)
≥ 70 years	84 (84–85)	60 (59–61)	92 (90–93)	74 (72–75)	93 (92–94)	81 (80–83)	96 (94–98)	80 (78–82)	94 (90–97)	67 (63–72)
3 months										
≤ 60 years	90 (90–91)	59 (58–60)	93 (91–94)	61 (59–63)	95 (93–96)	78 (75–80)	96 (93–98)	67 (63–70)	95 (90–98)	61 (55–67)
60–69 years	86 (85–87)	53 (53–54)	89 (87–91)	55 (53–57)	92 (91–94)	69 (67–71)	91 (88–94)	59 (56–62)	93 (88–96)	54 (48–59)
≥ 70 years	71 (71–72)	40 (39–40)	79 (77–81)	42 (41–44)	83 (81–84)	55 (53–56)	85 (82–88)	44 (42–47)	81 (75–86)	39 (35–44)
6 months										
≤ 60 years	81 (80–82)	41 (40–42)	83 (81–86)	36 (34–37)	90 (87–92)	59 (56–62)	88 (82–91)	43 (39–46)	92 (85–95)	44 (38–49)
60–69 years	74 (73–75)	35 (35–36)	79 (77–81)	32 (31–34)	86 (83–88)	50 (48–53)	79 (74–83)	37 (34–40)	82 (74–87)	40 (34–45)
≥ 70 years	57 (56–57)	24 (24–25)	63 (61–66)	22 (21–23)	67 (65–69)	34 (32–35)	67 (63–71)	22 (20–24)	70 (63–76)	19 (16–23)
12 months										
≤ 60 years	60 (58–61)	20 (20–21)	62 (59–65)	13 (12–15)	72 (69–76)	31 (28–34)	65 (58–71)	20 (17–23)	65 (56–72)	17 (13–22)
60–69 years	54 (52–55)	17 (17–18)	57 (54–59)	12 (11–13)	65 (62–68)	24 (22–26)	55 (49–60)	13 (11–15)	59 (50–66)	19 (15–24)
≥ 70 years	36 (35–36)	10 (10–11)	40 (38–42)	7 (7–8)	43 (40–45)	14 (13–15)	42 (37–46)	7 (6–9)	49 (42–56)	7 (5–10)
24 months										
≤ 60 years	36 (34–37)	7 (6–7)	31 (28–34)	4 (4–5)	47 (43–51)	10 (9–12)	39 (32–46)	7 (5–9)	35 (27–43)	6 (3–9)
60–69 years	30 (29–31)	5 (5–6)	30 (27–33)	3 (2–3)	38 (35–41)	6 (4–7)	30 (25–35)	3 (2–4)	24 (18–31)	4 (2–6)
≥ 70 years	18 (17–19)	3 (3–3)	20 (18–22)	2 (1–2)	21 (19–22)	3 (3–4)	19 (16–23)	2 (1–3)	25 (19–31)	2 (1–4)
36 months										
≤ 60 years	26 (24–27)	3 (3–4)	21 (18–24)	2 (2–3)	34 (30–37)	5 (4–7)	25 (19–32)	4 (2–6)	23 (16–30)	2 (1–4)
60–69 years	20 (19–21)	2 (2–3)	19 (17–22)	1 (1–2)	25 (22–28)	2 (1–3)	19 (14–24)	1 (< 1–2)	14 (9–20)	2 (1–3)
≥ 70 years	12 (11–12)	1 (1–2)	14 (12–16)	1 (< 1–1)	13 (11–14)	1 (1–2)	13 (10–17)	1 (< 1–1)	14 (9–19)	1 (< 1–2)
60 months										
≤ 60 years	19 (18–20)	2 (1–2)	14 (12–17)	1 (1–1)	23 (19–26)	2 (1–3)	16 (11–22)	1 (< 1–2)	15 (9–23)	2 (1–4)
60–69 years	13 (12–14)	1 (1–1)	12 (10–14)	< 1 (< 1–1)	16 (14–19)	1 (< 1–1)	13 (9–18)	< 1 (< 1–1)	8 (4–14)	1 (< 1–3)
≥ 70 years	7 (7–8)	1 (< 1–1)	7 (6–9)	< 1 (< 1–1)	7 (6–8)	1 (< 1–1)	8 (5–11)	< 1 (< 1–1)	8 (5–13)	< 1 (< 1–1)

OS overall survival, *CI* confidence interval
[a]Data are shown as survival proportion (95% confidence interval) [5]

Table 4 Unadjusted survival rates in overall and resected pancreatic cancer patients diagnosed in 2003–2005, 2006–2008, and 2009–2011

Survival	Period	Stage	USA		The Netherlands		Belgium		Norway		Slovenia	
			Overall	Resected	Overall	Resected	Overall	Resected	Overall	Resected	Overall	Resected
			OS (95% CI)[a]	OS (95% CI)	OS (95% CI)	OS (95% CI)	OS (95% CI)	OS (95% CI)	OS (95% CI)	OS (95% CI)	OS (95% CI)	OS (95% CI)
1 month	2003–2005	I–II	83 (82–84)	95 (94–96)	89 (87–91)	96 (93–97)	94 (92–96)	97 (94–98)	91 (88–94)	99 (94–100)	89 (84–93)	96 (90–98)
		III–IV	61 (60–62)	86 (82–89)	73 (71–75)	88 (74–95)	88 (85–90)	96 (86–99)	78 (75–80)	100 (100–100)	69 (65–74)	92 (71–98)
	2006–2008	I–II	84 (84–85)	96 (95–96)	92 (91–94)	97 (95–98)	95 (94–97)	97 (95–98)	90 (83–96)	99 (93–100)	93 (88–96)	99 (93–100)
		III–IV	62 (61–63)	89 (86–91)	77 (75–78)	100 (100–100)	86 (85–88)	98 (91–99)	79 (76–81)	96 (75–99)	75 (71–78)	97 (80–100)
	2009–2011	I–II	86 (85–87)	96 (96–97)	92 (90–93)	97 (96–98)	96 (95–97)	98 (97–99)	94 (91–96)	98 (95–99)	90 (85–94)	99 (94–100)
		III–IV	63 (62–64)	90 (88–92)	76 (75–78)	91 (81–96)	85 (84–87)	100 (100–100)	78 (75–80)	96 (77–100)	75 (72–79)	98 (86–100)
	Percent unit change,[b] P	I–II	**+ 3, 0.006**	**+ 2, 0.004**	**+ 3, 0.021**	+ 1, 0.257	+ 2, 0.116	+ 1, 0.577	+ 3, 0.175	–1, 0.473	+ 1, 0.851	+ 4, 0.083
		III–IV	**+ 2, 0.002**	+ 4, 0.989	**+ 3, 0.001**	+ 3, 0.635	–2, 0.086	+4, 0.189	+ < 1, 0.972	–4, 0.301	**+ 6, 0.024**	+ 6, 0.229
3 months	2003–2005	I–II	72 (71–73)	91 (90–92)	74 (71–76)	92 (89–94)	86 (83–89)	93 (90–96)	76 (71–80)	98 (93–99)	76 (69–82)	87 (79–92)
		III–IV	42 (41–43)	74 (69–78)	42 (40–43)	84 (69–92)	66 (62–69)	93 (82–97)	44 (41–47)	87 (68–95)	36 (31–40)	58 (36–75)
	2006–2008	I–II	73 (72–74)	92 (91–92)	78 (76–81)	93 (91–95)	87 (85–89)	92 (90–94)	72 (67–76)	94 (86–97)	80 (73–86)	92 (85–96)
		III–IV	44 (43–44)	79 (76–82)	46 (44–47)	98 (88–100)	63 (61–65)	85 (95–91)	48 (46–51)	84 (63–94)	43 (39–47)	85 (67–93)
	2009–2011	I–II	76 (75–77)	93 (92–94)	80 (78–82)	93 (91–95)	89 (87–91)	94 (92–96)	82 (78–85)	96 (92–98)	76 (70–82)	97 (91–99)
		III–IV	45 (44–46)	81 (78–84)	45 (43–46)	85 (74–92)	63 (60–65)	93 (85–96)	47 (44–49)	86 (66–94)	44 (40–48)	76 (61–86)
	Percent unit change,[b] P	I–II	**+ 4, < 0.001**	**+ 2, < 0.001**	**+ 6, 0.001**	+ 1, 0.546	+ 3, 0.118	+ 1, 0.508	**+ 6, 0.035**	– 1, 0.562	+ < 1, 0.909	**+ 10, 0.005**
		III–IV	**+ 3, < 0.001**	**+ 7, 0.017**	**+ 3, 0.001**	+ 1, 0.831	–3, 0.087	– < 1, 0.972	+ 3, 0.225	–1, 0.890	**+ 8, 0.007**	+ 18, 0.085
12 months	2003–2005	I–II	38 (36–39)	64 (62–66)	33 (30–36)	64 (59–68)	52 (48–57)	62 (56–67)	34 (29–39)	66 (57–74)	38 (30–45)	51 (41–60)
		III–IV	11 (11–12)	34 (29–39)	8 (7–9)	49 (33–63)	19 (17–22)	45 (31–57)	8 (6–10)	37 (20–53)	5 (3–8)	13 (3–29)
	2006–2008	I–II	40 (39–41)	65 (64–67)	36 (33–38)	64 (60–68)	56 (53–60)	69 (65–73)	33 (29–38)	71 (60–79)	51 (43–59)	67 (57–76)
		III–IV	12 (12–13)	35 (31–39)	8 (7–9)	53 (38–64)	19 (17–21)	47 (36–57)	11 (10–13)	56 (35–73)	12 (10–15)	39 (23–55)
	2009–2011	I–II	44 (43–45)	70 (68–71)	45 (43–48)	69 (65–72)	55 (52–57)	68 (65–71)	44 (39–49)	77 (70–83)	42 (35–48)	60 (50–68)
		III–IV	14 (14–15)	47 (42–51)	9 (8–10)	41 (29–52)	20 (18–22)	53 (42–62)	10 (8–11)	46 (28–63)	11 (9–14)	17 (8–30)
	Percent unit change,[b] P	I–II	**+ 6, < 0.001**	**+ 5, < 0.001**	**+ 12, < 0.001**	+ 5, 0.066	+ 3, 0.297	+ 6, 0.057	**+ 10, 0.003**	**+ 11, 0.025**	+ 4, 0.577	+ 9, 0.101
		III–IV	**+ 3, < 0.001**	**+ 13, < 0.001**	**+ 1, 0.001**	–8, 0.496	+ 1, 0.476	+ 8, 0.548	**+ 2, 0.027**	+ 10, 0.689	**+ 6, < 0.001**	+ 5, 0.238
Survival	Period	Stage	USA		The Netherlands		Belgium		Norway		Slovenia	
			Overall	Resected	Overall	Resected	Overall	Resected	Overall	Resected	Overall	Resected
			OS (95% CI)[1]	OS (95% CI)	OS (95% CI)	OS (95% CI)	OS (95% CI)	OS (95% CI)	OS (95% CI)	OS (95% CI)	OS (95% CI)	OS (95% CI)
36 months	2003–2005	I–II	13 (13–14)	27 (25–29)	8 (7–10)	18 (14–22)	17 (14–21)	24 (19–29)	12 (9–16)	28 (20–36)	9 (6–14)	11 (6–17)
		III–IV	2 (2–2)	7 (5–10)	1 (1–2)	14 (6–26)	2 (2–4)	8 (2–16)	1 (1–2)	10 (3–24)	1 (< 1–2)	NA
	2006–2008	I–II	14 (14–15)	29 (27–30)	12 (10–13)	24 (20–28)	21 (18–23)	28 (25–32)	10 (7–14)	32 (22–41)	19 (14–26)	27 (19–37)
		III–IV	2 (2–2)	9 (7–11)	1 (1–1)	11 (5–21)	2 (2–3)	7 (3–14)	2 (1–2)	24 (10–42)	2 (1–3)	12 (4–26)

Table 4 Unadjusted survival rates in overall and resected pancreatic cancer patients diagnosed in 2003–2005, 2006–2008, and 2009–2011 *(Continued)*

Survival	Period	Stage	USA		The Netherlands		Belgium		Norway		Slovenia	
			Overall	Resected	Overall	Resected	Overall	Resected	Overall	Resected	Overall	Resected
			OS (95% CI)[a]	OS (95% CI)	OS (95% CI)	OS (95% CI)	OS (95% CI)	OS (95% CI)	OS (95% CI)	OS (95% CI)	OS (95% CI)	OS (95% CI)
	2009–2011	I–II	17 (16–18)	33 (31–34)	16 (15–18)	29 (26–32)	20 (18–22)	30 (26–33)	15 (12–18)	30 (23–37)	12 (8–16)	17 (11–24)
		III–IV	2 (2–2)	11 (9–14)	1 (1–1)	12 (6–21)	2 (1–3)	10 (5–16)	1 (1–2)	14 (5–30)	1 (< 1–1)	NA
	Percent unit change,[b] P	I–II	**+4, < 0.001**	**+ 5, < 0.001**	**+ 8, < 0.001**	**+ 11, < 0.001**	+ 3, 0.076	**+ 5, 0.035**	**+ 2, 0.025**	+ 2, 0.205	+ 2, 0.468	+ 6, 0.069
		III–IV	**+ < 1, < 0.001**	**+ 5, < 0.001**	**+ < 1, 0.005**	−2, 0.886	−1, 0.285	+ 2, 0.317	− < 1, 0.062	+4, 0.785	**+ < 1, 0.002**	NA, NA
60 months	2003–2005	I–II	9 (8–10)	18 (17–20)	4 (3–5)	10 (7–13)	11 (8–14)	16 (12–21)	9 (6–12)	18 (12–25)	7 (3–11)	9 (5–15)
		III–IV	1 (1–1)	4 (2–5)	1 (< 1–1)	9 (3–20)	1 (< 1–2)	4 (1–11)	1 (< 1–1)	3 (< 1–15)	< 1 (< 1–1)	NA
	2006–2008	I–II	10 (9–11)	20 (19–21)	7 (6–9)	15 (12–19)	13 (11–15)	18 (15–21)	7 (4–9)	20 (12–28)	9 (5–14)	13 (7–21)
		III–IV	1 (1–1)	6 (5–9)	< 1 (< 1–1)	6 (2–14)	1 (1–2)	5 (2–11)	1 (< 1–1)	4 (< 1–17)	2 (1–3)	12 (4–26)
	2009–2011	I–II	NA	NA	10 (8–12)	18 (15–21)	12 (10–14)	18 (15–21)	10 (7–13)	20 (14–27)	8 (5–12)	11 (6–17)
		III–IV	NA	NA	1 (< 1–1)	12 (6–21)	1 (< 1–1)	2 (< 1–7)	< 1 (< 1–1)	NA	< 1 (< 1–1)	NA
	Percent unit change,[b] P	I–II	NA, NA	NA, NA	**+ 6, < 0.001**	**+ 8, < 0.001**	+ 1, 0.109	+ 2, 0.090	**+ 1, 0.043**	+ 2, 0.262	+ 2, 0.469	+ 2, 0.113
		III–IV	NA, NA	NA, NA	**+ < 1, 0.004**	+ 3, 0.935	−< 1, 0.290	−2, 0.409	- < 1, 0.069	NA, NA	**+ < 1, 0.002**	NA, NA

OS overall survival, *NA* not available as follow-up was not long enough
[a]Data are shown as survival rate (95% confidence interval) [%]
[b]Percent changes are shown by comparing average survival of patients diagnosed in 2009–2011 to those in 2003–2005. Significant changes according to *P* values calculated using the log-rank test are highlighted in bold

distressed, also generating great burdens to their caregivers, it would be important to show them the objective survival data, especially for the resected patients, potentially rebuilding hope of life.

Survival in patients with stages III–IV PaCs, the majority of the diagnosed cases, was much poorer than that in those with stages I–II tumors, especially in the long term. In locally advanced PaC, the average overall survival remains < 1 year [18], and in metastatic tumors, the median survival is < 6 months [19], with 5-year survival of only ~ 2% [5]. We showed that even for those < 60 years, the overall 3- and 5-year survival was as low as 2–5% and 1–4%, respectively. Most patients with stages III–IV PaCs are deemed unresectable [9, 11]. This may, however, improve in the years to come with the increasing use of FOLFIRINOX [20]. In many of the cases where patients with metastatic PaC underwent resection, the metastasis was unexpectedly detected only during surgery [21]. Although resection rates in advanced tumors were low, notably, in stages III–IV PaCs substantially higher survival was observed for resected compared to total patients in all age groups, and resected patients < 70 years could have a 3-year survival of 5–34%. Even in those ≥ 70 years old, higher survival estimates for the resected subgroup were observed (1-year, 16–42% vs. 5–14%; 3-year, 2–14% vs. 1%–1%). While this difference might again at least partly reflect patient selection, i.e., inclusion of healthier patients or those with more favorable tumor characteristics for resection, our results indicated that not all patients with stages III–IV PaC had such a dismal prognosis as suggested by the overall survival estimates. These strong differences again underline the importance of reporting respective outcomes for stratified resected patients for enhanced counseling of these patients.

The perioperative survival is noteworthy, especially for elderly patients. It is volume-dependent, and is mainly influenced by failure to rescue and surgical expertise [22]. While resection could be safely performed for some proportion of the typically more vulnerable elderly patients [23, 24], at the population level, we found that in stages III–IV PaCs, which are associated with poorer general status, the 1-month survival dropped from 94–99% for patients < 70 years to 81–96% for those ≥ 70 years, which was more dramatic compared to results for the stages I–II disease. Age was negatively associated with survival, necessitating it as a stratification factor when providing survival information. Increasing ages are associated with more frequent comorbidities and complications, decreasing the potential survival benefits of resection. However, some studies suggested that, compared to younger individuals, fit elderly patients might obtain similar survival benefits from resection [23, 24]. The better survival observed for the younger patients might be partly explained by the more aggressive therapeutic strategies applied, which might contribute to survival improvements in the fit elderly as well [4]. These possibilities highlight the importance of geriatric assessment before treatment.

No substantial survival changes (5-year, 5–6%) were reported in PaC in the EUROCARE-5 study [4] over the period 1999–2007. In the USA, 5-year survival improved from 6 to 8% between 1992 and 1996 and 2002–2006 [25] and from 8 to 12% between 2002 and 2004 and 2008–2010 [16]; especially for localized tumors, strong improvement in 5-year survival by 7% units from 1998 to 2003 was observed [17]. We observed modest but nevertheless encouraging improvements in survival in patients both with stages I–II and III–IV tumors from 2003 to 2005 to 2009–2011, which potentially reflects the advancement in surgical skill, technique, and perioperative care. In the USA, 3-year survival increased by 4% units in stages I–II PaCs overall, but only by < 1% units in stages III–IV cancers. For resected cancers, survival increased by 5% units among patients with stages I–II cancer. In Europe, 3-year survival for both overall and resected patients with stages I–II PaC increased in all investigated countries, and a large increment was observed in the Netherlands (overall, 8% units; resected, 11% units), where postoperative mortality is decreasing [26]. Notably, centralization agreements were implemented in the Netherlands since 2005, and promoted more resections [27], which might be associated with the continuous improvement in survival [28]. While further major survival advancement in resected patients could be limited even with surgical technique modification, improved outcomes are likely to come from more effective systemic treatments (e.g., FOLFIRINOX) combined with surgery. The different trends between overall and resected patients further highlight the need to offer survival data in specific subgroups.

This study covered the periods when the sixth and seventh TNM staging systems were in effect, and both are compatible/identical with each other [8]. While potentially improved imaging might result in a shift in stage classification, the proportions of each stage remained relatively stable in investigated countries (data not shown). In the era of the eighth TNM staging, where the definitions of the T4 and M1 categories indicating mostly unresectable cancers remain unchanged [29], our results would still be usable for prognosis counseling.

This study was limited by the small case numbers in some subgroups. Further potentially prognostically important factors (e.g., comorbidity) were not considered because they were unknown/unavailable in the national registries of most countries. Although older ages and more advanced tumor stages herein investigated were the most prominent negative prognostic factors and might contraindicate resection, precise and personalized factors should be considered for evaluation of an individual patient's prognosis. Some prognostic tools (e.g., the nomogram) might offer more precise prognostic information for a specific patient. Non-surgical treatment was not incorporated considering the low sensitivity in recording in some registries and the varying regimens used. Information from more countries would increase the comprehensiveness of the report. However, treatment or TNM staging data were mostly not readily available in the other national population-based registries. Our study was based on complete-case analysis. Differences in data recording, especially of TNM stage, should be noted, and the stages I–II cancer proportion varied from 25% in Norway and Slovenia to 38% in Belgium. There could be underreporting, especially of advanced-stage disease, with various extents, besides the potential impact of missing staging information. These differences highlight the need for standardization in the registration practice. Potential variation in registration practice, especially for stage, might affect outcomes, and inter-country comparisons were not made considering the possible heterogeneity. Results were only analyzed and interpreted independently in the respective country without pooling or comparison with other countries. Results from a specific national registry might not be generalizable to another country. For counseling of patients not in the studied countries, other aspects including treatment profiles and health care systems should be considered.

In the main analyses, we included PaC cases irrespective of microscopic confirmation, which is in accordance with the real-world situation [15] and which is also consistent with the approach in the EUROCARE studies [4, 14]. While resected cases were mostly microscopically confirmed, the confirmation rates for overall cases varied. The microscopic confirmation rates for PaC have been relatively low [4], and PaC has always been difficult to verify microscopically, especially unresectable PaC. In our complete-case study inclusion of patients with known stage might have an impact on the observed confirmation rates. After limiting the overall cases to the microscopically confirmed ones in sensitivity analyses, the survival estimates mostly became higher in all participating countries except in Belgium, where microscopic confirmation rates were high. Furthermore, the survival increase was the most prominent in patients ≥ 70 years old, who are generally more frail and for whom the selection of treatment is usually more cautious. While including microscopically confirmed cases only could help to further increase the chance of selecting real PaC patients, those not receiving any treatment and usually having poorer patient and/or tumor characteristics might be more likely excluded, potentially partly explaining the higher observed survival estimates in the sensitivity analyses.

We showed that it is important to provide survival estimates separately to resected patients for counseling, as the resected subgroup has substantially higher survival than the overall estimation. We did not show the results for unresected PaC patients and avoided direct comparisons between the resected and the unresected, as they may to a large extent reflect selection effects related to factors including patients' health status and hospital characteristics. In the resected subgroup, curative and palliative resections were not differentiated from each other, considering the greatly geographically and temporally varying standards for defining clear resection margins in PaC surgery.

Nevertheless, the multinational, population-based, large-scale character of this study with the country-specific respective analysis adds important novel survival data to the literature. In particular, results stratified by TNM stage and age for resected and overall patients will further aid patient counseling in clinical practice, providing more specific survival information for specific patient populations.

Conclusions

Our international population-based study provides comprehensive data on survival expectations of resected PaC patients which are substantially higher than the widely available and known dismal survival prognosis for total patients. The benefits of resection cannot be concluded from this observational study. However, the TNM stage- and age-stratified survival results might be helpful for clinical counseling. Estimated survival for advanced-stage disease should be interpreted with caution due to potential underreporting. Patients with advanced stage and/or old age should undergo careful assessment. Limited but encouraging survival improvement is observed.

Additional file

Additional file 1: Table S1. Selection of contacted national population-based cancer registries in Europe. **Table S2.** General information on participating population-based registries. **Table S3.** Inclusion codes according to International Classification of Diseases for Oncology, Third Edition. **Table S4.** Unadjusted survival proportions in patients with overall and resected stages III–IV PaC. **Figure S1.** Kaplan-Meier curves (*solid lines*) of age group-specific survival in overall (*upper panel*) and resected patients (*lower panel*) with TNM stages III–IV pancreatic cancers. The *dashed lines* indicate the 95% confidence limits, and the *shadows* represent the Hall-Wellner confidence bands. Numbers of patients at risk are also reported. Median survival is in months. *IQR* interquartile range. **Figure S2.** Kaplan-Meier curves (*solid lines*) of age group-specific survival in microscopically confirmed overall TNM stages I–II (*upper panel*) and stages III–IV pancreatic cancer patients (*lower panel*). The *dashed lines* indicate the 95% confidence limits, and the *shadows* represent the Hall-Wellner confidence bands. Numbers of patients at risk are also reported. Median survival is in months. *IQR* interquartile range. **Figure S3.** Changes in 1-month survival over calendar periods among overall and resected patients with stages I–II and III–IV pancreatic cancers. **Figure S4.** Changes in 3-month survival over calendar periods among overall and resected patients with stages I–II and III–IV pancreatic cancers. **Figure S5.** Changes in 12-month survival over calendar periods among overall and resected patients with stages I–II and III–IV pancreatic cancers. **Figure S6.** Changes in 36-month survival over calendar periods among overall and resected patients with stages I–II and III–IV pancreatic cancers. **Figure S7.** Changes in 60-month survival over calendar periods among overall and resected patients with stages I–II and III–IV pancreatic cancers. **Supplementary Results.** Patient characteristics. (DOCX 3259 kb)

Abbreviations

AJCC: American Joint Committee on Cancer; NCCN: National Comprehensive Cancer Network; PaC: Pancreatic cancer; SEER: Surveillance, Epidemiology, and End Results; UICC: Union for International Cancer Control

Acknowledgements

We are very grateful to the staff in Surveillance, Epidemiology, and End Results (SEER) Program, the Netherlands Cancer Registry (NCR), the Belgian Cancer Registry (BCR), the Cancer Registry of Norway (CRN), and the Cancer Registry of Slovenia (CRS) for their kind work in data collection and delivery. We would like to thank Dr. Dianne Pulte very much for her kind assistance with the English language.

Funding

This study was partly supported by the German Cancer Aid (Deutsche Krebshilfe, #111365). The funder played no role in study design; in collection, analysis, or interpretation of data; in writing of the paper; or in the decision to submit the paper for publication.

Authors' contributions

LH, LJ, YB, PSK, and HB conceived or designed the study. LH, LJ, YB, MB, LvdG, VL, LVE, HDS, TJ, MPŽ, VZ, MGB, PSK, and HB acquired, analyzed, or interpreted the data. LH drafted the manuscript. LJ, YB, MB, LvdG, VL, LVE, HDS, TJ, MPŽ, VZ, MGB, PSK, and HB critically revised the manuscript for important intellectual content. LH and YB performed the statistical analysis. LJ and HB provided supervision. All authors have approved the manuscript for publication.

Competing interests

The authors declare that they have no competing interests.

Author details

[1]Division of Clinical Epidemiology and Aging Research, German Cancer Research Center (DKFZ), Im Neuenheimer Feld 581, 69120 Heidelberg, Germany. [2]Medical Faculty Heidelberg, Heidelberg University, Heidelberg, Germany. [3]German Cancer Consortium (DKTK), German Cancer Research Center (DKFZ), Heidelberg, Germany. [4]Division of Preventive Oncology, DKFZ and National Center for Tumor Diseases (NCT), Heidelberg, Germany. [5]The Netherlands Cancer Registry, The Netherlands Comprehensive Cancer Organization (IKNL), Utrecht, the Netherlands. [6]Belgian Cancer Registry (BCR), Brussels, Belgium. [7]Cancer Registry of Norway (CRN), Oslo, Norway. [8]Cancer Registry of Slovenia (CRS), Ljubljana, Slovenia. [9]Dutch Pancreatic Cancer Group, Amsterdam UMC, University of Amsterdam, Amsterdam, the Netherlands.

References

1. Torre LA, Bray F, Siegel RL, Ferlay J, Lortet-Tieulent J, Jemal A. Global cancer statistics, 2012. CA Cancer J Clin. 2015;65(2):87–108.
2. Malvezzi M, Carioli G, Bertuccio P, Rosso T, Boffetta P, Levi F, La Vecchia C, Negri E. European cancer mortality predictions for the year 2016 with focus on leukaemias. Ann Oncol. 2016;27(4):725–31.
3. Ferlay J, Partensky C, Bray F. More deaths from pancreatic cancer than breast cancer in the EU by 2017. Acta Oncol. 2016;55(9–10):1158–60.
4. Lepage C, Capocaccia R, Hackl M, Lemmens V, Molina E, Pierannunzio D, Sant M, Trama A, Faivre J, Grouph E-W. Survival in patients with primary liver cancer, gallbladder and extrahepatic biliary tract cancer and pancreatic cancer in Europe 1999–2007: results of EUROCARE-5. Eur J Cancer. 2015; 51(15):2169–78.
5. Wolfgang CL, Herman JM, Laheru DA, Klein AP, Erdek MA, Fishman EK, Hruban RH. Recent progress in pancreatic cancer. CA Cancer J Clin. 2013; 63(5):318–48.
6. Ryan DP, Hong TS, Bardeesy N. Pancreatic adenocarcinoma. N Engl J Med. 2014;371(22):2140–1.
7. Tempero MA, Malafa MP, Behrman SW, Benson AB 3rd, Casper ES, Chiorean EG, Chung V, Cohen SJ, Czito B, Engebretson A, et al. Pancreatic adenocarcinoma, version 2.2014: featured updates to the NCCN guidelines. J Natl Compr Cancer Netw. 2014;12(8):1083–93.
8. Ducreux M, Cuhna AS, Caramella C, Hollebecque A, Burtin P, Goere D, Seufferlein T, Haustermans K, Van Laethem JL, Conroy T, et al. Cancer of the pancreas: ESMO Clinical Practice Guidelines for diagnosis, treatment and follow-up. Ann Oncol. 2015;26(Suppl 5):v56–68.
9. Sohal DP, Mangu PB, Khorana AA, Shah MA, Philip PA, O'Reilly EM, Uronis HE, Ramanathan RK, Crane CH, Engebretson A, et al. Metastatic pancreatic cancer: American Society of Clinical Oncology Clinical Practice Guideline. J Clin Oncol. 2016;34(23):2784–96.
10. Khorana AA, Mangu PB, Berlin J, Engebretson A, Hong TS, Maitra A, Mohile SG, Mumber M, Schulick R, Shapiro M, et al. Potentially curable pancreatic Cancer: American Society of Clinical Oncology Clinical Practice Guideline. J Clin Oncol. 2016;34(21):2541–56.
11. Balaban EP, Mangu PB, Khorana AA, Shah MA, Mukherjee S, Crane CH, Javle MM, Eads JR, Allen P, Ko AH, et al. Locally advanced, unresectable pancreatic cancer: American Society of Clinical Oncology Clinical Practice Guideline. J Clin Oncol. 2016;34(22):2654–68.
12. Evans DB, George B, Tsai S. Non-metastatic pancreatic cancer: resectable, borderline resectable, and locally advanced-definitions of increasing importance for the optimal delivery of multimodality therapy. Ann Surg Oncol. 2015;22(11):3409–13.
13. Huang L, Jansen L, Balavarca Y, Molina-Montes E, Babaei M, van der Geest L, Lemmens V, Van Eycken L, De Schutter H, Johannesen TB et al.: Resection of pancreatic cancer in Europe and USA: an international large-scale study highlighting large variations. Gut 2017. https://doi.org/10.1136/gutjnl-2017-314828. https://www.ncbi.nlm.nih.gov/pubmed/29158237. Accessed 10 Jan 2018.
14. De Angelis R, Sant M, Coleman MP, Francisci S, Baili P, Pierannunzio D, Trama A, Visser O, Brenner H, Ardanaz E, et al. Cancer survival in Europe 1999-2007 by country and age: results of EUROCARE--5-a population-based study. Lancet Oncol. 2014;15(1):23–34.
15. Asbun HJ, Conlon K, Fernandez-Cruz L, Friess H, Shrikhande SV, Adham M, Bassi C, Bockhorn M, Buchler M, Charnley RM, et al. When to perform a pancreatoduodenectomy in the absence of positive histology? A consensus statement by the International Study Group of Pancreatic Surgery. Surgery. 2014;155(5):887–92.
16. Sirri E, Castro FA, Kieschke J, Jansen L, Emrich K, Gondos A, Holleczek B, Katalinic A, Urbschat I, Vohmann C, et al. Recent trends in survival of patients with pancreatic Cancer in Germany and the United States. Pancreas. 2016;45(6):908–14.
17. Brenner H, Gondos A, Arndt V. Recent major progress in long-term cancer patient survival disclosed by modeled period analysis. J Clin Oncol. 2007; 25(22):3274–80.
18. Loehrer PJ Sr, Feng Y, Cardenes H, Wagner L, Brell JM, Cella D, Flynn P, Ramanathan RK, Crane CH, Alberts SR, et al. Gemcitabine alone versus gemcitabine plus radiotherapy in patients with locally advanced pancreatic cancer: an Eastern Cooperative Oncology Group trial. J Clin Oncol. 2011; 29(31):4105–12.
19. Hammel P, Huguet F, van Laethem JL, Goldstein D, Glimelius B, Artru P, Borbath I, Bouche O, Shannon J, Andre T, et al. Effect of chemoradiotherapy vs chemotherapy on survival in patients with locally advanced pancreatic cancer controlled after 4 months of gemcitabine with or without erlotinib: the LAP07 randomized clinical trial. JAMA. 2016;315(17):1844–53.
20. Suker M, Beumer BR, Sadot E, Marthey L, Faris JE, Mellon EA, El-Rayes BF, Wang-Gillam A, Lacy J, Hosein PJ, et al. FOLFIRINOX for locally advanced pancreatic cancer: a systematic review and patient-level meta-analysis. Lancet Oncol. 2016;17(6):801–10.
21. Kim Y, Kim SC, Song KB, Kim J, Kang DR, Lee JH, Park KM, Lee YJ. Improved survival after palliative resection of unsuspected stage IV pancreatic ductal adenocarcinoma. HPB (Oxford). 2016;18(4):325–31.
22. Krautz C, Nimptsch U, Weber GF, Mansky T, Grutzmann R. Effect of hospital volume on in-hospital morbidity and mortality following pancreatic surgery in Germany. Ann Surg. 2018;267(3):411–7.
23. van der Geest LG, Besselink MG, van Gestel YR, Busch OR, de Hingh IH, de Jong KP, Molenaar IQ, Lemmens VE. Pancreatic cancer surgery in elderly patients: balancing between short-term harm and long-term benefit. A population-based study in the Netherlands. Acta Oncol. 2016;55(3):278–85.
24. Barbas AS, Turley RS, Ceppa EP, Reddy SK, Blazer DG 3rd, Clary BM, Pappas TN, Tyler DS, White RR, Lagoo SA. Comparison of outcomes and the use of multimodality therapy in young and elderly people undergoing surgical resection of pancreatic cancer. J Am Geriatr Soc. 2012;60(2):344–50.

25. Pulte D, Redaniel MT, Brenner H, Jeffreys M. Changes in survival by ethnicity of patients with cancer between 1992-1996 and 2002-2006: is the discrepancy decreasing? Ann Oncol. 2012;23(9):2428–34.
26. de Wilde RF, Besselink MG, van der Tweel I, de Hingh IH, van Eijck CH, Dejong CH, Porte RJ, Gouma DJ, Busch OR, Molenaar IQ, et al. Impact of nationwide centralization of pancreaticoduodenectomy on hospital mortality. Br J Surg. 2012;99(3):404–10.
27. Lemmens VE, Bosscha K, van der Schelling G, Brenninkmeijer S, Coebergh JW, de Hingh IH. Improving outcome for patients with pancreatic cancer through centralization. Br J Surg. 2011;98(10):1455–62.
28. van der Geest LG, van Rijssen LB, Molenaar IQ, de Hingh IH, Groot Koerkamp B, Busch OR, Lemmens VE, Besselink MG. Volume-outcome relationships in pancreatoduodenectomy for cancer. HPB (Oxford). 2016; 18(4):317–24.
29. Shi S, Hua J, Liang C, Meng Q, Liang D, Xu J, Ni Q, Yu X. Proposed modification of the 8th edition of the AJCC staging system for pancreatic ductal adenocarcinoma. Ann Surg. 2018; https://doi.org/10.1097/SLA.0000000000002668.

8

Modelling population-level impact to inform target product profiles for childhood malaria vaccines

Alexandra B. Hogan[1*], Peter Winskill[1], Robert Verity[1], Jamie T. Griffin[1,2] and Azra C. Ghani[1]

Abstract

Background: The RTS,S/AS01 vaccine for *Plasmodium falciparum* malaria demonstrated moderate efficacy in 5–17-month-old children in phase 3 trials, and from 2018, the vaccine will be evaluated through a large-scale pilot implementation program. Work is ongoing to optimise this vaccine, with higher efficacy for a different schedule demonstrated in a phase 2a challenge study. The objective of our study was to investigate the population-level impact of a modified RTS,S/AS01 schedule and dose amount in order to inform the target product profile for a second-generation malaria vaccine.

Methods: We used a mathematical modelling approach as the basis for our study. We simulated the changing anti-circumsporozoite antibody titre following vaccination and related the titre to vaccine efficacy. We then implemented this efficacy profile within an individual-based model of malaria transmission. We compared initial efficacy, duration and dose timing, and evaluated the potential public health impact of a modified vaccine in children aged 5–17 months, measuring clinical cases averted in children younger than 5 years.

Results: In the first decade of delivery, initial efficacy was associated with a higher reduction in childhood clinical cases compared to vaccine duration. This effect was more pronounced in high transmission settings and was due to the efficacy benefit occurring in younger ages where disease burden is highest. However, the low initial efficacy and long duration schedule averted more cases across all age cohorts if a longer time horizon was considered. We observed an age-shifting effect due to the changing immunological profile in higher transmission settings, in scenarios where initial efficacy was higher, and the fourth dose administered earlier.

Conclusions: Our findings indicate that, for an imperfect childhood malaria vaccine with suboptimal efficacy, it may be advantageous to prioritise initial efficacy over duration. We predict that a modified vaccine could outperform the current RTS,S/AS01, although fourth dose timing will affect the age group that derives the greatest benefit. Further, the outcome measure and timeframe over which a vaccine is assessed are important when prioritising vaccine elements. This study provides insight into the most important characteristics of a malaria vaccine for at-risk groups and shows how distinct vaccine properties translate to public health outcomes. These findings may be used to prioritise target product profile elements for second-generation childhood malaria vaccines.

Keywords: RTS,S/AS01, Target product profile, *Plasmodium falciparum*, Malaria, Efficacy, Second-generation malaria vaccine

* Correspondence: a.hogan@imperial.ac.uk
[1]Department of Infectious Disease Epidemiology, MRC Centre for Global Infectious Disease Analysis, Imperial College London, School of Public Health, St Mary's Campus, Norfolk Place, London W2 1PG, UK
Full list of author information is available at the end of the article

Background

The success of modern vaccines has greatly reduced the global burden of infectious diseases, particularly for childhood infections [1, 2]. However, in sub-Saharan Africa, the childhood burden of malaria remains significant, even with the widespread use of vector control interventions and effective treatment, which have greatly reduced morbidity and mortality. As vaccines are being introduced for more complex diseases, the development of a vaccine for malaria has become a key global health priority. The first strategic goal in the World Health Organization's Malaria Vaccine Technology Roadmap is the development of malaria vaccines with protective efficacy against clinical malaria of at least 75% over 2 years, for administration to appropriate at-risk groups in malaria-endemic areas, with a booster dose administered no more frequently than annually [3].

The most advanced vaccine is currently the RTS,S/AS01 vaccine for *Plasmodium falciparum* malaria. The phase 3 trial of RTS,S/AS01 was conducted over the period 2009–2014, in two target age groups and for three- and four-dose schedules. In infants aged 6–12 weeks at enrolment who received four doses of the trial vaccine, efficacy was 27.8% (21.7–33.4 95% CI) over a 32-month follow-up period. In 5–17-month-old children who received four doses, efficacy against clinical malaria was 43.9% (39.7–47.8 95% CI) over the same time period [4]. The RTS,S/AS01 vaccine is unlikely to be pursued as a viable vaccine for infants, due to the low observed efficacy. However, RTS,S/AS01 will now be evaluated through a large-scale pilot implementation program in 5–17-month-old children in three sub-Saharan Africa settings: Ghana, Kenya and Malawi [5].

Work is ongoing to improve the efficacy of the RTS,S/AS01 vaccine, and recent evidence has indicated that varying the timing and amount of the fourth dose could lead to greater efficacy and improved public health outcomes [6, 7]. In an RTS,S/AS01 challenge study of healthy adults, with a fractional third dose and fractional booster, efficacy against clinical disease was 86.7% (66.8–94.6 95% CI) at the first challenge (3 weeks after the third dose) and 43% (− 9 to 70 95% CI) at the second challenge (8 months after the first challenge). In the group that received a fractional booster (fourth dose) 8 months after the first challenge, efficacy was 90% (36–98 95% CI) at the second challenge. The immunological reason for this difference is not fully understood, although it may in part be due to improved affinity of the antibodies [7].

Target product profiles (TPPs) have traditionally been used by industry to guide vaccine and drug development, by setting preferred criteria for product safety, indication, efficacy and cost-effectiveness. However, there is increasing focus on using TPPs as more adaptable, broader tools that capture the full public health value of a drug or vaccine, to help a wider range of stakeholders, such as policy-makers, design and evaluate vaccine formulations [8]. For diseases with complex epidemiological features, such as malaria, mathematical modelling can be particularly useful for informing the public health impact components of TPPs [9].

In this study, we used mathematical models of malaria transmission and vaccine efficacy to predict the impact of childhood vaccination with a modified RTS,S/AS01 vaccine and to inform TPPs for second-generation vaccines, focussing on the elements of initial efficacy, duration of protection, dosing schedules and coverage [10–13]. We determined the relative importance of initial vaccine efficacy versus duration of protection in a range of *P. falciparum* prevalence settings, in terms of clinical cases averted in children younger than 5 years, for the first decade following vaccine introduction. We also considered how the timing and efficacy of the fourth dose are likely to change the public health impact. Finally, we explored options for realistic vaccine efficacy profiles for a modified RTS,S/AS01 vaccine, in line with the results of a recent study by Regules et al. [6], and used these profiles to estimate the impact of an enhanced vaccine in different transmission settings.

Methods

Modelling approach

Our modelling approach comprised two steps. First, we simulated the changing anti-circumsporozoite (anti-CSP) antibody titre following vaccination, and we then used a mathematical model relating antibody titre to efficacy against infection to establish the corresponding efficacy profile. Second, assuming the vaccine was delivered to young children, we implemented this efficacy profile within an individual-based model of malaria transmission, as has been described previously [12].

White et al. used data from African infants and children to analyse the determinants of immunogenicity after inoculation with the RTS,S/AS01 malaria vaccine and to develop a model relating these determinants to vaccine efficacy [13]. There were two components to the model: (1) a biphasic exponential function that simulated the changing antibody titre over time after the third dose of the vaccine and (2) a Hill function that captured the relationship between antibody titre and vaccine efficacy. We used the same biphasic exponential function to describe the time-dependent anti-CSP antibody titre resulting from inoculation with a malaria vaccine. This function simulated the initial increase, and then decay, of antibody titres induced by the combined short-lived and long-lived B-cell responses to vaccination. We used the fitted parameters described by White et al., Table 3, for the 5–17-month age category [13]. For the peak observed antibody titre, we applied the median of the 11 site values in the phase 3 RTS,S/AS01 trial, which was 621 EU/mL [13].

The Hill function used to simulate vaccine efficacy is:

$$V(t) = V_{max}\left(1 - \frac{1}{1 + \left(\frac{CS(t)}{\beta}\right)^{\alpha}}\right),$$

where $CS(t)$ represents the modelled anti-CSP antibody titre (EU/mL) over time t, $V_{\max}$ represents the maximum efficacy against infection, α represents the shape parameter of the dose-response curve and β represents the scale parameter of the dose-response curve. In simple terms, α relates to the initial efficacy of the vaccine and β relates to the duration of protection (Fig. 1). Varying α and β allows us to model different antibody avidities for a given titre, resulting in different vaccine efficacy profiles (Additional file 1: Figure S10).

We used this formulation within a previously published mathematical transmission model for *P. falciparum* malaria transmission. The model pairs an individual-based model of the human transmission process with a stochastic compartmental model that captures mosquito biology. In the model, susceptible individuals are bitten by infectious mosquitoes at a rate driven by mosquito density and infectivity. Different disease states, treatment and temporary prophylaxis following a treated infection are incorporated, as are exposure-driven immunity and passive maternally derived immunity in the first 6 months of life. The individual-based transmission model has been previously validated using data on the relationship between the entomological inoculation rate and parasite prevalence, clinical disease, severe disease and deaths from multiple sites [14, 15]. Full details of the transmission model are available elsewhere [10, 11], with the key parameters summarised in Table 1.

We ran the simulations for generalised settings that were characteristic of malaria-endemic regions in Africa. The starting *P. falciparum* prevalence for 2–10-year-old individuals, denoted as $Pf\text{PR}_{2-10}$, was in the range 5 to 50%, and we selected four initial prevalence settings for comparison. This starting prevalence reflected the assumed existing levels of interventions in addition to treatment, with no scale-up of these interventions after vaccine implementation. We assumed that treatment coverage for clinical cases was 40%. Computation time is roughly proportional to the number of infected individuals; therefore, at higher prevalence levels, we reduced the simulation size for computational efficiency. All simulations were repeated for 50 transmission model parameter sets, drawn from the posterior distribution of the model fit, to account for underlying parameter uncertainty.

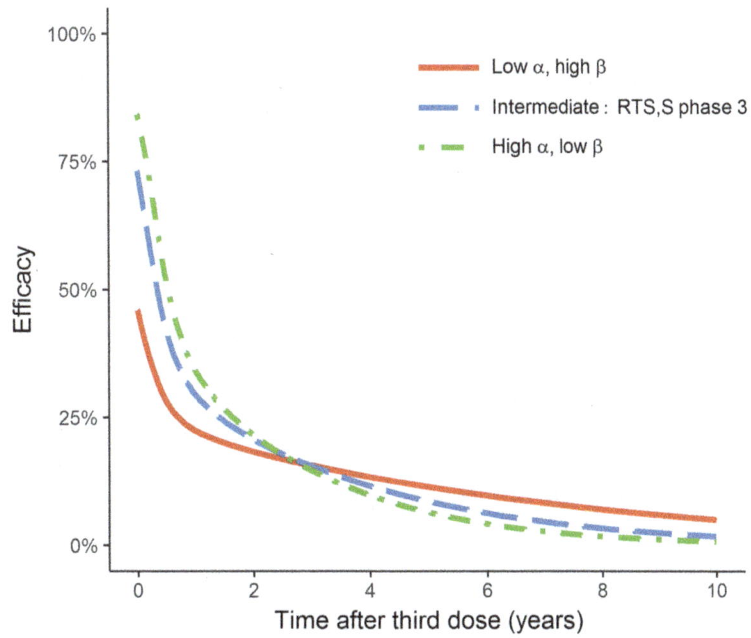

Fig. 1 Profiles for three points on the α-β curve, where the area under the efficacy-time curve is held constant. *Red solid line* α = 0.40, β = 615.06, V_{max} = 0.93 (lower initial efficacy, longer duration). *Blue dashed line* α = 0.74, β = 99.20, V_{max} = 0.93 (RTS,S/AS01 phase 3 trial modelled parameters). *Green dash-dotted line* α = 1.00, β = 60.56, V_{max} = 0.93 (higher initial efficacy, shorter duration). The corresponding antibody titre curve for the intermediate scenario is shown in Additional file 1: Figure S2, and the role of the shape parameter α and scale parameter β is illustrated in Additional file 1: Figure S10

Table 1 Summary of malaria transmission model parameters

Category	Settings
Prevalence settings	5–50% in 5% increments. Four distinct transmission settings, with $PfPR_{2-10}$ at start year set to 5%, 15%, 30% and 45%
Simulation size	30,000–65,000, depending on prevalence level
Seasonality	Perennial, with Fourier coefficients for the perennial setting as in Walker et al. [22]
Treatment	40% coverage of artemisinin-based combination therapy (ACT) treatment with 95% efficacy
Vaccine coverage	Default value of 80% coverage for the first three vaccine doses, with fourth dose coverage at 80% of the coverage for the first three doses in line with Penny et al. [12]. Varied in the range 50–90% in 5% increments
Vaccine dose timing	First three RTS,S/AS01 vaccine doses administered at 5, 6.5 and 8 months of age. Fourth dose administered at 26 months (default) and varied in the range 16–30 months

$PfPR_{2-10}$ represents *P. falciparum* parasite prevalence in 2–10-year-old children

Profile exploration with three vaccine doses

We first considered the time-dependent antibody profile for a three-dose vaccine schedule, using the parameters described in White et al. [13]. We varied the parameters in the corresponding Hill function to systematically explore the impact of varying the initial efficacy (α) and duration of protection (β) on the transmission model outcome. The objective of this analysis was to determine the relative importance of initial vaccine efficacy versus duration of protection, and how this relationship changed across age groups and prevalence settings, while keeping the overall efficacy constant. We therefore calculated the area under the curve for the efficacy profile in Additional file 1: Figure S2, which replicates the efficacy profile fitted by White et al. using the results of the phase 3 RTS,S/AS01 clinical trial [4, 13]. We then obtained a set of α-β parameter pairs where the area under the curve was held constant, by fixing α and calculating the fitted β value using the Nelder-Mead optimisation method in R [16]. We used this method to create two additional efficacy curves: one for low initial efficacy and long duration, and another for high initial efficacy and short duration. Finally, we ran the transmission model for the range of efficacy profiles produced by these α-β pairs, for each transmission setting.

Profile exploration with four vaccine doses

In the second analysis, we simulated the impact of a four-dose vaccine schedule administered to children aged 5–17 months. The results of the Regules et al. trial indicate that an enhanced RTS,S/AS01 vaccine could be obtained by varying dose timings and dosage amounts, and that efficacy can be improved without a significant increase in antibody concentration [6, 7]. In our vaccine model, antibody levels for the first three doses are fixed, and we vary the parameters of the function relating titre to efficacy to achieve different efficacy profiles. However, the fourth vaccine dose also assumes the same underlying relationship between titre and efficacy. Therefore, to determine the impact of varying efficacy following the fourth dose, we modified the titre at this dose to achieve different corresponding efficacy levels.

We first ran simulations for a range of values of the time interval between the third and fourth vaccine doses, and the antibody titre after the fourth dose. We then selected four titre-timing combinations for further analysis, and we derived the cumulative clinical cases averted in children younger than 5 years for these parameter pairs.

Public health impact of childhood vaccination

Finally, we explored the potential public health impact of a hypothetical enhanced RTS,S/AS01 vaccine profile designed to correspond to the early clinical trial results in this area, compared to the results of the phase 3 trial [4, 6]. We created a set of three possible vaccine efficacy scenarios, with one scenario corresponding to the phase 3 trial data [4, 13]; another scenario approximating the phase 2a challenge study results [6, 7]; and an intermediate scenario. In these scenarios, the initial efficacy, duration, fourth dose titre and fourth dose timing were all varied (Table 2). We calculated the number of clinical cases averted across a range of prevalence settings and vaccine coverage levels (Table 1).

Table 2 Antibody model parameters

Scenario	$t_{dose\ 4}$ (months)	$AB_{dose\ 4}$ (EU/mL)	V_{max}	α	β
A: RTS,S/AS01 phase 3	18	277	0.93	0.74	99.2
B: Intermediate	13	450	0.93	0.85	85.0
C: Modified	8	621	0.93	0.95	70.0

These parameters correspond to three vaccine scenarios: an RTS,S/AS01 phase 3 efficacy profile (A), a modified profile based on the phase 2a challenge study (C) [6, 7] and an intermediate profile (B). The antibody titre and efficacy profiles are provided in Additional file 1: Figure S6 and Fig. 4, respectively. The parameter ABdose 4 represents the antibody titre following the fourth vaccine dose at time tdose 4

Sensitivity to outcome measure

For each simulation run we calculated the number of clinical and severe cases averted in 1-year age bands, per 1000 population per year, for 40 years following vaccine introduction. To measure vaccine impact, we calculated the number of cases averted as the difference in number of cases between the vaccine and baseline scenarios, per 1000 population. For the main results, we presented our findings in terms of clinical cases averted in 0–5-year-old children, in the first 10 years following vaccine introduction. This outcome was selected based on the reference to clinical malaria episodes in the World Health Organization Malaria Vaccine Technology Roadmap [3] and the time horizon and age cohorts over which a childhood malaria vaccine is most likely to be assessed. However, using the three-dose schedule efficacy profiles, we also tested the sensitivity of these outputs to a longer follow-up period, broader age range and to severe rather than clinical cases. For the analysis of the public health impact of a modified vaccine versus the current RTS,S/AS01 (with all four doses administered), we used three different measures to quantify vaccine impact: cumulative cases averted per 1000 0–5-year-old children; cumulative cases averted per 1000 fully vaccinated with four vaccine doses; and percentage reduction in cumulative cases in 0–5-year-old children.

Results

Profile exploration with three vaccine doses

We derived three efficacy profiles where the overall efficacy (determined by the area under the efficacy-time curve) was held constant over a 10-year period following delivery of the third dose (Fig. 1). For the scenarios with higher initial efficacy, and in higher prevalence settings,

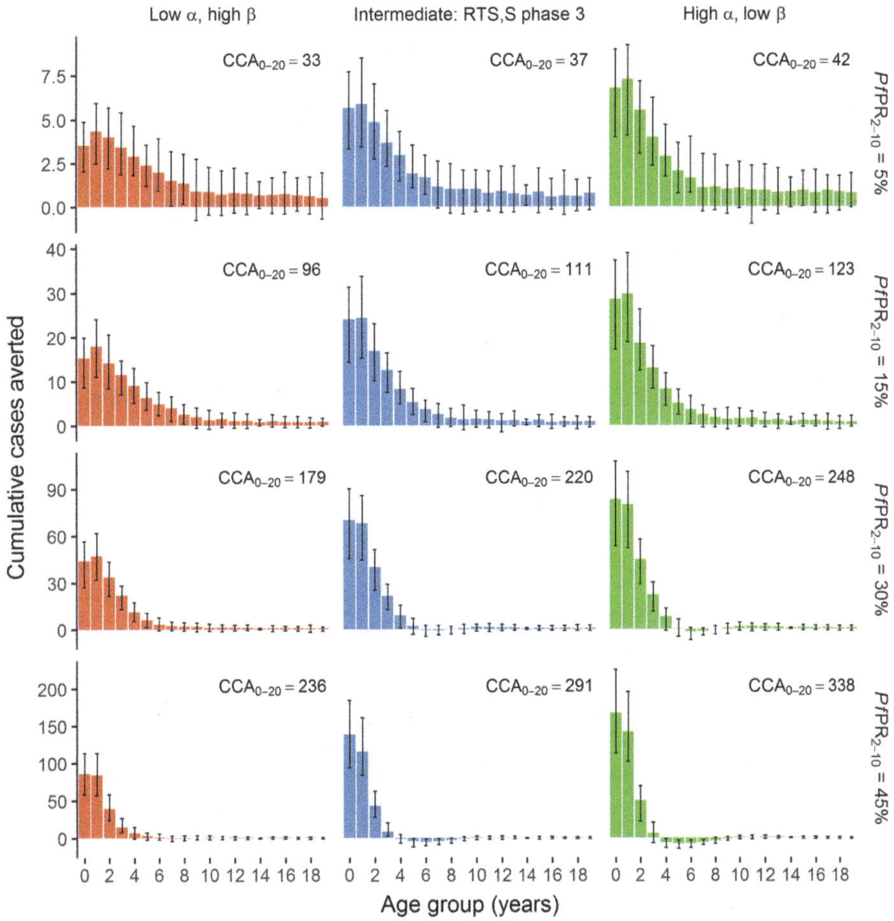

Fig. 2 Population-level impact of the three-dose vaccine schedule. These figures show the total number of clinical cases averted over 10 years, for 1-year age groups up to 20 years of age. The total cases averted are shown per 1000 individuals in each age group, stratified by transmission setting (*rows*) and efficacy profile (*columns*) of Fig. 1. The *bars* show the median estimates, and the *error bars* show 95% credible intervals, based on 50 parameter draws. CCA_{0-20} represents the cumulative number of clinical cases averted over a 10-year period following the introduction of vaccination, in individuals younger than 20 years, per 1000 individuals. $PfPR_{2-10}$ represents *P. falciparum* prevalence for 2–10-year-old individuals, prior to vaccination

the public health impact was more concentrated in younger age groups (Fig. 2). Further, the excess of cases in older children in the intervention group was more pronounced in these scenarios, compared to the lower transmission and longer duration scenarios, where the impact was more evenly spread across age cohorts. Overall the greatest number of clinical cases averted was obtained with a high initial efficacy, rather than a long duration of protection (Fig. 2). Additionally, we performed the same analysis with a fourth vaccine dose (Additional file 1: Figures S4 and S5) and for a wide range of α-β pairs (Additional file 1: Figure S3). In all transmission settings, the initial vaccine efficacy was the main determinant of the number of clinical cases averted.

Profile exploration with four vaccine doses

For the four-dose vaccine schedule, the greatest impact was achieved with a high antibody boosting at the fourth dose (which directly influenced efficacy) and a large interval between the third and fourth doses. Figure 3a shows the output for a transmission setting of $PfPR_{2-10}$ = 30%; however, the overall trend was consistent across all prevalence scenarios. In this part of the analysis, the area under the efficacy curve was not fixed, which resulted in the overall area under the curve of vaccine efficacy being higher when doses were spaced further apart, due to the primary series affording impact for a longer time. We found that the number of clinical cases averted correlated strongly with the overall area under the efficacy curve.

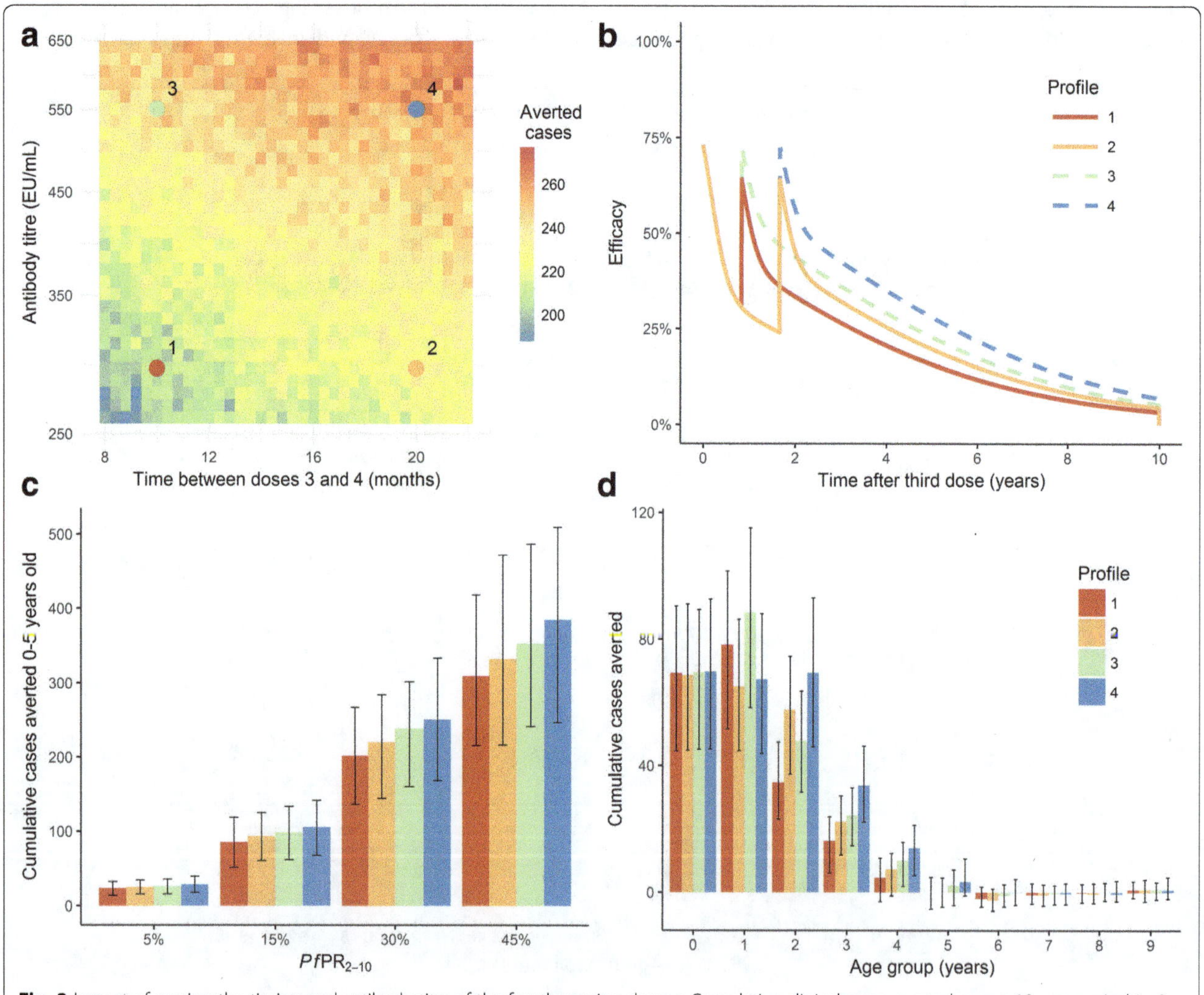

Fig. 3 Impact of varying the timing and antibody titre of the fourth vaccine dose. **a** Cumulative clinical cases averted over a 10-year period in 0–5-year-old children, for a range of antibody titre and fourth dose timing values, where $PfPR_{2-10}$ = 30%. **b** Efficacy curves corresponding to the timing-titre parameter pairs indicated in panel **a**. **c** Cumulative clinical cases averted over a 10-year period in 0–5-year-old children, stratified by prevalence setting and efficacy profile. **d** Cumulative clinical cases averted over a 10-year period per 1000 individuals for 1-year age groups, where $PfPR_{2-10}$ = 30%. In **c** and **d**, the *bars* show the median estimates and the *error bars* show 95% credible intervals, based on 50 parameter draws. $PfPR_{2-10}$ represents *P. falciparum* prevalence for 2–10-year-old individuals, prior to vaccination

We selected four titre-timing combinations to create four efficacy scenarios: low efficacy and short timing; low efficacy and long timing; high efficacy and short timing; and high efficacy and long timing (Fig. 3a and b). The higher fourth dose efficacy and longer timing scenario resulted in the highest number of averted cases, and this effect was more marked in higher transmission settings (Fig. 3c). While the two higher efficacy (driven by the higher antibody titre) scenarios resulted in more averted cases overall, the longer timing schedules resulted in more averted cases in older age groups (Fig. 3d).

Public health impact of childhood vaccination

Figure 4 shows the time-dependent vaccine efficacy over 10 years for the RTS,S/AS01 vaccine (Fig. 4a), a modified RTS,S/AS01 vaccine that approximately emulates the observations from the fractional third and fourth dose challenge study (Fig. 4c) and an intermediate efficacy scenario (Fig. 4b). The parameters used to create Fig. 4c were selected such that the efficacy following both the third and fourth doses was close to 90%, and the time between doses three and four was also reduced. To achieve a higher efficacy after dose four, we set the antibody titre following dose four to that observed after dose three in the phase 3 trial (i.e. 621 EU/mL). The parameters corresponding to the three scenarios are provided in Table 1, and the corresponding antibody titre plots are shown in Additional file 1: Figure S6.

Comparing these three profiles, we found that the modified RTS,S/AS01 outperformed the profile based on the RTS,S/AS01 phase 3 data, even though the fourth vaccine dose was timed at 8 months, compared to 18 months (Fig. 5). In terms of cumulative cases averted per 1000 0–5-year-old children over a 10-year period, the modified vaccine schedule averted between 21 and 25% more clinical cases than the current RTS,S/AS01, across the four transmission settings (Additional file 1: Table S1). We found that in the lowest transmission setting where $PfPR_{2-10} = 5\%$, the RTS,S/AS01 phase 3 vaccine averted more cases in older children. We also observed a stronger shifting of cases from younger to older ages in higher transmission settings with the modified vaccine profile (Fig. 5). Cumulative clinical cases averted increased approximately linearly with higher vaccine coverage (Additional file 1: Figure S7).

Sensitivity to outcome measure

We found that for the three-dose vaccine schedule analysis, measuring the cumulative clinical cases averted across all age groups, rather than children, and over a longer time horizon changed the results, with the low initial efficacy and long duration vaccine schedule becoming more advantageous at an earlier time point in low transmission settings (Additional file 1: Figure S8). However, where we used cumulative severe cases averted as the outcome measure, across all age groups there was almost no difference between the three efficacy profiles (Additional file 1: Figure S9).

For the analysis of the public health impact of three vaccine scenarios, where all four doses were administered, we included two additional outcome measures: clinical cases averted per 1000 fully vaccinated children, and percentage of clinical cases averted in 0–5-year-old children. The modified vaccine (scenario in Fig. 4c) was the most advantageous for all outcome measures, although the percentage reduction was higher in low malaria transmission settings.

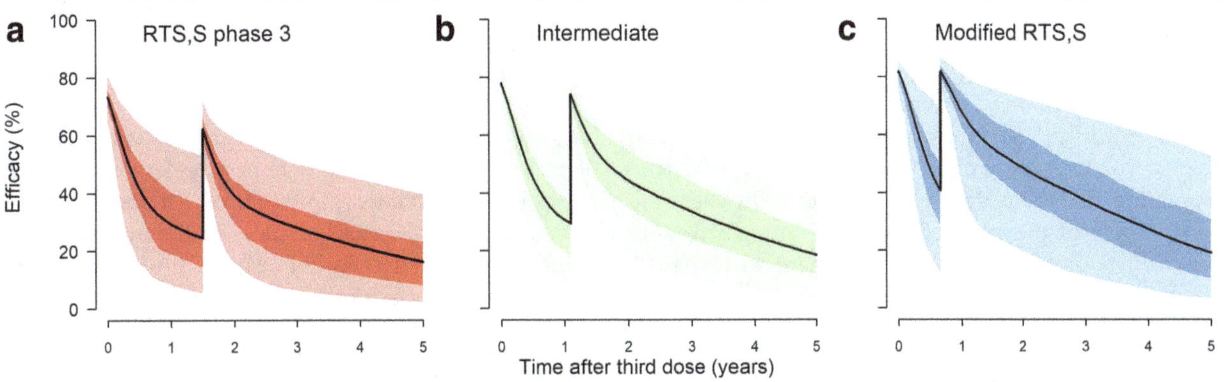

Fig. 4 Time after the third vaccine dose (years), versus vaccine efficacy, for a four-dose schedule. Three scenarios are shown. **a** Fourth dose at 18 months, corresponding to the phase 3 trial data; **b** intermediate scenario; **c** fourth dose at 8 months with a higher antibody titre (corresponding to higher efficacy), approximating observed efficacy in the Regules et al. study, and referred to as the 'modified' vaccine scenario [6]. The parameters are given in Table 1 and the corresponding antibody titre curves in Additional file 1: Figure S6. In each subplot, the *solid line* is the median of 2000 simulations, and the *dark* and *light shaded* regions represent the 50% and 95% predictive intervals, respectively. Other parameters are those described in White et al, Table 3, for the 5–17-month age category [13]

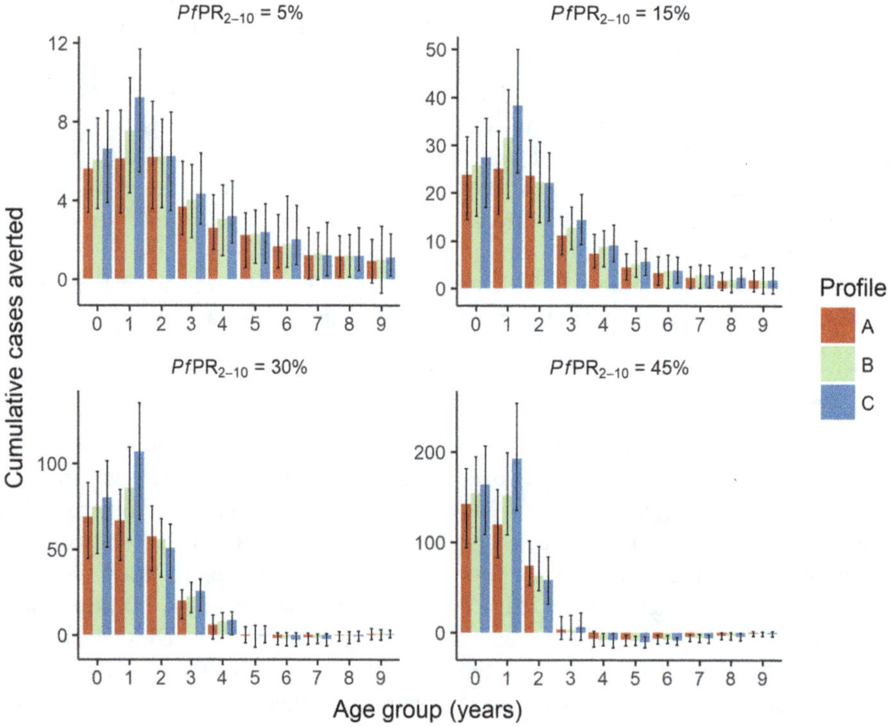

Fig. 5 Population-level impact of the three efficacy scenarios in Fig. 4. Cumulative clinical cases averted over a 10-year period, per 1000 individuals, stratified by prevalence setting and efficacy profile. The *bars* show the median estimates, and the *error bars* show 95% credible intervals, based on 50 parameter draws. $PfPR_{2-10}$ represents *P. falciparum* prevalence for 2–10-year-old individuals, prior to vaccination

Discussion

In our study we used a dynamic modelling approach to compare the relative contributions of vaccine characteristics, to inform a TPP for a second-generation malaria vaccine for young children. We first examined the characteristics of initial efficacy and duration in the context of a three-dose schedule before analysing the characteristics specific to the fourth vaccine dose. Our results demonstrated that, for the three-dose vaccine schedule, initial efficacy was associated with a higher reduction in childhood clinical cases compared to vaccine duration. This effect was more pronounced in high malaria transmission settings due to the concentration of clinical cases in younger age groups, and this finding held true when a fourth vaccine dose was incorporated (where the fourth dose had the same efficacy and timing across all scenarios). However, we found that there was a larger age-shifting effect in higher transmission settings, where the initial efficacy was higher, due to the delayed acquisition of clinical immunity [17].

Examining the characteristics of the fourth dose, we found that the largest benefit in terms of clinical cases averted always occurred when the efficacy at the fourth dose was highest, and that a longer timing between doses three and four was also advantageous. In the third part of the analysis, we created three scenarios where all of the vaccine parameters — initial efficacy, duration and fourth dose titre and timing — were varied, to replicate the RTS,S/AS01 phase 3 profile; a profile approximately corresponding to the fractional dose study (referred to as the modified profile); and an intermediate profile. This analysis showed that a modified malaria vaccine would likely outperform the current RTS,S/AS01, but that increasing the timing between doses three and four could further reduce the number of clinical cases in older children.

The World Health Organization has specified that a malaria vaccine for children younger than 5 years should reduce incidence of all clinical malaria episodes by at least 75% for at least 1 year and preferably at least 2 years [3]. Importantly, the Preferred Product Characteristics state that initial efficacy and duration will be jointly considered, and the duration of protection is assessed as being as important as the short-term efficacy for the target vaccine group, in medium to high transmission settings [18]. Our findings indicate that, for imperfect vaccines with suboptimal efficacy, it may be advantageous to prioritise initial efficacy over duration.

The results of our study should be interpreted in the context of the selected follow-up time window, age cohorts and outcome measure. We focussed on children younger than 5 years and a 10-year horizon following vaccine introduction as our primary outcome measure, given the circumstances in which a childhood vaccine is likely to be assessed in field studies, as well as the many other changes to malaria interventions likely to occur over longer time periods. We found that the low initial efficacy and long duration profile resulted in more clinical cases averted when measuring cases in all age groups, and over a longer time window; however, this is likely due to the functional form of this efficacy profile allowing the vaccine benefit to extend for far longer than expected in practice. We also found that measuring the severe cases averted across all ages meant little difference in impact of the three efficacy profiles considered, further justifying the focus on childhood impact. Finally, our main outcome measure was clinical cases averted, and we did not account for the implementation costs associated with different schedules, which may change how vaccine efficacy and duration are prioritised.

Our study had several limitations. First, we fixed the age at first vaccine delivery at 5 months and did not incorporate any reduction in susceptibility to infection until after the third vaccine dose. It is possible that some protection is afforded after the first vaccine dose, which would further increase the vaccine impact. Additional data on the protection between doses would be needed to capture this in the modelling framework. Second, our proxy for total efficacy, i.e. total area under the time-efficacy curve over a 10-year period, meant that some of the area under the efficacy curve was outside the measured time window. However, our study focussed on impact in the childhood age group, and so we do not expect this assumption to greatly influence our results.

Our method assumes that there is a non-linear but positively increasing relationship between antibody titre and vaccine efficacy. This is biologically plausible based on findings from the RTS,S/AS01 vaccine. However, in the phase 2a challenge study there was not a great change in antibody levels between the protected and non-protected groups, suggesting that factors other than antibody titre may influence efficacy [6]. By varying the antibody titre at the fourth dose, we were able to capture the observed challenge study efficacy, without explicitly incorporating other factors into our antibody model, and these efficacy curves in turn informed the estimates of population-level vaccine impact. However, the efficacy of a second-generation vaccine may need to be improved by enhancing antibody quality or avidity, rather than by solely increasing antibody titre (given that higher titres may not be achievable in African children). Fitting of dose-response relationships to data from challenge studies for other malaria vaccines could be undertaken to incorporate other factors such as antibody quality into this modelling framework, to consider the potential public health impact of candidate vaccines in phase 2 studies.

Our analysis was motivated by the findings of the fractional third dose and fractional booster dose study by Regules et al. [6], which provides an early indication that changing dosage and timing could improve vaccine efficacy. However, the fractional dose study was conducted in a relatively small sample of 30 healthy malaria-naïve adults, meaning there are limitations in comparing these results with those from the phase 3 trial. In addition, it is not clear from this single study whether the increased efficacy is due to the fractional third dose or to the delay in the third dose [7]. A phase 2 trial of RTS,S/AS01E compared 0, 1, 2 month and 0, 2, 7 month dosing schedules within the Expanded Programme on Immunization. The trial found that over the 19 month study period, efficacy was higher in the 0, 1, 2 month group, although when comparing malaria episodes in the 12-month period following the third dose, efficacy across the two schedules was similar (noting that this study was in infants only) [19]. Further characterisation of the dose-response relationship between antibody titre and efficacy within this and future challenge studies could help elucidate this mechanism and guide TPP development. Furthermore, in creating the 'intermediate' vaccine efficacy profile, with parameters approximately at midpoints between those selected for the phase 3 and modified efficacy profiles, we implicitly assumed a trade-off between the timing of and antibody titre at the fourth dose, where a later dose timing resulted in a lower antibody titre (and therefore efficacy) following the fourth dose. A more complex relationship between these factors is possible and could be quantified given further data on this relationship.

Despite the success in developing the RTS,S/AS01 vaccine, there have been challenges, many of which will impact the progress of a second-generation vaccine. A key issue is that we still do not have a full understanding of the immunological mechanisms by which the RTS,S/AS01 confers protection against malaria disease, and there is no widely accepted immune correlate of protection. While there is evidence that high anti-CSP antibodies are associated with protection, antibody titre is not an established protective correlate. Further, it is likely that a second-generation vaccine will need to be assessed relative to the first-generation vaccine, which presents feasibility issues in terms of community acceptance, trial design and trial sample size. The measures by which the success of a new vaccine is assessed will also need to be carefully considered [20, 21].

Conclusions

In vaccine development and evaluation, considerable focus is typically given to the durability, or half-life, of a vaccine. However, our findings show that these vaccine properties need to be considered in the context of the target population and immunological profile. In our study, we found that in the first decade of vaccine implementation the initial efficacy was more important than duration, based on our current understanding of the RTS,S/AS01 vaccine and in terms of childhood clinical cases averted. This study also emphasises the importance of considering the age distribution of incidence in a range of disease prevalence settings when predicting the impact of an age-targeted vaccine. Finally, our analysis demonstrates that the timing of the fourth RTS,S/AS01 dose can change the overall health benefit, which should be considered with the logistics of implementing a childhood malaria vaccine within the current Expanded Programme on Immunization framework. The findings from this analysis could provide insight for vaccine developers and policy-makers into how distinct properties of a malaria vaccine may translate to public health outcomes and how the importance of these characteristics changes across different malaria prevalence settings.

Funding
This work was funded by a grant from PATH. RV acknowledges fellowship support from the UK Medical Research Council, and PW and ACG acknowledge support from the Bill & Melinda Gates Foundation. We additionally acknowledge Centre support from the UK Medical Research Council and Department for International Development under the MRC/DfID concordat. The funders had no role in study design, data collection and analysis, decision to publish or preparation of the manuscript.

Authors' contributions
ABH, PW, RV and ACG designed the study. ABH prepared and performed the analysis, and PW, RV, JTG and ACG contributed to the analysis. All authors interpreted the results. ABH drafted the manuscript, and all authors contributed to and approved the final manuscript.

Competing interests
RV, JTG and ACG have collaborated with Glaxo SmithKline on analysis of the RTS,S malaria vaccine trial data. This was funded by the Malaria Vaccine Initiative/PATH, and no funding was received directly from Glaxo SmithKline. All other authors report that they have no competing interests.

Author details
[1]Department of Infectious Disease Epidemiology, MRC Centre for Global Infectious Disease Analysis, Imperial College London, School of Public Health, St Mary's Campus, Norfolk Place, London W2 1PG, UK. [2]School of Mathematical Sciences, Queen Mary University London, Mile End Road, London E1 4NS, UK.

References
1. Chan M, Elias C, Fauci A, Lake A, Berkley S. Reaching everyone, everywhere with life-saving vaccines. Lancet. 2017;389:777–9. https://doi.org/10.1016/S0140-6736(17)30554-8.
2. Andre FE, Booy R, Bock HL, Clemens J, Datta SK, John TJ, Lee BW, Lolekha S, Peltola H, Ruff TA, Santosham M, Schmitt HJ. Vaccination greatly reduces disease, disability, death and inequity worldwide. Bull World Health Organ. 2008;86:140–6. https://doi.org/10.2471/BLT.07.040089.
3. Malaria Vaccine Funders Group. Malaria vaccine technology roadmap: World Health Organization; 2013. http://www.who.int/immunization/topics/malaria/vaccine_roadmap/en/. Accessed 29 Jan 2018
4. RTSS Clinical Trials Partnership. Efficacy and safety of RTS,S/AS01 malaria vaccine with or without a booster dose in infants and children in Africa: final results of a phase 3, individually randomised, controlled trial. Lancet. 2015;6736:31–45. https://doi.org/10.1016/S0140-6736(15)60721-8
5. World Health Organization. Q&A on the malaria vaccine implementation programme (MVIP). 2018. http://www.who.int/malaria/media/malaria-vaccine-implementationqa/en/. Accessed 20 June 2018.
6. Regules JA, Cicatelli SB, Bennett JW, Paolino KM, Twomey PS, Moon JE, et al. Fractional third and fourth dose of RTS,S/AS01 malaria candidate vaccine: a phase 2a controlled human malaria parasite infection and immunogenicity study. J Infect Dis. 2016;214:762–71. https://doi.org/10.1093/infdis/jiw237.
7. Chaudhury S, Regules JA, Darko CA, Dutta S, Wallqvist A, Waters NC, et al. Delayed fractional dose regimen of the RTS,S/AS01 malaria vaccine candidate enhances an IgG4 response that inhibits serum opsonophagocytosis. Sci Rep. 2017;7:7998. https://doi.org/10.1038/s41598-017-08526-5.
8. Kaslow DC. The full public health value of vaccines: malaria. Spoken presentation at the 66th annual meeting of the American Society of Tropical Medicine and Hygiene (ASTMH). Baltimore: American Society of Tropical Medicine and Hygiene (ASTMH); 2017.
9. malERA Consultative Group on Modeling. A research agenda for malaria eradication: modeling. PLoS Med. 2011;8:e1000403.
10. Griffin JT, Hollingsworth TD, Okell LC, Churcher TS, White M, Hinsley W, et al. Reducing Plasmodium falciparum malaria transmission in Africa: a model-based evaluation of intervention strategies. PLoS Med. 2010;7:e1000324. https://doi.org/10.1371/journal.pmed.1000324.
11. Winskill P, Slater HC, Griffin JT, Ghani AC, Walker PGT. The US President's malaria initiative, Plasmodium falciparum transmission and mortality: a modelling study. PLoS Med. 2017;649:1–14. https://doi.org/10.1371/journal.pmed.1002448.
12. Penny MA, Verity R, Bever CA, Sauboin C, Galactionova K, Flasche S, et al. Public health impact and cost-effectiveness of the RTS,S/AS01 malaria vaccine: a systematic comparison of predictions from four mathematical models. Lancet. 2016;387:367–75. https://doi.org/10.1016/S0140-6736(15)00725-4.
13. White MT, Verity R, Griffin JT, Asante KP, Owusu-Agyei S, Greenwood B, et al. Immunogenicity of the RTS,S/AS01 malaria vaccine and implications for duration of vaccine efficacy: secondary analysis of data from a phase 3 randomised controlled trial. Lancet Infect Dis. 2015;15:1450–8. https://doi.org/10.1016/S1473-3099(15)00239-X.
14. Griffin JT, Ferguson NM, Ghani AC. Estimates of the changing age-burden of Plasmodium falciparum malaria disease in sub-Saharan Africa. Nat Commun. 2014;5:3136. https://doi.org/10.1038/ncomms4136.
15. Griffin JT, Hollingsworth TD, Reyburn H, Drakeley CJ, Riley EM, Ghani AC. Gradual acquisition of immunity to severe malaria with increasing exposure. Proc R Soc B Biol Sci. 2015;282:1–8.
16. R Core Team. R: a language and environment for statistical computing. Vienna: R Foundation for Statistical Computing; 2017. https://www.r-project.org/
17. Ghani AC, Sutherland CJ, Riley EM, Drakeley CJ, Griffin JT, Gosling RD, et al. Loss of population levels of immunity to malaria as a result of exposure-reducing interventions: consequences for interpretation of disease trends. PLoS One. 2009;4:e4383. https://doi.org/10.1371/journal.pone.0004383.
18. World Health Organization. WHO Preferred Product Characteristics (PPC) for Malaria Vaccines. Geneva; 2015. http://www.who.int/immunization/documents/innovation/WHO_IVB_14.09/en/. Accessed 29 Jan 2018
19. Asante KP, Abdulla S, Agnandji S, Lyimo J, Vekemans J, Soulanoudjingar S, et al. Safety and efficacy of the RTS,S/AS01Ecandidate malaria vaccine given with expanded-programme-on-immunisation vaccines: 19 month follow-up of a randomised, open-label, phase 2 trial. Lancet Infect Dis. 2011;11(10):741–9. https://doi.org/10.1016/S1473-3099(11)70100-1.
20. Ballou WR. The development of the RTS,S malaria vaccine candidate: challenges and lessons. Parasite Immunol. 2009;31:492–500.
21. Fowkes FJI, Simpson JA, Beeson JG. Implications of the licensure of a partially efficacious malaria vaccine on evaluating second-generation vaccines. BMC Med. 2013;11:1–8. https://doi.org/10.1186/1741-7015-11-232.
22. Walker PGT, Griffin JT, Ferguson NM, Ghani AC. Estimating the most efficient allocation of interventions to achieve reductions in Plasmodium falciparum malaria burden and transmission in Africa: a modelling study. Lancet Glob Health. 2016;4:e474–84. https://doi.org/10.1016/S2214-109X(16)30073-0.

9

Progress toward eliminating TB and HIV deaths in Brazil, 2001–2015: a spatial assessment

Jennifer M. Ross[1,2], Nathaniel J. Henry[2], Laura A. Dwyer-Lindgren[2], Andrea de Paula Lobo[3,4], Fatima Marinho de Souza[4], Molly H. Biehl[2], Sarah E. Ray[2], Robert C. Reiner Jr[2], Rebecca W. Stubbs[2], Kirsten E. Wiens[2], Lucas Earl[2], Michael J. Kutz[2], Natalia V. Bhattacharjee[2], Hmwe H. Kyu[2], Mohsen Naghavi[2] and Simon I. Hay[2*]

Abstract

Background: Brazil has high burdens of tuberculosis (TB) and HIV, as previously estimated for the 26 states and the Federal District, as well as high levels of inequality in social and health indicators. We improved the geographic detail of burden estimation by modelling deaths due to TB and HIV and TB case fatality ratios for the more than 5400 municipalities in Brazil.

Methods: This ecological study used vital registration data from the national mortality information system and TB case notifications from the national communicable disease notification system from 2001 to 2015. Mortality due to TB and HIV was modelled separately by cause and sex using a Bayesian spatially explicit mixed effects regression model. TB incidence was modelled using the same approach. Results were calibrated to the Global Burden of Disease Study 2016. Case fatality ratios were calculated for TB.

Results: There was substantial inequality in TB and HIV mortality rates within the nation and within states. National-level TB mortality in people without HIV infection declined by nearly 50% during 2001 to 2015, but HIV mortality declined by just over 20% for males and 10% for females. TB and HIV mortality rates for municipalities in the 90th percentile nationally were more than three times rates in the 10th percentile, with nearly 70% of the worst-performing municipalities for male TB mortality and more than 75% for female mortality in 2001 also in the worst decile in 2015. The same municipality ranking metric for HIV was observed to be between 55% and 61%. Within states, the TB mortality rate ratios by sex for municipalities in the worst decile versus the best decile varied from 1.4 to 2.9, and HIV varied from 1.4 to 4.2. The World Health Organization target case fatality rate for TB of less than 10% was achieved in 9.6% of municipalities for males versus 38.4% for females in 2001 and improved to 38.4% and 56.6% of municipalities for males versus females, respectively, by 2014.

Conclusions: Mortality rates in municipalities within the same state exhibited nearly as much relative variation as within the nation as a whole. Monitoring the mortality burden at this level of geographic detail is critical for guiding precision public health responses.

Keywords: Tuberculosis, HIV, Small area estimation, Geospatial, Geographic, Brazil, Case fatality, Mortality

* Correspondence: sihay@uw.edu
[2]Institute for Health Metrics and Evaluation, University of Washington, 2301 5th Ave Suite 600, Seattle, WA 98121, USA
Full list of author information is available at the end of the article

Background

Brazil is a high-burden country for tuberculosis (TB) and human immunodeficiency virus (HIV)-TB co-infection [1] and also characterised by high levels of inequality in social and health indicators [2–4]. The twin slogans of 'Leave no one behind' and 'Everybody counts' adopted for World Tuberculosis Day and World AIDS Day, respectively, in 2017, emphasise the importance of reducing inequality to end these leading epidemics [5]. TB and HIV inequalities may manifest in geographic patterns because the underlying risk factors for TB and HIV infection and death, such as poverty, incarceration, undernutrition, crowding and poor access to health services, vary across geographic areas and through time [6–10]. Additionally, the disease mechanisms of transmission between persons in close contact can lead to geographic clusters of disease burden [11–13]. Brazil has invested in massive social programmes to improve health and equality, such as the Family Health programme of free community-based healthcare, the Bolsa Familia programme of cash transfers conditional on education and health behaviours [14], and universal eligibility for free TB care and free antiretroviral therapy for HIV infection since its discovery in 1996 [15]. The national strategy to end TB in Brazil prescribes TB control strategies based on local epidemiology; fine-scale mapping of TB and HIV burden can provide information to prioritise additional programmatic investments toward improving health [16].

Prior investigations of the spatial distribution of TB and HIV burden in Brazil varied in their scope and level of geographic detail, but few achieved coverage of the entire nation at fine spatial resolution or for long time series. The Global Burden of Disease (GBD) study collaborators modelled mortality due to an exhaustive set of causes, including HIV and TB, at the state level for 1990 through to 2015 [4]. Other investigations modelled mortality or case notifications at finer spatial scale for portions of the country [17–20]. Harling et al. [21] completed a nationwide municipal-level analysis of case notifications in Brazil of a shorter time series, 2002 to 2009. Outside of Brazil, there are few national-level spatial modelling studies of TB incidence and, to our knowledge, no nationally comprehensive spatial models of TB mortality at fine spatial scale [22–24]. There are broader spatial modelling efforts for HIV, corresponding to the greater availability of spatially resolved data sources for HIV than for TB in high-burden countries [25, 26].

There are methodologic challenges associated with spatial modelling of TB and HIV mortality which are addressed by this analysis. First, despite being leading infectious causes of death globally, TB and HIV death counts are low in small areas, leading to instability in case counts and difficulty in separating true differences in risk from stochastic noise for individual geographic areas. A modelling approach that draws strength from neighbouring groups across space and time could stabilise these estimates. Second, TB and HIV deaths may be misclassified due to failure to recognise the cause of death as HIV or TB or stigma associated with reporting these conditions [27–29]. Furthermore, the International Statistical Classification of Diseases (ICD) convention is for TB deaths in persons living with HIV infection (PLHIV) to be assigned to HIV as the underlying cause, which can hide the contribution of TB to these deaths if only a single cause of death is reported in vital registration [30]. In this study, we address these challenges by utilising comprehensive cause of death assignment and small area estimation to conduct a nationwide analysis of TB and HIV mortality at fine geographic scale. We also estimate the TB case fatality ratio, defined as the proportion of persons with TB who die of TB, a key metric in the World Health Organization (WHO) End TB Strategy [1]. HIV case fatality ratios are not estimated due to a lack of data to inform HIV incidence.

Methods

Overview

GBD collaborators estimated mortality burden for 249 causes of death from 1990 to 2015 for the 26 states and Federal District in Brazil [4]. This study extended the modelling of deaths assigned to TB or HIV by GBD 2016 to the second administrative level (municipality) using the municipality of residence recorded in vital registration records. TB incidence was modelled at the second administrative level using TB case notification records. All rates presented are age-standardised unless otherwise stated. This study complies with the Guidelines for Accurate and Transparent Health Estimates Reporting (GATHER; http://gather-statement.org). Analyses were done with R version 3.2.4 [31].

Study design and data sources

This ecological study included all municipalities in Brazil. Mortality data included anonymised individual-level records from all deaths reported in the Brazil Mortality Information System occurring between January 1, 2001, and December 31, 2015. These records were tabulated according to the decedent's municipality of residence, age, sex, and cause of death coded according to the tenth revision of the ICD (ICD-10), which was adopted in Brazil in 1996 (Additional file 1: Table S1) [30]. Case notification data included all persons with new cases of tuberculosis reported to the Brazil national notification system (Sistema de Informacao de Agravos de Notificao; http://portalsinan.saude.gov.br/) between January 1, 2001, and December 31, 2015, and were tabulated by the municipality of residence at the time of case notification, by age, sex and HIV status. HIV incidence was not estimated from case notification because only a subset of HIV cases, persons with AIDS, were notifiable prior to 2014. An annual population series by age and sex for each municipality was obtained from the Brazilian Institute for Geography and Statistics [32].

To inform the model, we included covariates with a known or postulated epidemiologic relationship with HIV or TB infection, progression to active disease, or mortality (Additional file 1: Table S2). Covariates applied annually at the level of the municipality included population density, adjusted monthly income, literacy rate, outdoor air pollution, proportion of population in prison, ambient temperature, household crowding, night-time light brightness, and population-level coverage of Family Health programme teams. Data sources and processing are described in Additional file 1: Table S2. Model comparisons using different covariate sets are described in Additional file 1: Table S3. Additional covariates were estimated annually at the state level from the GBD 2016 study due to lack of available data at the municipality level. These included HIV prevalence, smoking prevalence, diabetes (fasting plasma glucose in mmol/L), alcohol consumption (litres of pure alcohol per capita per year), indoor air pollution prevalence, and a TB risk factor index [33]. However, the addition of these state-level covariates did not substantially alter TB or HIV mortality estimates (Additional file 1: Table S3); they were not included in the final model in an effort to simplify the model.

Municipality boundaries changed to accommodate new municipalities in a small number of cases between 2001 and 2015. Municipalities that had undergone a boundary change during the period of the analysis were merged to create a stable unit. Of the 5565 municipalities present in Brazil in 2015, boundary changes during the analysis period required merging to form 5477 geographic units for analysis. Details of these shifts are provided in Additional file 1: Table S4.

Cause of death attribution

Standardisation of vital registration data was done based on methods developed in GBD 2016 [34]. In this study, each death was attributed to a single underlying cause that fit within a hierarchy of mutually exclusive and collectively exhaustive causes. The portion of deaths coded with ICD-10 codes that could not be underlying causes of death or were non-specific causes were redistributed according to a framework for processing so-called garbage codes developed by Naghavi et al. [35].

Mortality rates for TB, HIV, and TB among PLHIV were estimated for this study. TB deaths among PLHIV were estimated as a subset of the burden of HIV/AIDS deaths to maintain consistency with GBD and ICD-10 convention [34]. The ICD-10 codes corresponding to each cause estimated here are listed in Additional file 1: Table S1. The patterns of death redistribution through the processing algorithm to each category of TB without HIV and HIV are shown in Additional file 1: Figures S2 and S3, respectively.

Statistical analysis

Mortality due to TB and HIV (including HIV/TB) was estimated separately by cause and sex using a small area estimation approach developed by Dwyer-Lindgren et al. [36]. This approach applies a Bayesian spatially explicit mixed effects regression model. Conditional autoregressive distributions were used to smooth over age, year and municipality. Covariates for each municipality and year were included as fixed effects (Additional file 1). One thousand draws (i.e. candidate maps) were sampled from the posterior distributions of modelled parameters. Point estimates were produced from the mean of these draws, and uncertainty intervals were generated from the 2.5th to 97.5th percentiles for each age, sex, year, municipality, and cause. Population-weighted municipal-level estimates for each cause and sex were aggregated to the level of the administrative state and Federal District ($n = 27$) for calibration to state-level estimates from GBD 2016 [4]. The posterior probability of a positive or negative association with the outcomes of TB and HIV mortality was estimated for each covariate.

Model validation

Separate model validation datasets were defined for TB and HIV mortality using municipalities with large numbers of deaths and small year-by-year variation in TB and HIV mortality rates [37]. Further details of statistical comparison between models are provided in the Additional file 1, including Additional file 1: Table S5.

Case fatality analysis

Case fatality ratios for TB were calculated jointly for persons with and without HIV infection due to unrecorded HIV status in nearly 40% of TB case notification records, with completeness of reporting improving during the period of analysis. Case fatality analysis was restricted to 2001 to 2014 due to an incomplete set of case notification data for 2015. For this analysis, TB mortality events in persons with and without HIV infection were summed for each age, sex, year and municipality. These combined TB and HIV-TB mortality events were modelled using the small area approach described above and calibrated to state-level estimates from GBD 2016. TB incidence in persons with and without HIV infection was modelled from TB case notifications using the same approach and calibrated to state-level TB incidence estimates from GBD 2016. Age-standardised, sex-specific TB and HIV-TB deaths were divided by the age-standardised TB incidence for the corresponding sex, year and municipality. While persons who die from TB may not die in the same year that their case is notified, this is the standard calculation for this TB metric [1].

Results

National-level geographic patterns by municipality and notable time trends

TB and HIV mortality rates varied substantially by municipality within the nation during 2001–2015 (Fig. 1). National age-standardised mortality due to TB in persons without HIV decreased by nearly 50% from 6.7 (95% uncertainty interval (UI) 6.5–6.9) deaths per 100,000 in 2001 to 3.5 (95% UI 3.4–3.6) deaths per 100,000 in 2015 among males, and from 2.3 (95% UI 2.2–2.4) deaths per 100,000 in 2001 to 1.2 (95% UI 1.1–1.2) deaths per 100,000 in 2015 among females. National age-standardised mortality due to HIV was 11.0 (95% UI 10.8–11.2) deaths per 100,000 in 2001 versus 8.7 (95% UI 8.5–8.8) deaths per 100,000 in 2015 among males, and 5.0 (95% UI 4.8–5.1) deaths per 100,000 in 2001 versus 4.4 (95% UI 4.2–4.5) deaths in 2015 among females. Despite national-level declines, the majority of

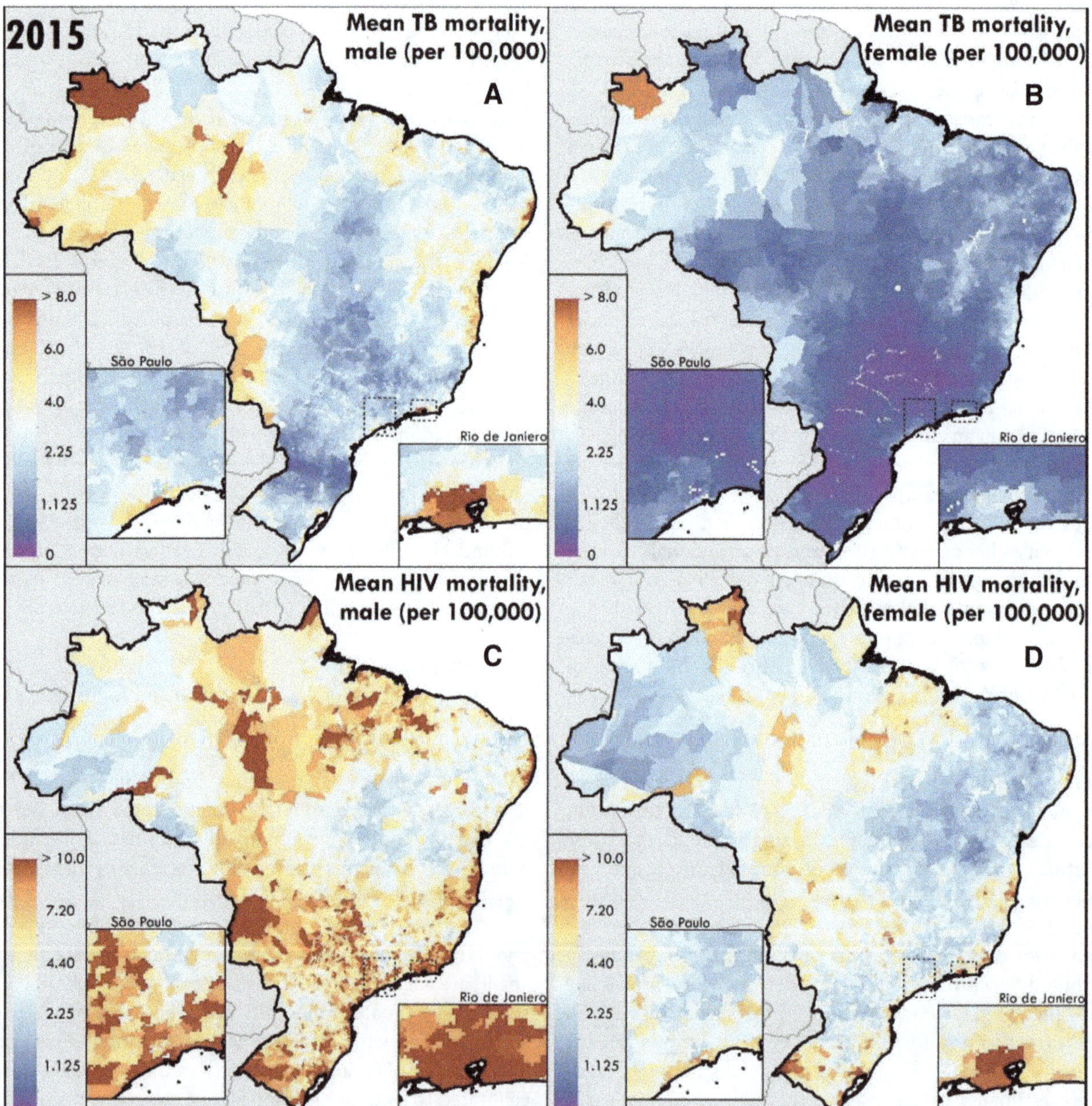

Fig. 1 Mean mortality rate per 100,000 population in 2015 for **a** TB among males, **b** TB among females, **c** HIV among males, and **d** HIV among females modelled by municipality in Brazil ($n = 5477$ stable units). All rates are age-standardised and calibrated to the Global Burden of Diseases Study 2016

municipalities demonstrated increases in HIV mortality during this period, while TB mortality declined in nearly all municipalities (Fig. 2).

The municipalities with mortality rates in the 90th percentile nationally for TB and HIV had mortality rates more than three times higher than those in the 10th percentile nationally (Additional file 1: Table S6). For TB, nearly 70% of municipalities with male mortality rates and more than 75% of municipalities with female mortality rates greater than the 90th percentile in 2001 remained in the 90th percentile in 2015 (Fig. 2, Additional file 1: Table S6). The highest-burden municipalities were less constant for HIV mortality; between 55% and 61% of the municipalities with male or female mortality rates greater than the 90th percentile in 2001 remained in the 90th percentile in 2015 (Fig. 2, Additional file 1: Table S6). TB mortality in persons without HIV and HIV mortality exhibited somewhat different spatial patterns in 2015, with high burdens of TB mortality in persons without HIV infection in the north-western Amazon regions. The joint burdens of TB in persons without HIV infection and HIV mortality were high in the large coastal cities, and the northern states of

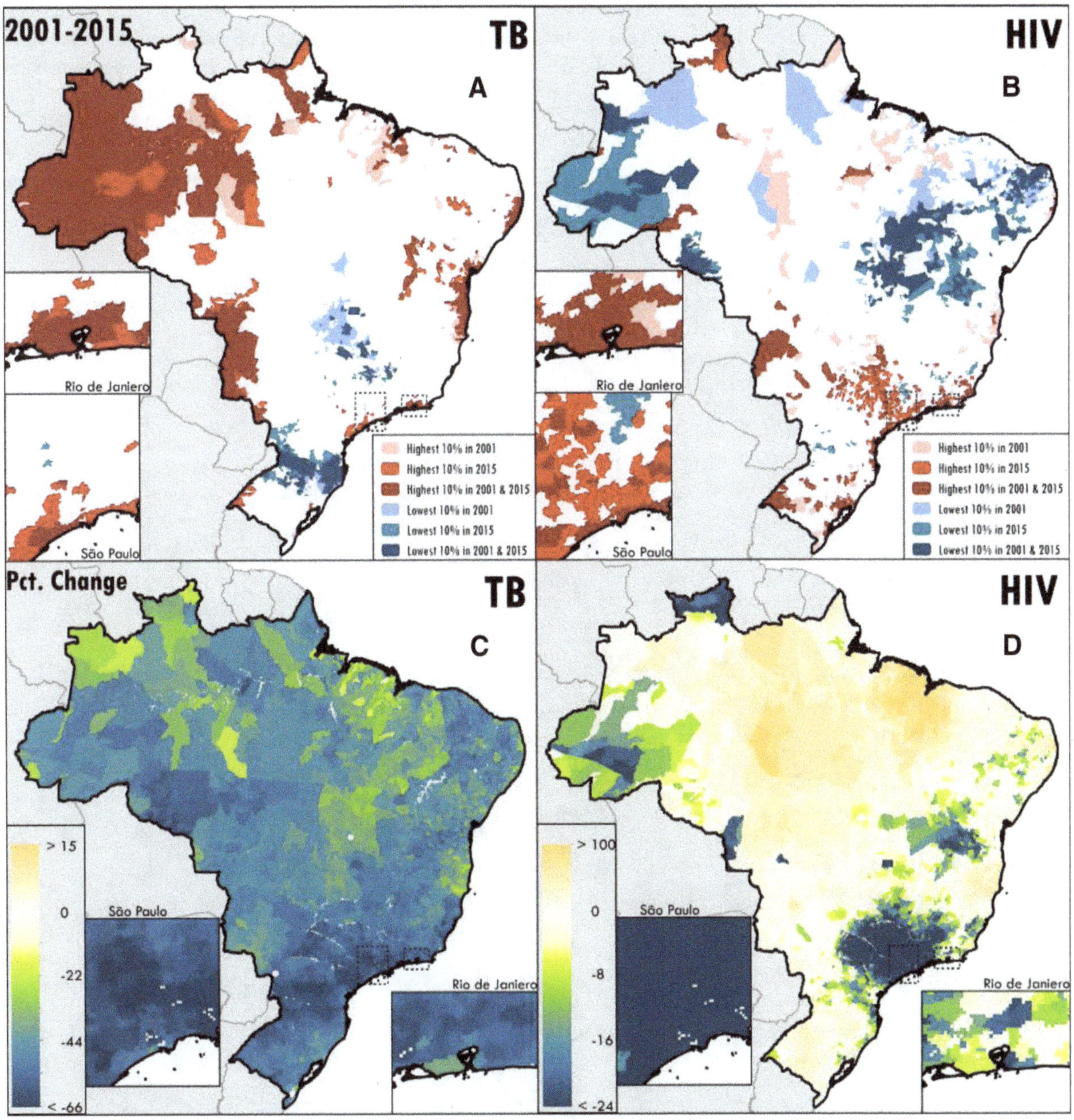

Fig. 2 Age-standardised mortality for **a** TB and **b** HIV in highest-burden versus lowest-burden municipalities in select years. Percent change in age-standardised mortality rate between 2001 and 2015 for **c** TB and **d** HIV by municipality in Brazil

Amapa and Maranhao (Fig. 3). HIV mortality was also high in inland municipalities in Sao Paulo state, which demonstrated relatively lower TB mortality burden in persons without HIV infection (Fig. 3).

Mortality variation by municipalities within states

TB and HIV mortality varied between municipalities located in the same state (Additional file 1: Figure S4). State-level TB mortality rate ratios for municipalities in the 90th percentile versus those in the 10th percentile varied from 1.4 in Acre to 2.9 in Minas Gerais for males and 1.4 in Rio Grande do Norte to 2.3 in Minas Gerais and Rio de Janeiro for females in 2001. They ranged from 1.6 in Piaui and Goias to 3.3 in Rio de Janiero for males and 1.5 in Amapa, Rio Grande do Norte, and Paraiba to 3.1 in Mato Grosso do Sul for females in 2015. There was an overall trend toward increasing inequality within states over time (Fig. 4a). State-level HIV mortality rate ratios for municipalities in the 90th percentile versus those in the 10th percentile varied from 1.8 in Piaui to 3.4 in Rio Grande do Sul for males and 1.4 in Rio Grande do Norte and Piaui to 3.1 in Santa Catarina for females in 2001. They ranged from 2.0 in Rio Grande do Norte to 4.2 in Pernambuco for males and from 1.4 in Amapa to 3.7 in Pernambuco for females in 2015. There was also increasing inequality within states over time for HIV (Fig. 4b).

Case fatality ratios for TB in all forms

National TB case fatality ratios, including TB in PLHIV, ranged from 11% to 17% for males and 8% to 11% for females with decreasing values over time (Additional file 1: Figure S7). The proportion of municipalities meeting the WHO End TB Strategy target of a case fatality less than 10%, for males versus females, respectively, was 15% and 40% aggregated over years 2001–2005, 28% and 48% over 2006–2010, and 36% and 54% over 2011–2014. Figure 5 shows the geographic pattern of TB case fatality ratios over this period.

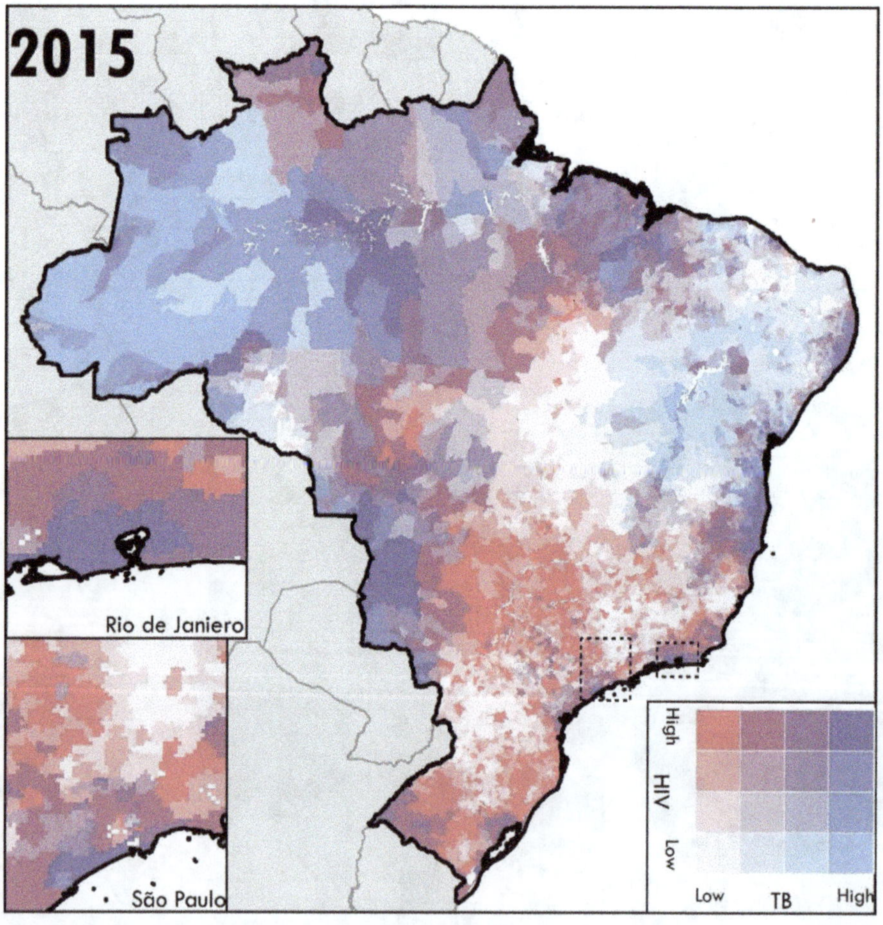

Fig. 3 Joint burdens of mortality due to HIV (including TB deaths in people living with HIV) and TB in persons without HIV infection by Brazilian municipality in 2015

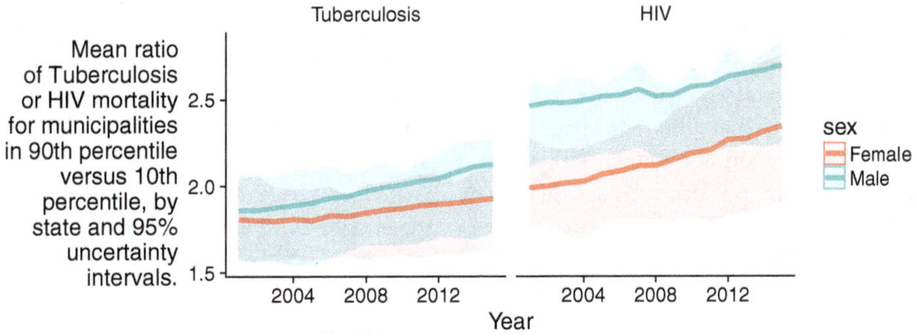

Fig. 4 Mean ratio of TB or HIV mortality for municipalities in 90th percentile versus 10th percentile, by state, with 95% uncertainty intervals

Relationships with covariates

Greater population coverage of Family Health programme teams was associated with lower TB and HIV mortality (Additional file 1: Table S7). Higher population income was associated with lower TB mortality but higher HIV mortality. Several covariates were associated with higher rates of TB and HIV mortality, including greater household crowding, population density, outdoor air pollution, population literacy, proportion of the male or female population in prison, and higher air temperature.

Discussion

Despite marked progress nationally in reducing deaths due to TB and concentrated gains for HIV, substantial inequality in TB and HIV burden are apparent at each geographic level of analysis. Trends in within-state variation for TB were driven by faster mortality reductions in the lowest-burden municipalities relative to slower improvement in the highest-burden areas, the majority of which remained in the highest-burden decile at the end of the 15-year interval. HIV mortality declines in highly populated, high-burden areas drove national-level declines, but the majority of municipalities demonstrated an increase in HIV mortality rate during this period, which was also observed in prior studies [38]. Evaluation of the municipalities with the greatest mortality improvements may identify successful strategies that could be extended to areas experiencing increases or slower declines.

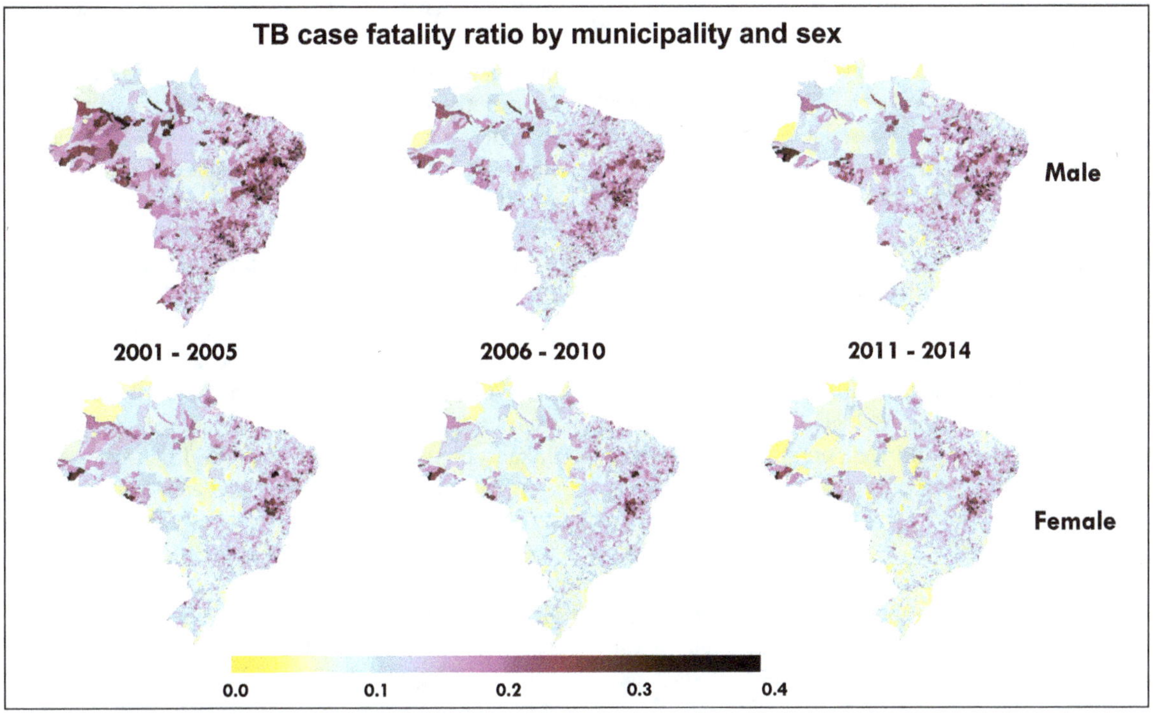

Fig. 5 Age-standardised TB all-forms case fatality ratio by municipality and sex. Mapped values are means per year bin. TB all-forms estimation includes persons with and without HIV infection. Estimates are calibrated to the Global Burden of Diseases Study 2016

Mortality estimates disaggregated by sex revealed differences in TB and HIV burden and geographic distribution. Consistent with known TB and HIV epidemiology, we found a greater burden of TB and HIV mortality in males than in females, but also somewhat different spatial patterns by sex [28, 39]. Incarceration is a known risk factor for TB infection, with prisoners (pessoas privadas de liberdade) in Brazil having an estimated TB notification rate more than 30 times that of the non-incarcerated population [40]. HIV prevalence is also higher in Brazilian inmates than in the non-incarcerated population [41–43]. Men comprise more than 90% of the Brazilian prison population. Municipalities with large prison populations, such as several in Sao Paulo state, stand out in the maps showing results for males as having a higher TB incidence and HIV mortality than neighbouring municipalities. In contrast, municipalities where females were at greatest risk for HIV and TB mortality were concentrated along the national border areas and in the interior Amazon.

National-level case fatality ratios for TB improved over the period of this analysis. However, broader efforts are also needed, as only half of municipalities achieved a WHO End TB Strategy case fatality ratio target of < 10% among females and just over one-third of municipalities achieved it among males in the final period of the analysis between 2011 and 2014. Nearly twice as many municipalities achieved the WHO target for females than for males, indicating a critical need for TB treatment completion strategies that successfully engage men. Underreporting of TB case notifications could bias these estimates downward; however, this effect is likely to be small in later years, when reporting completeness is estimated at more than 90% [1]. There was less apparent geographic patterning for case fatality than for TB or HIV mortality, but the burden of higher case fatality ratios appeared to shift from coastal areas to more inland areas over the analysis period.

While increased funds are required to maintain gains and further improve health and equality, congress approved Constitutional Amendment 95 in December 2016, restricting funds allocated to the health sector and providing no real increase in health funding for the next 20 years [44]. This austerity has also extended to other sectors impacting health and wellbeing, including education and public utilities such as sanitation. These policies could stall the important progress made in Brazil over the period of this study.

This work extends previous efforts to model subnational TB and HIV burden by generating estimates that are both nationally comprehensive and fine-scale. It supports calls to collect and analyse TB and HIV data with high spatial resolution in order to inform interventions that are most appropriate to the transmission dynamics in particular settings [45]. Knowledge of the local variation in TB and HIV burden can inform programmatic interventions to improve health outcomes [16]. TB interventions, such as active case finding and mobile testing units, can be resource-intensive and are utilised most effectively when prioritised to high-burden areas [46]. Subnational differences in HIV burden have also been used to develop locally tailored strategies for HIV prevention and elimination [25, 47–49]. However, the benefits of highly geographically resolved disease burden estimation should be weighed against the risk of potentially identifying individuals if analyses of exceptionally rare outcomes are carried out over very small areas.

Limitations

There are several limitations to this analysis. While adult mortality data in Brazil are assessed to be complete for the period of this analysis, child mortality data are estimated to be < 95% complete in the vital registration system [50]. Other national-level analyses have included additional data sources at a different spatial resolution such as household surveys [51]. Due to the complexity of integrating different data types, only vital registration data were included in this analysis. However, calibrating these estimates to GBD, which includes survey data in all-cause mortality estimation, reduces the undercounting of deaths. Deaths in children under the age of 15 constitute a small proportion of TB (1.6%) and HIV (7%) deaths in Brazil during this period, so the spatial effect of this difference in data sources is not expected to be large. Similarly, TB cases may be under-ascertained in the case notification system. While the overall completeness of TB case notification is estimated currently to be greater than 90%, completeness of reporting may vary spatially [1]. Future work may assess whether factors such as treatment-seeking behaviour and reporting completeness can be used to improve modelling of TB incidence from case notifications.

HIV and TB are under-ascertained as causes of death, and TB is under-ascertained as a contributing cause of death among persons with HIV infection [52]. The GBD mortality redistribution method attempts to correct for these biases. Other correction methods include linkage analysis of HIV and TB surveillance systems [27], or linkage of diagnoses made at health facility encounters with information recorded on death certificates. These could be pursued as additional methods to improve ascertainment of TB and HIV deaths.

Future directions

There are several additional future directions for this work. First, while the causes of TB mortality and TB incidence are further broken down in GBD analyses into drug-susceptible TB, multidrug-resistant TB and extensively drug-resistant TB, data were not available at the geographic scale of this study to inform analysis by drug resistance categories. Additional geographic detail in data sources would facilitate analysis by drug resistance categories. Second, climatologic variables were included in the TB models as an exploratory analysis due to postulated relationships between air temperature, wind speed and TB transmission [22, 53]. Relationships with these factors may be tested in future spatial models in order to potentially improve estimation of TB burden in areas with minimal health surveillance data. Third, a similar small area estimation approach could be used to estimate all-cause and cause-specific mortality due to other causes at the municipal level in Brazil. Finally, this small area estimation approach to spatial mapping of HIV and TB mortality could be extended to other nations with well-functioning vital registration systems.

Conclusion

Mortality due to TB and HIV exhibited nearly as much relative variation within Brazilian states as within the nation as a whole. This demonstrates the role for increasing geographic detail in burden estimation to guide precision public health responses. Fewer than half of municipalities met the WHO End TB Strategy target for a case fatality rate of < 10%, indicating priority areas for improvement in order to achieve international targets and improve health equity.

Abbreviations

GBD: Global Burden of Diseases; HIV: human immunodeficiency virus; ICD: International Statistical Classification of Diseases; PLHIV: people living with HIV; TB: tuberculosis; UI: uncertainty interval; WHO: World Health Organization

Funding

This study was supported by grant OPP1132415 from the Bill & Melinda Gates Foundation.

Authors' contributions

JMR, FMS and SIH conceived and planned the study. JMR, LE and NJH prepared tables and figures. MHB provided project coordination. All authors provided intellectual inputs into aspects of this study. JMR wrote the first draft of the manuscript, and all authors contributed to subsequent revisions. All authors read and approved the final manuscript.

Competing interests

The authors declare that they have no competing interests.

Author details

[1]Division of Allergy and Infectious Diseases, Department of Medicine, University of Washington, Seattle, Washington, USA. [2]Institute for Health Metrics and Evaluation, University of Washington, 2301 5th Ave Suite 600, Seattle, WA 98121, USA. [3]Department of Public Health, University of Brasilia, Distrito Federal, Brazil. [4]Department of Health Surveillance, Ministry of Health, Brasilia, Brazil.

References

1. World Health Organization. Global Tuberculosis Report 2017. Geneva: WHO; 2017.
2. de Andrade LOM, Pellegrini Filho A, Solar O, Rígoli F, de Salazar LM, Serrate PC-F, et al. Social determinants of health, universal health coverage, and sustainable development: case studies from Latin American countries. Lancet. 2015;385:1343–51.
3. Monteiro CA, Conde WL, Popkin BM. Income-specific trends in obesity in Brazil: 1975-2003. Am J Public Health. 2007;97:1808–12.
4. França EB, Passos VM de A, Malta DC, Duncan BB, ALP R, Guimarães MDC, et al. Cause-specific mortality for 249 causes in Brazil and states during 1990-2015: a systematic analysis for the global burden of disease study 2015. Popul Health Metr. 2017;15:39.
5. World Health Organization. World AIDS Day Around the World. http://www.who.int/campaigns/aids-day/2017/en/. Accessed 26 Jan 2018
6. Snyder RE, Jaimes G, Riley LW, Faerstein E, Corburn J. A comparison of social and spatial determinants of health between formal and informal settlements in a large metropolitan setting in Brazil. J Urban Health Bull N Y Acad Med. 2014;91:432–45.
7. de Almeida Wda S, Szwarcwald CL. Infant mortality and geographic access to childbirth in Brazilian municipalities. Rev Saude Publica. 2012;46:68–76.
8. Rasella D, Aquino R, Barreto ML. Impact of income inequality on life expectancy in a highly unequal developing country: the case of Brazil. J Epidemiol Community Health. 2013;67:661–6.
9. Ferreira DN, Matos DL, de Loyola Filho AI. Absence of routine medical consultation among hypertensive and/or diabetic elders: an epidemiological study based on the Brazilian National Household Survey 2008. Rev Bras Epidemiol Braz J Epidemiol. 2015;18:578–94.
10. Teixeira TRA, Gracie R, Malta MS, Bastos FI. Social geography of AIDS in Brazil: identifying patterns of regional inequalities. Cad Saude Publica. 2014;30:259–71.
11. Correia Sacchi FP, Tatara MB, Camioli de Lima C, Ferreia da Silva L, Cunha EA, Simonsen V, et al. Genetic clustering of tuberculosis in an indigenous community of Brazil. Am J Trop Med Hyg. 2018;98(2):372–5.
12. Bishai WR, Graham NM, Harrington S, Pope DS, Hooper N, Astemborski J, et al. Molecular and geographic patterns of tuberculosis transmission after 15 years of directly observed therapy. JAMA. 1998;280:1679–84.
13. Tanser F, Bärnighausen T, Cooke GS, Newell M-L. Localized spatial clustering of HIV infections in a widely disseminated rural South African epidemic. Int J Epidemiol. 2009;38:1008–16.
14. Rasella D, Aquino R, Santos CAT, Paes-Sousa R, Barreto ML. Effect of a conditional cash transfer programme on childhood mortality: a nationwide analysis of Brazilian municipalities. Lancet. 2013;382:57–64.
15. Hacker MA, Petersen ML, Enriquez M, Bastos FI. Highly active antiretroviral therapy in Brazil: the challenge of universal access in a context of social inequality. Rev Panam Salud Publica. 2004;16:78–83.
16. Ministry of Health. Brazil Free of Tuberculosis: National Plan for the End of Tuberculosis as a Public Health Problem. Brasilia DF, Brazil. 2017. http://portalarquivos2.saude.gov.br/images/pdf/2017/julho/05/af-miolo-plano-nac-tuberculose-29jun17-grafica.pdf. Accessed 15 Feb 2018.
17. Alves ATJ, Nobre FF. The acquired immunodeficiency syndrome in the state of Rio de Janeiro, Brazil: a spatio-temporal analysis of cases reported in the period 2001-2010. Geospat Health. 2014;8:437–43.
18. Vendramini SHF, Santos NSGMD, Santos M de LSG, Chiaravalloti-Neto F, Ponce MAZ, Gazetta CE, et al. Spatial analysis of tuberculosis/HIV coinfection: its relation with socioeconomic levels in a city in south-eastern Brazil. Rev Soc Bras Med Trop. 2010;43:536–41.
19. de Holanda ER, Galvão MTG, Pedrosa NL, Paiva S de S, de Almeida RLF. Spatial analysis of infection by the human immunodeficiency virus among pregnant women. Rev Lat Am Enfermagem. 2015;23:441–9.
20. Yamamura M, Santos Neto M, Chiaravalloti Neto F, Arroyo LH, Ramos ACV, de Queiroz AAR, et al. Areas with evidence of equity and their progress on mortality from tuberculosis in an endemic municipality of Southeast Brazil. Infect Dis Poverty. 2017;6:134.
21. Harling G, Castro MC. A spatial analysis of social and economic determinants of tuberculosis in Brazil. Health Place. 2014;25:56–67.
22. Cao K, Yang K, Wang C, Guo J, Tao L, Liu Q, et al. Spatial-temporal epidemiology of tuberculosis in mainland China: an analysis based on Bayesian theory. Int J Environ Res Public Health. 2016;13(5):E469.

23. Jafari-Koshki T, Arsang-Jang S, Raei M. Applying spatiotemporal models to study risk of smear-positive tuberculosis in Iran, 2001-2012. Int J Tuberc Lung Dis. 2015;19:469–74.
24. Sun W, Gong J, Zhou J, Zhao Y, Tan J, Ibrahim AN, et al. A spatial, social and environmental study of tuberculosis in China using statistical and GIS technology. Int J Environ Res Public Health. 2015;12:1425–48.
25. McGillen JB, Anderson S-J, Dybul MR, Hallett TB. Optimum resource allocation to reduce HIV incidence across sub-Saharan Africa: a mathematical modelling study. Lancet HIV. 2016;3:e441–8.
26. Cuadros DF, Li J, Branscum AJ, Akullian A, Jia P, Mziray EN, et al. Mapping the spatial variability of HIV infection in Sub-Saharan Africa: effective information for localized HIV prevention and control. Sci Rep. 2017;7:9093.
27. Carvalho CN, Dourado I, Bierrenbach AL. Underreporting of the tuberculosis and AIDS comorbidity: an application of the linkage method. Rev Saude Publica. 2011;45:548–55.
28. GBD Tuberculosis Collaborators. The global burden of tuberculosis: results from the Global Burden of Disease Study 2015. Lancet Infect Dis. 2018;18(3): 261–84.
29. GBD 2015 HIV Collaborators. Estimates of global, regional, and national incidence, prevalence, and mortality of HIV, 1980–2015: the Global Burden of Disease Study 2015. Lancet HIV. 2016;3:e361–87.
30. World Health Organization. International Statistical Classification of Diseases and Related Health Problems 10th Revision. 2016. http://www.who.int/classifications/icd/icdonlineversions/en/. Accessed 2 Feb 2018.
31. R Core Team. R: A Language and Environment for Statistical Computing. Vienna: Foundation for Statistical Computing; 2015.
32. Ministerio da Saude. Resident Population - Brazil. Ministerio da Saude. http://tabnet.datasus.gov.br/cgi/deftohtm.exe?ibge/cnv/popbr.def. Accessed 24 Apr 2017.
33. GBD 2016 Risk Factors Collaborators. Global, regional, and national comparative risk assessment of 84 behavioural, environmental and occupational, and metabolic risks or clusters of risks, 1990–2016: a systematic analysis for the Global Burden of Disease Study 2016. Lancet. 2017;390:1345–422.
34. GBD 2016 Causes of Death Collaborators. Global, regional, and national age-sex specific mortality for 264 causes of death, 1980–2016: a systematic analysis for the Global Burden of Disease Study 2016. Lancet. 2017;390:1151–210.
35. Naghavi M, Makela S, Foreman K, O'Brien J, Pourmalek F, Lozano R. Algorithms for enhancing public health utility of national causes-of-death data. Popul Health Metr. 2010;8:9.
36. Dwyer-Lindgren L, Bertozzi-Villa A, Stubbs RW, Morozoff C, Kutz MJ, Huynh C, et al. US county-level trends in mortality rates for major causes of death, 1980-2014. JAMA. 2016;316:2385–401.
37. Srebotnjak T, Mokdad AH, Murray CJ. A novel framework for validating and applying standardized small area measurement strategies. Popul Health Metr. 2010;8:26.
38. MDC G, Carneiro M, de Abreu DMX, França EB. HIV/AIDS Mortality in Brazil, 2000–2015: Are there reasons for concern? Rev Bras Epidemiol Braz J Epidemiol. 2017;20(Suppl 01).102–90.
39. Horton KC, MacPherson P, Houben RMGJ, White RG, Corbett EL. Sex differences in tuberculosis burden and notifications in low- and middle-income countries: a systematic review and meta-analysis. PLoS Med. 2016;13:e1002119.
40. Bourdillon PM, Gonçalves CCM, Pelissari DM, Arakaki-Sanchez D, Ko AI, Croda J, et al. Increase in tuberculosis cases among prisoners, Brazil, 2009-20141. Emerg Infect Dis. 2017;23:496–9.
41. Coelho HC, Perdoná GC, Neves FR, Passos ADC. HIV prevalence and risk factors in a Brazilian penitentiary. Cad Saude Publica. 2007;23:2197–204.
42. Catalan-Soares BC, Almeida RT, Carneiro-Proietti AB. Prevalence of HIV-1/2, HTLV-I/II, hepatitis B virus (HBV), hepatitis C virus (HCV), Treponema pallidum and Trypanosoma cruzi among prison inmates at Manhuaçu, Minas Gerais State, Brazil. Rev Soc Bras Med Trop. 2000;33:27–30.
43. Sgarbi RVE, Carbone A da SS, Paião DSG, Lemos EF, Simionatto S, MAM P, et al. A cross-sectional survey of HIV testing and prevalence in twelve Brazilian correctional facilities. PLoS One. 2015;10:e0139487.
44. Federal Legislature of Brazil. Constitutional Amendment Number 95. http://legislacao.planalto.gov.br/legisla/legislacao.nsf/Viw_Identificacao/emc%2095-2016?OpenDocument. Accessed 25 May 2018.
45. Theron G, Jenkins HE, Cobelens F, Abubakar I, Khan AJ, Cohen T, et al. Data for action: collection and use of local data to end tuberculosis. Lancet. 2015; 386:2324–33.
46. Bassett IV, Regan S, Mbonambi H, Blossom J, Bogan S, Bearnot B, et al. Finding HIV in hard to reach populations: mobile HIV testing and geospatial mapping in Umlazi township, Durban, South Africa. AIDS Behav. 2015;19: 1888–95.
47. Anderson S-J, Cherutich P, Kilonzo N, Cremin I, Fecht D, Kimanga D, et al. Maximising the effect of combination HIV prevention through prioritisation of the people and places in greatest need: a modelling study. Lancet. 2014;384:249–56.
48. Coburn BJ, Okano JT, Blower S. Using geospatial mapping to design HIV elimination strategies for sub-Saharan Africa. Sci Transl Med. 2017;9:383.
49. Gerberry DJ, Wagner BG, Garcia-Lerma JG, Heneine W, Blower S. Using geospatial modelling to optimize the rollout of antiretroviral-based pre-exposure HIV interventions in sub-Saharan Africa. Nat Commun. 2014;5:5454.
50. Queiroz BL, Freire FHM de A, Gonzaga MR, de Lima EEC. Completeness of death-count coverage and adult mortality (45q15) for Brazilian states from 1980 to 2010. Rev Bras Epidemiol Braz J Epidemiol. 2017;20(Suppl 01):21–33.
51. França EB, Lansky S, MAS R, Malta DC, França JS, Teixeira R, et al. Leading causes of child mortality in Brazil, in 1990 and 2015: estimates from the Global Burden of Disease study. Rev Bras Epidemiol Braz J Epidemiol. 2017;20(Suppl 01):46–60.
52. Pacheco AG, Saraceni V, Tuboi SH, Lauria LM, Moulton LH, Faulhaber JC, et al. Estimating the extent of underreporting of mortality among HIV-infected individuals in Rio de Janeiro, Brazil. AIDS Res Hum Retroviruses. 2011;27:25–8.
53. Fernandes FM de C, Martins E de S, Pedrosa DMAS, Evangelista M do SN. Relationship between climatic factors and air quality with tuberculosis in the Federal District, Brazil, 2003-2012. Braz J Infect Dis. 2017;21:369–75.

10

Changes in HbA1c and weight, and treatment persistence, over the 18 months following initiation of second-line therapy in patients with type 2 diabetes: results from the United Kingdom Clinical Practice Research Datalink

John Wilding[1*], Thomas Godec[2], Kamlesh Khunti[3], Stuart Pocock[2], Robin Fox[4], Liam Smeeth[2], Per Clauson[5], Peter Fenici[6], Niklas Hammar[5] and Jesús Medina[7]

Abstract

Background: Intensification of metformin monotherapy with additional glucose-lowering drugs is often required in patients with type 2 diabetes (T2D). This study evaluated changes in HbA1c and weight, as well as treatment persistence, associated with different second-line therapies used in UK clinical practice.

Methods: The UK Clinical Practice Research Datalink was used to identify patients with T2D who initiated second-line therapy after metformin monotherapy between 1 August 2013 and 14 June 2016. Treatment persistence and changes in HbA1c and weight were assessed at 6-month intervals up to 18 months.

Results: In total, 9097 patients (mean age 61.2 years, 57.2% men, mean [standard deviation] HbA1c 9.0% [1.8]/ 75 mmol/mol [19.7]) were included in the analysis, with a median 2.3 years between initiating metformin monotherapy and initiating second-line therapy. Patients were stratified according to second-line therapy: metformin in combination with sulfonylurea (SU; $n = 4655$ [51.2%]), a dipeptidyl peptidase-4 inhibitor (DPP-4 inhibitor; $n = 2899$ [31.9%]), or a sodium–glucose cotransporter-2 inhibitor (SGLT-2 inhibitor; $n = 441$ [4.9%]) or other therapies (all other second-line treatments; $n = 1102$ [12.1%]). At 18 months, the cumulative proportion of patients changing treatment was lowest for those who received metformin plus an SGLT-2 inhibitor (42.3%), followed by patients on metformin plus SU or metformin plus a DPP-4 inhibitor (46.8%). HbA1c reductions were seen with all second-line therapies, with an overall mean (standard error) reduction of −1.23% (0.05)/−13.4 mmol/mol (0.5). Changes were directly, but not linearly, related to baseline HbA1c and were greater in those with higher HbA1c at baseline. Weight loss from baseline was greatest in patients treated with metformin plus either an SGLT-2 inhibitor (−4.2 kg) or a DPP-4 inhibitor (−1.5 kg). The highest proportion of patients who achieved the composite outcome of HbA1c reduction ≥ 0.5%, body weight loss ≥ 2.0 kg and treatment persistence for 18 months was observed in those receiving metformin plus an SGLT-2 inhibitor (36.5%).

(Continued on next page)

* Correspondence: j.p.h.wilding@liverpool.ac.uk
[1]University of Liverpool, Liverpool, UK
Full list of author information is available at the end of the article

(Continued from previous page)
Conclusions: In this population-based cohort, all second-line therapies added to metformin monotherapy improved glycaemic control, but the lowest treatment change/discontinuation rate and most sustained weight loss was seen with patients receiving metformin plus an SGLT-2 inhibitor.

Keywords: Clinical practice research datalink (CPRD), Dipeptidyl peptidase-4 inhibitor (DPP-4 inhibitor), HbA1c, Metformin, Second-line therapy, Sodium-glucose cotransporter 2 inhibitor (SGLT-2 inhibitor), Sulfonylurea, Type 2 diabetes (T2D)

Background

Type 2 diabetes (T2D) is a complex chronic condition characterised by increased blood glucose levels and associated with micro- and macrovascular complications. In 2015, an estimated 415 million people globally had diabetes, with the vast majority (~ 90%) having T2D [1]. Optimal glycaemic control (i.e. attaining recommended treatment targets) has been shown to reduce the incidence of diabetes-related complications, microvascular disease and myocardial infarction in the large, long-term United Kingdom Prospective Diabetes Study [2, 3].

Along with lifestyle modifications, current guidelines recommend the use of metformin as the preferred first-line glucose-lowering therapy in patients with T2D [4]. Metformin has a low risk of hypoglycaemia and is weight neutral, with no increased risk of or benefit against adverse cardiovascular events [5, 6]. However, in view of its progressive nature, the majority of patients with T2D require treatment intensification from metformin monotherapy to achieve and maintain recommended HbA1c targets [6]. Second-line agents approved for dual therapy with metformin in the UK include sulfonylureas (SUs), thiazolidinediones (TZDs), dipeptidyl peptidase-4 (DPP-4) inhibitors, sodium–glucose cotransporter-2 (SGLT-2) inhibitors, glucagon-like peptide-1 (GLP-1) receptor agonists and basal insulin analogues. The National Institute for Health and Care Excellence (NICE) guidelines and the position statement of the American Diabetes Association and the European Association for the Study of Diabetes recommend that initial treatment intensification after failure of metformin monotherapy should consist of dual therapy with one of the following agents: DPP-4 inhibitors, pioglitazone, SUs or SGLT-2 inhibitors [4, 6]. The choice of second-line agent should be based upon patient-specific considerations to minimise side effects whilst reducing HbA1c levels [7].

Established agents such as SUs are highly efficacious but are associated with weight gain and may cause hypoglycaemia [8]. TZDs do not induce hypoglycaemia, but tend to cause weight gain and fluid retention, and have been associated with an increased risk of heart failure [6, 9]. Unlike SUs and TZDs, DPP-4 inhibitors do not lead to weight gain and a have minimal risk for hypoglycaemia, comparable to metformin [10, 11]. Likewise, SGLT-2 inhibitors do not induce hypoglycaemia and bring the added benefits of reductions in body weight and blood pressure [12–14]. Results from the EMPA-REG OUTCOME [15] and CANVAS [16] randomised controlled trials and the CVD-REAL observational studies [17–19] have shown a reduced risk for major adverse cardiovascular events, hospitalisation for heart failure or death in patients with T2D treated with SGLT-2 inhibitors, with additional studies ongoing [20]. GLP-1 receptor agonists are associated with low risk for hypoglycaemia and significant reductions in body weight [21]. GLP-1 receptor agonists are not generally recommended as a second-line therapy in the UK [22], and their effect on adverse cardiovascular outcomes is inconsistent. While liraglutide has been associated with a reduction in adverse cardiovascular outcomes in patients with T2D at high cardiovascular risk, a neutral effect on cardiovascular outcomes has been observed with other GLP-1 receptor agonists [23–26]. Of all the glucose-lowering agents, insulin has the greatest HbA1c-lowering potential, although it carries the highest risk of hypoglycaemia and is associated with weight gain [6, 21].

The NICE guidelines and the position statement of the American Diabetes Association and the European Association for the Study of Diabetes recommend that therapies should be reviewed every 3–6 months, and therapy escalated if HbA1c targets are not met. Despite these recommendations, therapeutic inertia is still common, with the average time to initiate second-line therapy in the UK being between 1.6 to 2.9 years after HbA1c levels had reached those recommended for treatment intensification (HbA1c > 7.5% [58 mmol/mol]) [27]. Likewise, in patients from North America, Europe and Israel receiving one oral anti-diabetic drug, second-line treatment intensification occurs a median of 0.3–2.7 years following above-target HbA1c levels [28]. This may carry grave consequences for patients who have poor glycaemic control for extended periods and may result in higher risk of cardiovascular events and other late-stage diabetes complications [29]. On the other hand, patients who receive earlier treatment intensification have greater HbA1c reductions and a higher probability of attaining target HbA1c levels, as well as a lower risk of micro- and macrovascular complications, compared with patients with delayed intensification [2, 3, 30–32].

Real-world clinical-practice data are an important source of evidence for clinicians considering second-line therapies for the treatment of T2D. This study assessed the clinical outcomes of patients initiated on second-line glucose-lowering therapies, using data from the UK Clinical Practice Research Datalink (CPRD). The impact of these second-line therapies on HbA1c, weight and treatment persistence was evaluated over 18 months in patients who had received first-line metformin monotherapy. The data in this manuscript were accepted as an abstract for - and presented at - the 53rd Annual Meeting of the European Association for the Study of Diabetes [33].

Methods

Data source

This retrospective study was performed using data retrieved from the UK CPRD, which contains anonymised longitudinal primary-care medical records from over 14 million patients and is broadly representative of the UK population [34]. The study protocol was approved by the independent scientific advisory committee of the UK CPRD (protocol 16_045R).

Study population

The cohort comprised patients with T2D aged ≥ 18 years who initiated a second-line therapy between 1 August 2013 and 14 June 2016. Only patients who received metformin monotherapy as first-line therapy were included in the analysis, irrespective of the duration of metformin treatment before initiation of second-line therapy and HbA1c values at the time of treatment initiation. Patients were grouped according to second-line therapy, which could include any glucose-lowering medication, oral or injectable, given either as an add-on to metformin or as a switch to a single agent or in combination with other agents after discontinuing metformin. For this analysis, patients were stratified into one of the following groups: metformin in combination with an SU (glibenclamide, glipizide, gliclazide, glimepiride, tolbutamide or chlorpropamide), metformin in combination with a DPP-4 inhibitor (sitagliptin, vildagliptin, saxagliptin, linagliptin or alogliptin), metformin in combination with an SGLT-2 inhibitor (canagliflozin, dapagliflozin or empagliflozin), or metformin in combination with any other second-line therapy (including pioglitazone, a GLP-1 receptor agonist, an insulin, repaglinide, natiglinide, acarbose) or another second-line therapy following metformin discontinuation.

Study design

This was an observational study comparing the use of second-line glucose-lowering agents in patients with T2D who received metformin as their first-line therapy. The index date was the date of second-line therapy initiation, and baseline measurements of HbA1c and weight closest to the index date (within 180 days prior to the index date and 2 weeks after the index date) were selected for analysis. The follow-up periods were defined as 6, 12 and 18 months, with measurements closest to each time point (±90 days) selected for the analysis. To represent an on-treatment population, data were analysed for patients who were receiving their index second-line treatment at each time point (i.e. had not intensified, switched or discontinued treatment) and who had data available for the variable of interest (HbA1c or weight) at baseline and the time point being analysed. Discontinuation of second-line therapy was defined as cessation of treatment for 184 days or more.

Study outcomes

Index treatment persistence over the 18-month study period was evaluated. HbA1c and weight were evaluated for all patients who were on-treatment and had data available at both baseline and the end of the corresponding follow-up period. A composite outcome assessed treatment success, defined as the number of patients who had not discontinued their index therapy, achieved HbA1c reductions ≥ 0.5% (5.5 mmol/mol) and weight reductions ≥ 2 kg at 18 months. The individual components of the composite endpoint were also evaluated for all patients who had HbA1c and weight data available at baseline and at 18 months.

Statistical analysis

The characteristics of the study population were summarised with descriptive statistics (number, mean, standard deviation [SD], standard error [SE], median and interquartile range [IQR]). Demographics and baseline characteristics, as well as changes in HbA1c and weight over time, are presented separately for the different second-line treatment groups. Mean (SE) HbA1c and weight at baseline and at the 6-, 12- and 18-month time points were used to calculate crude changes over each 6-month period. For each second-line therapy group, the change in HbA1c and weight at each time point was determined using analysis of covariance (ANCOVA) models, adjusted for baseline measurements using variance-weighted least-squares regression estimation.

The relationship between baseline measurements and the changes at each subsequent time point was explored to determine the best way to adjust for baseline measurements. The relationship between baseline HbA1c and change in HbA1c was not strictly linear and was modelled using linear splines as two straight lines connected at a baseline HbA1c of 9% (75 mmol/mol) [28]. The relationship between baseline body mass index (BMI) and change in BMI showed no evidence of departure from linearity and was, therefore, modelled in a linear manner.

The composite outcome (number [%] of patients who had not discontinued index therapy, achieved HbA1c reductions of ≥ 0.5% [5.5 mmol/mol] and weight reductions of ≥ 2 kg at 18 months) was tabulated by second-line treatment type.

Results

Patient populations

From the initial 407,700 patients screened, we identified 9097 patients with T2D who had received first-line metformin monotherapy and were initiated on second-line treatment (Additional file 1: Figure S1). The median (IQR) time between initiating metformin and initiating second-line therapy was 2.3 (0.85–4.72) years. The most common second-line treatments were metformin plus an SU ($n = 4655$; 51.2%), metformin plus a DPP-4 inhibitor ($n = 2899$; 31.9%) and metformin plus a SGLT-2 inhibitor ($n = 441$; 4.8%). The remaining 1102 patients (12.1%) were on a variety of second-line treatments and were combined into the other category. This included monotherapy with an SU ($n = 397$; 4.4%), monotherapy with a DPP-4 inhibitor ($n = 212$; 2.3%), monotherapy with any other agent ($n = 38$; 0.4%), insulin either as mono- or combination therapy ($n = 46$; 0.5%) or any other drug combinations not specified above ($n = 409$; 4.5%).

The baseline characteristics of the patients included in the analysis are shown in Table 1. Overall 57.2% of the patients were male, their mean age was 61.2 years and the mean HbA1c was 9.0% (75 mmol/mol). The baseline characteristics varied among the groups, with higher mean baseline HbA1c values observed for patients who received metformin plus an SU or metformin plus an SGLT-2 inhibitor, compared with patients who received metformin plus a DPP-4 inhibitor or other therapies. Patients who were initiated on second-line therapy with an SGLT-2 inhibitor had the highest mean BMI and body weight values, with patients who were initiated on second-line therapy with a DPP-4 inhibitor having the second highest values. Furthermore, patients who were initiated on second-line treatment with an SGLT-2 inhibitor were younger and had the shortest duration between initiation of metformin and initiation of second-line therapy. Patients in the other therapy group had the longest interval between initiation of first- and second-line therapies.

Persistence of second-line treatment

The proportion of patients who changed or discontinued their index second-line therapy over the 18-month follow-up period for each treatment group is shown in Fig. 1. Overall, the cumulative proportion changing therapy (including discontinuation, switch or intensification) was 21.6%, 34.8% and 47.3% at 6, 12 and 18 months of follow-up, respectively.

Across all time points, fewer patients receiving metformin plus an SGLT-2 inhibitor changed therapy, with 42.3% cumulative proportion of patients changing treatment by 18 months. For patients receiving metformin plus either an SU or a DPP-4 inhibitor, the cumulative proportion of patients changing treatment for both therapies was 46.8%. Patients receiving other regimens changed treatment most frequently, with 52.8% cumulative proportion of patients changing treatment at 18 months, a significantly higher incidence compared with that seen in patients receiving metformin plus either an SU or a DPP-4 inhibitor ($p = 0.003$).

Changes in HbA1c

For all patients initiated on second-line therapy (including those who subsequently discontinued, switched or intensified treatment), the mean unadjusted changes in HbA1c were −1.26% (−13.8 mmol/mol; $n = 6042$), −1.16% (−12.7 mmol/mol; $n = 4945$) and −0.99% (−10.8 mmol/mol; $n = 3665$) at 6, 12 and 18 months, respectively. When only patients who were on-treatment (i.e. had not intensified, switched or discontinued second-line treatment) were included in the analysis, the mean unadjusted changes in HbA1c were −1.38% (−15.1 mmol/mol; $n = 4480$), −1.32% (−14.4 mmol/mol; $n = 3080$) and – 1.20% (−13.1 mmol/mol; $n = 1755$) at 6, 12 and 18 months, respectively.

Analysis of HbA1c levels at 6 months shows that patients with lower baseline HbA1c levels experienced smaller changes from baseline, and fewer achieved HbA1c reductions ≥ 0.5% (5.5 mmol/mol) compared with patients with a higher baseline HbA1c (Table 2). The change in HbA1c levels at 6 and 18 months correlated with baseline HbA1c levels, and the changes were more marked in patients with baseline HbA1c levels ≥ 9.0% (75 mmol/mol; $p < 0.001$; Fig. 2). At 6 months, patients who had baseline HbA1c levels < 9.0% (75 mmol/mol), had an expected additional HbA1c decrease of 0.48% (5.2 mmol/mol) for every 1.0% (10.9 mmol/mol) increment in baseline HbA1c, whereas patients with baseline HbA1c levels ≥ 9.0% had an expected additional HbA1c decrease of 0.75% (8.2 mmol/mol) for every 1.0% increment. This correlation was maintained throughout the 18 months of therapy ($p = 0.015$).

The mean changes in HbA1c over 18 months, after adjustment for baseline values for each second-line treatment group, are shown in Table 3. At 6 months, patients receiving metformin plus an SU or metformin plus an SGLT-2 inhibitor had the greatest mean reductions in HbA1c (−1.33% [−14.5 mmol/mol] and – 1.26% [−13.8 mmol/mol], respectively), and, combined, these reductions were significantly greater ($p < 0.001$) than those observed in patients receiving metformin plus a DPP-4 inhibitor or other therapies

Table 1 Demographic and baseline characteristics

	MET + SU N = 4655	MET + DPP-4i N = 2899	MET + SGLT-2i N = 441	Other* N = 1102	Overall N = 9097
Male, *n* (%)	2679 (57.6)	1704 (58.8)	266 (60.3)	551 (50.0)	5200 (57.2)
Age (years), mean (SD)	61.54 (12.97)	60.81 (12.34)	55.05 (10.14)	62.81 (14.85)	61.15 (12.98)
<50	892 (19.2%)	544 (18.8%)	128 (29.0%)	210 (19.1%)	1774 (19.5%)
50 to <60	1150 (24.7%)	805 (27.8%)	165 (37.4%)	241 (21.9%)	2361 (26.0%)
60 to <70	1291 (27.7%)	842 (29.0%)	119 (27.0%)	275 (25.0%)	2527 (27.8%)
≥70	1322 (28.4%)	708 (24.4%)	29 (6.6%)	376 (34.1%)	2435 (26.8%)
HbA1c (%), mean (SD)	9.19 (1.88)	8.75 (1.50)	9.07 (1.58)	8.72 (1.91)	8.98 (1.77)[†]
<7	283 (6.2%)	147 (5.1%)	20 (4.6%)	164 (15.2%)	614 (6.9%)
7 to <8	971 (21.3%)	829 (28.8%)	100 (23.0%)	276 (25.5%)	2176 (24.3%)
8 to <9	1245 (27.3%)	923 (32.1%)	120 (27.7%)	254 (23.5%)	2542 (28.4%)
9 to <10	783 (17.2%)	468 (16.3%)	84 (19.4%)	152 (14.1%)	1487 (16.6%)
10 to <11	491 (10.8%)	244 (8.5%)	54 (12.4%)	92 (8.5%)	881 (9.8%)
≥11	787 (17.3%)	266 (9.3%)	56 (12.9%)	144 (13.3%)	1253 (14.0%)
HbA1c (mmol/mol), mean (SD)	77 (20.6)	72 (16.4)	76 (17.3)	72 (20.9)	75 (19.3)[†]
BMI (kg/m^2, mean (SD)	31.78 (6.50)	33.21 (6.56)	36.56 (6.98)	33.12 (7.93)	32.64 (6.82)[†]
<20	43 (0.9%)	8 (0.3%)	0	24 (2.2%)	75 (0.8%)
20 to <25	498 (10.9%)	194 (6.8%)	8 (1.8%)	106 (9.8%)	806 (9.0%)
25 to <30	1457 (31.9%)	795 (27.7%)	65 (14.8%)	273 (25.2%)	2590 (28.9%)
30 to <35	1366 (29.9%)	887 (31.0%)	129 (29.5%)	301 (27.8%)	2683 (30.0%)
≥35	1208 (26.4%)	982 (34.3%)	236 (53.9%)	379 (35.0%)	2805 (31.3%)
Weight (kg), mean (SD)	90.97 (21.00)	96.00 (21.50)	107.30 (22.87)	93.63 (25.55)	93.70 (22.18)[†]
<60	189 (4.1%)	63 (2.2%)	2 (0.5%)	51 (4.7%)	305 (3.4%)
60 to <80	1227 (26.6%)	578 (20.1%)	40 (9.1%)	298 (27.3%)	2143 (23.8%)
80 to <100	1837 (39.9%)	1133 (39.3%)	127 (28.9%)	361 (33.1%)	3458 (38.4%)
100 to <120	954 (20.7%)	728 (25.3%)	166 (37.7%)	232 (21.3%)	2080 (23.1%)
≥120	399 (8.7%)	378 (13.1%)	105 (23.9%)	149 (13.7%)	1031 (11.4%)
Time since diagnosis (years), median (IQR)	4.00 (1.57–7.20)	4.25 (1.88–7.21)	3.30 (1.47–5.55)	4.64 (1.94–8.05)	4.10 (1.70–7.22)
<6 months	542 (11.6%)	237 (8.2%)	40 (9.1%)	74 (6.7%)	893 (9.8%)
6 months to <1 year	283 (6.1%)	174 (6.0%)	35 (7.9%)	68 (6.2%)	560 (6.2%)
1 to <3 years	1076 (23.1%)	658 (22.7%)	129 (29.3%)	250 (22.7%)	2113 (23.2%)
3 to <5 years	839 (18.0%)	591 (20.4%)	104 (23.6%)	194 (17.6%)	1728 (19.0%)
≥5 years	1915 (41.1%)	1239 (42.7%)	133 (30.2%)	516 (46.8%)	3803 (41.8%)
Time since initiation of first-line therapy (years), median (IQR)	2.20 (0.72–4.65)	2.62 (1.02–4.89)	2.05 (0.85–4.02)	2.30 (0.89–4.84)	2.33 (0.85–4.72)
<6 months	953 (20.5%)	427 (14.7%)	71 (16.1%)	171 (15.5%)	1622 (17.8%)
6 months to <1 year	474 (10.2%)	280 (9.7%)	50 (11.3%)	124 (11.3%)	928 (10.2%)
1 to <3 years	1346 (28.9%)	884 (30.5%)	157 (35.6%)	346 (31.4%)	2733 (30.0%)
3 to <5 years	840 (18.1%)	613 (21.2%)	89 (20.2%)	199 (18.1%)	1741 (19.1%)
≥5 years	1042 (22.4%)	695 (24.0%)	74 (16.8%)	262 (23.8%)	2073 (22.8%)

BMI body mass index, *DPP-4i* dipeptidyl peptidase-4 inhibitor, *HbA1c* glycated haemoglobin, *IQR* interquartile range, *MET* metformin, *SD* standard deviation, *SGLT-2i* sodium-glucose cotransporter 2 inhibitor, *SU* sulfonylurea

*Includes all other add-on combinations to metformin, combinations without metformin and other monotherapies

†Baseline HbA1c, BMI and weight were missing for 144, 138 and 80 patients, respectively

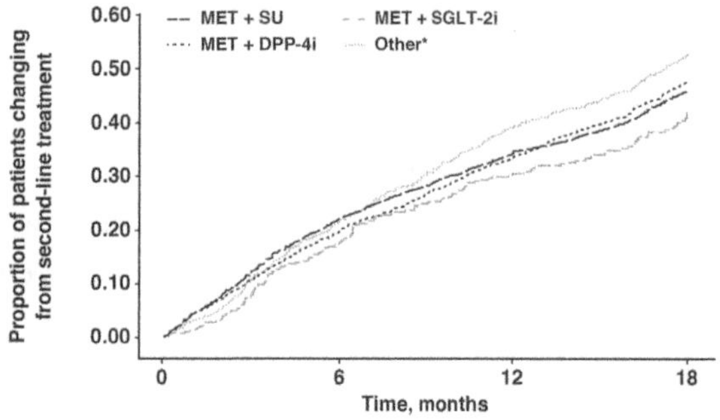

Numbers at risk	0	6	12	18
——	4655	3300	2419	1586
······	2899	2143	1585	969
– –	441	314	233	134
······	1102	789	541	342

Fig. 1 Cumulative proportion of patients changing second-line therapy over time according to treatment group. Frequency is shown as proportion of 1. DPP-4i dipeptidyl peptidase-4 inhibitor, MET metformin, SGLT-2i sodium–glucose cotransporter 2 inhibitor, SU sulfonylurea. *Includes all other add-on combinations to metformin, combinations without metformin and other monotherapies

(−1.11% [−12.1 mmol/mol] and − 1.03% [−11.3 mmol/mol], respectively). At 18 months, there was a trend for patients receiving metformin plus an SGLT-2 inhibitor to achieve greater mean reductions in HbA1c, compared with patients receiving any other treatment (−1.46% [−16 mmol/mol] versus −1.21% [−13.2 mmol/mol]; $p = 0.052$; Table 3).

Changes in weight

In all four treatment groups, weight loss from baseline at 18 months was directly correlated with baseline weight (Additional file 2: Figure S2). The mean baseline-adjusted changes in weight at 6, 12 and 18 months for each treatment group are shown in Fig. 3. The greatest mean reduction in weight from baseline was observed for patients who received metformin plus an SGLT-2 inhibitor (mean weight loss at 18 months, 4.2 kg; $p < 0.001$ versus baseline). A significant mean reduction in weight from baseline was also observed for patients receiving metformin plus a DPP-4 inhibitor (mean weight loss at 18 months, 1.5 kg; $p < 0.001$ versus baseline). In contrast, small but significant mean increases in weight from baseline ($p < 0.001$) were observed at all time points for patients receiving metformin plus an SU. Overall, no pattern of weight change was observed for patients receiving other second-line treatments.

Achievement of the composite outcome of treatment success according to second-line therapy

To evaluate treatment success, a composite outcome, defined as the number of patients who had not discontinued their index therapy, achieved HbA1c reductions ≥0.5% (5.5 mmol/mol) and weight reductions ≥ 2 kg at 18 months, was assessed for all patients with data available at baseline and 18 months (Table 4). A higher proportion of patients assigned to the metformin plus an SGLT-2 inhibitor treatment group achieved HbA1c reductions ≥0.5% (71.6%) or weight reductions ≥ 2.0 kg (71.6%) at 18 months, compared with all the other treatment groups analysed. Of patients who intensified metformin treatment with a DPP-4 inhibitor, 55.1% achieved HbA1c reductions ≥ 0.5% and 42.8% of patients had weight reductions ≥ 2.0 kg. By comparison, 66% of patients on metformin plus an SU group achieved HbA1c reductions ≥ 0.5%, although only 25.6% achieved weight loss ≥ 2.0 kg at 18 months. Treatment persistence at 18 months was highest for patients receiving metformin plus an SU (56.4%) and metformin plus an SGLT-2 inhibitor (55.4%).

Overall, 36.5% of patients receiving metformin plus an SGLT-2 inhibitor met the composite outcome for treatment success, compared with 17.1% of those who received metformin plus a DPP-4 inhibitor, 9.6% of those who received metformin plus an SU and 9.1% of patients who received other treatments. This pattern was confirmed after adjustment for baseline HbA1c, weight, age, sex and time since initiation of first-line treatment. Multivariate analysis showed that initiation of second-line therapy with an SGLT-2 inhibitor resulted in a significantly higher overall success rate, compared with all other second-line therapies combined ($p < 0.001$).

Table 2 Change in HbA1c at 6 months post-initiation of second-line treatment, stratified by baseline HbA1c category

Baseline HbA1c		*N*	Mean change at 6 months (standard error)		*N* (%) with fall ≥ 0.5% at 6 months
%	mmol/mol		%	mmol/mol	
<7.5	< 58	811	0.02 (0.04)	0.2 (0.4)	277 (34.2)
7.5 to <9.0	58 to <75	2751	−0.71 (0.02)	−7.8 (0.2)	1855 (67.4)
9.0 to <10.5	75 to <91	1325	−1.47 (0.04)	−16.1 (0.4)	1099 (82.9)
10.5 to <12.0	91 to <108	715	−2.48 (0.06)	−27.1 (0.7)	641 (89.7)
≥12.0	≥108	440	−4.40 (0.12)	−48.1 (1.3)	405 (92.1)
Overall		6042	−1.26 (0.02)	−13.8 (0.2)	4277 (70.8)

Data from patients who had available HbA1c measurements at 6 months and at baseline, and who were on-treatment at 6 months (i.e. had not switched, intensified or discontinued second-line treatment since the previous time point)

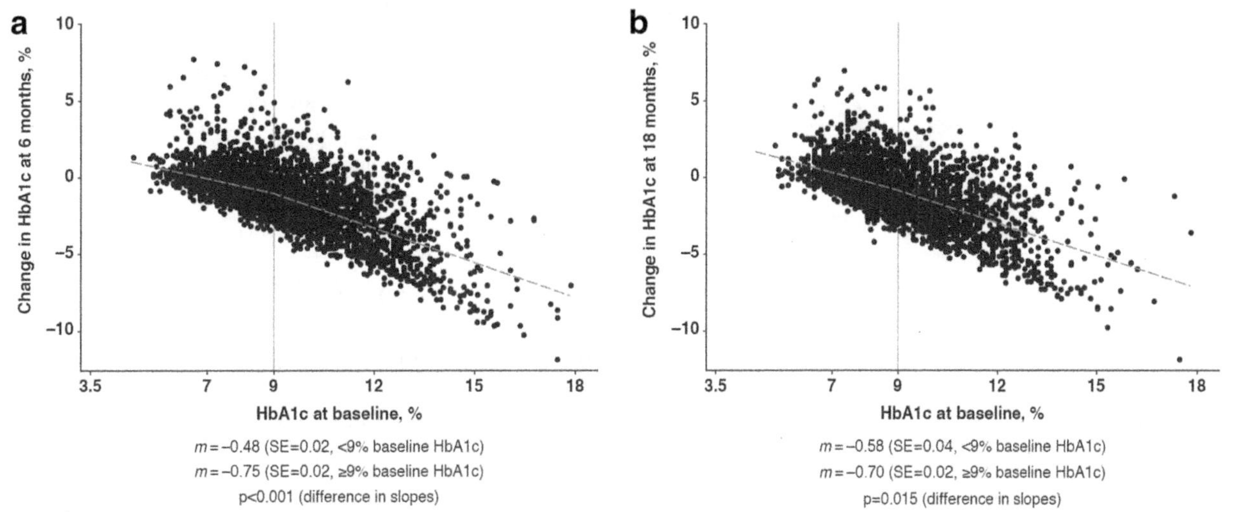

Fig. 2 Relationship between change in HbA1c and baseline HbA1c (patient-level data). Scatter plots of baseline (index) HbA1c against change in HbA1c at **a** 6 and **b** 18 months. Regression lines are shown as grey dashed lines, and their corresponding gradient slopes (*m*) were calculated for baseline HbA1c levels < 9% and ≥ 9%. SE standard error

Discussion

This study used a large, representative population of UK patients to evaluate the use of second-line therapies after metformin monotherapy in a real-world clinical practice setting.

Unlike most clinical trials, which have durations of 6–12 months, this observational study followed patients for 18 months, with 6-month follow-up intervals, and compared the effect of initiation of different second-line therapies on three clinically relevant criteria: changes in HbA1c and weight, and treatment persistence. When these three criteria were evaluated as a composite outcome representative of treatment success at 18 months, more patients (36.5%) on metformin plus an SGLT-2 inhibitor achieved HbA1c reductions of ≥ 0.5% (5.5 mmol/mol), body weight loss ≥ 2 kg and treatment persistence for 18 months, compared with all other therapies. Patients who received combination therapy with metformin plus a DPP-4 inhibitor achieved the second highest composite outcome, with 17.1% of patients achieving treatment success.

In this study, all second-line therapies reduced HbA1c levels, with a mean reduction of 1.2% (13.4 mmol/mol) at 18 months. HbA1c reductions achieved at 6 months following second-line treatment initiation correlated with HbA1c levels at baseline: patients with lower baseline levels experience smaller HbA1c reductions than patients who had higher baseline levels. This observation is in line with previous studies, which report a positive correlation between baseline HbA1c and subsequent changes in HbA1c levels [28, 35]. The greatest reductions in HbA1c at 6 months were observed in patients on metformin plus an SU or on metformin plus an SGLT-2 inhibitor, although at 18 months, these reductions were observed only in patients on metformin plus an SGLT-2 inhibitor. It is known that SUs are highly

Table 3 Change in HbA1c levels over 18 months after initiation of second-line treatment

Second-line treatment	6 months			12 months			18 months		
	N (%)	Mean change in HbA1c (SE)*		*N* (%)	Mean change in HbA1c (SE)*		*N* (%)	Mean change in HbA1c (SE)*	
		%	mmol/mol		%	mmol/mol		%	mmol/mol
MET + SU	2257 (50.38)	−1.33 (0.04)	−14.5 (0.4)	1571 (51.01)	−1.30 (0.04)	−14.2 (0.4)	907 (51.68)	−1.21 (0.05)	−13.2 (0.5)
MET + DPP-4i	1486 (33.17)	−1.11 (0.04)	−12.1 (0.4)	1044 (33.90)	−1.12 (0.05)	−12.2 (0.5)	572 (32.59)	−1.23 (0.06)	−13.4 (0.7)
MET + SGLT-2i	225 (5.02)	−1.26 (0.08)	−13.8 (0.9)	156 (5.06)	−1.32 (0.10)	−14.4 (1.1)	90 (5.13)	−1.46 (0.13)	−16.0 (1.4)
Other[†]	512 (11.43)	−1.03 (0.06)	−11.3 (0.7)	309 (10.03)	−1.20 (0.08)	−13.1 (0.9)	186 (10.60)	−1.18 (0.10)	−12.9 (1.1)
Overall	4480	−1.23 (0.03)	−13.4 (0.3)	3080	−1.24 (0.04)	−13.6 (0.4)	1755	−1.23 (0.05)	−13.4 (0.5)

Data from patients who had available HbA1c measurements at each time point and at baseline, and who were on-treatment at each time point (i.e. had not switched, intensified or discontinued second-line treatment since the previous time point)

*Baseline adjusted means using analysis of covariance

[†]Includes all other add-on combinations to metformin, combinations without metformin and other monotherapies

DPP-4i dipeptidyl peptidase-4 inhibitor, *MET* metformin, *SGLT-2i* sodium–glucose cotransporter 2 inhibitor, *SE* standard error, *SU* sulfonylurea

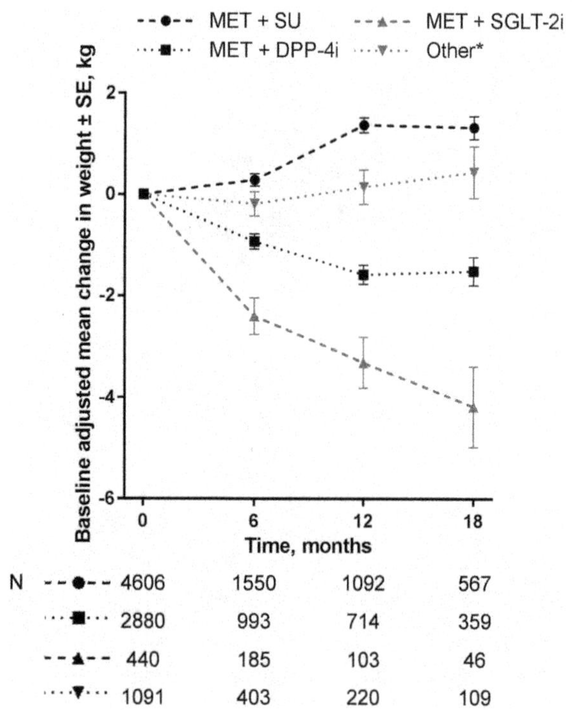

Fig. 3 Baseline-adjusted change in weight over 18 months in patients initiated on second-line therapies. Data are means ± SE. Data are from patients who had available weight measurements at each timepoint and at baseline, and who were on-treatment at each time-point (i.e. had not switched, intensified or ceased second-line treatment since the previous time-point). DPP-4i, dipeptidyl peptidase-4 inhibitor; MET, metformin; N, number of patients; SGLT-2i, sodium–glucose cotransporter 2 inhibitor; SE, standard error; SU, sulfonylurea. *Includes all other add-on combinations to metformin, combinations without metformin and other monotherapies

efficient at rapidly reducing HbA1c levels in patients with T2D, with only insulin acting on HbA1c faster [6]. However, many clinical trials comparing SU to other therapies have shown the effects of SUs on HbA1c to be short-lived [36–38]. The sustained reduction in HbA1c levels observed in patients receiving metformin plus an SGLT-2 inhibitor has been previously reported in a meta-analysis [39]. However, the higher HbA1c levels at baseline and the reduced number of patients who had HbA1c measurements at 18 months in the CPRD database may have contributed to the effect seen.

The effect of a particular treatment on weight is also an important factor when deciding upon an appropriate second-line agent, as obesity is often associated with T2D [40]. Overall, modest weight gain was seen in patients who received the combination of metformin plus an SU, whereas weight loss was observed for patients treated with metformin plus either a DPP-4 inhibitor or an SGLT-2 inhibitor, with significantly greater weight loss observed in patients receiving an SGLT-2 inhibitor. While DPP-4 inhibitors are generally considered to be weight neutral [6], reductions in BMI following treatment with a DPP-4 inhibitor have been observed in a previous database analysis in Italy [41]. Weight reductions comparable to those reported here following treatment with a DPP-4 inhibitor (mean −1.58 kg at 12 months) were also seen in a previous analysis of a US database, in which patients achieved a mean weight change from baseline of −1.26 kg at 12 months [42]. Previous studies have demonstrated the add-on benefit of SGLT-2 inhibitors by promoting weight loss via increased glucose excretion [43–46]. The weight reductions seen in this analysis following initiation with an SGLT-2 inhibitor were higher than those observed in clinical trials (mean weight reduction at 18 months of 4.2 kg versus 2.2–3.4 kg) [43] and continued at each time point up to 18 months, which may reflect a greater likelihood of treatment persistence in those who lose weight. Patients who received an SGLT-2 inhibitor-based treatment generally had a higher weight at baseline, suggesting selection of this therapy in more obese patients due to its established effects on weight, consistent with NICE guidelines [4, 47]. Given the demonstrated correlation between baseline weight and weight loss, this may also partly account for the greater weight loss observed with SGLT-2 inhibitors in this analysis. Additionally, the low number of patients who had weight measurements at 18 months in the SGLT-2 inhibitors group could be considered a possible confounder. Perhaps expectedly, no overall change in weight was observed in patients included in the other group, as this group included both

Table 4 Composite outcome representing treatment success after 18 months for each treatment group

Second-line treatment	*N*	HbA1c reduction ≥ 0.5% (≥ 5.5 mmol/mol)	Weight-loss ≥ 2 kg	No treatment change over 18 months	Overall success (i.e. attained all three endpoints)
MET + SU	847	559 (66.0)	217 (25.6)	478 (56.4)	81 (9.6)
MET + DPP-4i	608	335 (55.1)	260 (42.8)	300 (49.3)	104 (17.1)
MET + SGLT-2i	74	53 (71.6)	53 (71.6)	41 (55.4)	27 (36.5)
Other*	187	105 (56.2)	61 (32.6)	91 (48.7)	17 (9.1)
Overall	1716	1052 (61.3)	591 (34.4)	910 (53.0)	229 (13.3)

Data are in *n* (%). Data from all patients who had both HbA1c and weight measurements available at baseline and at 18 months
DPP-4i dipeptidyl peptidase-4 inhibitor, *MET* metformin, *SGLT-2i* sodium–glucose cotransporter 2 inhibitor, *SU* sulfonylurea
*Includes all other add-on combinations to metformin, combinations without metformin and other monotherapies

patients who received agents that are known to cause weight gain (including insulins and TZDs) and patients who received agents associated with weight loss (including GLP-1 receptor agonists). The weight changes presented in this analysis were adjusted for baseline values to allow comparisons between treatment groups. However, the effect of second-line treatment on weight has been associated with ethnicity, with Asian populations showing a greater response to agents such as DPP-4 inhibitors [48]. Despite information on ethnic groups not being available in the CPRD, the Asian population in the UK represents approximately 7% of the general population [49] and, thus, this population effect should not be considered a potential bias.

A pooled analysis of previous clinical and observational studies reported that treatment persistence in patients with T2D receiving oral anti-diabetic agents ranged from 41.0 to 81.1%, and treatment discontinuation estimates ranged from 9.9% to 60.1% [50]. In the current study, treatment persistence was highest in patients receiving treatment with metformin plus an SGLT-2 inhibitor at all time points, with 57.7% of patients continuing with the index treatment at 18 months. By comparison, 53.2% of patients who received metformin plus either an SU or a DPP-4 inhibitor and 47.2% of patients on other treatments continued with their index therapies, respectively. In line with this, a previous study has shown greater treatment persistence in patients receiving SGLT-2 inhibitors versus SU [51]. The higher rates of treatment persistence seen with an SGLT-2 inhibitor may be associated with the steady decrease in HbA1c levels and weight reductions and reflect increased patient satisfaction with these therapies. Although the reasons for patient discontinuation, switching or intensification of therapy were not reliably recorded in the UK CPRD, and information on adherence to medication and completion of each course of treatment were limited to the available records, in clinical practice common reasons for discontinuation or change of treatment include undesirable side effects (such as weight gain or risk of hypoglycaemia) and inefficacy of treatment requiring intensification or change of therapy [52].

The median time to initiation of second-line treatment did not differ substantially among the different treatment groups investigated, with patients initiating second-line therapy a median of 2.3 years after metformin initiation. Therapeutic inertia remains an issue in clinical practice, with a previous analysis of the UK CPRD database observing a delay of 1.6–2.9 years before second-line treatment intensification in patients with suboptimal glycaemic control (study cohort of 81,573 patients) [27]. Another analysis of the UK CPRD ($n = 6710$) observed that only 39.5% of patients had their treatment intensified within the year following metformin monotherapy treatment failure (HbA1c ≥ 7% [53 mmol/mol]), and 24% of patients had no evidence of treatment intensification throughout the ~4.3 years of the study [31]. In an analysis of a large US insurance claims database ($n = 11{,}525$), which included a cohort of patients with T2D and poor glycaemic control (HbA1c ≥ 8% [64 mmol/mol]), more than half (52%) of the patients did not receive treatment intensification within 12 months of treatment failure [53]. Another study using a US claims database that included patients with T2D identified a mean time to treatment intensification after HbA1c levels were above the target of over 700 days [54]. A recent systematic review that assessed data from patients with T2D from North America, Europe and Israel showed that the median time to treatment intensification after HbA1c levels were above target was 0.3–2.7 years and 1.3–4.9 years, in patients receiving one or two oral anti-diabetic drugs respectively [28].

As an observational study, this analysis had a number of limitations. Firstly, as it aimed to represent a population on-treatment, patients at each time point who discontinued, switched or intensified the index second-line treatment, as well as those who did not have HbA1c levels or body weight data available, were censored from the study. The number of patients evaluated for changes in HbA1c levels and weight were, therefore, smaller at later time points. This is particularly noticeable for the analysis at 18 months, which may limit the generalisability of the results. Secondly, only patients whose first-line therapy was metformin monotherapy were included. Although these patients accounted for the majority of those identified initiating a second-line therapy in the CPRD, consistent with guidelines and clinical practice [4, 6], this patient population may limit the generalisability of these findings to patients who receive a different first-line therapy. Thirdly, consideration should be given to the limited use of some of the more recent glucose-lowering therapies, such as DPP-4 inhibitors and SGLT-2 inhibitors, which have not been used as widely, as is the case for older, more established therapies. Moreover, these more recent therapies were not recommended by NICE guidelines as a treatment choice for treatment intensification after metformin until December 2015, close to the cut-off date for inclusion in this study. Consequently, fewer patients were exposed to these agents, limiting the analyses and interpretations of these results. And fourthly, given the low number of patients identified who received therapy combinations other than metformin plus an SU, a DPP-4 inhibitor or an SGLT-2 inhibitor or received second-line therapy without metformin, these patients were combined into the other treatment group, which prevented reliable analysis of clinical outcomes for each individual treatment strategies.

In addition to the above, observational studies using databases such as the UK CPRD inherently have a number of limitations, including potential issues relating to the quality of the data for key clinical measurements and possible misclassification of exposure and outcome. Hypoglycaemia events were not reliably captured in the UK CPRD, which prevents the assessment of risk of hypoglycaemia for second-line therapy in this analysis. The reports for events such as diabetic ketoacidosis or urinary tract infections are also limited and, therefore, not reported in this analysis. These safety events have been formally evaluated in other post-authorisation safety studies specifically designed to that end, and their incidence evaluated in an independent meta-analysis [55] and in clinical practice [56]. In addition, there is the possibility of confounding by indication, as patients were not randomised to receive the treatments; rather, treatments were selected by the physician based on clinical judgement according to specific patient characteristics. This non-random selection resulted in the differences between the baseline characteristics of the treatment groups. While multivariate regression was undertaken to adjust for the measured differences, the possibility of residual confounding contributing to the findings remains.

Conclusions

In this population-based cohort, all second-line therapies initiated after metformin monotherapy improved glycaemic control, with the greatest HbA1c reductions seen in patients with higher baseline HbA1c levels. In addition, significant reductions in weight were observed for patients treated with metformin plus either a DPP-4 inhibitor or an SGLT-2 inhibitor. The lowest incidence of second-line therapy change was seen in patients treated with metformin plus an SGLT-2 inhibitor. Patients treated with metformin plus an SGLT-2 inhibitor were most likely to achieve a composite of HbA1c reduction ≥ 0.5% (5.5 mmol/mol), weight reduction ≥ 2 kg and continued treatment at 18 months. This highlights the potential benefits of treating patients with more recent agents, including SGLT-2 inhibitors. The ongoing, randomised, pragmatic trial (DECIDE; NCT02616666) aims to evaluate the comparative effectiveness between the SGLT-2 inhibitor dapagliflozin and standard of care over 2 years in patients with T2D, and should provide further data on this therapeutic class [57].

Additional files

Additional file 1: Figure S1. Study attrition. (TIF 53 kb)

Additional file 2: Figure S2. Relationship between change in weight at 18 months and baseline weight according to second-line treatment. Scatter plots of baseline (index) weight against change in weight at 18 months in patients on metformin plus either an SU (**a**), a DPP-4 inhibitor, (**b**) an SGLT-2 inhibitor (**c**), or other therapies (**d**). Regression lines are shown as grey dashed lines, and their corresponding gradient slopes (*m*) were calculated for baseline weight. (TIF 3255 kb)

Abbreviations

BMI: Body mass index; CPRD: Clinical Practice Research Datalink; DPP-4: Dipeptidyl peptidase-4; GLP-1: Glucagon-like peptide-1; IQR: Interquartile range; MET: Metformin; NICE: National Institute for Health and Care Excellence; SD: Standard deviation; SE: Standard error; SGLT-2: Sodium–glucose cotransporter 2; SU: Sulfonylurea; T2D: Type 2 diabetes; TZD: Thiazolidinedione

Acknowledgements

This analysis was supported by AstraZeneca. Editorial support was provided by Nicola Truss and Diana Marouco of inScience Communications, Springer Healthcare Ltd, London, UK, funded by AstraZeneca. KK acknowledges support from the National Institute for Health Research Collaboration for Leadership in Applied Health Research and Care – East Midlands, and the National Institute for Health Research Leicester Biomedical Research Centre.

Funding

This study was funded by AstraZeneca.

Authors' contributions

JW, KK, SP, PF and JM contributed to the study design. TG and JM were involved in data acquisition. All authors were involved in data analysis and interpretation. All authors contributed to the drafting and critical review of the manuscript and approved the final draft.

Competing interests

JM, PC, PF and NH are employees of AstraZeneca.
KK has received honoraria and research support from AstraZeneca, Boehringer Ingelheim, Eli Lilly, Janssen, Merck Sharp & Dohme, Novartis, Novo Nordisk, Roche and Sanofi.
JW has received honoraria from Astellas, AstraZeneca, Boehringer Ingelheim, Janssen, Lilly, Novo Nordisk, Orexigen, and Sanofi; undertaken institutional consultancy with AstraZeneca, Boehringer Ingelheim, Janssen, Lilly, and Orexigen; and received institutional grants from Takeda, Novo Nordisk and AstraZeneca.
LS is supported by a senior clinical fellowship from The Wellcome Trust, UK.
TG and RF report no conflicts of interest.

Author details

[1]University of Liverpool, Liverpool, UK. [2]London School of Hygiene and Tropical Medicine, London, UK. [3]University of Leicester, Leicester, UK. [4]Bicester Health Centre, Bicester, UK. [5]AstraZeneca, Gothenburg, Sweden. [6]AstraZeneca, Luton, UK. [7]AstraZeneca Farmacéutica Spain, Madrid, Spain.

References

1. IDF Diabetes Atlas [http://www.diabetesatlas.org/across-the-globe.html]. Accessed 23 June 2017.
2. Group UpDSU. Intensive blood-glucose control with sulphonylureas or insulin compared with conventional treatment and risk of complications in patients with type 2 diabetes (UKPDS 33). UK Prospective Diabetes Study (UKPDS) Group. Lancet. 1998;352(9131):837–53.
3. Holman RR, Paul SK, Bethel MA, Matthews DR, Neil HA. 10-year follow-up of intensive glucose control in type 2 diabetes. N Engl J Med. 2008;359(15):1577–89.
4. National Institute for Health and Clinical Excellence: Type 2 diabetes in adults: management [https://www.nice.org.uk/guidance/ng28/chapter/1-Recommendations#blood-glucose-management-2]. Accessed 25 July 2017.
5. Metformin 500 mg tablets [http://www.medicines.org.uk/emc/medicine/23244/SPC#PHARMACODYNAMIC_PROPS]. Accessed 25 July 2017.
6. Inzucchi SE, Bergenstal RM, Buse JB, Diamant M, Ferrannini E, Nauck M, Peters AL, Tsapas A, Wender R, Matthews DR. Management of hyperglycemia in type 2 diabetes, 2015: a patient-centered approach:

update to a position statement of the American Diabetes Association and the European Association for the Study of diabetes. Diabetes Care. 2015;38(1):140 9.

7. Handelsman Y, Bloomgarden ZT, Grunberger G, Umpierrez G, Zimmerman RS, Bailey TS, Blonde L, Bray GA, Cohen AJ, Dagogo-Jack S, et al. American Association of Clinical Endocrinologists and American College of endocrinology–clinical practice guidelines for developing a diabetes mellitus comprehensive care plan–2015–executive summary. Endocr Pract. 2015;21(4):413–37.
8. Bennett WL, Balfe LM, Faysal JM. AHRQ's comparative effectiveness research on oral medications for type 2 diabetes: a summary of the key findings. J Manag Care Pharm. 2012;18(1 Suppl A):1–22.
9. Dormandy JA, Charbonnel B, Eckland DJ, Erdmann E, Massi-Benedetti M, Moules IK, Skene AM, Tan MH, Lefebvre PJ, Murray GD, et al. Secondary prevention of macrovascular events in patients with type 2 diabetes in the PROactive study (PROspective pioglitAzone clinical trial in macroVascular events): a randomised controlled trial. Lancet. 2005;366(9493):1279–89.
10. Marathe PH, Gao HX, Close KL. American Diabetes Association standards of medical Care in Diabetes 2017. J Diabetes. 2017;9:320–4.
11. Foroutan N, Muratov S, Levine M. Safety and efficacy of dipeptidyl peptidase-4 inhibitors vs sulfonylurea in metformin-based combination therapy for type 2 diabetes mellitus: systematic review and meta-analysis. Clin Invest Med. 2016;39(2):E48–62.
12. List JF, Woo V, Morales E, Tang W, Fiedorek FT. Sodium–glucose cotransport inhibition with dapagliflozin in type 2 diabetes. Diabetes Care. 2009;32(4):650–7.
13. Nauck MA. Update on developments with SGLT2 inhibitors in the management of type 2 diabetes. Drug Des Devel Ther. 2014;8:1335–80.
14. Mudaliar S, Henry RR, Boden G, Smith S, Chalamandaris AG, Duchesne D, Iqbal N, List J. Changes in insulin sensitivity and insulin secretion with the sodium glucose cotransporter 2 inhibitor dapagliflozin. Diabetes Technol Ther. 2014;16(3):137–44.
15. Zinman B, Wanner C, Lachin JM, Fitchett D, Bluhmki E, Hantel S, Mattheus M, Devins T, Johansen OE, Woerle HJ, et al. Empagliflozin, cardiovascular outcomes, and mortality in type 2 diabetes. N Engl J Med. 2015;373(22):2117–28.
16. Neal B, Perkovic V, Mahaffey KW, de Zeeuw D, Fulcher G, Erondu N, Shaw W, Law G, Desai M, Matthews DR. Canagliflozin and cardiovascular and renal events in type 2 diabetes. N Engl J Med. 2017;377(7):644–57.
17. Birkeland KI, Jorgensen ME, Carstensen B, Persson F, Gulseth HL, Thuresson M, Fenici P, Nathanson D, Nystrom T, Eriksson JW, et al. Cardiovascular mortality and morbidity in patients with type 2 diabetes following initiation of sodium–glucose co-transporter-2 inhibitors versus other glucose-lowering drugs (CVD-REAL Nordic): a multinational observational analysis. Lancet Diabetes Endocrinol. 2017;5(9):709–17.
18. Kosiborod M, Cavender MA, Fu AZ, Wilding JP, Khunti K, Holl RW, Norhammar A, Birkeland KI, Jorgensen M, Thuresson M, et al. lower risk of heart failure and death in patients initiated on SGLT-2 inhibitors versus other glucose-lowering drugs: the CVD-REAL study. Circulation. 2017;18(117):029190.
19. Persson F, Nystrom T, Jorgensen ME, Carstensen B, Gulseth HL, Thuresson M, Fenici P, Nathanson D, Eriksson JW, Norhammar A, et al. Dapagliflozin compared to DPP-4 inhibitors is associated with lower risk of cardiovascular events and all-cause mortality in type 2 diabetes patients (CVD-REAL Nordic): a multinational observational study. Diabetes Obes Metab. 2017;3(10):13077.
20. Raz I, Bonaca MP, Mosenzon O, Kato ET, Cahn A, Silverman MG, Bhatt DL, Leiter L, Mcguire DK, Wilding JPH, Gause-Nilsson IAM, Langkilde AM, Johansson PA, Sabatine MS, Wiviott SD DECLARE-TIMI 58: design and baseline characteristics. Diabetes Obes Metab. 2018;20(5):1102-10.
21. Thrasher J. Pharmacologic Management of Type 2 diabetes mellitus: available therapies. Am J Med. 2017;130(6S):S4–S17.
22. National Institure for Health and Clinical Excellence: Type 2 diabetes mellitus: medicines optimisation priorities [https://www.nice.org.uk/advice/ktt12/chapter/Evidence-context]. Accessed 25 July 2017.
23. Marso SP, Bain SC, Consoli A, Eliaschewitz FG, Jodar E, Leiter LA, Lingvay I, Rosenstock J, Seufert J, Warren ML, et al. Semaglutide and cardiovascular outcomes in patients with type 2 diabetes. N Engl J Med. 2016;375(19): 1834–44.
24. Marso SP, Daniels GH, Brown-Frandsen K, Kristensen P, Mann JF, Nauck MA, Nissen SE, Pocock S, Poulter NR, Ravn LS, et al. Liraglutide and cardiovascular outcomes in type 2 diabetes. N Engl J Med. 2016;375(4):311–22.
25. Holman RR, Bethel MA, Mentz RJ, Thompson VP, Lokhnygina Y, Buse JB, Chan JC, Choi J, Gustavson SM, Iqbal N, et al. Effects of once-weekly Exenatide on cardiovascular outcomes in type 2 diabetes. New ENgl J Med. 2017;377(13):1228–39.
26. Pfeffer MA, Claggett B, Diaz R, Dickstein K, Gerstein HC, Kober LV, Lawson FC, Ping L, Wei X, Lewis EF, et al. Lixisenatide in patients with type 2 diabetes and acute coronary syndrome. N Engl J Med. 2015;373(23):2247–57.
27. Khunti K, Wolden ML, Thorsted BL, Andersen M, Davies MJ. Clinical inertia in people with type 2 diabetes: a retrospective cohort study of more than 80,000 people. Diabetes Care. 2013;36(11):3411–7.
28. Khunti K, Gomes MB, Pocock S, Shestakova MV, Pintat S, Fenici P, Hammar N, Medina J. Therapeutic inertia in the treatment of hyperglycaemia in patients with type 2 diabetes: a systematic review. Diabetes Obes Metab. 2017;22(10):13088.
29. Paul SK, Klein K, Thorsted BL, Wolden ML, Khunti K. Delay in treatment intensification increases the risks of cardiovascular events in patients with type 2 diabetes. Cardiovasc Diabetol. 2015;14(100):015–0260.
30. Pantalone KM, Wells BJ, Chagin KM, Ejzykowicz F, Yu C, Milinovich A, Bauman JM, Kattan MW, Rajpathak S, Zimmerman RS. Intensification of diabetes therapy and time until A1C goal attainment among patients with newly diagnosed type 2 diabetes who fail metformin monotherapy within a large integrated health system. Diabetes Care. 2016;39(9):1527–34.
31. Watson L, Das R, Farquhar R, Langerman H, Barnett AH. Consequences of delaying treatment intensification in type 2 diabetes: evidence from a UK database. Curr Med Res Opin. 2016;32(9):1465–75.
32. Fu AZ, Sheehan JJ. Change in HbA1c associated with treatment intensification among patients with type 2 diabetes and poor glycemic control. Curr Med Res Opin. 2017;33(5):853–8.
33. Wilding JPH, Godec T, Khunti K., et al. Changes in HbA(1c) and weight after initiation of second-line therapy in patients with type 2 diabetes in clinical practice. In: 53 rd EASD Annual Meeting of the European Association for the Study of Diabetes. Diabetologia 2017;60(Suppl 1):1.
34. Herrett E, Gallagher AM, Bhaskaran K, Forbes H, Mathur R, van Staa T, Smeeth L. Data resource profile: clinical practice research datalink (CPRD). Int J Epidemiol. 2015;44(3):827–36.
35. DeFronzo RA, Stonehouse AH, Han J, Wintle ME. Relationship of baseline HbA1c and efficacy of current glucose-lowering therapies: a meta-analysis of randomized clinical trials. Diabet Med. 2010;27(3):309–17.
36. Kahn SE, Haffner SM, Heise MA, Herman WH, Holman RR, Jones NP, Kravitz BG, Lachin JM, O'Neill MC, Zinman B, et al. Glycemic durability of rosiglitazone, metformin, or glyburide monotherapy. N Engl J Med. 2006;355(23):2427–43.
37. Nauck MA, Del Prato S, Duran-Garcia S, Rohwedder K, Langkilde AM, Sugg J, Parikh SJ. Durability of glycaemic efficacy over 2 years with dapagliflozin versus glipizide as add-on therapies in patients whose type 2 diabetes mellitus is inadequately controlled with metformin. Diabetes Obes Metab. 2014;16(11):1111–20.
38. Goke B, Gallwitz B, Eriksson JG, Hellqvist A, Gause-Nilsson I. Saxagliptin vs. glipizide as add-on therapy in patients with type 2 diabetes mellitus inadequately controlled on metformin alone: long-term (52-week) extension of a 52-week randomised controlled trial. Int J Clin Pract. 2013;67(4):307–16.
39. Monami M, Liistro F, Scatena A, Nreu B, Mannucci E. Short and medium-term efficacy of sodium glucose co-transporter-2 (SGLT-2) inhibitors: a meta-analysis of randomized clinical trials. Diabetes Obes Metab. 2018;12(10):13221.
40. Global BMIMC, Di Angelantonio E, Bhupathiraju Sh N, Wormser D, Gao P, Kaptoge S, Berrington de Gonzalez A, Cairns BJ, Huxley R, Jackson Ch L, et al. Body-mass index and all-cause mortality: individual-participant-data meta-analysis of 239 prospective studies in four continents. Lancet. 2016;388(10046):776–86.
41. Saglietti G, Placentino G, Schellino A. Observational study on dipeptidyl peptidase-4 inhibitors: a real-life analysis on 360 patients from the ASL VCO territory in Italy. Clin Drug Investig. 2014;34(7):513–9.
42. Carls GS, Tan R, Zhu JY, Tuttle E, Yee J, Edelman SV, Polonsky WH. Real-world weight change among patients treated with glucagon-like peptide-1 receptor agonist, dipeptidyl peptidase-4 inhibitor and sulfonylureas for type 2 diabetes and the influence of medication adherence. Obes Sci Pract. 2017;3(3):342–51.
43. Fujita Y, Inagaki N. Renal sodium glucose cotransporter 2 inhibitors as a novel therapeutic approach to treatment of type 2 diabetes: clinical data and mechanism of action. J Diabetes Investig. 2014;5(3):265–75.

44. Stenlof K, Cefalu WT, Kim KA, Alba M, Usiskin K, Tong C, Canovatchel W, Meininger G. Efficacy and safety of canagliflozin monotherapy in subjects with type 2 diabetes mellitus inadequately controlled with diet and exercise. Diabetes Obes Metab. 2013;15(4):372–82.
45. Ferrannini E, Ramos SJ, Salsali A, Tang W, List JF. Dapagliflozin monotherapy in type 2 diabetic patients with inadequate glycemic control by diet and exercise: a randomized, double-blind, placebo-controlled, phase 3 trial. Diabetes Care. 2010;33(10):2217–24.
46. Kaku K, Watada H, Iwamoto Y, Utsunomiya K, Terauchi Y, Tobe K, Tanizawa Y, Araki E, Ueda M, Suganami H, et al. Efficacy and safety of monotherapy with the novel sodium/glucose cotransporter-2 inhibitor tofogliflozin in Japanese patients with type 2 diabetes mellitus: a combined phase 2 and 3 randomized, placebo-controlled, double-blind, parallel-group comparative study. Cardiovasc Diabetol. 2014;13(65):1475–2840.
47. Wilding JPH. Medication use for the treatment of diabetes in obese individuals. Diabetologia. 2017;14(10):017–4288.
48. Seino Y, Kuwata H, Yabe D. Incretin-based drugs for type 2 diabetes: focus on east Asian perspectives. J Diabetes Investig. 2016;1:102–9.
49. 2011 Census: Ethnic group, local authorities in the United Kingdom [https://www.ons.gov.uk/peoplepopulationandcommunity/culturalidentity/ethnicity/articles/ethnicityandnationalidentityinenglandandwales/2012-12-11#ethnicity-in-england-and-wales]. Accessed 9 Mar 2018.
50. Iglay K, Cartier SE, Rosen VM, Zarotsky V, Rajpathak SN, Radican L, Tunceli K. Meta-analysis of studies examining medication adherence, persistence, and discontinuation of oral antihyperglycemic agents in type 2 diabetes. Curr Med Res Opin. 2015;31(7):1283–96.
51. Bell KF, Cappell K, Liang M, Kong AM. Comparing medication adherence and persistence among patients with type 2 diabetes using sodium-glucose cotransporter 2 inhibitors or sulfonylureas. Am Health Drug Benefits. 2017;10(4):165–74.
52. Polonsky WH, Henry RR. Poor medication adherence in type 2 diabetes: recognizing the scope of the problem and its key contributors. Patient Prefer Adherence. 2016;10:1299–307.
53. Fu AZ, Sheehan JJ. Treatment intensification for patients with type 2 diabetes and poor glycaemic control. Diabetes Obes Metab. 2016;18(9):892–8.
54. Lin J, Zhou S, Wei W, Pan C, Lingohr-Smith M, Levin P. Does clinical inertia vary by personalized A1c goal? A study of predictors and prevalence of clinical inertia in a U.S. managed-care setting. Endocr Pract. 2016;22(2):151–61.
55. Monami M, Nreu B, Zannoni S, Lualdi C, Mannucci E. Effects of SGLT-2 inhibitors on diabetic ketoacidosis: a meta-analysis of randomised controlled trials. Diabetes Res Clin Pract. 2017;130:53–60.
56. Gadzhanova S, Pratt N, Roughead E. Use of SGLT2 inhibitors for diabetes and risk of infection: analysis using general practice records from the NPS MedicineWise MedicineInsight program. Diabetes Res Clin Pract. 2017;130:180–5.
57. Perkins BA, Cherney DZ, Soleymanlou N, Lee JA, Partridge H, Tschirhart H, Zinman B, Mazze R, Fagan N, Kaspers S, et al. Diurnal glycemic patterns during an 8-week open-label proof-of-concept trial of Empagliflozin in type 1 diabetes. PLoS One. 2015;10(11):e0141085.

11

The cost-effectiveness of oral HIV pre-exposure prophylaxis and early antiretroviral therapy in the presence of drug resistance among men who have sex with men in San Francisco

Mingwang Shen[1,2,3], Yanni Xiao[2*], Libin Rong[4], Lauren Ancel Meyers[3,5] and Steven E. Bellan[6,7]

Abstract

Background: Poor adherence to either antiretroviral treatment (ART) or pre-exposure prophylaxis (PrEP) can promote drug resistance, though this risk is thought to be considerably higher for ART. In the population of men who have sex with men (MSM) in San Francisco, PrEP coverage reached 9.6% in 2014 and has continued to rise. Given the risk of drug resistance and high cost of second-line drugs, the costs and benefits of initiating ART earlier while expanding PrEP coverage remain unclear.

Methods: We develop an infection–age-structured mathematical model and fit this model to the annual incidence of AIDS cases and deaths directly, and to resistance and demographic data indirectly. We investigate the impact of six various intervention scenarios (low, medium, or high PrEP coverage, with or without earlier ART) over the next 20 years.

Results: Low (medium, high) PrEP coverage with earlier ART could prevent 22% (42%, 57%) of a projected 44,508 total new infections and 8% (26%, 41%) of a projected 18,426 new drug-resistant infections, and result in a gain of 43,649 (74,048, 103,270) QALYs over 20 years compared to the status quo, at a cost of $4745 ($78,811, $115,320) per QALY gained, respectively.

Conclusions: High PrEP coverage with earlier ART is expected to provide the greatest benefit but also entail the highest costs among the strategies considered. This strategy is cost-effective for the San Francisco MSM population, even considering the acquisition and transmission of ART-mediated drug resistance. However, without a substantial increase to San Francisco's annual HIV budget, the most advisable strategy may be initiating ART earlier, while maintaining current strategies of PrEP enrollment.

Keywords: Cost-effectiveness, Pre-exposure prophylaxis, Earlier ART initiation, Drug resistance, Mathematical model

* Correspondence: yxiao@mail.xjtu.edu.cn
[2]School of Mathematics and Statistics, Xi'an Jiaotong University, Xi'an 710049, People's Republic of China
Full list of author information is available at the end of the article

Background

In July 2012, the US Food and Drug Administration (FDA) approved tenofovir/emtricitabine for use as oral pre-exposure prophylaxis (PrEP) [1]. Estimates of PrEP efficacy in preventing HIV infection range from 39% to 86% in randomized controlled trials [2–6]. PrEP consumer demand has accelerated since mid-2013 [7]. PrEP coverage among men who have sex with men (MSM) in San Francisco was estimated at 9.6% in 2014 [8]. In May 2016, more than 6000 MSM in San Francisco were reported to receive PrEP [9], suggesting a coverage of approximately 12% given that the HIV-negative MSM population is estimated at 50,000 [7, 10, 11]. In 2010, prior to this increased PrEP uptake, San Francisco was one of the first cities to institute guidelines to initiate antiretroviral therapy (ART) as early as possible post-infection rather than waiting for signs of disease progression, such as clinical symptoms or low CD4+ cell counts [12], given findings that early ART initiation improves survival while reducing the risks of transmission to others [13]. However, it has been hypothesized that early ART initiation might provide more time for the evolution of drug resistance and that subsequent transmission of drug-resistant HIV might reduce PrEP effectiveness [14–16].

Herein, we address the long-term population-level costs and health benefits of expanding PrEP coverage in combination with increasingly early ART initiation among the MSM population in San Francisco. We assess the effectiveness and cost-effectiveness of expanding PrEP coverage, with and without earlier ART guidelines, using an infection–age-structured model [17, 18]. The model tracks the transmission rate and life expectancy of individuals at each infection age, while accounting for ART-mediated drug resistance and the costs of treatment failure and second-line regimens. We fit this model to epidemiological data on the annual incidence of newly diagnosed AIDS cases and deaths amongst MSM in San Francisco (simultaneously matching prevalence, resistance, and demographic data [18]) and estimate the impact of various intervention scenarios over the next 20 years.

Several modeling studies have addressed the impact of PrEP in San Francisco, including estimates of coverage required to curtail transmission [7], an assessment of whether PrEP might increase the drug-resistant transmission [14], and a cost-effectiveness analysis of PrEP in combination with a partially effective HIV vaccine [19]. Our study differs from these prior analyses and others of PrEP cost-effectiveness [20–26] in the United States in several aspects. First, we analyze the expansion in PrEP coverage in conjunction with changing ART guidelines, rather than comparing initiation of PrEP to no PrEP [7, 14, 19–24, 27, 28]. Second, we model the acquisition and transmission of ART-mediated resistance and the indirect population-level effects of PrEP (i.e., by reducing the number of infected individuals, PrEP indirectly benefits other individuals in the population who could have otherwise been infected by individuals on PrEP), which have not been addressed in previous studies [7, 19–25]. While two prior analyses of PrEP [16, 26] considered ART-mediated resistance and subsequent treatment failure, one [16] did not address the impact of earlier ART initiation on PrEP cost-effectiveness, and the other [26] did not account for increased costs and effectiveness of second-line drugs. Third, we consider increasingly earlier initiation of ART and the consequent increases in survival. In contrast, many prior studies modeled early ART by assuming individuals initiate ART whilst their CD4+ T cell counts remain above 350 cells/mm^3 [29], by assuming ART eligibility occurs once their CD4+ T cell count drops below 500 cells/mm^3 [30, 31], or by assuming ART initiation occurs within 2 years of infection [32]. Two studies that modeled ART initiation at 1 year post-infection [33, 34] did not incorporate the increased survival times, which may cause underestimation of intervention cost-effectiveness.

Methods

We extended our previously developed infection–age-structured model [18] to include a PrEP class (see the schematic diagram of the model structure in Fig. 1a, Additional file 1: Figure S1 and Table S1). We modeled the MSM population in San Francisco aged 18–65 years old [10, 18], assuming that first- and second-line ART reduced infectivity by 96% [13] and 80% [18], respectively. Here, the effectiveness of second-line drugs for drug-resistant cases is assumed to be lower than that of first-line drugs for drug-sensitive cases due to lower adherence [35]. We assume that earlier ART initiation confers longer life expectancy, as indicated previously [18, 36], based on clinical data [37, 38] and that treated individuals with drug resistance have life expectancies that are 11 years (varying from 0 to 20 years in sensitivity analyses) shorter than drug-sensitive patients [18, 37, 38]. We estimate that the average period from infection to ART initiation in San Francisco has been 1.6 years, on average [18] ('early ART', see Additional file 1: Supplementary Material for details). We compared early ART to 'earlier' ART, i.e., treatment initiation at 1 year post-infection, on average. Of the 33% of treated MSM who are virally unsuppressed [10], 76% exhibit drug resistance [39]; we thus assume that 25% of treated MSM in San Francisco [18] have acquired drug resistance as our base case (varied from 0 to 100% in a sensitivity analysis). Resistance here is assumed to be resistant to one or more first-line ART drugs. Given local monitoring protocols, we assume that drug-resistant cases are quickly switched to second-line drugs. We do not differentiate drug combinations beyond the categorizations

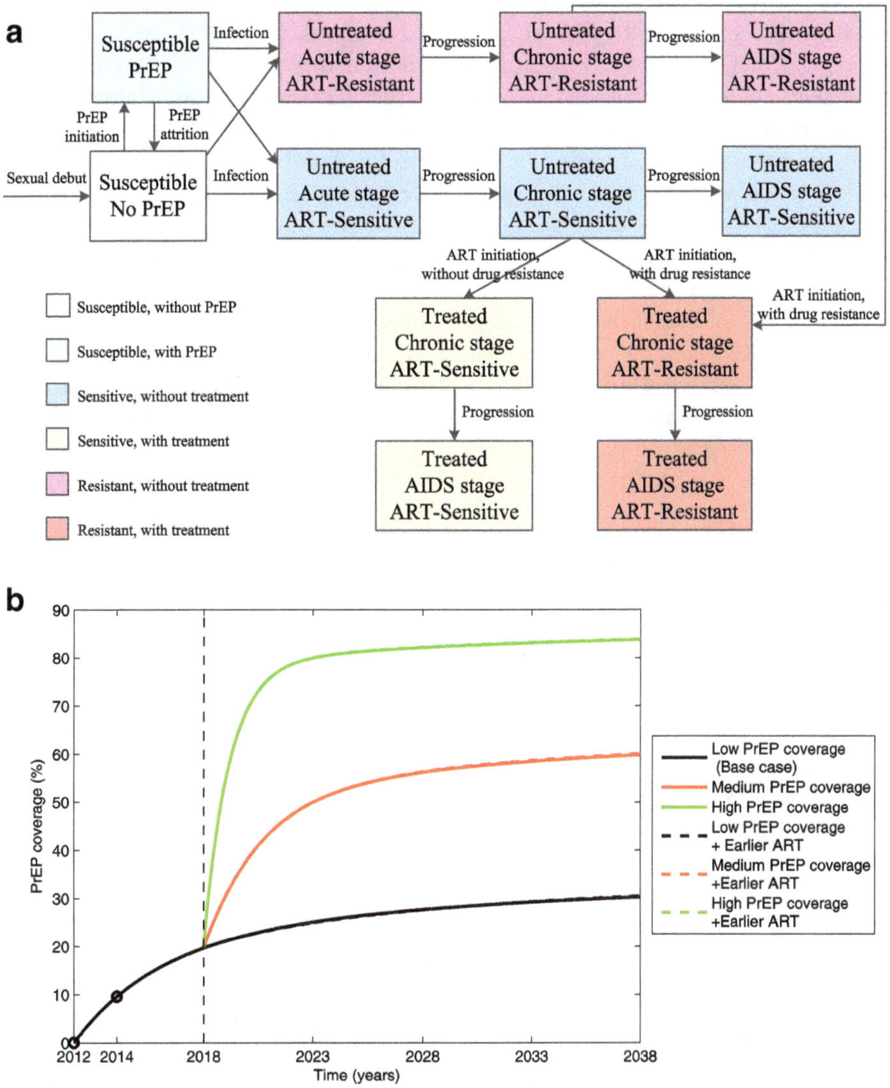

Fig. 1 **a** Flow diagram of the HIV transmission dynamics with PrEP and ART interventions, incorporating the acquisition and transmission of drug resistance following ART. **b** Low, medium, and high PrEP coverage scenarios in the San Francisco MSM population. PrEP coverage increased to an estimated 9.6% (blue circle) of San Francisco's MSM population by 2014 [8] after the Food and Drug Administration approved PrEP in 2012. Projection to 2023 of this rate of increase yields a PrEP coverage of 25% in 2023 (low PrEP scenarios). Efforts to further expand PrEP coverage were modelled by identifying a constant PrEP initiation rate that yielded coverage levels that saturated at 50% (medium PrEP coverage) and 80% (high PrEP coverage) by 2023. Earlier initiation of ART minimally affects PrEP coverage projections because, while it leads to increases in the number of susceptible individuals and, consequently, the numbers of PrEP users (Additional file 1: Figure S2), their ratio (i.e., PrEP coverage) remains relatively unchanged. *PrEP* pre-exposure prophylaxis, *ART* antiretroviral therapy, *MSM* men who have sex with men

of first- or second-line for two reasons. First, data to estimate drug-specific efficacies and adherence levels is not readily available. Second, drug-specific parameters are unnecessary to achieve our goal of estimating intervention cost-effectiveness when using these assumptions regarding the average relative effectiveness of first-line and second-line regimens.

We assumed PrEP effectiveness against drug-sensitive strains was 53% based on a meta-analysis [40], where this value reflects both biomedical efficacy and adherence. We assumed relative PrEP effectiveness against resistant strains was 50% (the ratio of PrEP effectiveness against drug-resistant versus drug-sensitive strains) [14–16]. In a sensitivity analysis, we varied PrEP effectiveness against drug-sensitive strains from 10% to 90% [21, 27] and relative effectiveness against drug-resistant strains from 0 to 1. We assumed an 8% annual rate of PrEP attrition, based on a cohort study in San Francisco [41], and varied it from 1% to 30% per year in sensitivity analyses. Based on low empirically observed dropout proportions [10], we assume that all individuals who initiate ART remain on ART until the end of life and do not drop out of care. We considered only ART-mediated and not PrEP-mediated resistance, because both clinical data [42, 43] and mathematical models [44, 45] suggest that PrEP contributes less than 5% to the total burden of resistance since PrEP-selected resistant phenotypes decay below detection by 6 months after drug cessation and remain undetectable for at least 2 years thereafter [46].

Model calibration

To achieve a realistic baseline scenario, we fitted our model to the annual incidence of diagnosed AIDS cases and deaths from 1980 to 2014 among MSM in San Francisco (Fig. 2a–c) using data from the San Francisco Department of Public Health HIV Epidemiology Section (see [18] for details). We modeled five distinct intervention eras, namely (1) no ART availability (1980–1995); (2) ART administered based on clinical symptoms or CD4 thresholds (1995–2006); (3) expanded ART and shortened time to begin ART based on name-based HIV reporting, which, without altering treatment guidelines, increased ART coverage [18, 47] (2006–2012); (4) initial PrEP roll out (2012–2018); and (5) expanded PrEP, with or without earlier ART (2018–2038). We estimated the parameters by fitting the model to data in eras 1–4, and then simulated various intervention scenarios in era 5. The detailed calibration of the first three eras has been previously provided [18] and the parameters of these eras in this study are the same as used therein. We calibrated the model to the fourth era by choosing a constant rate for PrEP initiation such that PrEP coverage rose from 0% in 2012 (post-Food and Drug Administration approval) to the most recent observed value of 9.6%

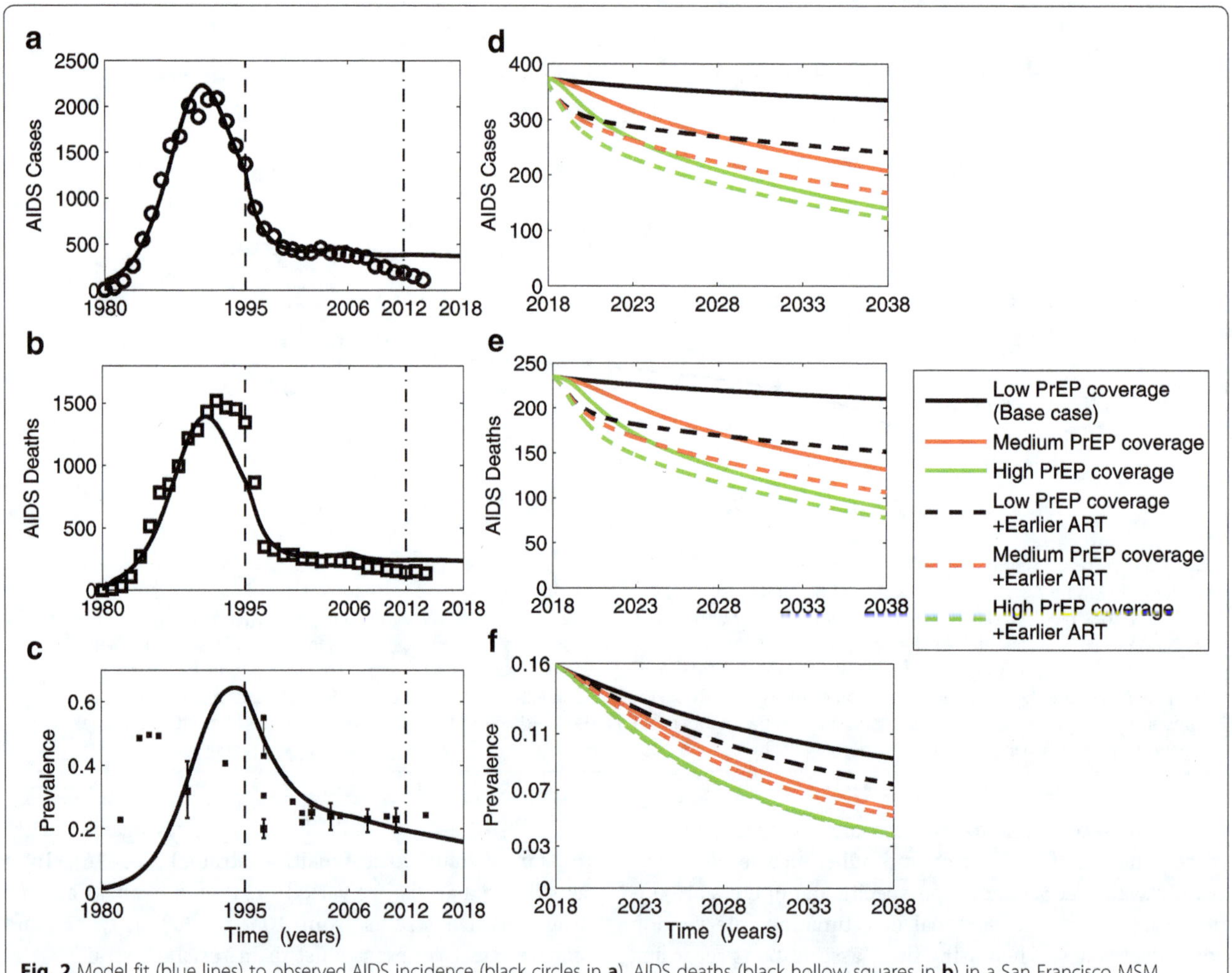

Fig. 2 Model fit (blue lines) to observed AIDS incidence (black circles in **a**), AIDS deaths (black hollow squares in **b**) in a San Francisco MSM cohort. **c** Comparing model-generated prevalence with observed HIV prevalence data among sampled MSM populations (black solid squares and 95% confidence interval if available). Dashed vertical black line divides the pre-treatment and post-treatment phases of our model, roughly approximating the increase in ART availability post-1995 in San Francisco. Dot-dashed vertical black lines show rollout of low coverage PrEP starting in 2012. AIDS cases (**d**), deaths (**e**), and prevalence (**f**) are projected for different PrEP coverage levels, with or without earlier ART (as shown in Fig. 1b) over the next 20 years (2018–2038) with the Y-axis rescaled relative to the left panels to clarify the differences between scenarios (blue lines in left and right panels correspond). *PrEP* pre-exposure prophylaxis, *ART* antiretroviral therapy, *MSM* men who have sex with men

in 2014 [8] (Fig. 1b). At this initiation rate (low PrEP coverage scenario), PrEP coverage would reach 25% (low coverage) after 5 years (2023). For the fifth era, we simulated various intervention scenarios, including continuation of PrEP initiation at this low level or increasing to 50% (medium) or 80% (high) PrEP coverage by 2023. We also considered how these PrEP scenarios interacted with the implementation of new, earlier ART guidelines (1 year post-infection versus the status quo of 1.6 years post-infection). We combined each of the three levels of PrEP intervention with each of the two timings of ART to model six different intervention strategies over the 2018–2038 period (Fig. 1b). The PrEP initiation rates were assumed to be constant for each of the low, medium, and high PrEP scenarios, with rates chosen such that PrEP coverage would saturate at the specified values for each scenario.

We predicted how the AIDS cases, deaths, prevalence (Fig. 2d–f), total new infections (incidence), and new drug-resistant infections (Fig. 3a, b), as well as the fraction of new infections that are drug resistant (Additoinal file 1: Figure S3) would change after 2018 under each of the six strategies, using the low PrEP and baseline ART strategy as our reference comparator. Additionally, we examined the potential for the incidence of drug-resistant infections to increase as a function of second-line drug effectiveness, PrEP coverage, and ART timing (Fig. 3c, d). All analyses were carried out in *Matlab*.

Economic model

We used published quality of life estimates for each health state (Additional file 1: Table S1) [23, 26, 48–51]. We assumed that PrEP did not reduce the quality of life [23, 26], but that the quality of life for drug-resistant

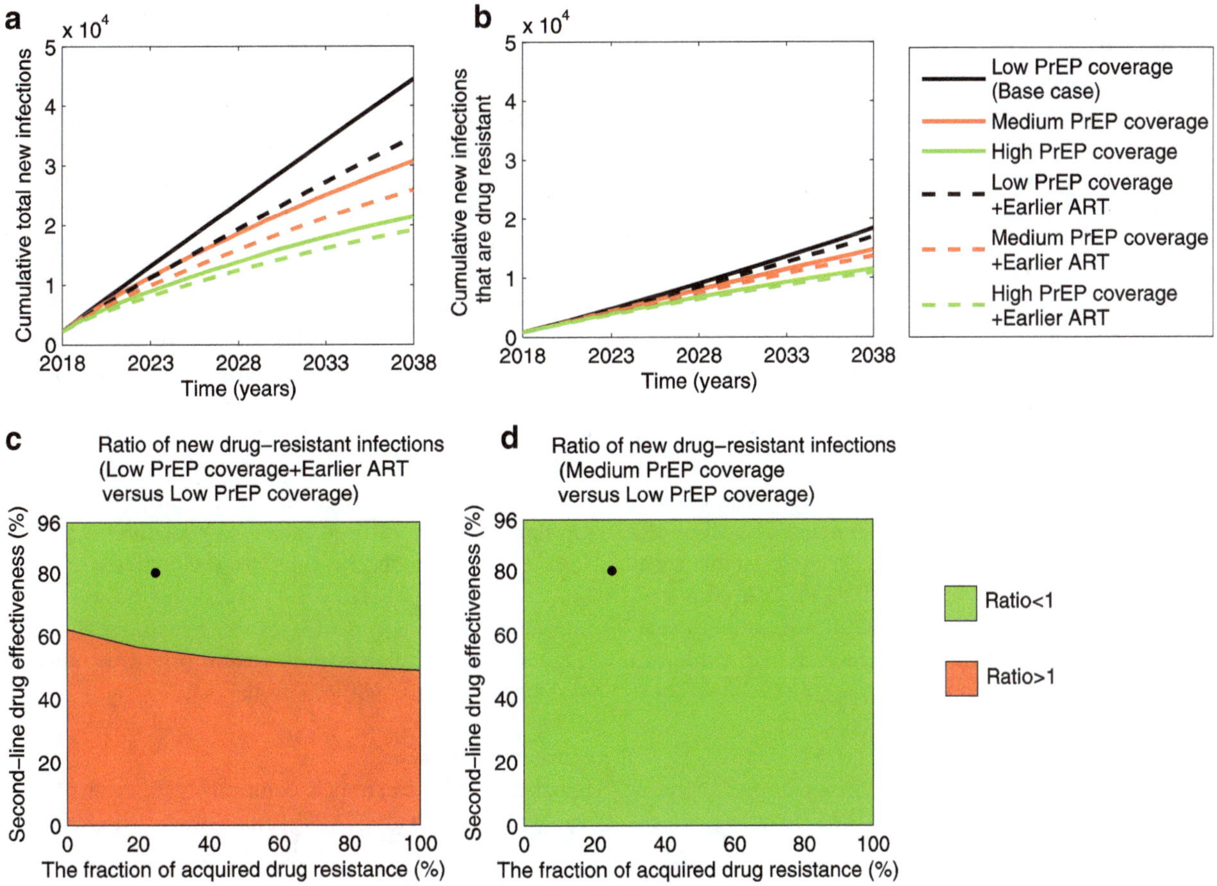

Fig. 3 The cumulative total incidence (**a**) and drug-resistant incidence (**b**) from 2018 to 2038 for different combinations of PrEP coverage and ART initiation time (as shown in Fig. 1b). The ratios of cumulative drug-resistant incidence over 20 years for low PrEP coverage plus earlier ART versus the status quo (**c**), and for medium PrEP coverage versus the status quo (**d**), respectively, where we consider the status quo as the low PrEP coverage scenario. The green and red areas in **c** indicate parameter combinations in which adding earlier ART to the status quo would decrease and increase the incidence of drug resistance, respectively. The drug-resistant incidence always decreases for medium PrEP coverage across all range of second-line drug effectiveness as shown in green area in **d**. The blue circles in **c** and **d** denote the base cases (the second-line drug effectiveness is 80% and 25% of treated cases have acquired drug resistance, and all of them switch to second-line drugs timely). All other parameters are fixed as shown in Additional file 1: Table S1. *PrEP* pre-exposure prophylaxis, *ART* antiretroviral therapy

cases decreases by 5% relative to drug-sensitive individuals at the same stage [26, 52] (varied from 0 to 10% in sensitivity analysis).

We also used published estimates of HIV-related healthcare costs, first- and second-line ART costs, the costs of antibody testing, genotype resistance testing, and counseling and diagnosis [23, 26, 49–51]. Our base case assumed that second-line drug costs for drug-resistant patients were 1.24 times higher than first-line drug costs for drug-sensitive individuals [53], and varied this multiplier from 1 to 5 in sensitivity analysis. Annual PrEP costs included ART medication, laboratory fees (i.e., HIV antibody test every 2–3 months, sexually transmitted infections test every 6 months), and professional fees for patient visits and consultations [54].

We discounted costs and quality-adjusted life years (QALYs) at 3% annually [55] and expressed costs in 2017 U.S. dollars. We calculated net health benefits (QALYs) and costs for various strategies over a 20-year time horizon assuming a public health perspective. The incremental cost-effectiveness ratio (ICER) for each strategy was calculated relative to both the status quo and the next best strategy. Using WHO standards [56], we denoted strategies with an ICER less than the per capita gross domestic product (GDP; $81,347 for San Francisco in 2015 [57]) as very cost-effective and those with an ICER less than three times the per capita GDP as cost-effective ($244,041).

Sensitivity analysis

We used sensitivity analyses to examine the impact of various model parameters on intervention cost-effectiveness, including the effectiveness of PrEP against drug-sensitive and drug-resistant strains, PrEP coverage, PrEP attrition rate, annual PrEP costs, ART effectiveness, and costs for first- and second-line drug regimens, as well as the reduction in lifespan of treated drug-resistant cases relative to treated drug-sensitive cases. We reported additional sensitivity analyses of ICER estimates to various combinations of PrEP coverage and ART timing in Additional file 1: Supplementary Material.

Results

Health outcomes

Under baseline levels of PrEP and ART coverage, we estimate that 44,508 total new HIV infections and 18,426 new drug-resistant infections would occur among MSM in San Francisco over the next 20 years (Table 1 and Fig. 3a, b). Assuming that ART timing remains unchanged, an increase in PrEP coverage to 50% of the MSM population is expected to prevent 13,798 total infections (31% of projected incidence under baseline PrEP and ART) and 3741 drug-resistant infections (20%), and yield 46,757 incremental QALYs (Table 1). An even greater increase in PrEP coverage (to 80%), would avert 23,138 total new infections (52%) and 6939 (38%) new drug-resistant infections, yielding an additional 87,411 QALYs relative to the status quo. Expanding PrEP coverage not only reduces AIDS cases (Fig. 2d) and deaths (Fig. 2e), but also decreases HIV prevalence (Fig. 2f). A 50% (or 80%) PrEP coverage would reduce the prevalence after 20 years from 9.26% in the base scenario to 5.67% (or 3.81%) (Table 1).

Relative to the base scenario, combining low or medium PrEP coverage and earlier ART is expected to avert an additional 9700 (22%) or 18,616 (42%) total new infections, 1457 (8%) or 4740 (26%) new drug-resistant infections, and add 43,649 or 74,048 QALYs, respectively. High PrEP coverage combined with earlier ART provides the most health benefits, with an additional 25,414 (57%) total new infections and 7559 (41%) new drug-resistant infections averted relative to the base scenario (Table 1 and Fig. 3a, b). HIV prevalence would drop to 7.43%, 5.14%, and 3.74% after 20 years when earlier ART is combined with low, medium, and high PrEP coverage, respectively.

Figure 3a, b shows that, in the base case, combining earlier ART and expanded PrEP coverage leads to reductions in drug-resistant incidence and even greater reductions in total incidence. For example, adding earlier ART reduces incidence of drug-resistant and total cases by 8% and 22%, respectively, and expansion to medium PrEP coverage leads to respective reductions of 20% and 31% (Table 1). However, the fraction of new infections that are drug resistant is expected to increase across all scenarios (Additional file 1: Figure S3b), in accordance with previous findings [14, 18]. Earlier ART combined with the low levels of PrEP coverage may also increase absolute drug-resistant incidence (i.e., not just the drug-resistant fraction of total incidence) relative to the base case only when second-line drug effectiveness is less than 60% (Fig. 3c). However, expansion to medium or high PrEP coverage decreases drug-resistant incidence (Fig. 3d) across all levels of second-line drug effectiveness both with and without earlier ART.

Economic outcomes

Expanding PrEP to either medium or high levels of coverage without changing ART timing was cost-effective by WHO standards [56], with an ICER of $117,130 or $132,520 per QALY gained, respectively, compared to the status quo (Table 1 and Fig. 4). Medium PrEP coverage would cost an additional $5477 million over 20 years ($5929 million for PrEP prevention minus $452 million in treatment savings; Additional file 1: Table S2), or $274 million annually, which is five times San Francisco's 2015–2016 annual HIV budget ($16.8 million for prevention and $37.6 million for care [58]).

Table 1 Benefits and costs of expanding PrEP coverage and earlier ART strategies over 20 years

Strategy	Total new Infections[a]	Total infections prevented (fraction)[a]	New infections with drug-resistant strains[a]	Drug-resistant infections prevented (fraction)[a]	HIV prevalence in 2038 (%)	Total costs of PrEP (million US $)[b,c]	Total costs (million US $)[c]	Total QALYs[c]	Incremental costs (million US $)[d]	Incremental QALYs[d]	ICER relative to the status quo	ICER relative to next best strategy
Status quo (Low PrEP coverage)	44,508	–	18,426	–	9.26	5648	9189	1,315,057	–	–	–	–
Medium PrEP coverage	30,710	13,798 (31%)	14,685	3741 (20%)	5.67	11,577	14,666	1,361,814	5477	46,757	117,130	Dominated[e]
High PrEP coverage	21,370	23,138 (52%)	11,487	6939 (38%)	3.81	18,056	20,773	1,402,468	11,584	87,411	132,520	Dominated[e]
Low PrEP coverage+Earlier ART	34,808	9700 (22%)	16,969	1457 (8%)	7.43	5914	9396	1,358,706	207	43,649	4745	4745
Medium PrEP coverage+Earlier ART	25,892	18,616 (42%)	13,686	4740 (26%)	5.14	11,905	15,025	1,389,105	5836	74,048	78,811	185,160
High PrEP coverage+Earlier ART	19,093	25,414 (57%)	10,867	7559 (41%)	3.74	18,307	21,098	1,418,327	11,909	103,270	115,320	207,830

PrEP pre-exposure prophylaxis, *ART* antiretroviral therapy, *ICER* incremental cost-effectiveness ratio, *QALY* quality-adjusted life-year

[a]Total new infections, new drug-resistant infections, total HIV infections prevented and drug-resistant infections prevented are undiscounted number from 2018 to 2038

[b]Includes the costs of antiretroviral drugs for PrEP, laboratory fees (such as HIV antibody test fee every 2–3 months, test fee for sexually transmitted infections every 6 months) and professional fees (such as visiting and consulting fees) [54]

[c]Costs and quality-adjusted life years (QALYs) are net present values (3% annual discount rate) over 20 years

[d]Incremental costs and QALYs are relative to the status quo

[e]The strategy that is dominated yields fewer QALYs at higher costs than the comparator and thus is not an effcient use of resources

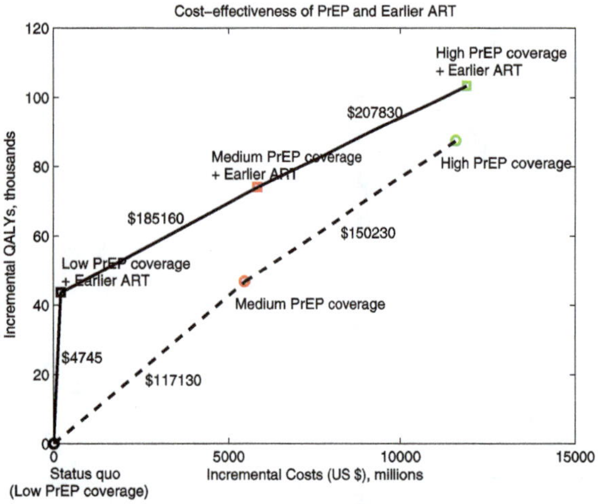

Fig. 4 Incremental costs and QALYs of expanded PrEP coverage with and without earlier ART (Fig. 1b), with the origin corresponding to the status quo of low PrEP coverage and baseline ART guidelines. The solid lines show the incremental cost-effectiveness ratio (ICER) relative to the next best strategy. The dashed lines show the ICER relative to the next best strategy when earlier ART is not implemented. These strategies are dominated by similar strategies with earlier ART, meaning that they are not an efficient use of resources. Incremental costs and QALYs are calculated over a 20-year time horizon (2018–2038) and are discounted to the present at 3% annually. *PrEP* pre-exposure prophylaxis, *ART* antiretroviral therapy, *ICER* incremental cost-effectiveness ratio, *QALY* quality-adjusted life-year

Adding earlier ART to baseline PrEP coverage is the most cost-effective strategy under our base assumptions, costing only $4745 per QALY gained relative to the status quo (Table 1 and Fig. 4). Combining earlier ART with expanded PrEP coverage (50% or 80%) provides more health benefits and costs $78,811 or $115,320 per QALY gained, respectively, compared to the status quo, costing an additional $5836 or $11,909 million, respectively, over 20 years relative to the status quo. However, incremental expansion of PrEP coverage when earlier ART is already in place is substantially more expensive. In particular, earlier ART with medium PrEP coverage costs $185,160 per QALY gained compared to earlier ART with low PrEP coverage level, and earlier ART with high PrEP coverage costs $207,830 per QALY gained compared to earlier ART with medium coverage. This is because earlier ART has already led to a substantial reduction in HIV infections (Fig. 2) and great gains in QALYs (Table 1), such that increased PrEP coverage provides protection only to individuals at a lower infection risk, yielding only modest gains in QALYs per unit cost (Table 1 and Fig. 4).

Sensitivity analysis

Our findings are qualitatively robust to parameter uncertainty. In sensitivity analysis, we found that the PrEP costs and coverage had the largest impact on PrEP cost-effectiveness for the combination of high PrEP coverage and earlier ART compared to the status quo (Fig. 5). If the annual costs of PrEP were 50% lower than the base case, the ICER would decrease from $115,320 to $54,027 per QALY gained. Increasing PrEP coverage from the low to high scenario in the presence of earlier ART would increase the ICER from $4745 to $115,320 per QALY gained. However, the ICER is less sensitive to other parameters (Additional file 1: Supplementary Material).

Discussion

We found that expanding PrEP while initiating ART earlier (at 1 year post-infection versus the status quo of 1. 6 years post-infection) could provide substantial, cost-effective health benefits to the San Francisco MSM population. However, the most cost-effective intervention is earlier ART without further PrEP expansion. This would prevent 9700 (22%) total new infections and 1457 (8%) new drug-resistant infections, and add 43,649 QALYs over the next 20 years; this is very cost-effective at $4745 per QALY gained. Expanding PrEP coverage in addition to earlier ART would further reduce incidence, but only add 1.7–2.4 times more QALYs while costing 28–58 times more than earlier ART alone (Table 1). Still, high PrEP coverage plus earlier ART ($115,320 per QALY gained) is cost-effective for San Francisco even considering the acquisition and transmission of ART-mediated drug resistance. For a budget under $470 million annually, the best strategy is to keep current strategies of PrEP enrollment while initiating ART earlier. This may be advisable for San Francisco, based on the city's 2015–2016 annual HIV/AIDS budget [58] (though this excludes private insurance and may therefore underestimate the total funding available). A higher budget would suggest that PrEP expansion in addition to earlier ART is advisable.

Our estimated ICER of expanding PrEP without earlier initiation of ART of $117,130–132,520 per QALY gained (Table 1) is far greater than estimates for targeted high-risk MSM interventions in New York City ($31,970 [20]) , Los Angeles County ($27,863–37,181 [26]), and nationwide US ($52,443 [23]), but lower than estimates for the general MSM population in New York City ($353,739 [22]) and nationwide US ($172,091–216,480 [23]). These discrepancies may stem from the different settings, PrEP targeting strategies, or model assumptions. For example, San Francisco has higher testing and treatment rates than New York City and the entire US [10, 18, 22, 23]. We assume two-fold higher life expectancy gains following treatment than Juusola et al. [23], based on more recent life expectancy estimates [37, 38]. Recent reviews discussed variation amongst ICER calculations in greater detail [28, 59].

Drabo et al. [26] conducted a similar study for high-risk MSM in Los Angeles, but used a different model

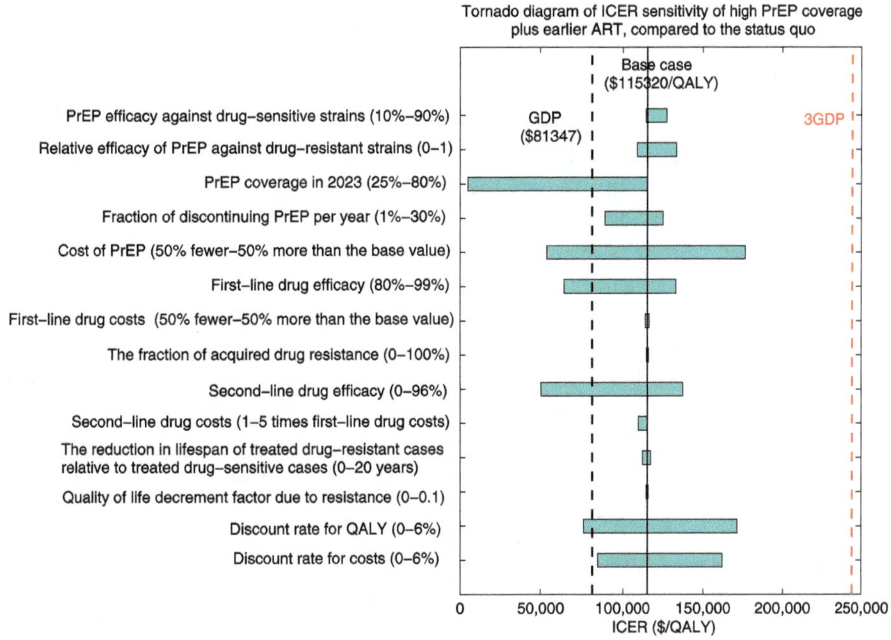

Fig. 5 One-way sensitivity analysis of the cost-effectiveness of high PrEP coverage plus earlier ART compared to the status quo. The horizontal bars represent the range of the incremental cost-effectiveness ratios (ICERs) as each variable is varied across its plausible range listed. The solid vertical black line indicates the base case ICER ($115,320 per QALY gained). The dashed vertical blue and red lines represent the per capita gross domestic product (GDP) for San Francisco ($81,347 in 2015 [57]) and three times the per capita GDP, respectively, two thresholds denoting a very cost-effective and cost-effective use of resources, by international standards [56]. *PrEP* pre-exposure prophylaxis, *ART* antiretroviral therapy, *ICER* incremental cost-effectiveness ratio, *QALY* quality-adjusted life-year, *GDP* gross domestic product

structure. Our infection–age-structured model allows us to track the life expectancy at different ART initiation times and among individuals with drug sensitive or resistant strains (the primary innovation of our model). In addition, their model initiated ART treatment at a CD4+ cell count ≤ 500 cells/mm^3, whereas we considered an even earlier ART strategy. Finally, we accounted for the switch to second-line drug treatment after treatment failure and its associated costs. Despite these differences, we concur that all combinations of earlier ART and PrEP coverage are cost-effective to varying degrees, and that the optimal strategy depends on budgetary constraints.

Our study has several limitations. First, to explore the cost-effectiveness of the above scenarios, we fit our model to multiple sources of data, including incidence of AIDS diagnoses and deaths, HIV prevalence, the fraction of drug-resistance amongst incident cases, and other demographic data [18]. Fitting to so many sources data has the advantage of integrating much of what is known about this epidemic but is ambitious in the sense that it is difficult to closely fit all data sets simultaneously. One possibility to solving this would have been to fit only a subset of these data such that model fits would have better reflected those datasets but not been informed by others. Second, we did not model PrEP-mediated acquired drug resistance. Our results should be robust to this exclusion, as recommended screening practices are thought to limit PrEP-acquired resistance via quick identification of breakthrough infections amongst individuals on PrEP [21, 43, 60]. Third, we assumed that sexual partners were assorted independent of PrEP or ART usage. If PrEP were targeted towards individuals whose partners, if infected, were less likely to be on ART, then PrEP would be expected to be more effective and cost-effective. Should individuals on PrEP be more likely to engage in sexual partnerships with infected individuals on ART than with those not on ART, then this would reduce the estimated cost-effectiveness of PrEP. Fourth, we assumed a homogenous PrEP coverage for the entire population irrespective of risk and age. We made this assumption for simplicity and due to the lack of information about age- and risk-group mixing contact patterns. If PrEP coverage is higher in individuals within the MSM population who are at higher risk of infection than the average (i.e., because of PrEP targeting to high-risk groups or high-risk individuals seeking out PrEP), then PrEP would be more cost-effective. In contrast, if high-risk groups also constitute groups that are hard to reach with PrEP, then PrEP cost-effectiveness would be lower than estimated. Similarly, the indirect effects of PrEP on the population would depend on the propensity to transmit of individuals on PrEP, should they have been infected if they were not on PrEP. Finally, while our results were qualitatively robust to parameter uncertainty, future changes in intervention costs or efficacy may affect our estimates.

Conclusions

In summary, expanding PrEP coverage and shifting ART initiation even earlier in San Francisco would reduce the total and drug resistant incidence, and add over 40,000 QALYs to the population over 20 years. Combining higher PrEP coverage and earlier ART is predicted to be cost-effective at three times the per capita GDP threshold. These results are robust across a wide range of assumptions regarding drug resistance and the effectiveness and cost of second-line drug regimens.

Abbreviations

ART: antiretroviral therapy; GDP: gross domestic product; ICER: incremental cost-effectiveness ratio; MSM: men who have sex with men; PrEP: pre-exposure prophylaxis; QALY: quality-adjusted life-year

Acknowledgements

We thank Ling Hsu for providing data from San Francisco Department of Public Health HIV Epidemiology Section. We also thank The University of Texas at Austin for hosting Mingwang Shen while the research was conducted.

Funding

This work was supported by the National Natural Science Foundation of China (NSFC, grant number 11631012 (YX) and 11571273 (YX)), by the National Mega-project of Science Research (grant number 2017ZX10201101-002-002 (YX)), and by the National Natural Science Foundation of China (NSFC, grant number 11701442(XS)).LR was supported by the National Science Foundation (DMS-1758290). LAM and SEB were supported by the US National Institute of General Medical Sciences Model of Infectious Disease Agent Study grant U01GM087719 to LAM and APG, and SEB was supported by a National Institute of Allergy and Infectious Diseases K01 award (K01AI125830).

Authors' contributions

MS, YX, LR, LAM, and SEB conceived and designed the study. MS analyzed the data, carried out the analysis, and performed numerical simulations. MS wrote the first draft of the manuscript. MS, YX, LR, LAM, and SEB contributed to writing the paper and agreed with manuscript results and conclusions. All authors read and approved the final manuscript.

Competing interests

The authors declare that they have no competing interests.

Author details

[1]Department of Epidemiology and Biostatistics, School of Public Health, Xi'an Jiaotong University Health Science Center, Xi'an, Shaanxi 710061, People's Republic of China. [2]School of Mathematics and Statistics, Xi'an Jiaotong University, Xi'an 710049, People's Republic of China. [3]Department of Integrative Biology, The University of Texas at Austin, Austin, TX 78712, USA. [4]Department of Mathematics, University of Florida, Gainesville, FL 32611, USA. [5]The Santa Fe Institute, Santa Fe, NM 87501, USA. [6]Department of Epidemiology and Biostatistics, College of Public Health, University of Georgia, Athens, GA 30602, USA. [7]Center for Ecology of Infectious Diseases, University of Georgia, Athens, GA 30602, USA.

References

1. Holmes D. FDA paves the way for pre-exposure HIV prophylaxis. Lancet. 2012;380:325.
2. Abdool Karim Q, Abdool Karim SS, Frohlich JA, et al. Effectiveness and safety of tenofovir gel, an antiretroviral microbicide, for the prevention of HIV infection in women. Science. 2010;329:1168–74.
3. Grant RM, Lama JR, Anderson PL, et al. Preexposure chemoprophylaxis for HIV prevention in men who have sex with men. N Engl J Med. 2010;363: 2587–99.
4. Molina JM, Capitant C, Spire B, et al. On-demand preexposure prophylaxis in men at high risk for HIV-1 infection. N Engl J Med. 2015;373:2237–46.
5. Grant RM, Anderson PL, McMahan V, et al. Uptake of pre-exposure prophylaxis, sexual practices, and HIV incidence in men and transgender women who have sex with men: a cohort study. Lancet Infect Dis. 2014;14:820–9.
6. McCormack S, Dunn DT, Desai M, et al. Pre-exposure prophylaxis to prevent the acquisition of HIV-1 infection (PROUD): effectiveness results from the pilot phase of a pragmatic open-label randomised trial. Lancet. 2016;387:53–60.
7. Grant RM, Liu A, Hecht J, et al. Scale-up of pre-exposure prophylaxis in San Francisco to impact HIV incidence. In: Conference on Retroviruses and Opportunistic Infections, Seattle, Washington. 2015. http://www.croiconference.org/sessions/scale-preexposure-prophylaxis-san-francisco-impact-hiv-incidence.
8. Chen YH, Snowden JM, McFarland W, Raymond HF. Pre-exposure prophylaxis (PrEP) use, seroadaptation, and sexual behavior among men who have sex with men, San Francisco, 2004-2014. AIDS Behav. 2016;20:2791–7.
9. Highleyman L. At least 6000 people thought to be on HIV PrEP in San Francisco. http://hivandhepatitis.com/hiv-prevention/hiv-prep/5730-at-least-6000-people-thought-to-be-on-hiv-prep-in-san-francisco.
10. San Francisco Department of Public Health Population Health Division HIV Epidemiology Section. HIV Epidemiology Annual Report. 2015. https://www.sfdph.org/dph/files/reports/RptsHIVAIDS/AnnualReport2015-20160831.pdf. Accessed 5 Nov 2016.
11. Grey JA, Bernstein KT, Sullivan PS, et al. Estimating the population sizes of men who have sex with men in US states and counties using data from the American community survey. JMIR Public Health Surveill. 2016;2:e14.
12. San Francisco Department of Public Health HIV Epidemiology Section. HIV/AIDS Epidemiology Annual Report. 2010. https://www.sfdph.org/dph/files/reports/RptsHIVAIDS/HIVAIDAnnlRpt2010.pdf. Accessed 5 November 2016.
13. Cohen MS, Chen YQ, McCauley M, et al. Prevention of HIV-1 infection with early antiretroviral therapy. N Engl J Med. 2011;365:493–505.
14. Supervie V, García-Lerma JG, Heneine W, Blower S. HIV, transmitted drug resistance, and the paradox of preexposure prophylaxis. Proc Natl Acad Sci U S A. 2010;107:12381–6.
15. Supervie V, Barrett M, Kahn JS, et al. Modeling dynamic interactions between pre-exposure prophylaxis interventions & treatment programs: predicting HIV transmission & resistance. Sci Rep. 2011;1:185.
16. Abbas UL, Anderson RM, Mellors JW. Potential impact of antiretroviral chemoprophylaxis on HIV-1 transmission in resource-limited settings. PLoS One. 2007;2:e875.
17. Shen MW, Xiao YN, Rong LB. Global stability of an infection-age structured HIV-1 model linking within-host and between-host dynamics. Math Biosci. 2015;263:37–50.
18. Shen MW, Xiao YN, Rong LB, Meyers LA, Bellan SE. Early antiretroviral therapy and potent second-line drugs could decrease HIV incidence of drug resistance. P Roy Soc B-Biol Sci. 2017;284:20170525.
19. Adamson BJ, Bounthavong M, Kublin JG, Garrison L. Cost-effectiveness analysis of a partially effective HIV vaccine in San Francisco. Value Health. 2015;18:A237.
20. Desai K, Sansom SL, Ackers ML, et al. Modeling the impact of HIV chemoprophylaxis strategies among men who have sex with men in the United States: HIV infections prevented and costeffectiveness. AIDS. 2008;22:1829–39.
21. Paltiel AD, Freedberg KA, Scott CA, et al. HIV preexposure prophylaxis in the United States: impact on lifetime infection risk, clinical outcomes, and cost-effectiveness. Clin Infect Dis. 2009;48:806–15.
22. Koppenhaver RT, Sorensen SW. The cost-effectiveness of pre-exposure prophylaxis in men who have sex with men in the United States: an epidemic model. J Acquir Immune Defic Syndr. 2011;58:e51–2.
23. Juusola JL, Brandeau ML, Owens DK, Bendavid E. The cost-effectiveness of

preexposure prophylaxis for HIV prevention in the United States in men who have sex with men. Ann Intern Med. 2012;156:541–50.
24. Kessler J, Myers JE, Nucifora KA, et al. Averting HIV infections in New York City: a modeling approach estimating the future impact of additional behavioral and biomedical prevention strategies. AIDS. 2014;28:2683–91.
25. Ross EL, Cinti SK, Hutton DW. Implementation and operational research: a cost-effective, clinically actionable strategy for targeting HIV preexposure prophylaxis to high-risk men who have sex with men. J Acquir Immune Defic Syndr. 2016;72:e61–7.
26. Drabo EF, Hay JW, Vardavas R, Wagner ZR, Sood N. A cost-effectiveness analysis of preexposure prophylaxis for the prevention of HIV among Los Angeles County men who have sex with men. Clin Infect Dis. 2016;63:1495–504.
27. Bernard CL, Brandeau ML, Humphreys K, et al. Cost-effectiveness of HIV preexposure prophylaxis for people who inject drugs in the United States. Ann Intern Med. 2016;165:10–9.
28. Gomez GB, Borquez A, Case KK, Wheelock A, Vassall A, Hankins C. The cost and impact of scaling up pre-exposure prophylaxis for HIV prevention: a systematic review of cost-effectiveness modelling studies. PLoS Med. 2013; 10:e1001401.
29. Anderson SJ, Cherutich P, Kilonzo N, et al. Maximising the effect of combination HIV prevention through prioritisation of the people and places in greatest need: a modelling study. Lancet. 2014;384:249–56.
30. Nichols BE, Baltussen R, van Dijk JH, et al. Cost-effectiveness of PrEP in HIV/AIDS control in Zambia: a stochastic league approach. J Acquir Immune Defic Syndr. 2014;66:221–8.
31. Hallett TB, Baeten JM, Heffron R, et al. Optimal uses of antiretrovirals for prevention in HIV-1 serodiscordant heterosexual couples in South Africa: a modelling study. PLoS Med. 2011;8:e1001123.
32. Kim SB, Yoon M, Ku NS, et al. Mathematical modeling of HIV prevention measures including pre-exposure prophylaxis on HIV incidence in South Korea. PLoS One. 2014;9:e90080.
33. Cremin I, Alsallaq R, Dybul M, Piot P, Garnett G, Hallett TB. The new role of antiretrovirals in combination HIV prevention: a mathematical modelling analysis. AIDS. 2013;27:447–58.
34. Smith JA, Anderson SJ, Harris KL, et al. Maximising HIV prevention by balancing the opportunities of today with the promises of tomorrow: a modelling study. Lancet HIV. 2016;3:e289–96.
35. Ramadhani HO, Bartlett JA, Thielman NM, et al. Association of first-line and second-line antiretroviral therapy adherence. Open Forum Infect Dis. 2014; 1(2):ofu079.
36. Dodd PJ, Garnett GP, Hallett TB. Examining the promise of HIV elimination by 'test and treat' in hyperendmic settings. AIDS. 2010;24:729–35.
37. May M, Gompels M, Sabin C. Life expectancy of HIV-1-positive individuals approaches normal, conditional on response to antiretroviral therapy: UK collaborative HIV cohort study. J Int AIDS Soc. 2012;15(Suppl 4):18078.
38. May M, Gompels M, Delpech V, et al. Impact on life expectancy of HIV-1 positive individuals of CD4+ cell count and viral load response to antiretroviral therapy. AIDS. 2014;28:1193–202.
39. Richman DD, Morton SC, Wrin T, et al. The prevalence of antiretroviral drug resistance in the United States. AIDS. 2004;18:1393–401.
40. Jiang J, Yang X, Ye L, et al. Pre-exposure prophylaxis for the prevention of HIV infection in high risk populations: a meta-analysis of randomized controlled trials. PLoS One. 2014;9:e87674.
41. Liu A, Cohen S, Follansbee S, et al. Early experiences implementing preexposure prophylaxis (PrEP) for HIV prevention in San Francisco. PLoS Med. 2014;11:e1001613.
42. Lehman DA, Baeten JM, McCoy CO, et al. Risk of drug resistance among persons acquiring HIV within a randomized clinical trial of single- or dual-agent preexposure prophylaxis. J Infect Dis. 2015;211:1211–8.
43. Grant RM, Liegler T, Defechereux P, et al. Drug resistance and plasma viral RNA level after ineffective use of oral pre-exposure prophylaxis in women. AIDS. 2015;29:331–7.
44. van de Vijver DA, Nichols BE, Abbas UL, et al. Preexposure prophylaxis will have a limited impact on HIV-1 drug resistance in sub-Saharan Africa: a comparison of mathematical models. AIDS. 2013;27:2943–51.
45. Abbas UL, Glaubius R, Mubayi A, Hood G, Mellors JW. Antiretroviral therapy and preexposure prophylaxis: combined impact on HIV-1 transmission and drug resistance in South Africa. J Infect Dis. 2013;208:224–34.
46. Weis JF, Baeten JM, McCoy CO, et al. Preexposure prophylaxis-selected drug resistance decays rapidly after drug cessation. AIDS. 2016;30:31–5.
47. Zetola NM, Bernstein K, Ahrens K, et al. Using surveillance data to monitor entry into care of newly diagnosed HIV-infected persons: San Francisco, 2006-2007. BMC Public Health. 2009;9:17.
48. Tengs TO, Lin TH. A meta-analysis of utility estimates for HIV/AIDS. Med Decis Mak. 2002;22:475–81.
49. Long EF, Brandeau ML, Owens DK. Potential population health outcomes and expenditures of HIV vaccination strategies in the United States. Vaccine. 2009;27:5402–10.
50. Long EF, Brandeau ML, Owens DK. The cost-effectiveness and population outcomes of expanded HIV screening and antiretroviral treatment in the United States. Ann Intern Med. 2010;153:778–89.
51. Juusola JL, Brandeau ML, Long EF, Owens DK, Bendavid E. The costeffectiveness of symptom-based testing and routine screening for acute HIV infection in men who have sex with men in the USA. AIDS. 2011;25: 1779–87.
52. Nichols BE, Sigaloff KC, Kityo C, et al. Increasing the use of second-line therapy is a cost-effective approach to prevent the spread of drug-resistant HIV: a mathematical modelling study. J Int AIDS Soc. 2014;17:19164.
53. Solem CT, Snedecor SJ, Khachatryan A, et al. Cost of treatment in a US commercially insured, HIV-1-infected population. PLoS One. 2014;9:e98152.
54. Horberg M, Raymond B. Financial policy issues for HIV pre-exposure prophylaxis: cost and access to insurance. Am J Prev Med. 2013;44(Suppl 2): S125–8.
55. Drummond M, Sculpher M, Torrance G, O'Brien B, Stoddart G. Methods for the economic evaluation of health care programmes. New York: Oxford University Press; 2005.
56. World Health Organization. The World Health Report 2002. Reducing Risks, Promoting Healthy Life. http://www.who.int/whr/2002/en. Accessed 5 Nov 2016.
57. Bureau of Economic Analysis US Department of Commerce. Per capita real GDP by metropolitan area. San Francisco-Oakland-Hayward, CA (Metropolitan Statistical Area). http://www.bea.gov/iTable/iTable.cfm?reqid=70&step=1&isuri=1&acrdn=2#reqid=70&step=10&isuri=1&7003=1000&7035=1&7004=naics&7005=1&7006=41860&7036=-1&7001=21000&7002=2&7090=70&7007=2015&7093=levels. Accessed 5 Nov 2016.
58. Lee EM. Mayor Lee Announces HIV/AIDS Funding in City's Budget. http://sfmayor.org/article/mayor-lee-announces-hivaids-funding-citys-budget. Accessed 5 Nov 2016.
59. Schackman BR. Cost-effectiveness of pre-exposure prophylaxis for HIV: a review. Curr Opin HIV AIDS. 2012;7:587–92.
60. Centers for Disease Control and Prevention, U.S. Public Health Service. Preexposure prophylaxis for the prevention of HIV infection in the United States-2014: A Clinical Practice Guideline. 2014. www.cdc.gov/hiv/pdf/prepguidelines2014.pdf. Accessed 5 Nov 2016.

12

Registration of published randomized trials

Ludovic Trinquart[1*], Adam G. Dunn[2] and Florence T. Bourgeois[3,4]

Abstract

Background: Prospective trial registration is a powerful tool to prevent reporting bias. We aimed to determine the extent to which published randomized controlled trials (RCTs) were registered and registered prospectively.

Methods: We searched MEDLINE and EMBASE from January 2005 to October 2017; we also screened all articles cited by or citing included and excluded studies, and the reference lists of related reviews. We included studies that examined published RCTs and evaluated their registration status, regardless of medical specialty or language. We excluded studies that assessed RCT registration status only through mention of registration in the published RCT, without searching registries or contacting the trial investigators. Two independent reviewers blinded to the other's work performed the selection. Following PRISMA guidelines, two investigators independently extracted data, with discrepancies resolved by consensus. We calculated pooled proportions and 95% confidence intervals using random-effects models.

Results: We analyzed 40 studies examining 8773 RCTs across a wide range of clinical specialties. The pooled proportion of registered RCTs was 53% (95% confidence interval 44% to 58%), with considerable between-study heterogeneity. A subset of 24 studies reported data on prospective registration across 5529 RCTs. The pooled proportion of prospectively registered RCTs was 20% (95% confidence interval 15% to 25%). Subgroup analyses showed that registration was higher for industry-supported and larger RCTs. A meta-regression analysis across 19 studies (5144 RCTs) showed that the proportion of registered trials significantly increased over time, with a mean proportion increase of 27%, from 25 to 52%, between 2005 and 2015.

Conclusions: The prevalence of trial registration has increased over time, but only one in five published RCTs is prospectively registered, undermining the validity and integrity of biomedical research.

Keywords: Randomized controlled trials, Registration, Reporting bias

Abbreviations: ANZCTR, Australian New Zealand Clinical Trials Registry; CT.gov, ClinicalTrials.gov; FDA, Food and Drug Administration; FDAAA, Food and Drug Administration Amendments Act; ICMJE, International Committee of Medical Journal Editors; ISCRCTN, International Standard Randomised Controlled Trials Number; IF, impact factor; PEDro, Physiotherapy Evidence Database; RCT, randomized controlled trial; SR, systematic review; WHO ICTRP, World Health Organization International Clinical Trials Registry Platform

* Correspondence: ludovic@bu.edu
[1]Department of Biostatistics, Boston University School of Public Health, Boston, Massachusetts, USA
Full list of author information is available at the end of the article

Background

Prospective clinical trial registration is at the foundation of research transparency [1, 2]. By documenting the existence of clinical trials and providing a summary of protocol details before patients are enrolled and trial results become known, registries can prevent unnecessary duplication of trials, facilitate the identification of research gaps, and support coordination of study efforts for a disease [3]. As registration allows public scrutiny of the availability of trial results, it also provides means to identify and monitor biased reporting of trials. Several cases have highlighted how selective reporting can lead to considerable harm to patients. Rofecoxib, a nonsteroidal anti-inflammatory drug, was found to be associated with increased risk of myocardial infarction as early as 2000, but the primary trial publication selectively omitted findings on cardiovascular safety, and rofecoxib was not withdrawn from the market until several years later, in 2004 [4, 5]. Incomplete trial reporting can also lead to considerable waste of resources, as has been seen in the case of oseltamivir [6] or gabapentin [7, 8] with billions of dollars spent despite poor evidence of efficacy. Prospective trial registration—if universally implemented—can serve as a powerful tool to detect and prevent this type of publication bias and selective outcome reporting [3, 9–11].

The International Committee of Medical Journal Editors (ICMJE) announced in 2004 a requirement for prospective registration of clinical trials as a pre-requisite for consideration for publication in its member journals, beginning the following year [2]. In the USA, the Food and Drug Administration Amendments Act (FDAAA) has mandated prospective trial registration with ClinicalTrials.gov since 2007 for drugs, biologics, and devices subject to Food and Drug Administration (FDA) regulation. The requirements for registration and result posting have recently been expanded with the FDAAA Final Rule and a similar policy by the National Institutes of Health [12, 13]. Other countries and funders have implemented similar policies [14, 15].

The clinical trial research community has widely adopted trial registration, and trial registries have been leveraged to monitor research activity and integrity [16–18]. For example, trial registration data have been used to show that the results of registered trials are frequently not disseminated, either through reporting in biomedical journals or posting on ClinicalTrials.gov [19, 20]. However, several studies in specific medical specialties have suggested that many published trials are not registered or not registered prospectively, raising concerns that long-standing efforts have not succeeded in achieving universal trial registration [21–23]. Our objective in this systematic review was to determine the extent to which published randomized controlled trials (RCTs) were registered and registered prospectively.

Methods

Search and study selection

Studies were eligible if they were based on a sample of RCTs identified in published reports in medical journals and evaluated their registration status. All eligible studies across medical specialties were included. Studies not limited to RCTs were not eligible, unless they provided relevant data on registration of the subgroup of RCTs. Studies that determined trial registration only through mention of trial registration in the published article (i.e., the article included the trial registration number in the abstract or main text), but did not further search for information on registration status with either a search for trial records in registries or by contacting the trial investigators to inquire about registration status, were excluded. Lastly, studies that covered a majority of trials published prior to 2005 (i.e., the middle of the range of years covered was prior to 2005) were excluded.

We did not register a protocol for the review. We searched MEDLINE via PubMed and EMBASE without language restriction for studies published between January 1, 2005, and October 31, 2017. The search strategy was (trial[tiab] OR trials[tiab]) AND (registration[ti] OR registered[ti] OR unregistered[ti]) in MEDLINE and (trial:ti OR trial:ab OR trials:ti OR trials:ab) AND (registration:ti OR registered:ti OR unregistered:ti) in EMBASE. Additionally, we screened all articles that were cited by or that cited any of the included studies and studies excluded after full-text screening, and we screened the reference lists of related reviews [24–26] for additional eligible studies.

Two investigators screened the titles and abstracts of all records, independently and in duplicate, to identify potentially eligible studies for further assessment. Discrepancies were discussed to reach consensus. All authors then independently assessed each remaining full-text article for inclusion. We again reviewed all discrepancies, and the final list of included studies was determined by consensus among all authors.

To eliminate overlapping samples of RCTs, we compared the medical specialties, journals searched for published RCTs, and time periods covered by the studies. In cases of complete overlap (i.e., when a study sample was included in a more recent, larger study), we discarded the smaller study encompassed in the larger one. When RCTs were identified based on a specific clinical topic (e.g., RCTs of cognitive behavioral therapy and new-generation antidepressants), we considered that the study was unlikely to overlap with another study based on a search of journals of a relevant medical specialty (e.g., journals in psychology), after consideration of years and journals searched. We could not exclude the possibility that some studies that searched for RCTs across multiple specialties or in general medicine journals would not overlap with other studies. To address this, we discarded studies for which we could not completely ensure that there was no overlap from the primary analysis but included the totality of the available data in a secondary analysis.

Data extraction

Two investigators independently extracted data from each included study using a standardized data collection form. Discrepancies were resolved by consensus. For each included study, we extracted the medical specialty, the publication years of included RCTs, the number of journals searched for RCTs, the list of journals (when provided), the number of identified RCTs, and the number of registered RCTs. We also assessed how trial registration was assessed (i.e., through the reporting of a trial registration number in the article, by searching for trial records in trial registries [27], and/or by contacting corresponding authors). We noted which registries were searched and assessed whether studies had included trials that started enrolment before 2005, as the ICMJE policy was implemented in September 2005. Moreover, we noted if each study assessed if the trial registration was prospective. In that case, we also extracted the number of trials registered prospectively. According to the ICMJE, trials must register at or before the onset of patient enrollment as a condition of consideration for publication. According to FDAAA, Applicable Clinical Trials must be registered no later than 21 days after enrollment of the first participant. We considered trials to be registered prospectively, as defined by the authors of the review.

Lastly, we also extracted the number of registered trials in certain subgroups, when this information was available: in trials that started enrolment after 2005, according to publication year and trial size, and in industry-supported trials. We defined industry support as direct or indirect financial support by a company that produces drugs or medical devices.

Data synthesis

For each included study, we calculated the proportion of registered RCTs with the 95% Clopper-Pearson exact confidence interval. We assessed the heterogeneity across studies through a visual examination of a forest plot and heterogeneity statistics (Cochran's chi-square test and between-study variance τ^2). We estimated pooled proportions by using arcsine transformations and a beta-binomial random-effects model with Anscombe continuity correction [28, 29]. We examined potential small-study effects by using a funnel plot showing the relationship between the log odds of being registered and the associated standard error. Similar methods were used for the synthesis of prospective registration data. For the latter analysis, we first calculated the proportion of RCTs registered prospectively out of the total number of identified RCTs. We also calculated the proportion of RCTs registered prospectively among registered RCTs.

To examine the effect of time on registration prevalence, we conducted three analyses. We synthesized data for RCTs that started enrolment exclusively after 2005. Because the RCT start dates were frequently unclear, we also performed an analysis limited to RCTs published in 2010 or later in order to capture RCTs that were likely to have all been initiated after the implementation of the ICMJE registration policy. The year 2010 was chosen based on data indicating that the time from start of study enrollment to publication is approximately 5 years [30, 31]. Finally, in order to detect changes in registration over the study period, we examined the proportion of registered trials by publication year, within studies and across studies, by using meta-regression models. We fitted the models on the log odds scale and back transformed the fitted lines to produce a plot showing the proportion of registered trials against publication year. We also analyzed the proportion of prospectively registered trials by publication year through a meta-regression.

To further explore sources of heterogeneity in registration prevalence, we performed a subgroup analysis in trials (fully or partially) supported with funding from industry. We also examined the prevalence of registration according to the sample size of RCTs. Because different thresholds were used across studies, we reported the extracted data without meta-analysis. Finally, we examined the subset of studies that identified published RCTs from a sample of high-impact factor journals. Analyses were performed using R v3.4.1 (R Development Core Team, Vienna, Austria) with the metafor package for meta-analysis. The data and R code are provided in Additional files 1 and 2.

Results

Characteristics of included studies

We identified 40 eligible studies reported in 43 articles [21, 22, 32–72]. Figure 1 shows the selection process. We screened 2180 records and 91 full-text articles. The most common reason for excluding articles was that the assessment of trial registration was based solely on mention of a trial registration number in the article (Additional file 3: Table S1). In addition, we excluded two articles [73, 74] because the data were completely included in two other, larger studies [34, 35]. Finally, for one study [37], we excluded data for a subset of RCTs which were also covered in another study [35].

Table 1 shows the characteristics of included studies. The 40 studies covered a wide range of clinical specialties. To identify RCTs, 17 (43%) studies searched a sample of high-impact factor journals, while 10 (25%) studies performed a systematic review of RCTs on a specific clinical topic. Among 27 studies that identified RCTs based on publication in a specific sample of

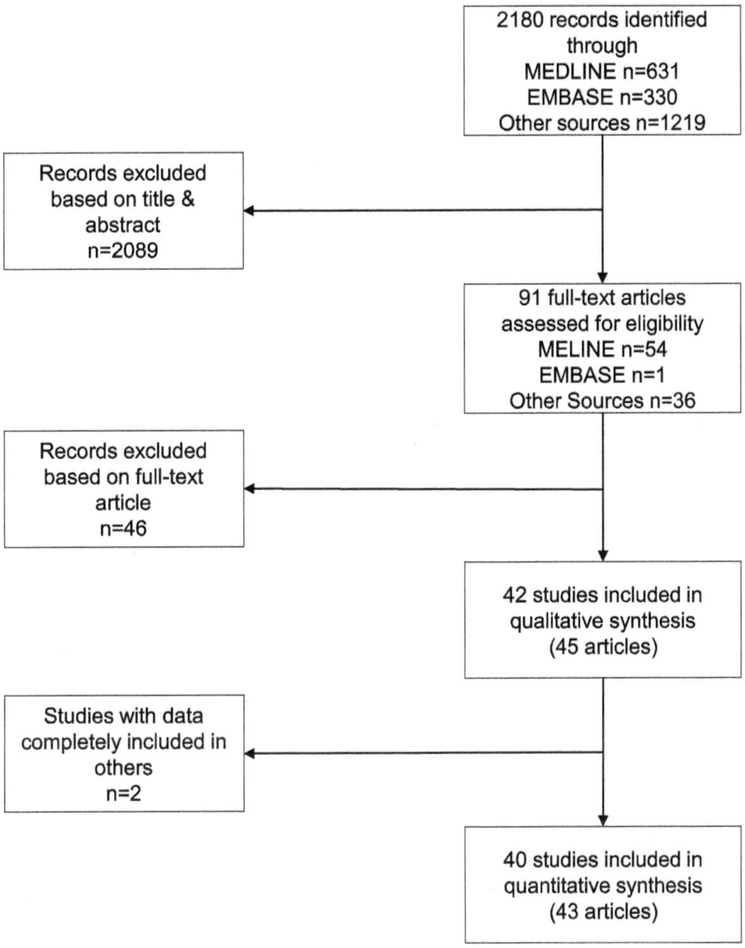

Fig. 1 Flow diagram of study selection

journals, the median number of included journals was 5 (Q1–Q3 4–10). Each study examined a median of 187 RCTs (Q1–Q3 103–301). Studies examined RCTs published over a median of 3 years (Q1–Q3 1–5 years), with a median starting year of 2009. To assess the registration status of published RCTs, all studies examined if a trial registration number was reported in the published article, except four studies. All studies except one searched trial registries, 28 (70%) searched ClinicalTrials.gov, and 29 (73%) searched the World Health Organization International Clinical Trials Registry Platform (WHO ICTRP). Finally, 19 (48%) studies contacted trial investigators to inquire about registration status. In all, 18 (45%) studies used all three methods (reporting of registration number, search in registries, and contact of authors).

Prevalence of registration

We included 31 non-overlapping studies in the main analysis. The studies examined a total of 6788 RCTs, among which 3267 (48%) RCTs had been registered. The proportion of registered trials varied considerably across studies, ranging from 21 to 100% (Q statistic 1126, $df = 30$, $p < 0.001$, between-study variance 0.17). In a random-effects meta-analysis, the pooled proportion of registered RCTs was 51% (95% confidence interval 44 to 58%) (Fig. 2). In a secondary analysis, we included an additional nine studies examining 1985 RCTs, which potentially overlapped in part with the primary sample. Among these, 924 (47%) RCTs were registered. When combining all 40 studies, totaling 8773 RCTs, the pooled proportion of registered RCTs was 53% (95% confidence 46 to 59%) with considerable between-study heterogeneity. A funnel plot did not show evidence of small-study effects (Additional file 3: Figure S1).

Among the 31 non-overlapping studies, 19 also reported the number of trials that were registered prospectively. The studies included a total of 4272 RCTs, among which 676 (16%) RCTs were registered prospectively. There was a considerable heterogeneity across studies, with the proportion of prospectively registered RCTs ranging from 4 to 90% (Q statistic 380, $df = 18$, $p < 0.001$, between-study variance 0.09). The pooled proportion of prospectively

Table 1 Characteristics of included studies

Reference	Medical specialty	Time period for RCT publication	Identification of trials	Journals (*N*)	Trials (*N*)	Assessment of registration			Registries searched				
						Reporting	Search	Email	CT.gov	ISRCTN	WHO ICTRP	ANZCTR	National registries
Ostervig [59]	Anesthesiology	2009–2014	Single journal	1	200	Yes	Yes	No	Yes	Yes	No	No	Yes
Jones [49]	Anesthesiology	2007; 2010; 2013; 2010	Selection of high IF journals	6	860	Yes	Yes	Yes	Yes	Yes	Yes	No	No
Nankervis [56]	Atopic dermatitis	01/2007–07/2011	SR of eczema RCTs	–	109	Yes	Yes	No	No	No	Yes	No	No
Mathieu [22]	Cardiology, rheumatology, gastroenterology	2008	SR of RCTs in cardiology, rheumatology, and gastroenterology	22	323	Yes	Yes	Yes	Yes	Yes	Yes	No	Yes
Wiebe [71]	Cardio-thoracic surgery	2008–2015	Selection of high IF journals	4	287	Yes	Yes	Yes	Yes	Yes	Yes	No	Yes
Emdin [42, 58]	Cardiovascular disease	12/2012	SR of cardiovascular disease RCTs	–	191	Yes	Yes	No	No	No	Yes	No	No
Cybulski [37]	Clinical psychology	2013	Selection of high IF journals	25	101	Yes	Yes	Yes	Yes	No	Yes	No	No
Anand [32]	Critical care	01/2005–03/2011	SR of RCTs in critical care	–	90	Yes	Yes	Yes	Yes	No	No	Yes	No
Shinohara [66]	Depression	2011–2013	SR of RCTs of cognitive behavioral therapy and new-generation antidepressants	–	170	Yes	No	Yes	Unclear				
Jones [48]	Emergency medicine	2008–2011	Selection of high IF journals	5	123	Yes	Yes	No	Yes	Yes	Yes	No	No
Farquhar [43, 44]	Fertility medicine	2010–2014	SR of RCTs of fertility treatments	NA	693	Yes	Yes	Yes	Yes	No	Yes	No	No
Li [52]	Gastroenterology and hepatology	2009–2012	Selection of high IF journals	10	305	Yes	Yes	No	Yes	Yes	Yes	Yes	No
Mann [53]	Geriatrics	2008–2012	Selection of high IF journals	5	220	Yes	Yes	No	No	No	Yes	No	No
McGee [54]	Kidney transplantation	10/2005–12/2010	SR of kidney transplantation RCTs	–	307	No	Yes	No	No	No	Yes	No	No
Gray [46]	Nursing	11/2011–09/2016	Key general and mental health journals in nursing	3	135	Yes	Yes	Yes	Yes	Yes	No	No	Yes
Byrne [36]	Obesity	01/2011–06/2016	Selection of specialty journals	4	223	Yes	Yes	Yes	Yes	Yes	Yes	Yes	Yes
You [33, 72]	Oncology	2005–2009	Journals thought to publish majority of oncology RCTs	10	366	Yes	Yes	No	Yes	Yes	No	No	No
Smail-Faugeron [68]	Oral health	2013	Selection of high IF journals	15	317	Yes	Yes	No	No	No	Yes	No	No
Hamm [21]	Pediatrics	2007	SR of pediatric RCTs	–	300	Yes	Yes	No	Yes	Yes	Yes	No	Yes
Gates [45]	Pediatrics	2012	SR of pediatric RCTs	–	300	Yes	Yes	No	Yes	Yes	No	No	No
Rosati [64]	Pediatrics	07/2013–11/2013	Single journal	1	20	Yes	Yes	No	Yes	Yes	No	Yes	Yes
Pinto [61]	Physical therapy	2009	Indexed in PEDro	–	200	Yes	Yes	Yes	Yes	Yes	Yes	Yes	Yes
Pidgeon [60]	Plastic surgery	04/2014–03/2015	Selection of high IF journals	3	24	No	Yes	No	Yes	Yes	Yes	No	No

Table 1 Characteristics of included studies *(Continued)*

Reference	Medical specialty	Time period for RCT publication	Identification of trials	Journals (*N*)	Trials (*N*)	Assessment of registration			Registries searched				
						Reporting	Search	Email	CT.gov	ISRCTN	WHO ICTRP	ANZCTR	National registries
Scott [65]	Psychiatry	2009–2013	Selection of high IF journals	5	181	Yes	Yes	Yes	Yes	Yes	No	No	Yes
Milette [55]	Psychosomatic and behavioral medicine	01/2008–09/2009	Selection of high IF journals	4	63	Yes	Yes	Yes	Yes	Yes	Yes	No	Yes
Riehm [63]	Psychosomatic and behavioral medicine	01/2013–10/2014	Selection of high IF journals	4	76	Yes	Yes	Yes	Yes	Yes	Yes	No	Yes
Bradley [35]	Psychotherapy	2010–2014	Selection of high IF journals	5	112	Yes	Yes	Yes	Yes	Yes	Yes	No	Yes
Sims [67]	Shoulder arthroplasty	2005–2015	SR of shoulder arthroplasty RCTs	10	37	Yes	Yes	Yes	Yes	Yes	Yes	No	No
Killeen [50]	Surgery	2009–2010	Selection of high IF journals	10	246	Yes	Yes	Yes	Yes	Yes	Yes	No	Yes
Hardt [47]	Surgery	06/2012–12/2012	Selection of high IF journals	10	103	Yes	Yes	No	No	No	Yes	No	No
Kunath [51]	Urology	2009	Selection of high IF journals	10	106	Yes	Yes	No	No	No	Yes	No	No
Potentially overlapping studies													
Bonnot [34]	Anesthesiology	2013	Selection of high IF journals	12	183	Yes	Yes	Yes	No	No	Yes	No	No
El-Boghdadly [41]	Anesthesiology	01/201412/2016	Single journal	1	90	Yes	Yes	No	Yes	Yes	No	Yes	Yes
Norris [57]	Diabetes, osteoporosis, lip-modifying agents	2005–2010	Comparative effectiveness reviews	–	299	No	Yes	No	No	No	Yes	No	No
Dekkers [40]	Multiple	2004–2012	Trial protocols submitted to ethics committee	–	54	Yes	Yes	No	No	No	Yes	No	No
Dechartres [38]	Multiple	2006–2014	Cochrane reviews	–	322	Yes	Yes	Yes	Yes	No	Yes	No	No
Dekkers [39]	Multiple	02/2009	SR of non-inferiority RCTs in Core Clinical Journals	121	133	Yes	Yes	No	Yes	Yes	No	No	No
Reveiz [62]	Multiple	2010	SR of RCTs from Latin America and Caribbean	–	526	No	Yes	No	No	No	Yes	No	No
Van de Wetering [70]	Multiple	11/2010	Core Clinical Journals	121	302	Yes	Yes	Yes	Yes	Yes	Yes	No	No
Walker [69]	Multiple	05/2011–05/2012	Selection of high IF journals	2	76	Yes	Yes	No	Yes	Yes	No	No	Yes

SR systematic review, *RCT* randomized controlled trial, *IF* impact factor, *PEDro* Physiotherapy Evidence Database, *CT.gov* ClinicalTrials.gov, *ISCRCTN* International Standard Randomised Controlled Trials Number, *WHO ICTRP* World Health Organization International Clinical Trials Registry Platform, *ANZCTR* Australian New Zealand Clinical Trials Registry

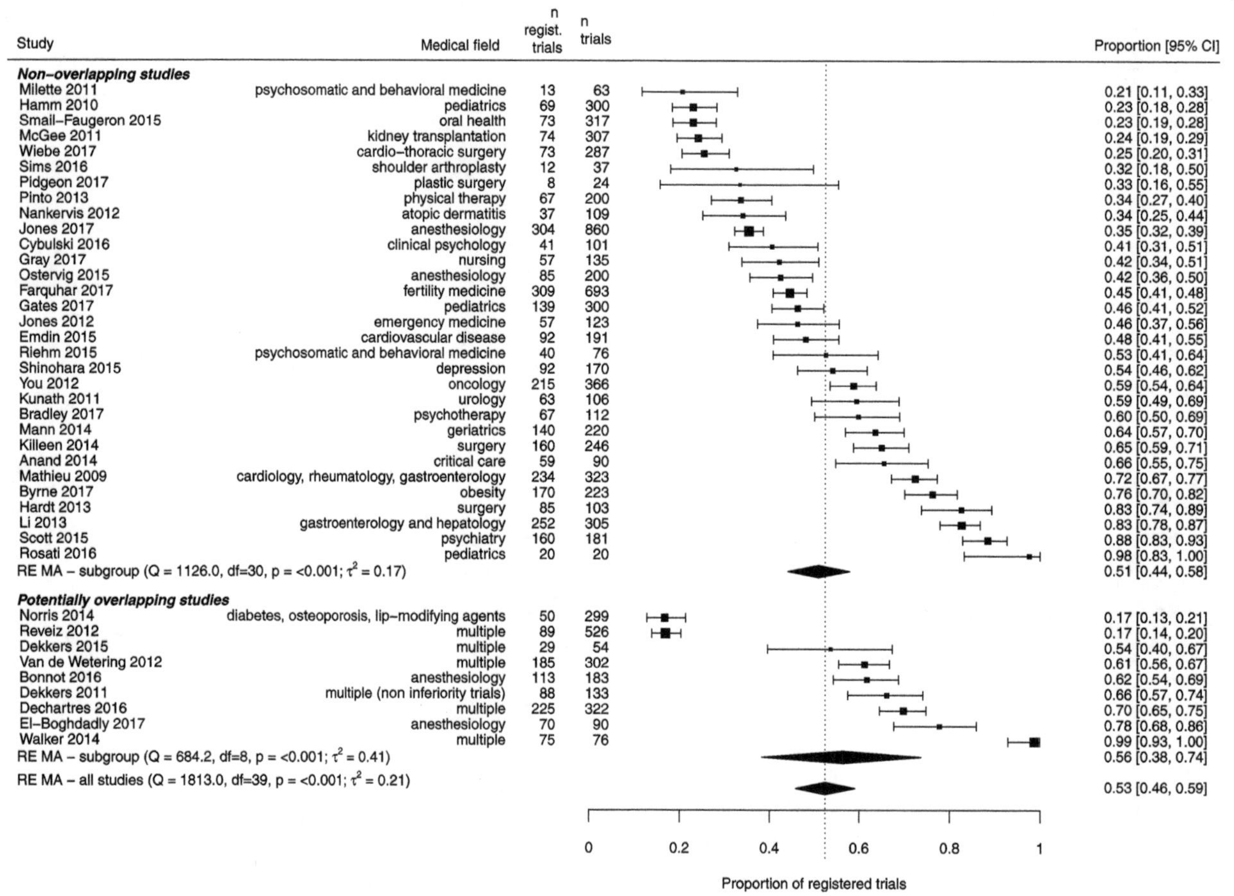

Fig. 2 Combined estimates of the prevalence of trial registration

registered RCTs was 21% (95% confidence interval 15 to 27%) (Fig. 3). Of the additional nine potentially overlapping studies included in the secondary analysis, five examined prospective registration across 1257 RCTs. When combining all 24 studies totaling 5529 RCTs, the pooled proportion of prospectively registered RCTs was 20% (95% confidence interval 15 to 25%). In addition, across these 24 studies, 1734 (67%) RCTs among 2588 registered RCTs were registered retrospectively, for a pooled proportion of 65% (95% confidence interval 59 to 71%).

Prevalence of registration over time in study subgroups

Four studies [32, 35, 65, 66] included only studies that started to enroll participants exclusively after 2005, and another four studies [38, 47, 51, 59] included sub-analyses based on studies enrolling only after 2005. Across these eight studies totaling 938 RCTs, 622 (66%) were registered, and the pooled proportion was 65% (95% confidence interval 50 to 78%) (Additional file 3: Figure S2).

Seven studies reported data on registration according to RCT publication year (Fig. 4). Separate meta-regression models showed that the proportion of registered trials increased over time in five of these studies. Moreover, 12 studies examined RCTs published in a single year ($n = 1$ for 2007 [21], $n = 3$ for 2009 [39, 51, 61], $n = 2$ for 2010 [62, 70], $n = 2$ for 2012 [42, 45]; $n = 4$ for 2013 [34, 37, 64, 68]) (Additional file 3: Table S2). When combining all 19 studies, totaling 5144 RCTs, a meta-regression model showed that the proportion of registered trials increased significantly over time ($p = 0.03$), with a mean absolute proportion increase of 27% between 2005 and 2015, from 25 to 52%. In addition, 7 of the 12 studies that examined RCTs published in a single year reported data on prospective registration (Additional file 3: Table S2). A meta-regression model suggested that the proportion of prospectively registered trials increased as well, from 3% in 2009 to 21% in 2013 (18% increase, $p = 0.04$) (Additional file 3: Figure S3). Finally, in an analysis limited to studies published in 2010 or after, 26 studies reported data on 5401 RCTs. Of these, 2550 (47%) were registered, for a pooled proportion of 54% (95% confidence interval 47 to 60%).

Prevalence of registration based on certain trial features

Nine studies examined registration of published RCTs according to industry funding. Across the nine studies, 778 of 2306 RCTs (34%) were supported fully or partially

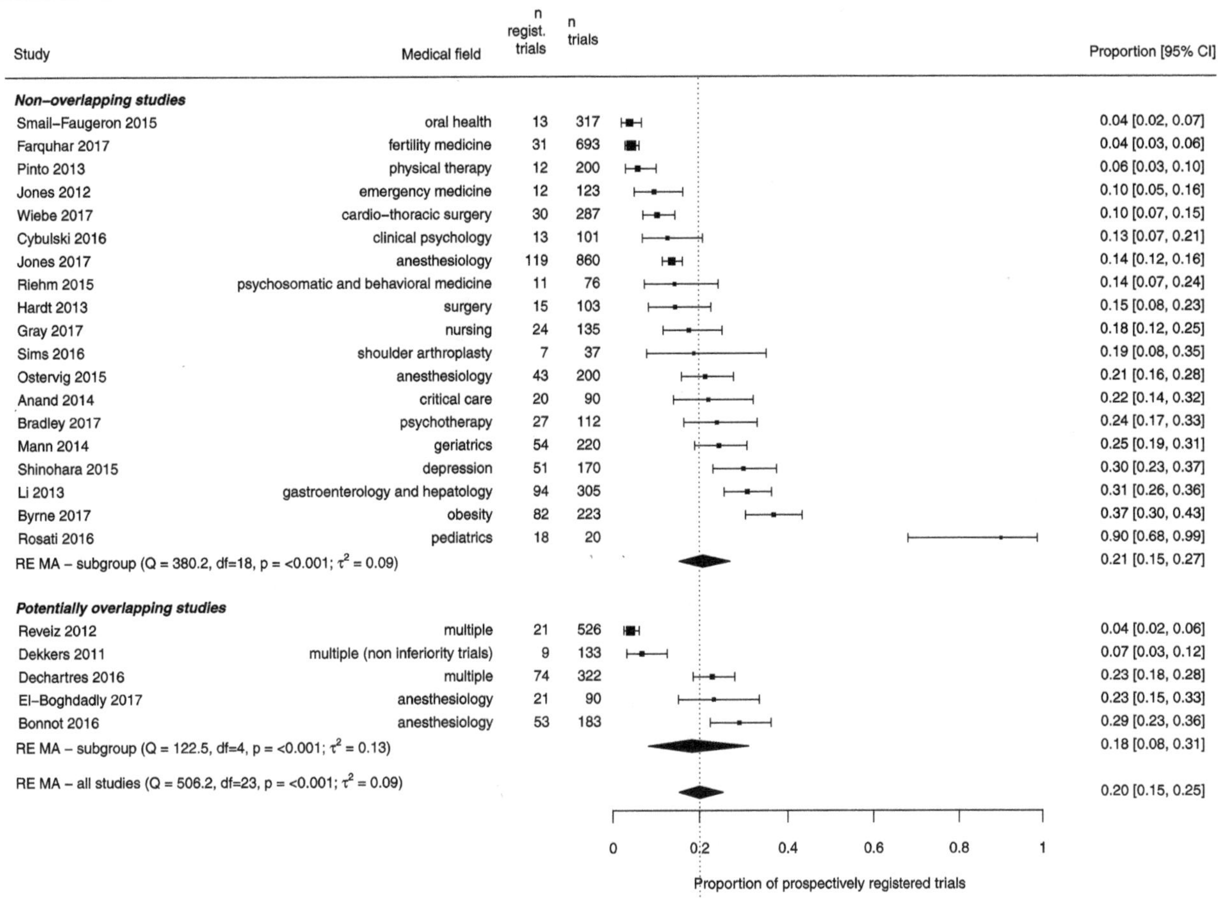

Fig. 3 Combined estimates of the prevalence of prospective trial registration

by industry sources. Of the 778 RCTs, 475 (61%) were registered. The pooled proportion was 59% (95% confidence interval 47 to 71%), as compared to 43% (95% confidence interval 30 to 58%) among trials not supported by industry. Five studies examined the prevalence of registration according to the trial sample size (Table 2). In all studies, there was evidence of higher registration prevalence among larger RCTs. Finally, 17 studies identified published RCTs from high-impact factor journals only. Out of 3383 RCTs, 1724 (51%) were registered. The pooled proportion was 55% (95% confidence interval 44 to 66%) as compared to 50% (95% confidence interval 42 to 59%) in the other 23 studies (5390 RCTs).

Discussion

In this systematic review, we found that, among published RCTs, the proportion of registered and prospectively registered RCTs has increased over time but lack of registration and retrospective registration are still common. In analyses of more than 8000 RCTs published in medical journals, half of the RCTs published in recent years had not been registered, and 4 in 5 published RCTs had not been registered prospectively. Registration prevalence was higher in trials supported by industry funding, in larger trials, and in trials published in high-impact factor journals. While sharing of individual participant data has recently garnered much attention, our findings highlight the need for renewed efforts to address the first step on the continuum of research transparency and make prospective trial registration a top priority. Without prospective registration, our ability to monitor and resolve issues in trial reporting is substantially diminished.

Our synthesis shows that publication of unregistered trials and of trials registered retrospectively in medical journals persists. Many journals do not endorse the ICMJE registration policy and continue to support the publication of unregistered trials [75, 76]. In a mixed-methods analysis, editors and publishers reported several reasons for why journals do not reject unregistered or retrospectively registered articles, including concerns about losing submissions or preventing publication of studies from developing countries. Conducting trials without making all the results publicly available is unethical [77, 78]. Publishing the results of unregistered trials may be considered an ethical imperative as it does ensure that the research community has access

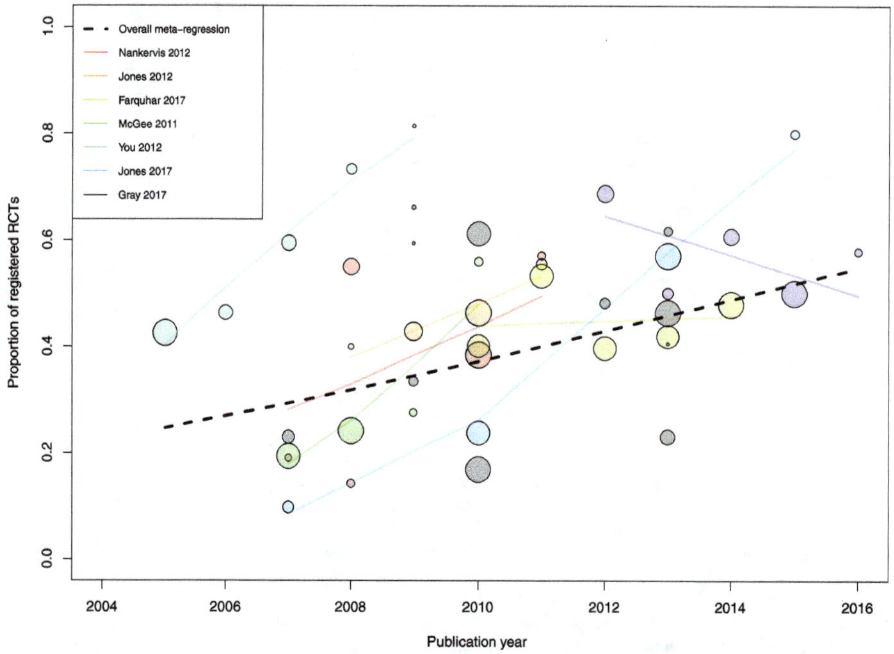

Fig. 4 Meta-regression analysis of the prevalence of trial registration in relation to publication year. Each circle represents one study, and the size of each circle represents the weight given to the study in meta-regression. Separate meta-regression models were fitted in 7 studies that reported trial registration data by publication year. The black dashed line corresponds to an overall meta-regression model across these 7 studies with 11 studies that examined RCTs published in a single year. It showed that the proportion of registered trials increased over time, from 23% in 2005 to 52% in 2015 (29% increase, $p = 0.03$)

Table 2 Prevalence of registration among published randomized trials according to trial size

Reference	Sample size	Number of trials	Number of registered trials	Proportion of registered trials (95% CI)	*p* value*
Jones [48]	< 100	48	17	0.35 (0.22; 0.51)	0.009
	100–199	36	14	0.39 (0.23; 0.57)	
	200–499	30	21	0.70 (0.51; 0.85)	
	≥ 500	9	5	0.56 (0.21; 0.86)	
Mann [53]	< 100	71	33	0.46 (0.35; 0.59)	0.0009
	100–499	117	83	0.71 (0.62; 0.79)	
	500–999	13	10	0.77 (0.46; 0.95)	
	≥ 1000	15	12	0.80 (0.52; 0.96)	
McGee [54]	< 200	235	40	0.17 (0.12; 0.22)	< 0.0001
	≥ 200	72	34	0.47 (0.35; 0.59)	
Pinto [61]	≤ 25	34	5	0.15 (0.05; 0.31)	< 0.0001
	26–50	53	13	0.25 (0.14; 0.38)	
	51–100	61	19	0.31 (0.20; 0.44)	
	101–499	42	23	0.55 (0.39; 0.70)	
	≥ 500	10	7	0.70 (0.35; 0.93)	
Reveiz [62]	≤ 100	442	59	0.13 (0.10; 0.17)	< 0.0001
	> 100	84	30	0.36 (0.26; 0.47)	

*Chi-squared test for trend in proportions in studies with three or more categories or chi-squared test for studies with two categories

to the results of these trials. But the large prevalence of unregistered trials published in medical journals raises concerns about persistent lack of transparency, underreporting or misreporting of trials, and biases in the resulting scientific literature. It directly undermines the first key objective of registries, which is to form a public "denominator" of all initiated trials, so that trials left unpublished can be identified and the available evidence interpreted in the context of unreported trials [79, 80].

Moreover, permitting publication of retrospectively registered trials defeats the second key objective of trial registration, which is to provide timestamped amendments to trial protocols. If a trial is registered after the enrollment of the first participants, it is no longer possible to compare reported results to the original trial record in order to identify selective reporting of outcomes and analyses [81, 82]. Among published RCTs that were registered, we found that 65% had been registered retrospectively. Zarin et al. [18] found a lower proportion; among 49 751 RCTs registered in ClinicalTrials.gov between 2012 and 2014, 33% had been registered more than 3 months after the trial start. Possible reasons for the difference is that our results concern only published RCTs; in contrast, most registered trials on ClinicalTrials.gov do not report results in a timely fashion [19]. In addition, we examined studies that assessed prospective registration according to the ICMJE or FDAAA definitions, which stipulates registration prior to the onset of patient enrollment or no later than 21 days after enrollment of the first participant. A higher proportion of trials may have been classified as prospectively registered had the cutoff been 3 months. Another reason for the difference is that we included trials registered in other registries and that practices with regard to prospective registration might be different among trials registered in these. Lastly, among 123 trials rejected by the BMJ between June 2013 and June 2017 because they did not comply with ICMJE trial registration requirements, 89% were retrospectively registered and 7% were unregistered [83].

Our findings have implications for systematic reviewers. Roberts et al. have suggested that systematic reviews include only prospectively registered trials, under the premise that such trials are the only ones not affected by reporting bias. Registered and unregistered trials have been found to differ in their risk of bias in studies examining 326 RCTs from Latin America and the Caribbean and 693 RCTs of fertility treatments [44, 62]. Other investigations have examined the impact of registration status on positive study findings and have not found differences between registered and non-registered trials [38, 42, 58]. We do not endorse restricting a systematic review to only registered trials but, given the large number of unregistered trials in the current medical literature and the potential difference from registered trials, systematic review authors should conduct subgroup analyses in cases where both registered and unregistered trials contribute to a meta-analysis. Such analyses should ideally distinguish between unregistered trials, retrospectively registered trials, prospectively registered trials with potential outcome reporting bias, and prospectively registered trials with no outcome reporting bias.

Our findings also have implications for a range of stakeholder groups focused on improving trial registration. Many actions have already been implemented by journal editors, regulatory agencies, and funding organizations to tackle the lack of prospective registration [18]. Because of the inherent lag between registration and publication, we could see substantial changes in upcoming years in response to the Final Rule and the new National Institutes of Health policy. However, existing laws and policies may not be sufficient and novel interventions may be required to increase trial registration. Many organizations in the USA do not have policies, staff, or other resources needed to ensure their trials are registered and reported in a timely fashion [84]. Twenty stakeholders have recently affirmed that prospective registration is of critical importance and that they will implement policies with monitoring systems to improve registration and reporting of results. In a recent commentary, Loder suggested treating unregistered or retrospectively registered trials as medical "never events." Such events should trigger drastic responses, similar to specified events in clinical medicine. For example, Dr. Loder argues that journal editors and peer reviewers should verify that trial registration occurred before the trial enrolment began and, according to the ICMJE policy, reject trials registered retrospectively. If not published in medical journals, trial results could still be posted online. Most importantly, we believe that multiple entities, including funding agencies, ethics committees, and academic institutions should continue to enforce standards of universal trial registration [85–88]. For example, these stakeholders could take prospective registration into account when considering full grant payments or academic promotions.

Our systematic review has limitations. First, some included studies examined RCTs that started prior to 2005 when registration requirements were implemented. However, we conducted analyses limited to RCTs started after 2005 and to RCTs published after 2010 that suggest that the low prevalence of registration among published RCTs has persisted among recent trials. Second, we could not rule out the possibility that some study samples overlapped with others among the 40 included studies. However, our primary analysis was restricted to 31 non-overlapping studies. The secondary analysis, which included all 40 studies, showed the same average prevalence of registration as in the primary analysis. Third, we were not able to fully explore sources of variability in the prevalence of registration, though we found that trial registration varied substantially across clinical fields and journals. Moreover, registration prevalence was higher among trials supported by the industry, larger trials, and trials in high-impact factor journals. Data were not available on trial location, and compliance with trial registration is likely to vary across countries. Viergever and Li [14] have shown that trends in registration on WHO ICTRP did not take place equally in all parts of the world. Fourth, our results apply to RCTs, while registration requirements apply broadly to all types of clinical trials. We therefore cannot ascertain whether the prevalence of registration we report here would be the same across all clinical study designs. Fifth, the included studies used different methods to ascertain whether published RCTs were registered. Some included studies might have missed registered RCTs and thus possibly underestimate the proportion of registered RCTs. Conversely, we excluded studies that assessed trial registration based solely on the mention of a trial registration number in the article, because such studies would underestimate the proportion of registered RCTs. However, trial registration is useful if end users can identify trial records. In this regard, the proportion of registered RCTs we found might be larger than the proportion of "useful" registrations. Sixth, data on the proportion of prospectively registered RCTs according to publication year were limited. Finally, in our systematic review, we have not assessed the quality of the registration of outcomes. The lack of a detailed specification of outcomes may also introduce reporting biases [89].

Conclusions

Non-registration and retrospective registration of clinical trials remain common, undermining the validity and integrity of biomedical research. Given long-standing policies mandating registration, enforcing prospective registration will likely require novel interventions and greater endorsement by a range of stakeholders in the research community, including investigators, funding entities, ethical oversight bodies, and journal editors. Universal, prospective trial registration should be a top priority in the endeavors to improve research transparency and ensure rigorous, high-quality evidence is available to inform patient care.

Additional files

Additional file 1: abstracted data. (CSV 2 kb)
Additional file 2: R code. (HTML 1110 kb)
Additional file 3: PRISMA checklist. (DOCX 149 kb)

Funding
FTB and AGD have received grant support from the Agency for Healthcare Research and Quality (R03HS024798 developing methods to improve systematic reviews using clinical trial registries). FTB has received grant support from the National Institutes of Health and holds an Innovation in Regulatory Science Award from the Burroughs Wellcome Fund. AGD has received grant support from the National Health and Medical Research Council (Australia) for unrelated research.

Authors' contributions
LT and FTB conceived and designed the study. LT, AGD, and FTB selected the studies and collected the data. LT analyzed data, and all authors interpreted the results. LT drafted and revised the paper. AGD and FTB revised the draft paper. All authors read and approved the final manuscript.

Competing interests
The authors declare that they have no competing interests.

Author details
[1]Department of Biostatistics, Boston University School of Public Health, Boston, Massachusetts, USA. [2]Centre for Health Informatics, Australian Institute of Health Innovation, Macquarie University, Sydney, Australia. [3]Department of Pediatrics, Harvard Medical School, Boston, Massachusetts, USA. [4]Center for Pediatric Therapeutics and Regulatory Science, and Computational Health Informatics Program, Boston Children's Hospital, Boston, MA, USA.

References

1. Zarin DA, Tse T. Medicine. Moving toward transparency of clinical trials. Science. 2008;319(5868):1340–2.
2. De Angelis C, Drazen JM, Frizelle FA, Haug C, Hoey J, Horton R, Kotzin S, Laine C, Marusic A, Overbeke AJ, et al. Clinical trial registration: a statement from the International Committee of Medical Journal Editors. N Engl J Med. 2004;351(12):1250–1.
3. Chan AW, Song F, Vickers A, Jefferson T, Dickersin K, Gotzsche PC, Krumholz HM, Ghersi D, van der Worp HB. Increasing value and reducing waste: addressing inaccessible research. Lancet. 2014;383(9913):257–66.
4. Topol EJ. Failing the public health--rofecoxib, Merck, and the FDA. N Engl J Med. 2004;351(17):1707–9.
5. Juni P, Nartey L, Reichenbach S, Sterchi R, Dieppe PA, Egger M. Risk of cardiovascular events and rofecoxib: cumulative meta-analysis. Lancet. 2004; 364(9450):2021–9.
6. Jefferson T, Jones MA, Doshi P, Del Mar CB, Hama R, Thompson MJ, Spencer EA, Onakpoya I, Mahtani KR, Nunan D, et al. Neuraminidase inhibitors for preventing and treating influenza in healthy adults and children. Cochrane Database Syst Rev. 2014;(4):CD008965.
7. Vedula SS, Bero L, Scherer RW, Dickersin K. Outcome reporting in industry-sponsored trials of gabapentin for off-label use. N Engl J Med. 2009;361(20): 1963–71.
8. Vedula SS, Goldman PS, Rona IJ, Greene TM, Dickersin K. Implementation of a publication strategy in the context of reporting biases. A case study based on new documents from Neurontin litigation. Trials. 2012;13:136.
9. Krleza-Jeric K, Chan AW, Dickersin K, Sim I, Grimshaw J, Gluud C. Principles for international registration of protocol information and results from human trials of health related interventions: Ottawa statement (part 1). BMJ. 2005;330(7497):956–8.
10. Bourgeois FT, Murthy S, Mandl KD. Outcome reporting among drug trials registered in ClinicalTrials.gov. Ann Intern Med. 2010;153(3):158–66.
11. Chan AW, Pello A, Kitchen J, Axentiev A, Virtanen JI, Liu A, Hemminki E. Association of Trial Registration With Reporting of Primary Outcomes in Protocols and Publications. JAMA. 2017;318(17):1709-1711. https://doi.org/10.1001/jama.2017.13001.
12. Zarin DA, Tse T, Williams RJ, Carr S. Trial reporting in ClinicalTrials.gov - the Final Rule. N Engl J Med. 2016;375(20):1998–2004.
13. Hudson KL, Lauer MS, Collins FS. Toward a new era of trust and transparency in clinical trials. JAMA. 2016;316(13):1353–4.
14. Viergever RF, Li K. Trends in global clinical trial registration: an analysis of numbers of registered clinical trials in different parts of the world from 2004 to 2013. BMJ Open. 2015;5(9):e008932.
15. Trial Registration, Organizations with Policies. http://www.who.int/ictrp/trial_reg/en/index2.html. Accessed 9 Sept 2018.

16. Laine C, Horton R, DeAngelis CD, Drazen JM, Frizelle FA, Godlee F, Haug C, Hebert PC, Kotzin S, Marusic A, et al. Clinical trial registration: looking back and moving ahead. Lancet. 2007;369(9577):1909–11.
17. Weber WE, Merino JG, Loder E. Trial registration 10 years on. BMJ. 2015;351:h3572.
18. Zarin DA, Tse T, Williams RJ, Rajakannan T. Update on trial registration 11 years after the ICMJE policy was established. N Engl J Med. 2017;376(4):383–91.
19. Chen R, Desai NR, Ross JS, Zhang W, Chau KH, Wayda B, Murugiah K, Lu DY, Mittal A, Krumholz HM. Publication and reporting of clinical trial results: cross sectional analysis across academic medical centers. BMJ. 2016;352:i637.
20. Ross JS, Tse T, Zarin DA, Xu H, Zhou L, Krumholz HM. Publication of NIH funded trials registered in ClinicalTrials.gov: cross sectional analysis. BMJ. 2012;344:d7292.
21. Hamm MP, Hartling L, Milne A, Tjosvold L, Vandermeer B, Thomson D, Curtis S, Klassen TP. A descriptive analysis of a representative sample of pediatric randomized controlled trials published in 2007. BMC Pediatr. 2010;10:96.
22. Mathieu S, Boutron I, Moher D, Altman DG, Ravaud P. Comparison of registered and published primary outcomes in randomized controlled trials. JAMA. 2009;302(9):977–84.
23. Missing trial data – briefing notes. http://www.alltrials.net/wp-content/uploads/2013/01/Missing-trials-briefing-note.pdf. Accessed 9 Sept 2018.
24. Dal-Re R, Marusic A. Prevention of selective outcome reporting: let us start from the beginning. Eur J Clin Pharmacol. 2016;72(10):1283–8.
25. Jones CW, Keil LG, Holland WC, Caughey MC, Platts-Mills TF. Comparison of registered and published outcomes in randomized controlled trials: a systematic review. BMC Med. 2015;13:282.
26. Bashir R, Bourgeois FT, Dunn AG. A systematic review of the processes used to link clinical trial registrations to their published results. Syst Rev. 2017;6(1):123.
27. Glanville JM, Duffy S, McCool R, Varley D. Searching ClinicalTrials.gov and the International Clinical Trials Registry Platform to inform systematic reviews: what are the optimal search approaches? J Med Libr Assoc. 2014; 102(3):177–83.
28. Trikalinos TA, Trow P, Schmid CH. Simulation-based comparison of methods for meta-analysis of proportions and rates. Rockville: Agency for Healthcare Research and Quality (US); 2013.
29. Bakbergenuly I, Kulinskaya E, Morgenthaler S. Inference for binomial probability based on dependent Bernoulli random variables with applications to meta-analysis and group level studies. Biom J. 2016;58(4):896–914.
30. Haidich AB, Ioannidis JP. Effect of early patient enrollment on the time to completion and publication of randomized controlled trials. Am J Epidemiol. 2001;154(9):873–80.
31. Ioannidis JP. Effect of the statistical significance of results on the time to completion and publication of randomized efficacy trials. JAMA. 1998;279(4): 281–6.
32. Anand V, Scales DC, Parshuram CS, Kavanagh BP. Registration and design alterations of clinical trials in critical care: a cross-sectional observational study. Intensive Care Med. 2014;40(5):700–22.
33. Boespflug A, Gan H, Chen EX, Pond G, You B. Consistency in the analysis and reporting of PEPs in oncology randomized controlled trials from registration to publication: a systematic review. Bull Cancer. 2012;99(10):943–52.
34. Bonnot B, Yavchitz A, Mantz J, Paugam-Burtz C, Boutron I. Selective primary outcome reporting in high-impact journals of anaesthesia and pain. Br J Anaesth. 2016;117(4):542–3.
35. Bradley HA, Rucklidge JJ, Mulder RT. A systematic review of trial registration and selective outcome reporting in psychotherapy randomized controlled trials. Acta Psychiatr Scand. 2017;135(1):65–77.
36. Byrne JL, Yee T, O'Connor K, Dyson MP, Ball GD. Registration status and methodological reporting of randomized controlled trials in obesity research: a review. Obesity (Silver Spring). 2017;25(4):665–70.
37. Cybulski L, Mayo-Wilson E, Grant S. Improving transparency and reproducibility through registration: the status of intervention trials published in clinical psychology journals. J Consult Clin Psychol. 2016;84(9): 753–67.
38. Dechartres A, Ravaud P, Atal I, Riveros C, Boutron I. Association between trial registration and treatment effect estimates: a meta-epidemiological study. BMC Med. 2016;14(1):100.
39. Dekkers OM, Soonawala D, Vandenbroucke JP, Egger M. Reporting of noninferiority trials was incomplete in trial registries. J Clin Epidemiol. 2011; 64(9):1034–8.
40. Dekkers OM, Cevallos M, Buhrer J, Poncet A, Ackermann Rau S, Perneger TV, Egger M. Comparison of noninferiority margins reported in protocols and publications showed incomplete and inconsistent reporting. J Clin Epidemiol. 2015;68(5):510–7.
41. El-Boghdadly K, Wiles M, Atton S, Bailey C. Analysis of registration rigour of randomised controlled trials published in anaesthesia. Anaesthesia. 2017;72:17.
42. Emdin C, Odutayo A, Hsiao A, Shakir M, Hopewell S, Rahimi K, Altman DG. Association of cardiovascular trial registration with positive study findings: epidemiological Study of Randomized Trials (ESORT). JAMA Intern Med. 2015;175(2):304–7.
43. Farquhar CM, Showell MG, Showell EAE, Beetham P, Baak N, Mourad S, Jordan VMB. Clinical trial registration in fertility trials - a case for improvement? Hum Reprod. 2017;32(9):1827–34.
44. Farquhar CM, Showell MG, Showell EAE, Beetham P, Baak N, Mourad S, Jordan VMB. Clinical trial registration was not an indicator for low risk of bias. J Clin Epidemiol. 2017;84:47–53.
45. Gates A, Hartling L, Vandermeer B, Caldwell P, Contopoulos-Ioannidis DG, Curtis S, Fernandes RM, Klassen TP, Williams K, Dyson MP. The conduct and reporting of child health research: an analysis of randomized controlled trials published in 2012 and evaluation of change over 5 years. J Pediatr. 2018;193:237–244.e37.
46. Gray R, Badnapurkar A, Hassanein E, Thomas D, Barguir L, Baker C, Jones M, Bressington D, Brown E, Topping A. Registration of randomized controlled trials in nursing journals. Res Integr Peer Rev. 2017;2:8. https://doi.org/10.1186/s41073-017-0036-9.
47. Hardt JL, Metzendorf MI, Meerpohl JJ. Surgical trials and trial registers: a cross-sectional study of randomized controlled trials published in journals requiring trial registration in the author instructions. Trials. 2013;14:407.
48. Jones CW, Platts-Mills TF. Quality of registration for clinical trials published in emergency medicine journals. Ann Emerg Med. 2012;60(4):458–464.e1.
49. Jones PM, Chow JTY, Arango MF, Fridfinnson JA, Gai N, Lam K, Turkstra TP. Comparison of registered and reported outcomes in randomized clinical trials published in anesthesiology journals. Anesth Analg. 2017;125(4):1292–300.
50. Killeen S, Sourallous P, Hunter IA, Hartley JE, Grady HL. Registration rates, adequacy of registration, and a comparison of registered and published primary outcomes in randomized controlled trials published in surgery journals. Ann Surg. 2014;259(1):193–6.
51. Kunath F, Grobe HR, Keck B, Rucker G, Wullich B, Antes G, Meerpohl JJ. Do urology journals enforce trial registration? A cross-sectional study of published trials. BMJ Open. 2011;1(2):e000430.
52. Li XQ, Yang GL, Tao KM, Zhang HQ, Zhou QH, Ling CQ. Comparison of registered and published primary outcomes in randomized controlled trials of gastroenterology and hepatology. Scand J Gastroenterol. 2013;48(12): 1474–83.
53. Mann E, Nguyen N, Fleischer S, Meyer G. Compliance with trial registration in five core journals of clinical geriatrics: a survey of original publications on randomised controlled trials from 2008 to 2012. Age Ageing. 2014;43(6):872–6.
54. McGee RG, Su M, Kelly PJ, Higgins GY, Craig JC, Webster AC. Trial registration and declaration of registration by authors of randomized controlled trials. Transplantation. 2011;92(10):1094–100.
55. Milette K, Roseman M, Thombs BD. Transparency of outcome reporting and trial registration of randomized controlled trials in top psychosomatic and behavioral health journals: a systematic review. J Psychosom Res. 2011;70(3):205–17.
56. Nankervis H, Baibergenova A, Williams HC, Thomas KS. Prospective registration and outcome-reporting bias in randomized controlled trials of eczema treatments: a systematic review. J Invest Dermatol. 2012;132(12): 2727–34.
57. Norris SL, Holmer HK, Fu R, Ogden LA, Viswanathan MS, Abou-Setta AM. Clinical trial registries are of minimal use for identifying selective outcome and analysis reporting. Res Synth Methods. 2014;5(3):273–84.
58. Odutayo A, Emdin CA, Hsiao AJ, Shakir M, Copsey B, Dutton S, Chiocchia V, Schlussel M, Dutton P, Roberts C, et al. Association between trial registration and positive study findings: cross sectional study (Epidemiological Study of Randomized Trials-ESORT). BMJ. 2017;356:j917.
59. Ostervig RM, Sonne A, Rasmussen LS. Registration of randomized clinical trials--a challenge. Acta Anaesthesiol Scand. 2015;59(8):986–9.
60. Pidgeon TE, Limb C, Agha RA, Whitehurst K, Chandrakumar C, Wellstead G, Fowler AJ, Orgill DP. The use of study registration and protocols in plastic surgery research: a systematic review. Int J Surg. 2017;44:215–22.
61. Pinto RZ, Elkins MR, Moseley AM, Sherrington C, Herbert RD, Maher CG, Ferreira PH, Ferreira ML. Many randomized trials of physical therapy interventions are not adequately registered: a survey of 200 published trials. Phys Ther. 2013;93(3):299–309.
62. Reveiz L, Bonfill X, Glujovsky D, Pinzon CE, Asenjo-Lobos C, Cortes M, Canon

M, Bardach A, Comande D, Cardona AF. Trial registration in Latin America and the Caribbean's: study of randomized trials published in 2010. J Clin Epidemiol. 2012;65(5):482–7.
63. Riehm KE, Azar M, Thombs BD. Transparency of outcome reporting and trial registration of randomized controlled trials in top psychosomatic and behavioral health journals: a 5-year follow-up. J Psychosom Res. 2015;79(1):1–12.
64. Rosati P, Porzsolt F, Ricciotti G, Testa G, Inglese R, Giustini F, Fiscarelli E, Zazza M, Carlino C, Balassone V, et al. Major discrepancies between what clinical trial registries record and paediatric randomised controlled trials publish. Trials. 2016;17(1):430.
65. Scott A, Rucklidge JJ, Mulder RT. Is mandatory prospective trial registration working to prevent publication of unregistered trials and selective outcome reporting? An observational study of five psychiatry journals that mandate prospective clinical trial registration. PLoS One. 2015;10(8):e0133718.
66. Shinohara K, Tajika A, Imai H, Takeshima N, Hayasaka Y, Furukawa TA. Protocol registration and selective outcome reporting in recent psychiatry trials: new antidepressants and cognitive behavioural therapies. Acta Psychiatr Scand. 2015;132(6):489–98.
67. Sims MT, Sanchez ZC, Herrington JM, Hensel JB, Henning NM, Scheckel CJ, Vassar M. Shoulder arthroplasty trials are infrequently registered: a systematic review of trials. PLoS One. 2016;11(10):e0164984.
68. Smail-Faugeron V, Fron-Chabouis H, Durieux P. Clinical trial registration in oral health journals. J Dent Res. 2015;94(3 Suppl):8S–13S.
69. Walker KF, Stevenson G, Thornton JG. Discrepancies between registration and publication of randomised controlled trials: an observational study. JRSM Open. 2014;5(5):2042533313517688.
70. van de Wetering FT, Scholten RJ, Haring T, Clarke M, Hooft L. Trial registration numbers are underreported in biomedical publications. PLoS One. 2012;7(11):e49599.
71. Wiebe J, Detten G, Scheckel C, Gearhart D, Wheeler D, Sanders D, Vassar M. The heart of the matter: outcome reporting bias and registration status in cardio-thoracic surgery. Int J Cardiol. 2017;227:299–304.
72. You B, Gan HK, Pond G, Chen EX. Consistency in the analysis and reporting of primary end points in oncology randomized controlled trials from registration to publication: a systematic review. J Clin Oncol. 2012;30(2):210–6.
73. Azar M, Riehm KE, McKay D, Thombs BD. Transparency of outcome reporting and trial registration of randomized controlled trials published in the journal of consulting and clinical psychology. PLoS One. 2015;10(11):e0142894.
74. De Oliveira GS Jr, Jung MJ, McCarthy RJ. Discrepancies between randomized controlled trial registry entries and content of corresponding manuscripts reported in anesthesiology journals. Anesth Analg. 2015;121(4):1030–3.
75. Wager E, Williams P, Project Overcome failure to Publish nEgative fiNdings C. "Hardly worth the effort"? Medical journals' policies and their editors' and publishers' views on trial registration and publication bias: quantitative and qualitative study. BMJ. 2013;347:f5248.
76. Hooft L, Korevaar DA, Molenaar N, Bossuyt PM, Scholten RJ. Endorsement of ICMJE's Clinical Trial Registration Policy: a survey among journal editors. Neth J Med. 2014;72(7):349–55.
77. Moorthy VS, Karam G, Vannice KS, Kieny MP. Rationale for WHO's new position calling for prompt reporting and public disclosure of interventional clinical trial results. PLoS Med. 2015;12(4):e1001819.
78. Pica N, Bourgeois F. Discontinuation and Nonpublication of Randomized Clinical Trials Conducted in Children. Pediatrics. 2016;138(3). pii: e20160223. https://doi.org/10.1542/peds.2016-0223.
79. Zarin DA, Tse T, Williams RJ, Califf RM, Ide NC. The ClinicalTrials.gov results database--update and key issues. N Engl J Med. 2011;364(9):852–60.
80. Dickersin K, Rennie D. The evolution of trial registries and their use to assess the clinical trial enterprise. JAMA. 2012;307(17):1861–4.
81. Dwan K, Gamble C, Williamson PR, Kirkham JJ, Reporting Bias G. Systematic review of the empirical evidence of study publication bias and outcome reporting bias - an updated review. PLoS One. 2013;8(7):e66844.
82. Dwan K, Altman DG, Clarke M, Gamble C, Higgins JP, Sterne JA, Williamson PR, Kirkham JJ. Evidence for the selective reporting of analyses and discrepancies in clinical trials: a systematic review of cohort studies of clinical trials. PLoS Med. 2014;11(6):e1001666.
83. Loder E, Loder S, Cook S. Characteristics and publication fate of unregistered and retrospectively registered clinical trials submitted to The BMJ over 4 years. BMJ Open. 2018;8(2):e020037.
84. Mayo-Wilson E, Heyward J, Keyes A, Reynolds J, White S, Atri N, Alexander GC, Omar A, Ford DE, National Clinical Trials R, et al. Clinical trial registration and reporting: a survey of academic organizations in the United States. BMC Med. 2018;16(1):60.
85. O'Reilly EK, Hassell NJ, Snyder DC, Natoli S, Liu I, Rimmler J, Amspacher V, Burnett BK, Parrish AB, Berglund JP, et al. ClinicalTrials.gov reporting: strategies for success at an academic health center. Clin Transl Sci. 2015;8(1):48–51.
86. Goldacre B. How to get all trials reported: audit, better data, and individual accountability. PLoS Med. 2015;12(4):e1001821.
87. Meerpohl JJ, Schell LK, Bassler D, Gallus S, Kleijnen J, Kulig M, La Vecchia C, Marusic A, Ravaud P, Reis A, et al. Evidence-informed recommendations to reduce dissemination bias in clinical research: conclusions from the OPEN (Overcome failure to Publish nEgative fiNdings) project based on an international consensus meeting. BMJ Open. 2015;5(5):e006666.
88. Doernberg SN, Wendler D. Ensuring respect for human research participants: institutional review boards and sharing results from research. JAMA. 2016;316(11):1149–50.
89. The COMPare Trials Project. www.COMPare-trials.org. Accessed 9 Sept 2018.

13

How can we teach medical students to choose wisely? A randomised controlled cross-over study of video-versus text-based case scenarios

Sascha Ludwig[1], Nikolai Schuelper[2], Jamie Brown[3], Sven Anders[4] and Tobias Raupach[1,3*]

Abstract

Background: The *Choosing Wisely* campaign highlights the importance of clinical reasoning abilities for competent and reflective physicians. The principles of this campaign should be addressed in undergraduate medical education. Recent research suggests that answering questions on important steps in patient management promotes knowledge retention. It is less clear whether increasing the authenticity of educational material by the inclusion of videos further enhances learning outcome.

Methods: In a prospective randomised controlled cross-over study, we assessed whether repeated video-based testing is more effective than repeated text-based testing in training students to choose appropriate diagnostic tests, arrive at correct diagnoses and identify advisable therapies. Following an entry exam, fourth-year undergraduate medical students attended 10 weekly computer-based seminars during which they studied patient case histories. Each case contained five key feature questions (items) on the diagnosis and treatment of the presented patient. Students were randomly allocated to read text cases (control condition) or watch videos (intervention), and assignment to either text or video was switched between groups every week. Using a within-subjects design, student performance on video-based and text-based items was assessed 13 weeks (exit exam) and 9 months (retention test) after the first day of term. The primary outcome was the within-subject difference in performance on video-based and text-based items in the exit exam.

Results: Of 125 eligible students, 93 provided data for all three exams (response rate 74.4%). Percent scores were significantly higher for video-based than for text-based items in the exit exam (76.2 ± 19.4% vs. 72.4 ± 19.1%, $p = 0.026$) but not the retention test (69.2 ± 20.2% vs. 66.4 ± 20.3%, $p = 0.108$). An additional Bayesian analysis of this retention test suggested that video-based training is marginally more effective than text-based training in the long term (Bayes factor 2.36). Regardless of presentation format, student responses revealed a high prevalence of erroneous beliefs that, if applied to the clinical context, could place patients at risk.

Conclusion: Repeated video-based key feature testing produces superior short-term learning outcome compared to text-based testing. Given the high prevalence of misconceptions, efforts to improve clinical reasoning training in medical education are warranted. The *Choosing Wisely* campaign lends itself to being part of this process.

Keywords: Medical education, Clinical reasoning, Choosing wisely, Test-enhanced learning, Video

* Correspondence: raupach@med.uni-goettingen.de
[1]Department of Cardiology and Pneumology, Göttingen University Medical Centre, Robert-Koch-Straße 40, D-37075 Göttingen, Germany
[3]Health Behaviour Research Centre, University College London, 1-19 Torrington Place, London WC1E 7HB, UK
Full list of author information is available at the end of the article

Background

One of the most important aims of undergraduate medical education is to enable future physicians to arrive at correct diagnoses and treatment recommendations based on the results of appropriate diagnostic tests. Making correct decisions is at least as important as avoiding unnecessary tests and incorrect diagnoses, and both need to be considered in the context of clinical reasoning [1]. Recently, the *Choosing Wisely* campaign has added another important feature to the professional approach to patient management [2, 3]. In order to avoid unnecessary or potentially harmful diagnostic and therapeutic procedures, recommendations compiled by medical societies in various countries across the globe [4] advise a more thorough consideration of the specific merits and limitations of these interventions and discourage the use of some in specific circumstances [5, 6]. Clinical reasoning abilities are a prerequisite for making 'wise choices' in clinical medicine, thus suggesting that teaching interventions aimed at fostering clinical reasoning may also enhance performance with regard to the recommendations derived from the *Choosing Wisely* campaign. Vice versa, these recommendations result from a stringent application of the principles of clinical reasoning. Thus, the choice of teaching formats that lend themselves to the discussion of these recommendations should be guided by a discussion of instructional formats used to address clinical reasoning itself. One effective approach to enhancing the complex cognitive functions related to clinical reasoning is case-based learning [7], which is traditionally facilitated in small groups [8] or at the bedside [9]. Given the limitations of these formats regarding resource intensity and availability of patients with rare but important diseases, computer-assisted case-based learning with virtual patients [10] has been proposed as a viable approach to teaching clinical reasoning [11, 12].

Digital interventions in medical education need to be informed by educational and psychological research. One recent example of this type of 'translational research' in medical education is the growing body of evidence showing that test-enhanced learning enhances knowledge and skills retention in undergraduate medical students. The basic idea is that questions can be used to stimulate learning processes [13, 14]. Thus far, a number of studies have shown that tests can in fact be used as learning tools in medical education [15]. For example, in one study involving 47 first-year medical students, repeated testing of factual knowledge in neurology elicited greater long-term retention than repeated study of the same material [16]. Another randomised study yielded a similar effect for the retention of practical (resuscitation) skills [17]. However, none of these studies focussed on clinical reasoning. One potential reason for this is that rote memory can easily be tested using multiple choice questions while testing clinical reasoning is more complex. One test format suited for this purpose is the so-called key feature question. A key feature is defined as a significant step in patient management. Key feature questions were designed to test the knowledge needed to avoid common errors occurring at these decisive points. For example, the key features in one of the cases used in this study referred to the management of a potentially life-threatening condition. First, students were prompted to provide the most likely diagnosis (key feature 1: pulmonary embolism) for a 44-year-old female patient who had been immobilised with lumbago for a week and who experienced sudden chest pain and shortness of breath following defaecation. In the second question, students were expected to identify calculation of the Wells Score as the next key feature in patient management. Following this, students were informed that this score was 6, and they were asked to name the most appropriate next step for the patient who was haemodynamically stable (key feature 3: CT scan). Upon confirmation of the diagnosis, students were asked about a diagnostic procedure that can inform risk stratification for this particular patient (key feature 4: PESI score, cardiac ultrasound or troponin measurement). In the fifth section of the case, the patient is no longer haemodynamically stable and requires catecholamine therapy, and students were asked to indicate the therapeutic action required (key feature 5: thrombolysis). A recent review [18] confirmed that key feature questions lend themselves to the assessment of clinical reasoning, and it has been suggested they could be used in a test-enhanced learning paradigm [19]. We recently reported the findings of a randomised study of repeated testing with key feature questions on outcomes related to clinical reasoning [20], wherein 6 months after the intervention, students retained significantly more content that had been presented in key feature questions compared to content that had been presented in a didactic format but without interspersed questions (56% vs. 19%; $p < 0.001$).

While this study showed that repeated case-based testing with key feature questions is more effective than repeated case-based study of the same material, the overall retention of procedural knowledge related to clinical reasoning at the 6-month follow-up was suboptimal. One reason might be that all the case-based material used in that study was presented as text on computer screens. While text can easily be scanned for relevant information, students might have found it harder to immerse in the clinical problem presented. This assumption is supported by psychological research dating back to 1975, when Godden and Baddeley demonstrated the importance of similarities between the learning environment and situations in which the learnt material needs to be recalled [21]. In addition, according to the dual-coding theory [22] and supporting original research [23], simultaneous presentation of audio-visual material is more likely to enhance retention of information than verbal material alone. Despite the increasing use of videos in undergraduate medical education, we are not aware of any studies addressing their value when used as part of exams focussing on clinical reasoning.

In summary, test-enhanced learning with video-based, computer-assisted exams could be an efficient way of enhancing student performance with regard to making the right choices about diagnostic tests and taking appropriate therapeutic action. In addition, the avoidance of unnecessary interventions as set out in the *Choosing Wisely* recommendations can ideally be addressed in key feature questions. To our knowledge, no previous study has reported student performance in this context. In addition, incorrect answers to key feature questions have rarely been analysed although they may reveal specific shortcomings in teaching that could be easily remedied.

This randomised cross-over study was designed to test the hypothesis that repeated testing with video-based key feature questions produces superior retention of procedural knowledge related to clinical reasoning compared to repeated testing with text-based key feature questions. The second aim was to investigate the effects of (non) alignment between presentation formats in the learning phase and subsequent exams on student performance. The third aim of this study was to identify common errors evident in student responses to key feature questions.

Methods

Study design

This was a randomised, controlled, non-blinded cross-over study involving fourth-year undergraduate medical students. At Göttingen Medical School, clinical reasoning is mainly addressed in study years 4 and 5. In addition to small-group case-based discussions and bedside teaching, students work on predefined patient case histories in computer-based 'electronic seminars' (e-seminars) lasting up to 45 min each. E-seminars are facilitated at the institution's e-learning resource centre.

Students enrolled in the first term of the fourth year were eligible for study participation during the summer of 2015. During the first 14 weeks of term ('learning phase'), students attended three thematic modules on cardiology, pulmonology, nephrology, rheumatology, haematology and oncology. Following stratification by sex and prior performance levels, they were randomised to one of two groups (A and B). Students in both groups attended weekly e-seminars during which they were presented with three patient case histories related to teaching content of the previous week. Case histories ('virtual patients') were adapted from an earlier study [20]; they had been designed according to a set of principles identified in a previous focus group study among German medical students [24]. Each patient case was broken up into five sections, and at the end of each section, students answered a key feature question on the most appropriate next diagnostic/therapeutic step by entering at least three letters in a box and choosing from a long menu of options provided by the exam software. An example of a key feature question is included in Additional file 1: Methods. Throughout this manuscript, the word 'item' refers to one key feature question, i.e. each case was made up of five items.

Case content was identical for all students but the format varied each week between 'text cases' or 'video cases'. In text cases, content was presented on the computer screen in written format while dealing with video cases involved watching five short films (mean duration 68 s), and answering a question (i.e. one item) after each film. Films were scripted based on written cases that had been piloted in two consecutive student cohorts. Wherever possible, videos were closely aligned to text cases. However, inevitably, minor differences arose in the exact wording of content, which are fundamental to the difference between written information and audio-visual material showing a true interaction between a patient and a physician. For a sample video, please refer to Additional file 2.

During the learning phase, students in the two study groups were alternately exposed to video-based or text-based e-seminars with all students being exposed to the same content in any given week. For example, in week 2, students in group A worked on video cases (Fig. 1, orange boxes) while students in group B were exposed to text cases presenting the same content (Fig. 1, blue boxes). The presentation format then alternated systematically for each group across 10 sessions. No specific measures were taken to prevent students from discussing e-seminar content outside the sessions.

Given that there were three cases per week, each containing five key feature questions (i.e. items), students answered a total of 150 items during the learning phase. Of these, 14 items in group A were predefined as intervention items which meant that these items were presented as video-based questions. The same items were used as control items (i.e. text-based questions) in group B. Conversely, 14 intervention items for students in group B were used as control items in group A. Item assignment to the two study groups was balanced with regard to item difficulty as derived from an earlier study using the same items [20]. Intervention and control items were scattered across cases, i.e. some cases did not contain any intervention/control item (these cases referred to important teaching content that was, however, not targeted in this study) while other cases contained up to five intervention/control items. All analyses (see below) were carried out on the (aggregated) item level, irrespective of the cases in which they had been embedded.

Each of the 28 intervention/control items was presented in two out of the 10 e-seminars during the learning phase.

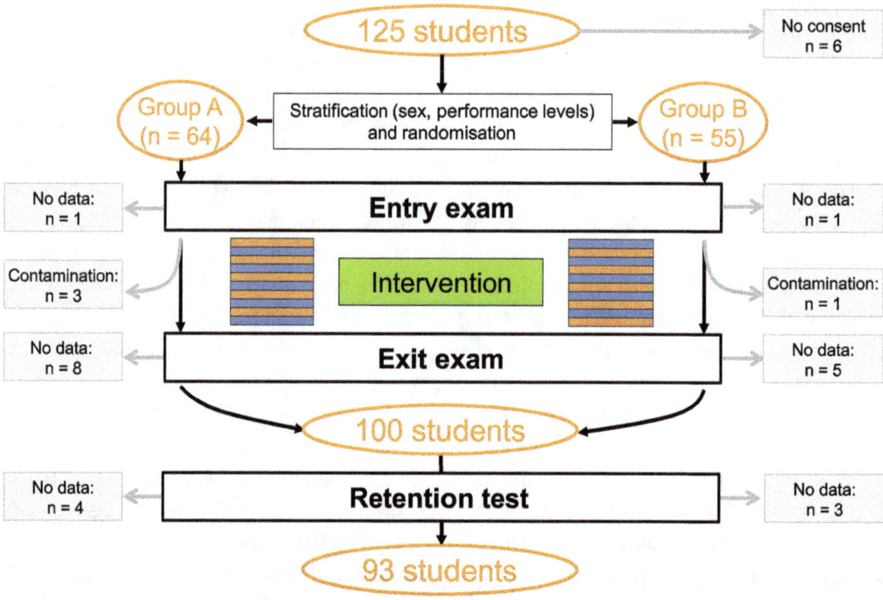

Fig. 1 Flow of participants through the study. Orange boxes, video cases; blue boxes, text cases. Contamination occurred when students were erroneously exposed to the wrong presentation format (by reporting to the computer room assigned to the other group) at least once

As a result, any student – regardless of group assignment – was exposed to 14 intervention (video) items in two e-seminars and to 14 control (text) items in two different e-seminars. During the final week of term, students took a formative exit exam consisting of these 28 items that had been arranged into four new cases containing 6 or 8 key features each. Again, cases were only used to provide a structure to accommodate the items, and analyses were done on the item level. A formative retention test was taken 6 months later.

Given the impact of context and format on exam performance with regard to the learning environment [21], presentation of items in the exit exam and retention test was balanced in that seven out of 14 intervention (video) items for both groups were presented as video items in these exams while the other seven were presented as text items and vice versa. This was done to address the second aim of the study outlined above. Item assignment to presentation format was balanced by item difficulty as derived from the previous study [20]. Thus, from the outset, item difficulty was expected to be similar for the 14 intervention and control items in the two study groups as well as for the 7 video and the 7 text items derived from these (respectively) in the exit exam and retention test. As a consequence, any differences in student performance were more likely to be caused by the intervention than by pre-existing differences in item difficulties.

Data analysis

Descriptive analyses involved calculation of student mean scores achieved for intervention and control items in the three exams as well as in the first and second occurrence of an item in an e-seminar. The primary outcome for this study was the within-subject difference in percent scores in the exit exam for those 14 items that had been presented in video format during the learning phase compared to those 14 items that had been presented in text format. The difference was assessed in a paired T-test. Based on an expected sample size of 90 and the results of a previous study [20], the study was adequately powered ($1 - \beta = 0.8$) to detect a performance difference between video and text items of 8% on an α level of 5%. Performance on items in the retention test was assessed as a function of the number of correct retrievals for the same items during e-seminars and the exit exam. Performance differences as a function of presentation format during the learning phase and the formative exams was assessed using Friedman and Wilcoxon tests. According to the statistical analysis plan, an additional Bayesian approach was scheduled in case one of these analyses yielded a non-significant result. The Bayes factor was to be calculated based on the assumption that the effect of using videos instead of text would be half the size of the effect observed in the mentioned previous study comparing repeated testing to repeated study of clinical cases.

With regard to the third aim of this study, common errors were addressed by calculating the proportion of students making incorrect choices in e-seminars (learning phase) and the exit exam and retention test, respectively.

Statistical analysis was performed using SPSS 22.0 (SPSS Inc., Chicago, Illinois, USA) and the Bayes factor calculator provided by Dienes [25]. Data are presented as mean ± SD or percentages unless otherwise stated. Significance levels were set to $p < 0.05$. This study was approved by the local Ethics Committee (application number 22/4/15), and all participants provided written consent.

Results

Student characteristics

The flow of participants through the study is displayed in Fig. 1. Of the 125 students eligible for study participation, six did not provide written consent. Following exclusion of students due to missing data or contamination (due to exposure to the wrong presentation format at least once), complete data were available for 93 students (effective response rate 74.4%). The mean age of study participants was 25.8 ± 3.9 years, and 64.5% ($n = 60$) were female.

Learning outcome

Mean percent scores in the entry, exit and retention exams were 28.5 ± 13.5%, 74.3 ± 17.4% and 67.8 ± 18.5%, respectively (Fig. 2). With regard to the primary endpoint, exit exam scores in items that had been presented as videos during the learning phase were significantly higher than in text items (76.2 ± 19.4% vs. 72.4 ± 19.1%, $T = 2.263$; df = 92; $p = 0.026$). A similar but non-significant difference was found in the retention test (69.2 ± 20.2% vs. 66.4 ± 20.3%, $T = 1.624$; df = 92; $p = 0.108$). Using the mean difference of 2.8% and the corresponding standard error (1.7%) yielded a Bayes factor of 2.36, supporting the hypothesis that video items were more effective than text items. In the aggregate sample, the probability of correctly answering an item in the retention test following three failed retrievals in preceding e-seminars and the exit exam was 27.7%; the corresponding percentage for one, two and three correct retrievals were 51.3%, 70.2% and 87.5%, respectively. A descriptive analysis of all exam results on the level of individual items is presented in Additional file 1: eTable1.

Association between presentation format during learning and in the formative exams

With regard to the different combinations between presentation format during e-seminars and in the formative exams, student performance in the four item types differed significantly for both the exit exam and the retention test ($p < 0.001$ for both). A detailed analysis revealed that, while video items were more beneficial for learning purposes than text items, the opposite was true for presentation format in the formative exams in that students achieved higher scores in text items than in video items (exit exam: 78.2 ± 18.5% vs. 70.4 ± 18.9%, $T = 5.485$; df = 92; $p < 0.001$; retention test: 72.2 ± 18.4% vs. 63.4 ± 21.2%, $T = 5.845$; df = 92; $p < 0.001$) (Table 1).

Common errors observed in e-seminars and formative exams

Given the small differences between video and text items, data from the two study groups were collapsed for the analysis of common errors. Table 2 presents proportions of correct and incorrect answers averaged across the two e-seminars, the exit exam and the retention test. Frequent errors included mechanical ventilation for isolated hypoxemia (24.2%), thrombolytic treatment without confirmation of a diagnosis of pulmonary embolism (17.7%), oxygen supplementation for CO_2 poisoning (16.9%), ECG diagnosis of a conduction block instead of atrial fibrillation (13.7%), rapid sodium supplementation for chronic hyponatremia (11.0%),

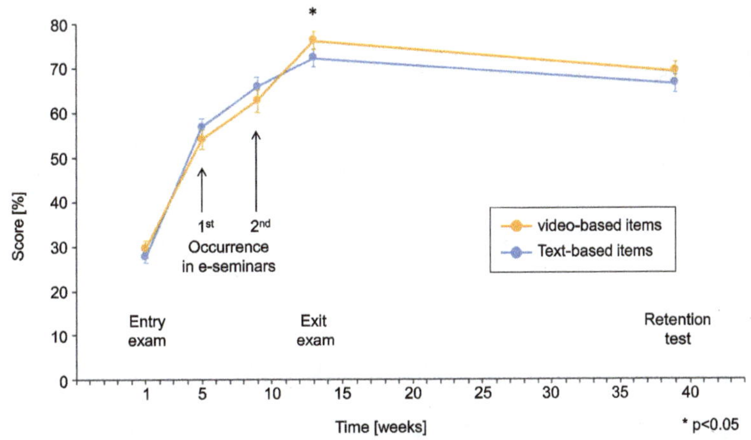

Fig. 2 Trajectories of student performance in video-based and text-based items, respectively. The first presentation ('1st occurrence') of a particular item in an e-seminar occurred between week 3 and week 9; the second item presentation occurred between week 5 and week 11 ('2nd occurrence'). In order to increase legibility, data collected during first and second occurrences, respectively, were collapsed into two data collection points although data were actually collected over a period of 6 weeks for each occurrence

Table 1 Impact of alignment between presentation format during e-seminars and formative exams on student performance

Presentation format		Percent scores achieved in the formative exams	
E-seminars	Formative exam	Exit exam	Retention test
Text	Text	77.4 ± 21.0^{a}	$71.6 \pm 20.4^{d,e}$
Text	Video	$67.3 \pm 22.2^{a,b}$	$61.3 \pm 25.4^{d,f}$
Video	Text	$79.0 \pm 20.2^{b,c}$	$72.8 \pm 23.1^{f,g}$
Video	Video	73.4 ± 22.3^{c}	$65.6 \pm 22.5^{e,g}$

The Friedman test was significant for both the exit exam and the retention test. Different pairs of superscript letters indicate a significant difference between two groups in Wilcoxon signed-rank tests after Bonferroni correction for multiple comparisons

and medical or surgical treatment for hyperthyroidism in a patient still receiving amiodarone (17.2%). A detailed analysis by item type (video or text) and data collection point is included in Additional file 1: eTable 2.

Discussion

This randomised cross-over study yielded two main findings. First, repeated testing with video-based key feature questions elicited higher short-term learning outcomes than testing with text-based questions regarding diagnostic accuracy and initial management issues with only weak evidence in the long-term. Second, we found a high prevalence of erroneous beliefs in medical students irrespective of item format (video or text). These misconceptions have the potential to negatively impact the quality of patient care unless corrected before graduation.

Choosing Wisely – a perspective on medical education

Clinical reasoning abilities are essential for competent and reflective physicians. Undergraduate medical education needs to equip students with a solid knowledge base and train them to apply that knowledge in a given clinical context. The *Choosing Wisely* recommendations emerged from clinical reasoning processes. Thus, the initiative could serve as a paradigm of quality assurance in clinical care that should be addressed in medical education. Albeit not having been specifically designed to match any of the top five lists, some of the key feature questions embedded in the patient cases presented to our students alluded to current *Choosing Wisely* recommendations. For example, the lists of both the American College of Chest Physicians and the American College of Emergency Physicians cover the treatment of pulmonary embolism, and our results (Table 2) show that some fourth-year medical students struggle with basic concepts such as confirming the diagnosis before initiating treatment or skipping D-dimer testing in patients with a high probability of pulmonary embolism. Our data also shed light on other misconceptions that may have fatal consequences (e.g. sole oxygen supplementation without ventilator support in CO_2 poisoning). Medical education research preferentially focuses on correct responses and aggregate scores. In the light of the *Choosing Wisely* campaign, a more thorough assessment of misconceptions and frequent errors appears promising in that it could guide improvements in the way clinical reasoning is being taught. This process should be informed by educational research. The present study suggests that repeated testing with key feature questions is effective in enhancing clinical reasoning performance.

Test-enhanced learning for clinical reasoning: a proof of concept

Since the introduction of test-enhanced learning to the field of medical education research, a number of studies on undergraduate medical [17], dental [26] and nursing [27] education have confirmed that repeated testing can be used to enhance retention of knowledge and skills relevant to preclinical [28] and clinical [29] medicine. The performance retention rates observed in our study are close to or exceed the upper bound of results reported in previous studies. In two prospective randomised trials involving medical students and residents, respectively, percent scores in retention tests 6 months after a test-based intervention approached 40% [16, 29]. Our study adds to the growing body of literature supporting the principle of test-enhanced learning in medical education by demonstrating that a resource-saving, computer-based intervention can have a beneficial impact on outcomes related to clinical reasoning.

Use of videos in medical education

There is a strong rationale for using audio-visual material in higher education as learning resources that are more closely aligned to the context in which knowledge will be applied is likely to produce more favourable learning outcomes [21]. However, high-quality studies on the effective use of videos in medical education are scarce, and only very few have assessed their potential to enhance clinical reasoning. If anything, the available evidence is apt to raise concerns regarding the validity of effectiveness claims. While video triggers are preferred by students in the context of problem-based learning [30, 31], recent research suggests that video-based problem-based learning cases may disrupt deep critical thinking [32], and that increased authenticity of instructional formats does not necessarily improve clinical reasoning performance in learners [33]. Our current study lends support to the notion that, when used for key feature testing, videos can enhance short-term retention of knowledge relevant to clinical reasoning. Our finding of a greater performance increase between the first e-seminar and the exit exam for video than for text items may be explained by the

Table 2 Proportions of correct and incorrect answers for the 28 key feature items, calculated across the two e-seminars, and exit exam and the retention test

Diseases	Key features (Items)	Proportion of correct answers	Frequent or relevant incorrect answers (proportion)
Pulmonary embolism	Diagnosis of *pulmonary embolism*	58.6%	Acute coronary syndrome (8.0%); aortic dissection (3.9%)
	Wells Score to assess likelihood of PE	74.0%	Assessment of hemodynamic stability (5.2%)
	Thorax CT scan to confirm PE in a patient with high clinical probability	50.0%	Thrombolysis without confirmation (17.7%); other imaging (9.7%); D-dimer testing (9.7%)
	Right ventricular strain for risk stratification	51.9%	
	Fibrinolysis for unstable pulmonary embolism	66.6%	Other medical treatment (10.2%)
Arterial hypertension	Diagnosis of *secondary hypertension*	49.6%	Essential hypertension (11.5%); cardiac disease (10.4%)
	Diagnosis of *diastolic dysfunction*	17.5%	Other myocardial disease (60.8%)
	Discontinuation of ACE inhibitors due to typical cough	93.7%	
Hyponatremia	*Hospital admission* for chronic symptomatic hyponatremia	70.5%	Rapid sodium supplementation (11.0%)
	Thiazide diuretics as cause of hyponatremia	83.0%	Hypovolemia (3.4%)
	Diagnosis of *central pontine myelinolysis* following rapid sodium supplementation	64.9%	Cerebral oedema (13.6%)
Atrial fibrillation	*Orthostatic challenge* after syncope	72.5%	Tilt testing (22.8%)
	ECG diagnosis of *tachyarrhythmia*	61.8%	Conduction blocks (13.7%); myocardial infarction (1.9%)
	CHA_2DS_2-VASc score for anticoagulation	83.6%	
Lupus erythematosus	Diagnosis of *nephrotic syndrome*	80.3%	Nephritic syndrome (8.0%)
	Diagnosis of *systemic lupus erythematosus*	83.8%	Non-specific glomerulonephritis (4.3%)
	Renal *biopsy* to confirm lupus nephritis	79.8%	Imaging (4.6%)
COPD	Diagnosis of *COPD*	91.1%	
	Confirmation of COPD by *$FEV_1/VC < 70\%$*	64.7%	FEV_1 (13.6%); FEV_1/VC % predicted (15.8%)
	ABG analysis for suspected CO_2 intoxication	67.2%	Imaging (7.2%)
	Treatment of CO_2 intoxication by *non-invasive ventilation*	53.3%	Oxygen (16.9%); CPAP (11.4%); buffering (6.7%)
Pneumonia	Diagnosis of *left apical pneumonia* in a chest X-ray	72.8%	Incorrect or no localisation (23.3%)
	Decision on hospitalisation based on the *CRB-65 score*	75.9%	Decision based on additional laboratory tests (5.6%)
Hyperthyroidism	Diagnosis of *hyperthyroidism* from lab results	88.8%	Hypothyroidism (4.1%)
	Stopping amiodarone in a pt. with hyperthyroidism	66.2%	other medical (11.4%) or surgical (5.7%) treatment
Pulmonary fibrosis	Diagnosis of *pulmonary fibrosis*	53.8%	Pulmonary oedema (12.5%); pneumonia (9.4%)
	Amiodarone as cause of pulmonary fibrosis	78.9%	Atrial fibrillation (4.8%)
	Indication for *long-term oxygen therapy*	47.6%	Mechanical ventilation (24.2%)

ABG arterial blood gases, *ACE* angiotensin converting enzyme, *CAD* coronary artery disease, *CHA_2DS_2-VASc* congestive heart failure, hypertension, age ≥75 (doubled), diabetes, stroke (doubled), vascular disease, age 65–74, and sex category (female), CO_2 carbon dioxide, *COPD* chronic obstructive pulmonary disease, *CPAP* continuous positive airway pressure, *CRB* confusion/respiratory rate/blood pressure, *CT* computed tomography, *ECG* electrocardiogram, *FEV_1* forced expiratory volume in 1 s, *NIV* non-invasive ventilation, *PAD* peripheral artery disease, *PE* pulmonary embolism, *VC* vital capacity

Italics indicate the key feature assessed in each item; answers that were frequently entered instead of these are shown in the last column of the table fact that videos are most effective in situations where sensory information (that cannot be provided in a text) helps to solve a problem [34]. For example, in a patient with suspected pulmonary fibrosis, the video contained an audio recording of the auscultation. Students watching the video were less likely to incorrectly diagnose this patient as having pulmonary oedema and more likely to spot the right diagnosis (Additional file 1: eTable 2). On the other hand, the wealth of information contained in videos increases cognitive load for learners [35] and may also increase the effort associated with retrieval in the context of test-enhanced learning. Our data support the theory that effortful retrieval produces superior retention [14]. The results of the Bayesian analysis with regard to long-term retention can be used to inform future studies in terms of priors for future analyses. This is particularly helpful when evaluating costly interventions.

Strengths and limitations

Test-enhanced learning is an emerging concept in medical education, and this is one of the first studies using video-based key feature questions to enhance clinical reasoning performance. The questions used during the learning phase and in formative exams referred to highly prevalent or important clinical problems, and all questions were piloted extensively [20]. The response rate was favourable, and randomisation minimised any effects potentially related to self-selection of students.

Despite these strengths, the generalisability of our findings is limited by the monocentric nature of the study. Given that the cases used focussed on internal medicine, we cannot draw conclusions on the potential of test-enhanced learning with key feature questions for other medical specialties. Finally, this study did not assess whether repeated testing with key feature questions impacts on actual student performance in the clinical setting. Although one study suggests such a link [36], more research is needed to establish a causal relation between repeated testing and more favourable patient outcomes.

Conclusions

Repeated video-based key feature testing was associated with significantly better clinical reasoning performance compared to text-based testing in the short term. However, student responses revealed a high prevalence of erroneous beliefs that – if applied to the clinical context – are potentially harmful to patients. Efforts to improve clinical reasoning training in medical education are warranted, and the *Choosing Wisely* campaign lends itself to being part of this process aimed at supporting students to become reflective and competent physicians.

Additional files

Additional file 1: Methods. Description and example of a key feature question. **eTable 1.** Proportions of correct answers for the 28 key feature items in the exit exam and the retention test. **eTable 2.** Frequent or relevant incorrect answers (proportion). (DOCX 59 kb)

Additional file 2: Sample video. Example of a video key feature item. This MP4-file is an example of a video key feature item featuring a 74 year-old simulated patient called "Mr. Teschke" (fictional name) with increasing shortness of breath. The interaction was scripted and both the patient and the doctor were played by actors who were not affiliated to the study team. Both individuals consented to participate in the research project and to be shown in this sample video. (MP4 7365 kb)

Acknowledgements

We would like to thank all medical students who devoted their time to this study.

Funding

This study was funded by a grant issued by Göttingen Medical School, Georg-August-University Göttingen.

Authors' contributions

SL helped to design the study, co-ordinated and facilitated video productions, uploaded cases, and helped to collect and analyse data. NS provided comments on all video scripts, participated in filming sessions, helped interpret the data and commented on various versions of the manuscript. JB was involved in Bayesian data analysis and contributed to the Background and Discussion section. SA helped to design the study, provided advice on data presentation and commented on various versions of the manuscript. TR conceived of the study, developed its design, drafted key feature cases, analysed the data and wrote the manuscript. All authors read and approved the final manuscript.

Competing interests

The authors declare that they have no competing interests.

Author details

[1]Department of Cardiology and Pneumology, Göttingen University Medical Centre, Robert-Koch-Straße 40, D-37075 Göttingen, Germany. [2]Department of Haematology and Medical Oncology, Göttingen University Medical Centre, Robert-Koch-Straße 40, D-37075 Göttingen, Germany. [3]Health Behaviour Research Centre, University College London, 1-19 Torrington Place, London WC1E 7HB, UK. [4]Department of Legal Medicine, University Medical Centre Hamburg-Eppendorf, Butenfeld 34, D-22529 Hamburg, Germany.

References

1. Croskerry P. A universal model of diagnostic reasoning. Acad Med. 2009;84(8):1022–8.
2. Cassel CK, Guest JA. Choosing wisely: helping physicians and patients make smart decisions about their care. JAMA. 2012;307(17):1801–2.
3. Brody H. Medicine's ethical responsibility for health care reform–the top five list. N Engl J Med. 2010;362(4):283–5.
4. Jung N, Lehmann C, Fatkenheuer G. The "choosing wisely" initiative in infectious diseases. Infection. 2015;45(3):263–8.
5. Hicks LK, Bering H, Carson KR, Haynes AE, Kleinerman J, Kukreti V, Ma A, Mueller BU, O'Brien SH, Panepinto JA, et al. Five hematologic tests and treatments to question. Blood. 2014;124(24):3524–8.
6. Langer-Gould AM, Anderson WE, Armstrong MJ, Cohen AB, Eccher MA, Iverson DJ, Potrebic SB, Becker A, Larson R, Gedan A, et al. The American Academy of Neurology's top five choosing wisely recommendations. Neurology. 2013;81(11):1004–11.
7. Kassirer JP. Teaching clinical reasoning: case-based and coached. Acad Med. 2010;85(7):1118–24.
8. Dequeker J, Jaspaert R. Teaching problem-solving and clinical reasoning: 20 years experience with video-supported small-group learning. Med Educ. 1998;32(4):384–9.

9. Spencer J. Learning and teaching in the clinical environment. BMJ. 2003;326(7389):591–4.
10. Cook DA, Triola MM. Virtual patients: a critical literature review and proposed next steps. Med Educ. 2009;43(4):303–11.
11. Wahlgren CF, Edelbring S, Fors U, Hindbeck H, Stahle M. Evaluation of an interactive case simulation system in dermatology and venereology for medical students. BMC Med Educ. 2006;6:40.
12. Berman NB, Durning SJ, Fischer MR, Huwendiek S, Triola MM. The role for virtual patients in the future of medical education. Acad Med. 2016;91(9):1217–22.
13. Karpicke JD, Roediger HL 3rd. The critical importance of retrieval for learning. Science. 2008;319(5865):966–8.
14. Roediger HL, Karpicke JD. The power of testing memory - basic research and implications for educational practice. Perspect Psychol Sci. 2006;1(3):181–210.
15. McConnell MM, St-Onge C, Young ME. The benefits of testing for learning on later performance. Adv Health Sci Educ Theory Pract. 2015;20(2):305–20.
16. Larsen DP, Butler AC, Roediger HL 3rd. Comparative effects of test-enhanced learning and self-explanation on long-term retention. Med Educ. 2013;47(7):674–82.
17. Kromann CB, Jensen ML, Ringsted C. Test-enhanced learning may be a gender-related phenomenon explained by changes in cortisol level. Med Educ. 2011;45(2):192–9.
18. Hrynchak P, Takahashi SG, Nayer M. Key-feature questions for assessment of clinical reasoning: a literature review. Med Educ. 2014;48(9):870–83.
19. Larsen DP, Butler AC, Roediger HL 3rd. Test-enhanced learning in medical education. Med Educ. 2008;42(10):959–66.
20. Raupach T, Andresen JC, Meyer K, Strobel L, Koziolek M, Jung W, Brown J, Anders S. Test-enhanced learning of clinical reasoning: a crossover randomised trial. Med Educ. 2016;50(7):711–20.
21. Godden DR, Baddeley A. Context-dependent memory in two natural environments: on land and underwater. Br J Psychol. 1975;66(3):325–31.
22. Paivio A. Imagery and Verbal Processes. New York: Holt, Rinehart and Winston; 1971.
23. Mayer RE, Sims VK. For whom is a picture worth a thousand words? Extensions of a dual-coding theory of multimedia learning. J Educ Psychol. 1994;86(3):389–401.
24. Huwendiek S, Reichert F, Bosse HM, de Leng BA, van der Vleuten CP, Haag M, Hoffmann GF, Tonshoff B. Design principles for virtual patients: a focus group study among students. Med Educ. 2009;43(6):580–8.
25. Dienes Z. Understanding Psychology as a Science: An Introduction to Scientific and Statistical Inference. Hampshire: Palgrave Macmillan; 2008.
26. Baghdady M, Carnahan H, Lam EW, Woods NN. Test-enhanced learning and its effect on comprehension and diagnostic accuracy. Med Educ. 2014;48(2):181–8.
27. Dobson JL, Linderholm T. Self-testing promotes superior retention of anatomy and physiology information. Adv Health Sci Educ Theory Pract. 2015;20(1):149–61.
28. Logan JM, Thompson AJ, Marshak DW. Testing to enhance retention in human anatomy. Anat Sci Educ. 2011;4(5):243–8.
29. Larsen DP, Butler AC, Roediger HL 3rd. Repeated testing improves long-term retention relative to repeated study: a randomised controlled trial. Med Educ. 2009;43(12):1174–81.
30. Chan LK, Patil NG, Chen JY, Lam JC, Lau CS, Ip MS. Advantages of video trigger in problem-based learning. Med Teach. 2010;32(9):760–5.
31. de Leng B, Dolmans D, van de Wiel M, Muijtjens A, van der Vleuten C. How video cases should be used as authentic stimuli in problem-based medical education. Med Educ. 2007;41(2):181–8.
32. Basu Roy R, McMahon GT. Video-based cases disrupt deep critical thinking in problem-based learning. Med Educ. 2012;46(4):426–35.
33. La Rochelle JS, Durning SJ, Pangaro LN, Artino AR, van der Vleuten CP, Schuwirth L. Authenticity of instruction and student performance: a prospective randomised trial. Med Educ. 2011;45(8):807–17.
34. Woodham LA, Ellaway RH, Round J, Vaughan S, Poulton T, Zary N. Medical student and tutor perceptions of video versus text in an interactive online virtual patient for problem-based learning: a pilot study. J Med Internet Res. 2015;17(6):e151.
35. Sweller J, van Merrienboer J, Paas F. Cognitive architecture and instructional design. Educ Psychol Rev. 1998;10:251–96.
36. Larsen DP, Butler AC, Lawson AL, Roediger HL 3rd. The importance of seeing the patient: test-enhanced learning with standardized patients and written tests improves clinical application of knowledge. Adv Health Sci Educ Theory Pract. 2013;18(3):409–25.

14

Spatio-temporal mapping of Madagascar's Malaria Indicator Survey results to assess *Plasmodium falciparum* endemicity trends between 2011 and 2016

Su Yun Kang[1], Katherine E. Battle[1], Harry S. Gibson[1], Arsène Ratsimbasoa[2,3], Milijaona Randrianarivelojosia[4,5], Stéphanie Ramboarina[2,3,6], Peter A. Zimmerman[6], Daniel J. Weiss[1], Ewan Cameron[1], Peter W. Gething[1] and Rosalind E. Howes[1,6*]

Abstract

Background: Reliable measures of disease burden over time are necessary to evaluate the impact of interventions and assess sub-national trends in the distribution of infection. Three Malaria Indicator Surveys (MISs) have been conducted in Madagascar since 2011. They provide a valuable resource to assess changes in burden that is complementary to the country's routine case reporting system.

Methods: A Bayesian geostatistical spatio-temporal model was developed in an integrated nested Laplace approximation framework to map the prevalence of *Plasmodium falciparum* malaria infection among children from 6 to 59 months in age across Madagascar for 2011, 2013 and 2016 based on the MIS datasets. The model was informed by a suite of environmental and socio-demographic covariates known to influence infection prevalence. Spatio-temporal trends were quantified across the country.

Results: Despite a relatively small decrease between 2013 and 2016, the prevalence of malaria infection has increased substantially in all areas of Madagascar since 2011. In 2011, almost half (42.3%) of the country's population lived in areas of very low malaria risk (<1% parasite prevalence), but by 2016, this had dropped to only 26.7% of the population. Meanwhile, the population in high transmission areas (prevalence >20%) increased from only 2.2% in 2011 to 9.2% in 2016. A comparison of the model-based estimates with the raw MIS results indicates there was an underestimation of the situation in 2016, since the raw figures likely associated with survey timings were delayed until after the peak transmission season.

Conclusions: Malaria remains an important health problem in Madagascar. The monthly and annual prevalence maps developed here provide a way to evaluate the magnitude of change over time, taking into account variability in survey input data. These methods can contribute to monitoring sub-national trends of malaria prevalence in Madagascar as the country aims for geographically progressive elimination.

Keywords: Madagascar, *Plasmodium falciparum*, Geostatistical model, Map, Malaria Indicator Surveys

* Correspondence: rosalind.howes@bdi.ox.ac.uk
[1]Malaria Atlas Project, Oxford Big Data Institute, Nuffield Department of Medicine, University of Oxford, Oxford, UK
[6]Center for Global Health and Diseases, Case Western Reserve University, Cleveland, OH, USA
Full list of author information is available at the end of the article

Background

Malaria remains an important public health problem in Madagascar despite concerted efforts over decades to control transmission. At times, these interventions, which have been primarily focussed on targeted vector control, have successfully reduced transmission to very low levels [1–3]. The island's malaria epidemiology is highly varied, reflecting a diverse ecological environment, with differing seasonal trends across the country [4], which can be further affected by unpredictable cyclonic activity that impedes malaria control efforts. Epidemics have punctuated the history of malaria in Madagascar [5]. They are closely associated with the spread of rice production [6] and remain an important component of the disease epidemiology [7]. Domestic political support and international investment following the turn of the century led to impressive reductions in transmission up to 2008, but were followed by a period of stagnation and subsequent reversal of progress in the aftermath of political instability in 2009 and funding disbursement delays [4].

The National Malaria Control Programme (NMCP) of Madagascar has recently entered a new phase, marked by the inauguration of the 2018–2022 National Strategic Plan for Malaria, which includes ambitious targets for progress towards elimination during this period [8]. Central to optimising the intervention policy strategy for the coming 5 years is a thorough understanding of the current epidemiological situation across the country and of the impact of investments in recent years. While routinely reported clinical case data can provide insight into general tendencies in the burden of malaria in Madagascar [4], important uncertainties associated with this stream of data present difficulties with robustly quantifying spatio-temporal trends. Madagascar has benefited from three Malaria Indicator Surveys (MIS 2011, 2013 and 2016), which provide standardised and rigorous measures of malaria endemicity at high spatial resolution from representative population samples from across the island [9–11].

A recent overview of Madagascar's routine malaria case data from 2010 to 2015 described the trends in reported case data across eight ecozones, which are programmatically relevant clusters of spatially contiguous districts that share similar malaria epidemiological characteristics [4] (Fig. 1). This sub-national perspective offered insight into important variation in malaria burden across the island's different environmental zones. The overview identified an increase in numbers of confirmed malaria cases. This is explained in part by increased access to rapid diagnostic tests, but also by a growing malaria burden, which is indicated by a significant rate of increase in the diagnostic positivity rate between 2010 (33%) and 2015 (50%) ($p < 0.0001$). The routine reported case data, therefore, indicate there was an increasing malaria burden from 2010 to 2015.

The quality of data reporting through a country's routine health information system, however, can vary, potentially impacting the reliability of the nationally aggregated health statistics as malariometric indicators, especially in a resource-limited setting such as Madagascar, which has a fragile health and communications infrastructure [12]. At

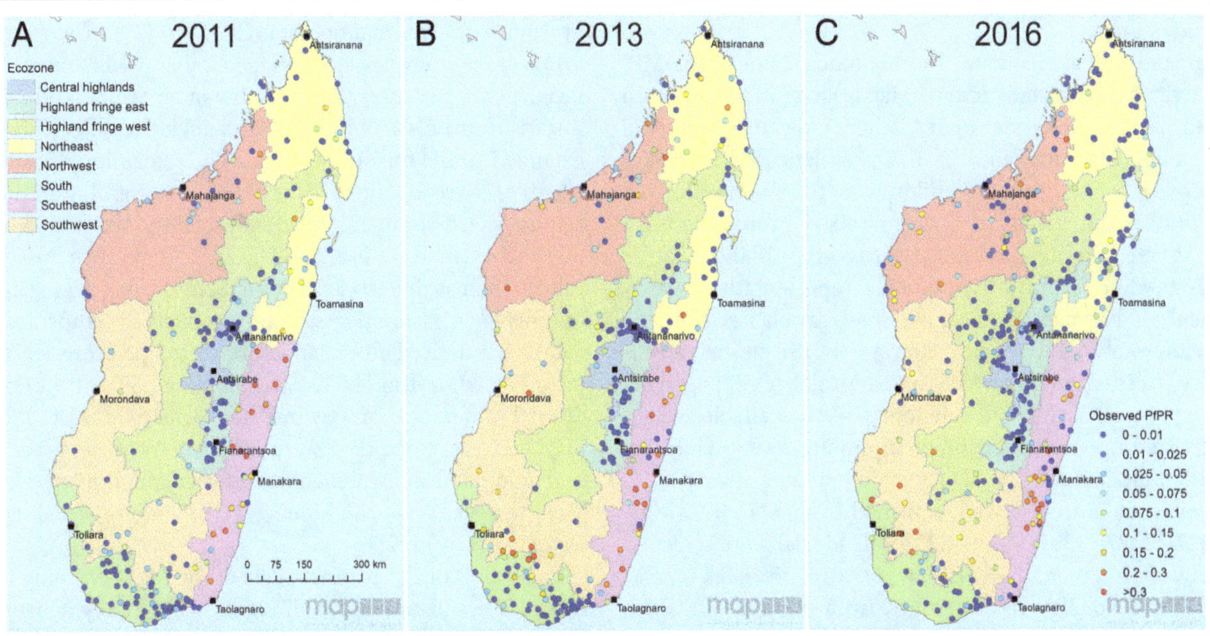

Fig. 1 Malaria Indicator Survey screening sites for (**a**) 2011, (**b**) 2013 and (**c**) 2016. The coloured regions represent the country's eight malaria ecozones [4]

every step of the data reporting chain, cases are lost from the system [13], for example from patients not interacting with public health facilities during malaria episodes [14], rapid diagnostic test stock-outs resulting in unconfirmed infections, or accessibility difficulties for health workers submitting monthly activity reports to the centralised database etc. [4]. Reported numbers can, therefore, be strongly influenced by factors external to the true underlying epidemiology.

MIS datasets provide a complementary perspective on recent trends in malaria endemicity, free from the intrinsic limitations of reported case data. Their strength lies in their standardised methodology applied repeatedly over multiple years across nationally representative sites. This present study uses the MIS data to map the prevalence of infection by *Plasmodium falciparum* in those under 5 years old (6 to 59 months in age: $Pf\mathrm{PR}_{6-59\mathrm{mo}}$) to obtain a deeper insight into epidemiological trends than that available from the published MIS overview analyses, which reported aggregated national prevalence rates of 6.2% for 2011 [9], 9.1% for 2013 [10] and 7.0% for 2016 [11]. This study aims to generate spatially continuous prevalence maps that account for disparities in sample collection dates between the different MIS years. This variation in the time window is not otherwise accounted for in the published MIS analyses [9–11]. The maps provide a benchmark of transmission intensity, free from the nuances of the datasets of routinely reported case data. These can support strategic resource allocation and allow progress towards the current strategic plan goals to be monitored.

Methods

Study data

Parasite prevalence data for this study came from MIS activities conducted across Madagascar in 2011, 2013 and 2016. Alongside many other indicators, an MIS includes measurements of the prevalence of *P. falciparum* infection among children 6 to 59 months old ($Pf\mathrm{PR}_{6-59\mathrm{mo}}$), based on a standardised protocol with a stratified sampling strategy across the island that is designed to capture a nationally representative assessment of prevalence. Data are freely available from the Demographic and Health Surveys (DHS) online repository. Across the three MIS years, a total of 898 spatially unique geo-positioned datapoints were available, which reported prevalence of infection among 19,986 children. The initial survey in 2011 included 266 sites (29.6% overall; 6827 individuals), screened from March to May. In 2013, 274 sites (30.5%; 6232 individuals) were screened between April and June. Finally, in 2016, 358 sites (39.9%; 6927 individuals) were screened from April to July. The diagnostic outcomes used here were from microscopy, read by the Institut Pasteur de Madagascar and NMCP parasitology teams. Survey locations are plotted by year in Fig. 1 and by month in Additional file 1: Figure S1. The maps reveal a west to east longitudinal gradient in the cluster sampling in both 2013 and 2016, with the high endemicity east coast sampled later than western and central populations. This sampling bias, with the east coast sampled later in the transmission season, reinforced the need to account for this in the model structure. Full details of the MIS protocols are available in the original published reports [9–11].

Environmental and socio-demographic variables known to interact with and influence *P. falciparum* prevalence [15] were assembled as 30 arcsecond spatial grids (Table 1). Among the suite of covariates, eight were temporally static covariates. The socio-demographic variables included stable night-time lights in 2010 [16], which indicated the presence of cities or towns [17], and accessibility to cities, which quantified travel time to cities larger than 50,000 people [18]. Static environmental variables included elevation as measured from the Shuttle Radar Topography Mission (SRTM) [19], slope, which was calculated from that elevation in ArcGIS 10.5.1 [20], and a measure of distance to water, which indicates the Euclidean distance to permanent and semi-permanent water based on the presence of lakes, wetlands, rivers and streams, and accounts for slope and precipitation [21, 22]. Also included were indices of aridity [23], potential evapotranspiration [23] and topographic wetness (which was calculated from the SRTM elevation surface).

Temporally dynamic covariates are those for which data were available at monthly intervals, or, for population density, annual intervals [24]. Precipitation data were obtained from the Climate Hazards Group Infrared Precipitation with Station data (CHIRPS) [25]. A *P. falciparum*-specific covariate developed by the Malaria Atlas Project that measures the suitability of air temperature for malaria transmission [26, 27] was included after it was extended to the full study period. The remaining dynamic variables were obtained from Moderate Resolution Imaging Spectroradiometer (MODIS) satellite data [28]. Note that these data were first gap-filled [29] to remove missing values, such as due to cloud cover, before being aggregated to monthly measurements. Three products of temperature data were derived from land surface temperature (LST), including (i) daytime LST, (ii) night-time LST and (iii) the diurnal difference of daytime to night-time LST [30]. MODIS reflectance data were used for measurements of vegetation and moisture: enhanced vegetation index (EVI) [31], tasselled cap brightness (TCB) and tasselled cap wetness (TCW) [32].

The values of the covariate data at the MIS screening locations were extracted for all points. Temporally dynamic covariates were matched to the same month as the survey, as well as 1, 2 and 3 months prior to the survey (lags).

Table 1 List of environmental and socio-demographic covariates

Covariate	Description	Dynamic	Round 1 selection	Round 2 selection	Source
Accessibility	Distance to cities with population >50,000	Static	Yes	Yes	Nelson [18]
AI	Aridity index	Static	Yes	Yes	World Clim [23]
DistToWater	GIS-derived surface that measures distance to permanent and semi-permanent water based on presence of lakes, wetlands, rivers and streams, and accounting for slope and precipitation	Static	Yes	Yes	MAP (from WWF surfaces [21, 22])
Elevation	Elevation as measured by the Shuttle Radar Topography Mission (SRTM)	Static	Yes	Yes	SRTM derivative [19]
PET	Potential evapotranspiration	Static	Yes	Yes	Trabucco & Zomer [23]
Slope	GIS-derived surface calculated from SRTM elevation surface	Static	Yes	Yes	MAP (from SRTM [19])
Stable_Lights_2010	Index that measures the presence of lights from towns, cities and other sites with persistent lighting	Static	Yes	Yes	NOAA [16]
TWI	Topographic wetness index	Static	Yes	Yes	MAP (from SRTM [19])
Population size	Estimated population per 1 km × 1 km pixel	Annual	Yes		Linard et al. [24]
EVI	Enhanced vegetation index	Monthly	Lag 0, 3	Lag 3	MODIS derivative [31]
LST_day	Daytime land surface temperature	Monthly			MODIS derivative [30]
LST_delta	Diurnal difference in land surface temperature	Monthly	Lag 0, 1, 2, 3	Lag 0, 1, 2, 3	MODIS derivative [30]
LST_night	Night-time land surface temperature	Monthly			MODIS derivative [30]
TCB	Tasselled cap brightness; measure of land reflectance	Monthly	Lag 0, 2	Lag 2	MODIS derivative [32]
TCW	Tasselled cap wetness	Monthly	Lag 3	Lag 3	MODIS derivative [32]
TSI	Temperature suitability index	Monthly	Lag 0, 1, 2, 3		MAP [26]
CHIRPS	Climate Hazards Group Infrared Precipitation with Station Data	Monthly	Lag 0, 1, 2, 3	Lag 0, 1, 3	CHIRPS [25]

CHIRPS Climate Hazards Group Infrared Precipitation with Station Data, *GIS* geographic information system, *MAP* Malaria Atlas Project, *MODIS* Moderate Resolution Imaging Spectroradiometer, *NOAA* National Oceanic and Atmospheric Administration, *SRTM* Shuttle Radar Topography Mission, *WWF* World Wildlife Fund

Bayesian spatio-temporal model

Parasite prevalence data (PfPR$_{6-59\text{mo}}$) were modelled via a Bayesian binomial logistic regression model with spatio-temporal random effects accounting for a spatial latent process varying with time. An integrated nested Laplace approximation [33] was adopted for model inference and prediction. The spatio-temporal random effects were modelled using stochastic partial differential equations [34], which represent a Matérn spatio-temporal Gaussian field as a Gaussian Markov random field via triangulation.

Let Y_{lt}, n_{lt} and p_{lt} be the number of infected individuals, the number of individuals screened and the prevalence of infection by *P. falciparum* at geocoded location l (l = 1, ..., N) for time t (t = 1, ..., T). Y_{lt} is assumed to follow a binomial distribution:

$$Y_{lt} \sim \text{Bin}(p_{lt}, n_{lt}).$$

The prevalence of infection, p_{lt}, is modelled via a linear regression on the logit scale:

$$\text{logit}(p_{lt}) = X_{lt}^T\boldsymbol{\beta} + f(\text{Year}) + \phi_{lt}.$$

The matrix X includes an intercept and a list of environmental and socio-demographic covariates known to affect prevalence. β is the vector of regression coefficient, f(Year) is a temporal random effect accounting for differences in years in the prevalence data and ϕ_{lt} is the spatio-temporally structured random effects. The temporal random effect, f(Year), is assigned a first-order autoregressive prior distribution (AR1). Monthly variations in the data are captured via the spatio-temporal process ϕ_{lt}, which changes in time with an AR1 process modelled at two semi-annual scales, as follows:

$$\begin{aligned} \phi_{l,t} &= \varepsilon_{l1}, & \text{if } t = 1, \\ \phi_{l,t} &= a\phi_{l,t-1} + \varepsilon_{l,t}, & \text{if } t = 2, \end{aligned}$$

where a ($|a| < 1$) is a temporal autoregressive coefficient and $\phi_{l,\,t}$ is the vector of the spatio-temporally structured effect, which follows a multivariate normal distribution with zero mean and a spatio-temporal covariance function of the Matérn family. See [34] for more details of the specification of the spatio-temporal random field. Since the prevalence data were only available for certain months each year, the AR1 process (time effect) of $\phi_{l,\,t}$ is modelled at two half-year intervals to ensure continuity: December to May and June to November.

As part of the variable selection procedure, collinearity among the environmental covariates was examined by calculating variance inflation factors (VIFs) prior to fitting the statistical model to the prevalence data. A stepwise selection of covariates using VIFs was undertaken to make sure all VIF values are below a desired threshold (VIF < 10 in this case). Put simply, using the full set of covariates, a VIF for each variable was calculated. The variable with the single highest value was removed and all VIF values with the new set of variables were recalculated. Then, the variable with the next highest value was removed, and so on, until all VIF values were below the threshold of 10. This resulted in a set of 26 covariates being considered for model fitting (Table 1, Round 1 selection). Subsequently, variable selection was performed using bidirectional elimination by running stepwise regressions on all model combinations using the 26 chosen covariates. The best-fitting (final) model had the smallest deviance information criterion value and included 18 covariates (Table 1, Round 2 selection).

Using the final model, the prevalence of infection by *P. falciparum* ($Pf\mathrm{PR}_{6-59\mathrm{mo}}$) was predicted over a 30 arcsecond spatial grid of 1,602,342 pixels (approximately 1 km × 1 km spatial resolution) for each month of 2011, 2013 and 2016. The final covariates were available at monthly intervals and this allowed us to make monthly predictions of prevalence. The resulting predictions included the monthly mean prevalence and the monthly interquartile range (IQR) of prevalence as a measure of the associated prediction uncertainty. The annual mean prevalence ($Pf\mathrm{PR}_{6-59\mathrm{mo}}$) and mean IQR were obtained by averaging across the 12 monthly predictions.

This Bayesian model-based geostatistical approach allows the smoothing of extreme rates due to small sample sizes by borrowing strength across neighbouring pixels to improve local estimates. Essentially, the approach assumes a positive spatial correlation between observations, borrows more information from neighbouring pixels than from pixels far away (in both space and time), and smooths local rates toward local, neighbouring values. The resulting smoothed prevalence estimates are robust and reliable while circumventing the issue of sparse data [35]. The inherently hierarchical structure of the current modelling framework permits the model-based estimation of covariate effects, the prediction of missing data and the estimation of spatio-temporal covariance structures [36]. Model predictions are presented at the pixel level and also summarised by ecozone [4].

A range of model validation analyses were used to assess the model's goodness of fit and predictive accuracy, including the Pearson correlation of observed and predicted data, and validation runs with incremental hold-out validation data subsets.

Results

The model framework

The Bayesian spatio-temporal model was developed in an integrated nested Laplace approximation framework to map the prevalence of *P. falciparum* malaria infection among children aged 6 to 59 months in age ($Pf\mathrm{PR}_{6-59\mathrm{mo}}$) across Madagascar for 2011, 2013 and 2016. Validation of the final model gave Pearson correlation coefficients of 0.96, 0.94 and 0.83 for each prediction year, respectively, between month-specific predicted and observed prevalence (Additional file 2: Figure S2), justifying a good fit of the Bayesian spatio-temporal model to the observed prevalence data. To assess the predictive power of the specified model, prevalence data were split into two sets: a training set (D_t) and a validation set (D_v) [37]. After being trained on D_t, the model accuracy was determined by its ability to predict D_v as well as the entire prevalence dataset. A percentage of D_v was chosen to be a random sample of 10%, 20%, 30% and 40% of the overall dataset. Each validation was repeated 100 times and the model accuracy was averaged across the 100 fitted models. The box plots of cross-validated correlations appeared satisfactory (Additional file 3: Figure S3a). The cross-validated R^2 had a mean of 0.78 and a range of (0.70, 0.83) for 10% D_v; a mean of 0.72 and a range of (0.62, 0.79) for 20% D_v; a mean of 0.65 and a range of (0.55, 0.74) for 30% D_v; and a mean of 0.58 and a range of (0.45, 0.68) for 40% D_v (Additional file 3: Figure S3b). The model was deemed accurate in its ability to predict a wide range of validation sets (Additional file 4: Figure S4).

Covariates

The combination of covariates that together best explained the spatio-temporal variation in the *Pf*PR datapoints were selected for inclusion in the spatio-temporal model and are listed in Tables 1 (Round 2 selection) and 2. Out of the 18 predictors which informed the statistical model, eight predictors were significant based on their 95% Bayesian credible intervals, namely LST_delta_2, TWI, PET, CHIRPS_1, Accessibility, Elevation, CHIRPS_0 and TCW_3. Of these eight predictors, LST_delta_2 (diurnal variation in land surface temperature 2 months prior to the prediction month) had a positive effect on the odds of risk with odds ratio OR = 1.1987. The odds of *P. falciparum* infection were negatively associated with TCW_3 (an index of surface wetness 3 months prior to the prediction month) with OR = 0.0025. The remaining six covariates had OR slightly

Table 2 Regression coefficients and odds ratios of the predictors selected by the final model and their associated 95% Bayesian credible intervals (CI)

Covariate	Regression coefficient	95% CI of regression coefficient	Odds ratio	95% CI of odds ratio
EVI_3	1.5872	(− 0.3861, 3.5926)	4.8913	(0.6799, 36.3362)
LST_delta_2	0.1812	(0.1098, 0.2527)*	1.1987	(1.1161, 1.2876)*
TWI	0.0535	(0.0048, 0.1017)*	1.0550	(1.0048, 1.1071)*
PET	0.0028	(0.0009, 0.0048)*	1.0028	(1.0009, 1.0048)*
CHIRPS_1	0.0023	(0.0010, 0.0037)*	1.0023	(1.0010, 1.0037)*
Accessibility	0.0020	(0.0009, 0.0031)*	1.0020	(1.0009, 1.0031)*
CHIRPS_3	0.0004	(−0.0010, 0.0018)	1.0004	(0.9990, 1.0018)
AI	0.0001	(0.0000, 0.0002)	1.0001	(1.0000, 1.0002)
DistToWater	0.0000	(0.0000, 0.0001)	1.0000	(1.0000, 1.0001)
Slope	0.0000	(0.0000, 0.0000)	1.0000	(1.0000, 1.0000)
Elevation	−0.0015	(−0.0022, − 0.0009)*	0.9985	(0.9978, 0.9991)*
CHIRPS_0	−0.0020	(−0.0036, − 0.0004)*	0.9980	(0.9964, 0.9996)*
LST_delta_1	−0.0111	(−0.0944, 0.0721)	0.9889	(0.9099, 1.0748)
Stable_Lights_2010	−0.0274	(−0.0801, 0.0218)	0.9730	(0.9231, 1.0221)
LST_delta_3	−0.0532	(−0.1173, 0.0106)	0.9482	(0.8894, 1.0106)
LST_delta_0	−0.0540	(−0.1360, 0.0281)	0.9475	(0.8729, 1.0285)
TCB_2	−1.7339	(−5.2983, 1.8037)	0.1765	(0.0050, 6.0672)
TCW_3	−5.9884	(−10.7712, − 1.2680)*	0.0025	(0.0000, 0.2813)*
Intercept	−11.5150	(−15.6992, −7.5190)	0.0000	(0.0000, 0.0005)

CI credible interval
*Significant based on 95% Bayesian credible interval

above or below 1, indicating that they did not have a large influence on the odds of risk. Note that the final model also included several predictors with OR being roughly one, namely aridity index, distance to water and slope, which suggests that they did not affect the odds of *P. falciparum* infection. However, the model selection procedure that optimised the deviance information criterion value justified the need to retain these predictors in the model.

Monthly variation in the key predictors is summarised at the national level in Fig. 2 and by the previously defined ecozones [4] in Additional file 5: Figure S5. These box plots include the temporally dynamic environmental predictors that informed the statistical model over different time lags. For example, EVI with a 3-month lag indicates that the malaria prevalence prediction for January 2011 was informed by the EVI level in October 2010. LST_delta, or the diurnal variation in land surface temperature, was influential across the whole time window up to 3 months prior to the prediction months. Predictions for January 2011, for example, were influenced by the difference in daytime and night-time temperatures (LST_delta) in October, November and December 2010, as well as January 2011. Seasonal variation in the different dynamic predictors differed in amplitude, with the most extreme being the CHIRPS dataset (a precipitation indicator), which dropped to very low between May and September. In contrast, the tasselled cap wetness (a remotely sensed transformed index of land surface water availability) remained relatively constant over time, with no significant monthly variation when summarised to the national level. At the higher-resolution ecozone level, ecological predictors show more extreme temporal variation, emphasising the country's environmental diversity. Put together, these constellations of monthly dynamic explanatory variables combined with the static predictors explained the spatio-temporal variation in the input data and informed extrapolation to locations and time points that were not represented in the MIS input datasets.

Spatio-temporal trends in malaria endemicity

This paper's primary objective was to assess changes in the prevalence of *P. falciparum* malaria infection among those under 5 years old ($Pf\mathrm{PR}_{6-59\mathrm{mo}}$) in Madagascar between the three surveyed years of 2011, 2013 and 2016. The published MIS reports gave national prevalence estimates for the 6–59 month age group of 6.2% [9], 9.1% [10] and 7.0% [11], respectively. The geostatistical model developed here generated 36 monthly prediction maps of endemicity (Additional file 5: Figure S5 and Additional file 6: Figure S6), which are summarised into three annual mean predictions (Fig. 3a–c), with ecozone-level box plot

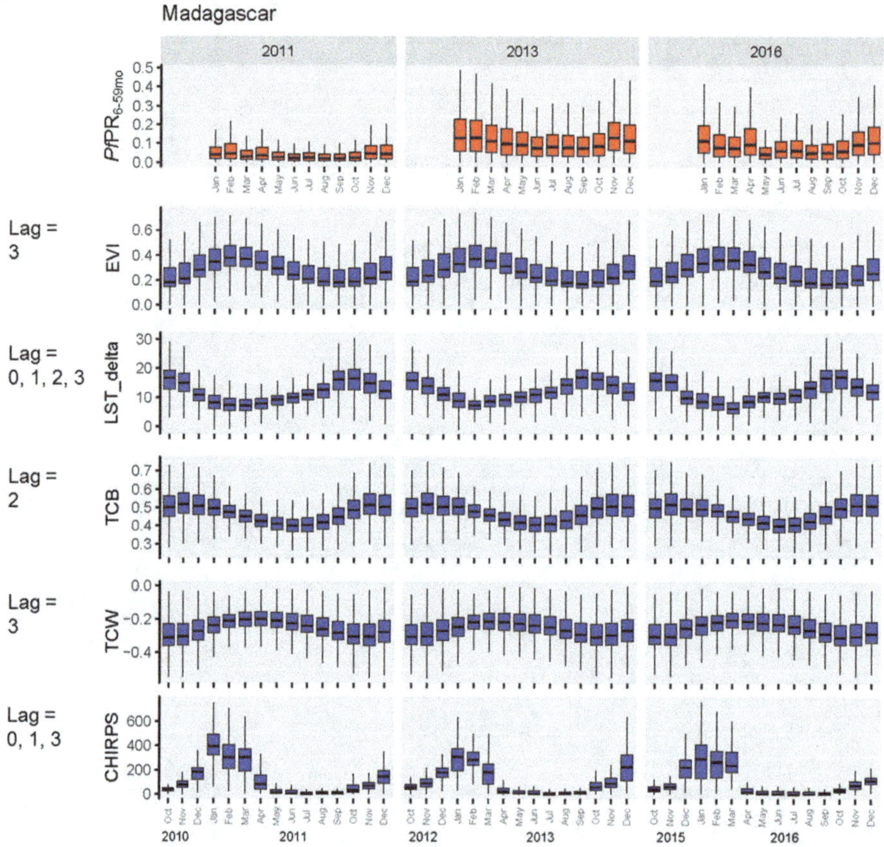

Fig. 2 National-level mean monthly PfPR$_{6-59mo}$ predictions, plotted alongside temporally variable predictor values. The box plot rectangles indicate the first to third quartiles (interquartile range), with the median shown as the dark line inside the box. Vertical lines correspond to the minimum and maximum values. Specified lags indicate the time points that were selected by the model as explanatory variables of PfPR$_{6-59mo}$. A time lag of 0 indicates that the covariate values in the concurrent month were predictive of PfPR$_{6-59mo}$, while a time lag of 3 indicates that the covariate value 3 months prior to the PfPR$_{6-59mo}$ prediction was predictive of PfPR$_{6-59mo}$

summaries of trends across the country's eight ecozones given in Fig. 4. Together, these model outputs allow spatio-temporal trends to be examined at different spatial and temporal scales: national, ecozone or pixel level, and monthly or annually. Model uncertainty is mapped alongside the mean PfPR$_{6-59mo}$ prediction surfaces as the IQR of the model posterior distribution (Fig. 3d–f and Additional file 6: Figure S6b, d, f), quantifying confidence in the model predictions. Coefficients of variation (standard deviation/mean) for each annual prediction are plotted in Additional file 7: Figure S7 to reflect the relative variability of the predictions. Together, these uncertainty maps show that while the absolute uncertainty (represented by the IQR) is lower in the central highlands where prevalence is lowest, when adjusted to the mean prediction values, confidence in the prediction is strongest in coastal areas where prevalence is higher.

Malaria endemicity remains spatially heterogeneous across Madagascar (Figs. 3 and 4), with the central highlands consistently having the lowest endemicity across the 3 years evaluated (<1% mean annual PfPR$_{6-59mo}$). To the east, a sharp transition towards the coast culminates in high prevalence regions, with pockets along the south-east coast with >30% mean annual prevalence, expanding in extent from 2011 into subsequent years. High prevalence in this ecozone is not homogeneous however, being interspersed with pockets of lower endemicity (<7.5% PfPR$_{6-59mo}$). The island's west coast is similarly high in prevalence, almost universally with PfPR$_{6-59mo}$ > 10% and with areas >30% mean annual PfPR$_{6-59mo}$ prevalence. The northern and southern tips have lower prevalence, typically under 5% endemicity. Confidence in the model predictions was variable across the country and between years. The low-prevalence data-rich highlands were modelled with greater confidence than the more heterogeneous coastal regions, where survey data indicated spatially variable rates of infection (Figs. 1 and 3d–f). The highest model uncertainty in all 3 years was in the north-eastern region of Sava, an area previously characterised as a malaria parasite transmission hotspot [38]. As seen across the whole

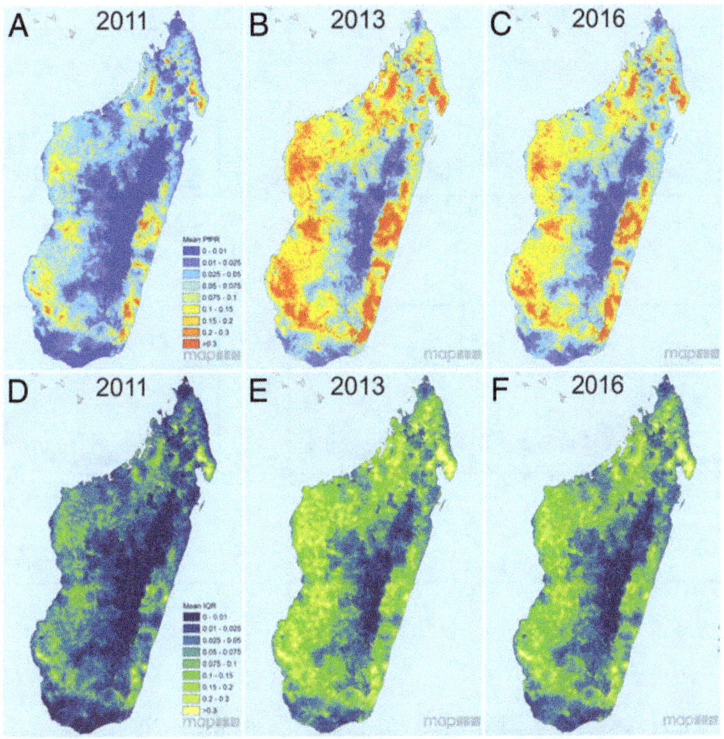

PfPR$_{6\text{-}59mo}$ class	G Pop 2011		H Pop 2013		I Pop 2016	
0-0.01	9,418,509	42.3%	5,278,699	22.3%	6,858,851	26.7%
0.01-0.025	4,200,124	18.8%	3,447,711	14.6%	4,105,352	16.0%
0.025-0.05	3,500,705	15.7%	3,279,490	13.9%	3,739,115	14.6%
0.05-0.075	1,911,174	8.6%	2,171,036	9.2%	2,599,709	10.1%
0.075-0.1	1,165,043	5.2%	1,767,207	7.5%	1,870,732	7.3%
0.1-0.15	1,103,066	5.0%	2,623,407	11.1%	2,605,211	10.2%
0.15-0.2	494,655	2.2%	1,768,446	7.5%	1,526,205	5.9%
0.2-0.3	361,505	1.6%	1,883,372	8.0%	1,457,138	5.7%
>0.3	128,619	0.6%	1,413,874	6.0%	898,141	3.5%

Fig. 3 Predicted annual mean *Pf*PR among children 6 to 59 months in age for 2011 (**a**), 2013 (**b**) and 2016 (**c**). **d**–**f** The corresponding map uncertainty (quantified as the prediction interquartile range). Values are mapped at 1 × 1 km pixel resolution. **g**–**i** National population breakdown by endemicity class, using population values based on WorldPop's Whole Continent UN-adjusted Population Count datasets for Africa for 2010, 2015 and 2020. Estimates for 2011, 2013 and 2016 were created by linear interpolation of the bookending quinquennial rasters

country after 2011, the higher observed prevalence was associated with a larger IQR, reflecting the wider range of potential prevalence values.

At the national level, the three mean annual maps were all significantly different from one another (Wilcoxon rank sum test, $p < 2.2 \times 10^{-16}$). PfPR$_{6-59mo}$ more than doubled between 2011 and 2016 (127% increase across the mean annual maps; Fig. 5a and c), despite a 23% decrease within that window between 2013 and 2016 (Fig. 5b and d). Changes in endemicity were spatially variable across the period examined. The magnitude of change across the country between 2011 and 2016 was highly heterogeneous, with a standard deviation of 34.0% around the 127% mean increase. All ecozones experienced at least a doubling in prevalence of PfPR$_{6-59mo}$ between 2011 and 2016, with the smallest proportional change being in the south-east (100.4%; Fig. 4 and Additional file 5: Figure S5d) and the highest up to 157.4% in the central highlands, where prevalence nevertheless remained the lowest (Fig. 4 and Additional file 5: Figure S5h). The south ecozone also saw an important increase of 142.5% over the 6-year period (Fig. 4 and Additional file 5: Figure S5g). The 23% mean fall in prevalence from 2013 to 2016 was fairly consistent across the whole country

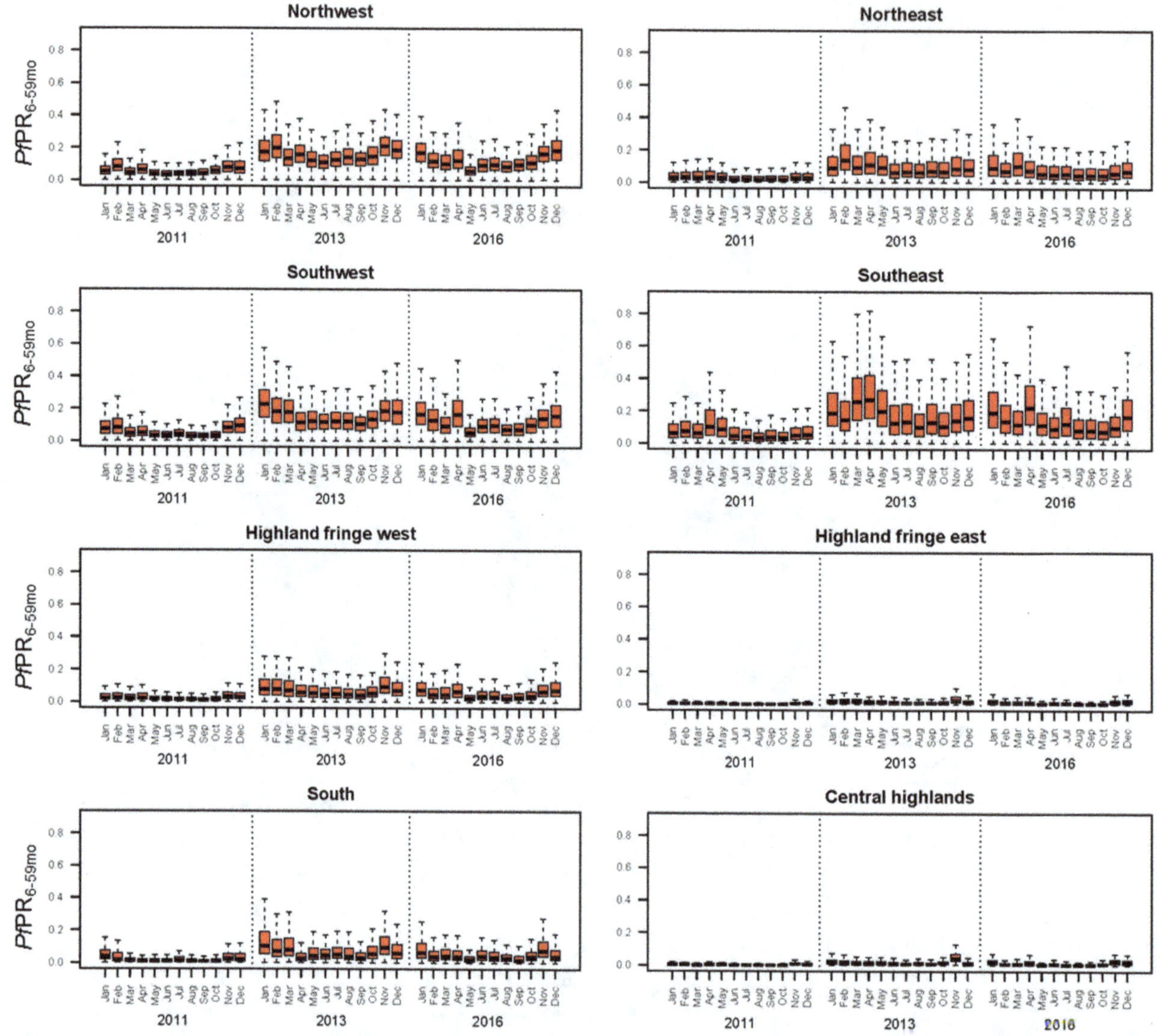

Fig. 4 Box plots of predicted monthly $Pf\mathrm{PR}_{6-59\mathrm{mo}}$ by ecozone for 2011, 2013 and 2016. Ecozone extents are shown in Fig. 1 [4]

(standard deviation 7.4%), and at the ecozone level, ranged from a 20.7% decrease in the central highlands to a 27.4% decrease in the eastern highland fringe zone. At the pixel level, 96% of pixels experienced a decrease of 10% to 50% between 2013 and 2016. In contrast, 27% of pixels increased between 0% and 100%, and 71% more than doubled in prevalence over the full study period from 2011 to 2016.

Trends in population exposure

Converting the geographic maps into population exposure rates offers insight into the relative intensity of infection prevalence across the population. The density of which is highly variable across the island [4]. Fig. 3g–i summarises the population numbers resident in each of the different endemicity categories. These show that the majority of the Malagasy population lives in the lowest endemicity areas, with almost half (42%) of the population in very low endemicity areas (<1% mean annual $Pf\mathrm{PR}_{6-59\mathrm{mo}}$) and less than 10% in areas where $Pf\mathrm{PR}_{6-59\mathrm{mo}}$ was >10% in 2011. The highest endemicity year, 2013, was predicted to have 32.5% of the population in areas where endemicity was >10%, a threefold increase from 2011. By 2016, this had dropped to 25.3% of the population being in areas of >10% prevalence, with a corresponding increase in the proportion living in very low (<1%) prevalence areas to 26.7%. Finally, the proportion of the population with infection prevalence greater than 20% rose from 2.2% in 2011 (an estimated 0.5 million individuals) to 14.0% in 2013 (3.3 million individuals) and 9.2% (2.4 million individuals) in 2016. Trends in endemicity across the population, therefore, reflect the overall tendencies in the geographic maps, with sharp increases in infection prevalence in the

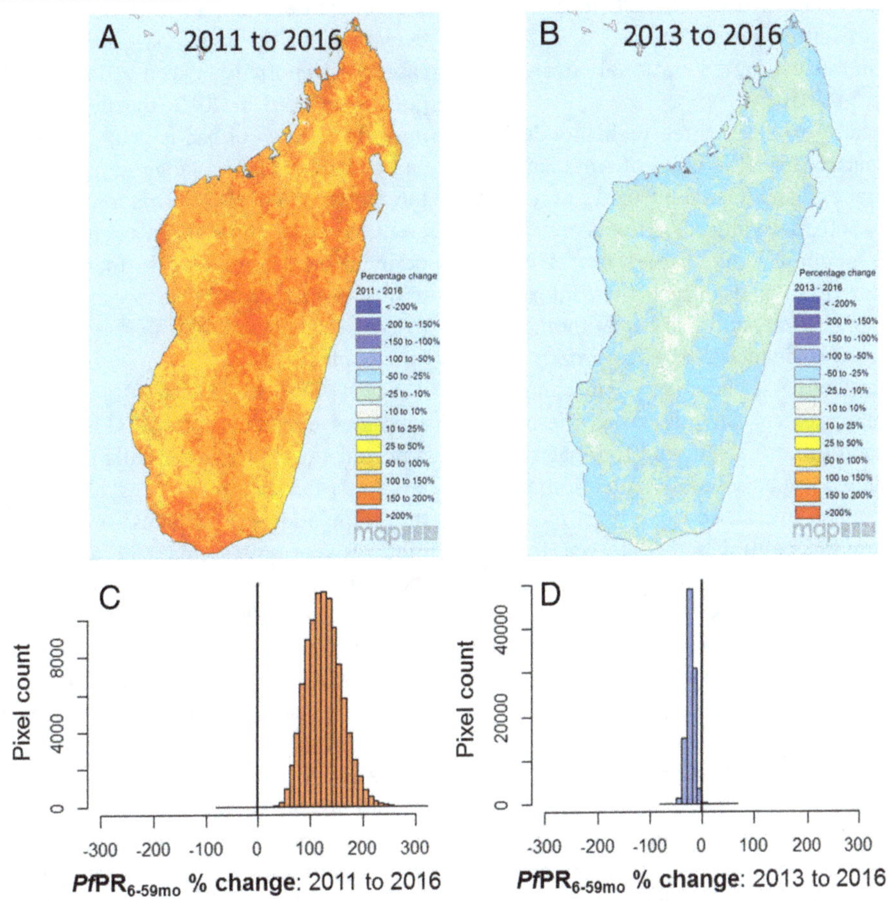

Fig. 5 Percentage changes in predicted *Pf*PR among children 6 to 59 months old across the three MIS time points: **a** from 2011 to 2016 and **b** from 2013 to 2016. Histograms of pixel-level change **c** from 2011 to 2016 and **d** from 2013 to 2016. Positive % change indicates an increase in prevalence, while negative % change is a decrease

low endemicity areas where most of the population lives, and notable increases in the population exposed to the highest end of the endemicity spectrum. A decrease of exposure levels from 2013 to 2016 was evident, but much less pronounced than the increase between 2011 and 2013, meaning that the exposure levels in 2016 were considerably worse than in 2011.

Discussion

Three MIS studies have taken place in Madagascar since 2011, providing a valuable source of information about the status of malaria from a standardised data collection protocol applied across a nationally representative set of locations. A broad range of indicator metrics are included in the MIS reports. This present study looks at the parasitology data in particular to assess how the prevalence of malaria infection in children 6 to 59 months old has changed in recent years. Given the limitations of the routine health data reporting chain discussed previously [4], this study provides a complementary perspective into the recent status of malaria endemicity in Madagascar, identifying important increasing trends since 2011 despite a relatively small fall in prevalence between 2013 and 2016.

Comparison with reported MIS results

The results presented in MIS reports are summaries of the raw survey data, with individuals weighted in such a way as to ensure appropriate national representation in the overall summary statistics. However, the results are not adjusted for the temporal lag in survey dates across years (Additional file 1: Figure S1). By 2016, the survey time window was pushed to 2 months later than in 2011, corresponding to a delay away from the peak transmission period in most regions (Additional file 3: Figure S3 and Additional file 4: Figure S4). The model presented here specifically accounts for this temporal lag, allowing for meaningful comparisons between years. Seasonal trends in transmission [4] mean that a delayed survey period will underestimate endemicity relative to the original survey time period. This is reflected in the raw MIS results, which suggest a 6.2% national $Pf\mathrm{PR}_{6-59\mathrm{mo}}$ in 2011 and 7% in 2016, a 13%

increase over that period. In contrast, the spatio-temporal model presented here identifies a 127% increase, resulting in an estimated national mean 9.3% annual $PfPR_{6-59mo}$ in 2016.

The MIS specifically excludes three highland districts considered to be malaria-free (the cities of Antananarivo-Renivohitra, Antsirabe I and Fianarantsoa I) as well as communes above 1500 m in altitude. Despite not being represented in the mapping input dataset, model predictions are derived for these areas, which then inform the ecozone- and national-level summaries. Without prior exclusion of these zones, the model-based approach risked over-inflating the estimates of endemicity. Environmental covariates, however, appear to have discerned the unsuitability of the highland urban habitat, and the malaria-free districts are predicted to have <0.5% infection prevalence in all 3 years. The overall ecozone-level mean annual $PfPR_{6-59mo}$ for the central highlands was 0.6% in 2011, 2.0% in 2013 and 1.6% in 2016, which were of the same order of magnitude as those in the MIS summaries of 0.8%, 1.1% and 0.9%, respectively. The excluded MIS sampling zones do not, therefore, seem to have impacted the spatio-temporal model predictions.

Comparison with previous prevalence maps

While geostatistical methods have been previously applied to infection prevalence datasets to predict spatially continuous prevalence maps of Madagascar, this has been within the context of continental or global-level mapping [37, 39]. The country-specific modelling approach applied here allows more freedom to the environmental covariates to adapt to Madagascar's specific ecological context, with the model selecting those covariates most pertinent to the island's environmental diversity. The continent-level spatio-temporal prediction cube developed by Bhatt et al. ([39], reproduced for Madagascar [4]), indicates a much coarser granularity than the present predictions, with little variation between years. Nevertheless, the continental maps do allow malaria endemicity in Madagascar to be viewed in its broader context, showing the relatively low prevalence of infection in Madagascar relative to many countries in sub-Saharan Africa (incidence rate ranked 13th lowest out of 43 countries in 2015 [39]). Prevalence mapping analyses are also valuable in evaluating trends in malaria prevalence over time.

Comparison with health metrics information system data

In this study, we map the parasite reservoir, as detectable by microscopy. In parallel, clinical case numbers are collated by the routine health metrics information system [4, 40, 41]. While the two metrics report different characteristics of malaria, spatio-temporal trends from both are similar, with a comparable geographic distribution of the burden of disease and an important increase in burden particularly along the west coast. A major increase in clinical cases was reported between 2014 and 2015, which subsequently reduced in 2016 (the third MIS year) following a mass distribution of bed nets treated with insecticide at the end of 2015 [41]. The longitudinal nature of the data from the health metrics information system allows extreme events to be identified, such as epidemics, which may drastically affect the annual case totals, as in 2015, but which may not be distinguishable as exceptional, or even captured by cross-sectional surveys that assess prevalence at isolated time points.

A 2017 World Health Organization (WHO) report estimates that only around 31% of all clinical cases are reported through the surveillance system to the central level in Madagascar. This is likely primarily driven by the population's low rates of seeking treatment. Of mothers seeking treatment in 2016 for their febrile children aged 6 to 59 months, 35.8% did so at public health facilities and 46.2% did so at any source (including public health facilities) [11]. Such low capture of the overall case burden, therefore, throws into question the system's capacity to adequately quantify changes in the malaria burden over time.

The two indicators, therefore, have their strengths and limitations, but together corroborate general trends of an increased burden between 2011 and 2016, punctuated with reductions, such as those identified between the 2013 and 2016 MIS surveys, or between 2015 and 2016 by the routinely reported case data [40, 41]. This temporal heterogeneity may be partly attributable to reductions in NMCP activities caused by Global Fund disbursement delays in 2014 [40]. In addition, recent evidence of the variable quality and durability of the insecticide-treated bed-net brands distributed across the country means that over their 3-year lifespans (mass distribution campaigns in Madagascar are triennial), protection from nets will be inconsistent [42]. MIS campaigns in Madagascar have all been timed to take place in the transmission season following mass bed-net distribution campaigns, which may, therefore, capture snapshots of prevalence at its lowest.

Limitations to the approach

In this study, we have used data on the prevalence of infection to assess the current spatio-temporal trends of malaria infection in Madagascar. This metric is independent of clinical symptoms, and instead quantifies the extent of the parasite reservoir across the population. The value of such a metric lies in its simplicity and standardised collection methods, and, in the context of the MIS, repeated national representation. A recent review by Cohen and colleagues [43], however, has argued for a multi-component mapping process that will adequately identify the underlying drivers of transmission, to enable

NMCP to target control measures optimally. Elimination requires both the reduction of the parasite reservoir and the prevention of transmission. Prevalence data alone cannot fully characterise the local epidemiology without a parallel understanding of a site's historical context, the significance of imported cases, the impact of recent control efforts, entomological and host behavioural/genetic factors, and so on [43]. A practical interpretation of the prevalence map, therefore, requires insight into the underlying factors driving the observed infection rates. The map suite presented here is one component in understanding malaria in Madagascar, but ought to be interpreted in association with a broader set of malariometric data when used to determine control intervention policy. Malaria transmission is also highly dynamic both spatially and temporally, meaning that predicted maps based on single time-point snapshots of prevalence may simplify the true underlying situation. Maps such as those presented here provide insight into general trends, and the validation statistics presented in Additional file 2: Figure S2, Additional file 3: Figure S3 and Additional file 4: Figure S4 indicate the level of variability that might be expected around these predictions.

Malaria prevalence is strongly influenced by intervention coverage levels, including rates of insecticide-treated net (ITN) ownership [39] and treatment seeking [13, 14]. Including these covariates in the modelling framework could help inform the model about the patterns of endemicity but this was not considered feasible in this present analysis. The coverage of indoor residual spraying and ITN use rates, for instance, have complex non-linear relationships with malaria prevalence. For example, indoor residual spraying in Madagascar is carefully targeted to the highest (as an emergency response to reduce mortality during outbreaks) and lowest (prevention of reintroduction and subsequent autochthonous transmission) endemicity districts only [8]. ITN coverage is strongly skewed to areas where malaria is endemic. The highland areas into which malaria is mainly imported are not covered by routine ITN distribution. The limited temporal window considered in this present study does not allow for the protective effect of high ITN coverage to be learnt by the model, and instead the coarse learnt association is that ITN coverage increases as prevalence increases. Treatment seeking was excluded for reasons of sample sizes. MIS data on treatment seeking from individual cluster locations are limited to mothers with infants who suffered from fever in the 2 weeks preceding the MIS interviews. Sample sizes at the cluster level are, therefore, very small, producing spurious results when analysed at the high resolution of the present analysis. Despite these barriers to including intervention covariates in the model, the suite of environmental and socio-demographic variables that were used allowed robust predictions of malaria prevalence, so this was not considered a major limitation to the mapping model presented here.

Madagascar is noted for its mosaic landscape of ecological habitats, with land cover varying across short distances [44]. The critical importance of the environmental covariates in the modelling process is evident from the methods described here, with a strong predictive role associated with vegetation cover that explains differences in malaria prevalence between different areas (Table 2). The covariates associated with each MIS site describe the local conditions associated with the observed malaria prevalence at the time and location of sampling. However, MIS datasets are geopositioned with a deliberate degree of spatial uncertainty (displacement) to promote anonymity of up to 2 km in urban areas, 5 km in rural areas and 10 km for 1% of rural points [45]. This spatial displacement, therefore, introduces uncertainty into the associations between reported *Pf*PR and their attributed covariate values, which could impact the model's predictions. For this study, we assumed that while the island is ecologically heterogeneous, the impact of this spatial uncertainty will be acceptably low (with ecological conditions similar for most points even at a distance of 5 km or 10 km), and similar enough to allow a prevalence signal to be identified. The model validation statistics corroborate this assumption.

A further limitation of the MIS datasets that informed the current mapping analysis stems from their sampling design and sample sizes. The broad range of indicators included in the MIS activities present conflicting demands on sample sizes, which are further constrained by financial and logistical considerations. Sample sizes cannot, therefore, be optimised for all indicators, but instead are focussed on a limited number of these. A recent retrospective model-based analysis of the 2011 and 2013 Madagascar MIS datasets estimated that sample sizes were under-powered by 17% and 36%, respectively, to reach effective sizes for infection prevalence rates [46]. This was based on rapid diagnostic test results and not microscopy (as considered in this present study), meaning that it may be a slight overestimate. The approach followed here, namely to consider samples from the three MIS datasets within a common Bayesian hierarchical modelling framework and to draw on a broad range of associated covariate surfaces, provides a solution to sample size limitations.

Furthermore, at very low transmission levels, such as in the central highlands and parts of the central fringe regions of Madagascar, microscopy-based cross-sectional surveys of parasite prevalence risk are underpowered to detect rare and low parasitaemia infections adequately [47]. In these areas, higher sensitivity diagnostics (such as nucleic-acid amplification-based approaches) and alternative indicators (such as serological markers) are required to monitor malaria epidemiological trends more effectively [47–50]. Particular interest is in the use of serological panels targeting both short- and long-lasting antigenic responses [51]. When applied to appropriate sentinel populations [52, 53], these tools can be powerful probes of changing transmission intensity or reintroduction events in the pre-elimination setting where the majority of infections at the time of survey may be microscopically sub-patent [54].

Conclusions

Malaria remains an important health problem in Madagascar, with the prevalence of infection more than doubling between 2011 and 2016 (a mean increase of 127%). Across the three survey time points, 2011 to 2013 saw the greatest $Pf\mathrm{PR}_{6\text{–}59\mathrm{mo}}$ increase, followed by a reduction to 2016 (mean reduction of 23%). However, while the whole population is at risk of infection, prevalence was lower in higher density areas, with 26.7% of the population in 2016 living in pre-elimination areas, where prevalence was <1% (a notable reduction from 42.3% of the population in 2011, however).

Presidential elections in December 2013 marked an optimistic turning point for Madagascar, with the return to democracy ending the country's 5-year isolation from the international community. The 2009–2013 political crisis placed a heavy burden on the country's socio-economic situation, with a deterioration in infrastructure and public services [55]. The sharp increase in malaria prevalence observed from 2011 to 2013 is likely a consequence of the country's wider economic situation and associated health infrastructure breakdown.

Madagascar is not alone in suffering losses with malaria control, with most countries in the African WHO region also experiencing stalling progress [40]. Madagascar's new strategic plan for 2018–2022, however, offers an opportunity to strengthen control with a policy shift away from blanket coverage of intervention commodities, towards a more locally targeted programme responsive to specific epidemiological contexts [56]. The current government's strong support for malaria elimination is reflected by a move towards closer integration of the NMCP into the Ministry of Health's core structures and activities rather than being a quasi-independent programme, coupled with the objective of partially devolving responsibilities for control planning to regional officers. New policies include the reintroduction of entomological control interventions, targeted seasonal chemoprophylaxis in epidemic-prone south-western communities, expanding household insecticide residual spraying to the highest and lowest risk areas, and specific consideration of high-risk populations [8].

Ambitious targets are being set for the end of the next National Strategic Plan in 2022, with a view towards geographically progressive elimination. Prevalence maps, as presented here, represent one component of monitoring progress towards those goals.

Additional files

Additional file 1: Figure S1. Sample screening during the three MIS events in Madagascar, showing the progressive delay in the sampling time window. a Overall bar plots of sampling months. b–d Maps by sampling month by cluster location. (PNG 1353 kb)

Additional file 2: Figure S2. Month-specific correlations between observed raw MIS prevalence values and the model predictions for each annual map. Pearson correlation coefficients are shown on each plot. (PNG 32 kb)

Additional file 3: Figure S3. Box plots of a cross-validated Pearson correlation coefficients and b cross-validated R^2, based on 100 randomly sampled validation sets. (PNG 26 kb)

Additional file 4: Figure S4. Observed prevalence against predicted prevalence averaged across 100 randomly sampled validation sets. (PNG 63 kb)

Additional file 5: Figure S5. Summary box plots of predicted monthly $Pf\mathrm{PR}_{6\text{–}59\mathrm{mo}}$ by ecozone, plotted alongside temporally variable predictor values. The box plot rectangles indicate the first to third quartiles (interquartile range), with the median shown as the dark line inside the box. Vertical lines correspond to the minimum and maximum values. Specified lags indicate the time points that were selected by the model as explanatory variables of $Pf\mathrm{PR}_{6\text{–}59\mathrm{mo}}$. A time lag of 0 indicates that the covariate values in the concurrent month were predictive of $Pf\mathrm{PR}_{6\text{–}59\mathrm{mo}}$, while a time lag of 3 indicates that the covariate value 3 months prior to the prediction was predictive of $Pf\mathrm{PR}_{6\text{–}59\mathrm{mo}}$. (ZIP 1859 kb)

Additional file 6: Figure S6. Predicted monthly mean $Pf\mathrm{PR}_{6\text{–}59\mathrm{mo}}$ maps for a 2011, c 2013 and e 2016, with associated uncertainty (interquartile range) for b 2011, d 2013 and f 2016. (ZIP 48310 kb)

Additional file 7: Figure S7. Maps of the coefficient of variation in the annual mean maps (standard deviation/annual mean) showing the relative confidence in the predictions across the country for a 2011, b 2013 and c 2016. (PNG 535 kb)

Abbreviations

AR1: First-order autoregressive prior distribution; CHIRPS: Climate Hazards Group Infrared Precipitation with Station Data; CI: Credible interval; DHS: Demographic and Health Surveys; EVI: Enhanced vegetation index; GIS: Geographic information system; IQR: Interquartile range; ITN: Insecticide-treated net; LST: Land surface temperature; MAP: Malaria Atlas Project; MIS: Malaria Indicator Survey; MODIS: Moderate Resolution Imaging Spectroradiometer; NMCP: National Malaria Control Programme; NOAA: National Oceanic and Atmospheric Administration; OR: Odds ratio; *P.*: *Plasmodium*; SRTM: Shuttle Radar Topography Mission; TCB: Tasselled cap brightness; TCW: Tasselled cap wetness; VIF: Variance inflation factor; WHO: World Health Organization; WWF: World Wildlife Fund

Acknowledgments

The authors thank the two reviewers for their helpful feedback and suggestions for improvements to the manuscript.

Funding

SYK receives support from the Bill and Melinda Gates Foundation (OPP1159934). KEB, HSG, DJW and EC are funded through Bill and Melinda Gates Foundation grants to PWG (OPP1106023 and OPP1152978). SR, AR, PAZ and REH are funded from a National Institutes of Health grant to PAZ (R01 AI097366). The funding bodies had no role in the study design, analysis, interpretation or decision to publish this manuscript.

Authors' contributions

REH, SYK, KEB, and PWG conceived the study. KEB and HG prepared the input data and covariate surfaces. SYK developed the statistical model. DW,

EC and PWG advised on the analysis. AR and MR were involved with the original MIS activities and generation of parasite prevalence data. REH wrote the first draft of the manuscript with SYK and KEB. All authors contributed to the interpretation of results. All authors read and approved the final manuscript.

Competing interests
The authors declare that they have no competing interests.

Author details
[1]Malaria Atlas Project, Oxford Big Data Institute, Nuffield Department of Medicine, University of Oxford, Oxford, UK. [2]National Malaria Control Programme, Ministry of Health, Antananarivo, Madagascar. [3]University of Antananarivo, Antananarivo, Madagascar. [4]Institut Pasteur de Madagascar, Antananarivo, Madagascar. [5]Faculté des Sciences, Université de Toliara, Toliara, Madagascar. [6]Center for Global Health and Diseases, Case Western Reserve University, Cleveland, OH, USA.

References

1. Joncour G. The fight against malaria in Madagascar. Bull World Health Organ. 1956;15:711–23.
2. Mouchet J, Blanchy S. Particularités et stratification du paludisme à Madagascar. Santé. 1995;5:386–8.
3. Randrianarivelojosia M, Raveloson A, Randriamanantena A, Juliano JJ, Andrianjafy T, Raharimalala LA, et al. Lessons learnt from the six decades of chloroquine use (1945-2005) to control malaria in Madagascar. Trans R Soc Trop Med Hyg. 2009;103:3–10.
4. Howes RE, Mioramalala SA, Ramiranirina B, Franchard T, Rakotorahalahy AJ, Bisanzio D, et al. Contemporary epidemiological overview of malaria in Madagascar: operational utility of reported routine case data for malaria control planning. Malar J. 2016;15:502.
5. Albonico M, De Giorgi F, Razanakolona J, Raveloson A, Sabatinelli G, Pietra V, et al. Control of epidemic malaria on the highlands of Madagascar. Parassitologia. 1999;41:373–6.
6. Laventure S, Mouchet J, Blanchy S, Marrama L, Rabarison P, Andrianaivolambo L, et al. Rice: source of life and death on the plateaux of Madagascar. Sante. 1996;6:79–86.
7. Girond F, Randrianasolo L, Randriamampionona L, Rakotomanana F, Randrianarivelojosia M, Ratsitorahina M, et al. Analysing trends and forecasting malaria epidemics in Madagascar using a sentinel surveillance network: a web-based application. Malar J. 2017;16:72.
8. National Malaria Control Programme of Madagascar. National strategic plan for malaria control in Madagascar 2018–2022. Progressive malaria elimination from Madagascar. (2017).
9. Institut National de la Statistique (INSTAT), Programme National de Lutte contre le Paludisme (PNLP), and ICF International. Madagascar Malaria Indicator Survey 2011 [Enquête sur les Indicateurs du Paludisme (EIPM)]. Calverton: INSTAT, PNLP, and ICF International; 2011.
10. Institut National de la Statistique (INSTAT), Programme National de Lutte contre le Paludisme (PNLP), Institut Pasteur de Madagascar (IPM), and ICF International. Madagascar Malaria Indicator Survey 2013 [Enquête sur les Indicateurs du Paludisme (EIPM)]. Calverton: INSTAT, PNLP, IPM and ICF International; 2013.
11. Institut National de la Statistique (INSTAT), Programme National de Lutte contre le Paludisme (PNLP), Institut Pasteur de Madagascar (IPM), and ICF International. Madagascar Malaria Indicator Survey 2016 [Enquête sur les Indicateurs du Paludisme (EIPM)]. Calverton: INSTAT, PNLP, IPM and ICF International; 2016.
12. Barmania S. Madagascar's health challenges. Lancet. 2015;386:729–30.
13. Cibulskis RE, Aregawi M, Williams R, Otten M, Dye C. Worldwide incidence of malaria in 2009: estimates, time trends, and a critique of methods. PLoS Med. 2011;8:e1001142.
14. Battle KE, Bisanzio D, Gibson HS, Bhatt S, Cameron E, Weiss DJ, et al. Treatment-seeking rates in malaria endemic countries. Malar J. 2016;15:20.
15. Weiss DJ, Mappin B, Dalrymple U, Bhatt S, Cameron E, Hay SI, et al. Re-examining environmental correlates of *Plasmodium falciparum* malaria endemicity: a data-intensive variable selection approach. Malar J. 2015;14:68.
16. National Oceanic and Atmospheric Administration (NOAA) National Centers for Environmental Information. Defense Meteorological Satellite Program (DMSP): Data Archive, Research, and Products. http://ngdc.noaa.gov/eog/dmsp.html. Accessed Sept 2017.
17. Noor AM, Alegana VA, Gething PW, Tatem AJ, Snow RW. Using remotely sensed night-time light as a proxy for poverty in Africa. Popul Health Metrics. 2008;6:5.
18. Nelson A. Travel time to major cities: A global map of Accessibility. Ispra: Global Environmental Monitoring Unit - Joint Research Centre of the European Commission; 2008. http://forobs.jrc.ec.europa.eu/products/gam/. Accessed Sept 2017.
19. Farr TG, Rosen PA, Caro E, Crippen R, Duren R, Hensley S, et al. The Shuttle Radar Topography Mission. Rev Geophys. 2007;45:RG2004.
20. ESRI. ArcGIS Desktop 10.5.1. Redlands: Environmental Systems Resource Institute; 2017.
21. HydroSHEDS database. http://hydrosheds.org/. Accessed Sept 2017.
22. World Wildlife Fund (WWF). Global Lakes and Wetlands Database. Washington, DC; 2004. https://www.worldwildlife.org/pages/global-lakes-and-wetlands-database. Accessed Sept 2017.
23. Trabucco A, Zomer RJ. Global aridity index (global-aridity) and global potential evapo-transpiration (global-PET) geospatial database. CGIAR Consortium for Spatial Information ed. 2009. Available online from the CGIAR-CSI GeoPortal at: http://www.cgiar-csi.org/. Accessed Sept 2017.
24. Linard C, Gilbert M, Snow RW, Noor AM, Tatem AJ. Population distribution, settlement patterns and accessibility across Africa in 2010. PLoS One. 2012;7:e31743.
25. Funk CC, Peterson PJ, Landsfeld MF, Pedreros DH, Verdin JP, Rowland JD, et al. A quasi-global precipitation time series for drought monitoring: U.S. Geological Survey Data Series, vol. 832; 2014. https://doi.org/10.3133/ds832.
26. Weiss DJ, Bhatt S, Mappin B, Van Boeckel TP, Smith DL, Hay SI, et al. Air temperature suitability for *Plasmodium falciparum* malaria transmission in Africa 2000-2012: a high-resolution spatiotemporal prediction. Malar J. 2014;13:171.
27. Gething PW, Van Boeckel TP, Smith DL, Guerra CA, Patil AP, Snow RW, et al. Modelling the global constraints of temperature on transmission of *Plasmodium falciparum* and *P. vivax*. Parasit Vectors. 2011;4:92.
28. NASA. Moderate Resolution Imaging Spectroradiometer (MODIS). https://modis.gsfc.nasa.gov/. Accessed Sept 2017.
29. Weiss DJ, Atkinson PM, Bhatt S, Mappin B, Hay SI, Gething PW. An effective approach for gap-filling continental scale remotely sensed time-series. ISPRS J Photogramm Remote Sens. 2014;98:106–18.
30. NASA Earth Observations (NEO). Average land surface temperature. http://neo.sci.gsfc.nasa.gov/view.php?datasetId=MOD_LSTD_CLIM_M. Accessed Sept 2017.
31. NASA Earth Data. MODIS (MOD 13) - Gridded Vegetation Indices (NDVI and EVI). http://modis.gsfc.nasa.gov/data/dataprod/dataproducts.php?MOD_NUMBER=13. Accessed Sept 2017.
32. NASA Earth Data. Land Processes Distributed Active Archive Center. https://lpdaac.usgs.gov/dataset_discovery/modis/modis_products_table/mcd43b5. Accessed Sept 2017.
33. Rue H, Martino S, Chopin N. Approximate Bayesian inference for latent Gaussian models by using integrated nested Laplace approximations. J Royal Stat Soc Series B Stat Methodo. 2009;71:319–92.
34. Cameletti M, Lindgren F, Simpson D, Rue H. Spatio-temporal modeling of particulate matter concentration through the SPDE approach. Adv Stat Ana. 2013;97:109–31.
35. Clayton D, Kaldor J. Empirical Bayes Estimates of Age-Standardized Relative Risks for Use in Disease Mapping. Biometrics. 1987;43:671–81.
36. Waller L, Carlin B. Disease mapping. In: Gelfand AE, Diggle P, Guttorp P, Fuentes M, editors. Handbook of Spatial Statistics. Boca-Raton: CRC Press; 2010.
37. Gething PW, Patil AP, Smith DL, Guerra CA, Elyazar IR, Johnston GL, et al. A new world malaria map: *Plasmodium falciparum* endemicity in 2010. Malar J. 2011;10:378.
38. Rice BL, Golden CD, Anjaranirina EJ, Botelho CM, Volkman SK, Hartl DL. Genetic evidence that the Makira region in northeastern Madagascar is a hotspot of malaria transmission. Malar J. 2016;15:596.
39. Bhatt S, Weiss DJ, Cameron E, Bisanzio D, Mappin B, Dalrymple U, et al. The effect of malaria control on *Plasmodium falciparum* in Africa between 2000 and 2015. Nature. 2015;526:207–11.

40. WHO. World Malaria Report 2017. Geneva: World Health Organization; 2017.
41. National Malaria Control Programme of Madagascar. Malaria Programme Review 2017 [Revue du Programme National de Lutte contre le Paludisme]. Antananarivo: Ministry of Health of Madagascar; 2017.
42. Randriamaherijaona S, Raharinjatovo J, Boyer S. Durability monitoring of long-lasting insecticidal (mosquito) nets (LLINs) in Madagascar: physical integrity and insecticidal activity. Parasit Vectors. 2017;10:564.
43. Cohen JM, Le Menach A, Pothin E, Eisele TP, Gething PW, Eckhoff PA, et al. Mapping multiple components of malaria risk for improved targeting of elimination interventions. Malar J. 2017;16:459.
44. Virah-Sawmy M, Gillson L, Willis KJ. How does spatial heterogeneity influence resilience to climatic changes? Ecological dynamics in southeast Madagascar. Ecol Monogr. 2009;79:557–74.
45. Burgert CR, Colston J, Roy T, Zachary B. Geographic displacement procedure and georeferenced data release policy for the demographic and health surveys. In: DHS Spatial Analysis Reports No 7. Calverton: ICF International; 2013. https://dhsprogram.com/pubs/pdf/SAR7/SAR7.pdf.
46. Alegana VA, Wright J, Bosco C, Okiro EA, Atkinson PM, Snow RW, et al. Malaria prevalence metrics in low- and middle-income countries: an assessment of precision in nationally-representative surveys. Malar J. 2017;16:475.
47. Dalrymple U, Mappin B, Gething PW. Malaria mapping: understanding the global endemicity of falciparum and vivax malaria. BMC Med. 2015;13:140.
48. Yalew WG, Pal S, Bansil P, Dabbs R, Tetteh K, Guinovart C, et al. Current and cumulative malaria infections in a setting embarking on elimination: Amhara, Ethiopia. Malar J. 2017;16:242.
49. Corran P, Coleman P, Riley E, Drakeley C. Serology: a robust indicator of malaria transmission intensity? Trends Parasitol. 2007;23:575–82.
50. Zimmerman PA, Howes RE. Malaria diagnosis for malaria elimination. Curr Opin Infect Dis. 2015;28:446–54.
51. Helb DA, Tetteh KK, Felgner PL, Skinner J, Hubbard A, Arinaitwe E, et al. Novel serologic biomarkers provide accurate estimates of recent *Plasmodium falciparum* exposure for individuals and communities. Proc Natl Acad Sci U S A. 2015;112:E4438–47.
52. Ray K, Upreti HB, Yadav RN, Sharma MC, Mukherjee AK, Sharma GK. Evaluation of serology as a tool for malaria surveillance in East Champaran District of Bihar, India. Ann Trop Med Parasitol. 1988;82:225–8.
53. Elliott SR, Fowkes FJ, Richards JS, Reiling L, Drew DR, Beeson JG. Research priorities for the development and implementation of serological tools for malaria surveillance. F1000Prime Rep. 2014;6:100.
54. Stresman GH, Stevenson JC, Ngwu N, Marube E, Owaga C, Drakeley C, et al. High levels of asymptomatic and subpatent *Plasmodium falciparum* parasite carriage at health facilities in an area of heterogeneous malaria transmission intensity in the Kenyan highlands. Am J Trop Med Hyg. 2014;91:1101–8.
55. The World Bank. Madagascar: Measuring the Impact of the Political Crisis. Washington DC; 2013. http://www.worldbank.org/en/news/feature/2013/06/05/madagascar-measuring-the-impact-of-the-political-crisis. Accessed 31 Jan 2016.
56. Baird JK. Malaria control by commodities without practical malariology. BMC Public Health. 2017;17:590.

15

Efficacy, effectiveness and safety of vaccination against human papillomavirus in males

Thomas Harder[1*], Ole Wichmann[1], Stefanie J. Klug[2], Marianne A. B. van der Sande[3] and Miriam Wiese-Posselt[1]

Abstract

Background: Human papillomavirus (HPV) vaccination is safe and effective in preventing cervical cancer in females. As HPV infections can also induce cancers of the anus, penis and oral cavity, male vaccination is also advocated, but systematic reviews on efficacy and safety in males are lacking.

Methods: We performed a systematic review on the efficacy, effectiveness and safety of HPV vaccination in males of any age. MEDLINE, Embase, the Cochrane Central Register of Controlled Trials and ClinicalTrials.gov were searched from inception to April 2017.

Results: We identified 5196 articles and seven studies (four randomized controlled trials (RCTs), three non-randomized studies) were included, comprising a total of 5294 participants. Vaccine efficacy against at least 6-month persisting anogenital HPV 16 infections was 46.9% (95% confidence interval (CI) 28.6–60.8%), whereas efficacy against persisting oral infections was 88% (2–98%). A vaccine efficacy of 61.9% (21.4–82.8%) and 46.8% (− 20 to −77.9%) was observed against anal intraepithelial neoplasia grade 2 and grade 3 lesions, respectively. No meaningful estimates were available on vaccine efficacy or effectiveness against penile intraepithelial neoplasia grade 2 or 3, and no data were identified for anal, penile or head and neck squamous cell cancer. In participants who were HPV-seronegative and PCR-negative at enrolment, efficacy against all outcomes was higher as compared to seropositive and/or PCR-positive individuals. Risk of bias was low in three RCTs and high in one, while the three non-randomized studies were at serious to critical risk of bias. Grading of Recommendations Assessment, Development and Evaluation evidence quality was moderate to low for most outcomes.

Conclusions: HPV vaccination in males is moderately effective against persistent anogenital HPV infection and high-grade anal intraepithelial lesions in studies where the population consists mainly of HPV-infected males. Vaccine effectiveness was high in study groups comprising HPV-naïve males. This supports a recommendation for vaccination of boys before the onset of sexual activity with the goal of establishing optimal vaccine-induced protection. Mathematical modelling studies will still be needed to assess the effects of adding males to existing HPV vaccination programs in females.

Trial registration: Prospective Register for Systematic Reviews (PROSPERO) registration CRD42016038965.

Keywords: Human papillomavirus, Systematic review, Efficacy, Effectiveness, Safety

* Correspondence: hardert@rki.de

[1]Robert Koch Institute, Immunization Unit, Seestrasse 10, 13353 Berlin, Germany

Full list of author information is available at the end of the article

Background

Human papillomavirus (HPV) is the most common sexually transmitted microorganism. The skin and mucosa of the anogenital tract, oral cavity, oropharynx and larynx are frequently affected by this virus [1]. The initial HPV infection is asymptomatic, and the virus is cleared in the majority of cases [2, 3]. About 10% of HPV infections persist, and less than 3% result in epithelial dysplasia or even cancer (1%) if the infection is due to an oncogenic HPV type [4–6]. Presently, more than 200 different HPV types have been described. They are classified as high risk (HR) and low risk (LR) viruses. While LR types such as HPV 6 and HPV 11 can cause genital warts, infections due to HR HPV types can induce cancer. The International Agency for Research on Cancer (IARC) classifies 12 HPV types as HR cancer-causing types, of which HPV 16 and HPV 18 are the most common [7, 8]. In females, nearly 100% of cervical cancers are attributable to HR HPV types [9]. In males, approximately 33% of penile cancers and up to 90% of anal cancers are attributed to HR HPV infections, primarily with HPV type 16 [10–12]. The HPV attributable fraction in cancers of the oral cavity, oropharynx and larynx was estimated to be 22.4%, 4.4% and 3.5%, respectively [13].

Anogenital HPV infections are common in men. In a population-based survey in the USA, 23% of participants had a penile infection with a high-risk HPV type [14]. In men who have sex with men (MSM) and in HIV-positive men, even higher prevalences were observed. A Dutch study reported that 45% of HIV-negative MSM and 65% of HIV-positive MSM had an anal infection by a high--risk HPV type [15]. HPV infections of the oral cavity are less prevalent: a systematic review reported a pooled prevalence of 4.5%, with no significant differences between men and women [16]. According to the German Centre for Cancer Registry Data, in 2013 a total of 1358 male cancer cases in Germany were attributable to HPV [17]. The life-time risk of HPV-associated genital warts has been estimated to be 5–10% [18].

To date, three different vaccines against HPV have been licensed [19]. They contain virus-like particles (VPLs) that induce immunity against certain HPV types. The bivalent vaccine protects against HR HPV types 16 and 18, and the quadrivalent vaccine protects against HR HPV types 16 and 18 as well as LR HPV types 6 and 11. A nonavalent vaccine was approved by the US and European regulatory authorities in 2015 and 2016, respectively, adding protection against five additional HR HPV types. Based on epidemiological data, it has been estimated that 85–90% of all cervical cancer cases could be prevented by vaccination with the nonavalent HPV vaccine if it is administered to girls before their sexual debut [20]. By targeting HPV 16 and 18 alone, 60–70% of all cervical cancers could be prevented.

While most industrialized countries have introduced routine female HPV vaccination into their national immunization programs, routine vaccination of boys and men is currently implemented in only a few countries, such as Australia, Canada, the USA and Austria. Vaccination of boys and men may further reduce the incidence of cervical cancer and its precursors via herd protection, and reduce the incidence of anal and penile as well as head and neck cancers [21, 22]. The aim of this systematic review was to assess the currently available evidence on the efficacy, effectiveness and safety of HPV vaccination in males.

Methods

Search strategy and selection criteria

This systematic review followed a protocol published in the Prospective Register for Systematic Reviews (PROSPERO; registration no. CRD42016038965) and was reported according to the guidelines in the Preferred Reporting Items for Systematic Reviews and Meta-analyses (PRISMA) statement [23]. To be eligible, a study had to investigate the efficacy, effectiveness and/or safety of vaccination (with a licensed vaccine) against HPV in males of any age. The control group had to be males who were either unvaccinated or had received placebo or a vaccine not directed against HPV. An eligible study had to report on at least one of the following predefined outcomes: (1) incident oral infection with an HR HPV type; (2) incident anogenital (or anal) infection with an HR HPV type; (3) persisting oral infection with an HR HPV type (≥ 6 months); (4) persisting anogenital (or anal) infection with an HR HPV type (≥ 6 months); (5) condyloma acuminatum (genital or anal) due to HPV 6 or 11; (6) anal intraepithelial neoplasia (AIN) grade 2; (7) AIN grade 3 or carcinoma; (8) penile intraepithelial neoplasia (PIN) grade 2, (9) PIN grade 3 or carcinoma; (10) squamous cell carcinoma of the head and neck region, including the oropharynx, larynx and oral cavity; (11) epithelial dysplasia related to (10); and (12) any severe adverse event following immunization. As we were primarily interested in clinical relevance, we did not restrict ourselves to vaccine-type specific lesions only.

The electronic databases searched were MEDLINE, Embase and the Cochrane Central Register of Controlled Trials (date of initial search 4 November 2016; last update 18 April 2017). For details on the complete search strategy, see Additional file 1. Additionally, ClinicalTrials.gov was searched systematically for unpublished or ongoing trials. Electronic searches were complemented by manually screening conference abstract books of major international HPV conferences (EUROGIN 2016, International HPV Conference 2017) as well as reference lists of all identified studies and those of identified reviews. Search results (titles, abstracts, full texts) were independently assessed by two investigators (TH, MWP). Differences were discussed until a consensus was reached.

We did not make any restrictions with regard to setting, language or publication status (published/unpublished). Potential indirect effects of male HPV vaccination on the incidence of clinical outcomes in females were not considered in this review.

Data extraction

From the eligible studies, two independent reviewers (TH, MWP) used standardized forms to extract study characteristics and assess methodological quality. In case of disagreement, a final decision was made by consensus. The corresponding authors or principal investigators of three studies were contacted for additional data and information [24–26]. The following data were extracted: study location, study design, study period, inclusion criteria, exclusion criteria, age at enrolment, duration of follow-up, vaccine used, comparator, study sponsorship, conflict of interests, number (proportion) of vaccinated participants with outcome, number (proportion) of control participants with outcome, unadjusted estimates, adjusted estimates, confounders.

Assessment of risk of bias and quality of evidence

For randomized controlled trials (RCTs), the Cochrane risk of bias tool was used to assess the following domains: random sequence generation, allocation concealment, blinding of participants and personnel, blinding of outcome assessment, incomplete outcome data, selective reporting, other bias [27]. Studies were categorized as being at "high risk", "low risk" or "unclear risk" of bias. For non-randomized studies, the Risk Of Bias in Non-randomized Studies - of Interventions (ROBINS-I) tool was used, comprising the following domains: bias due to confounding, bias in selection of participants into the study, bias in classification of interventions, bias due to deviations from intended interventions, bias due to missing data, bias in measurement of outcomes, bias in selection of the reported results [28]. Risk of bias was categorized as being "low risk", "moderate risk", "serious risk" or "critical risk".

The methodology of the Grading of Recommendations, Assessment, Development and Evaluation (GRADE) working group was used to assess the quality of the evidence [29, 30].

Statistical analysis

Abstracted data were aggregated in tables. Risk ratios, odds ratios, risk differences and corresponding 95% confidence intervals (95% CI) were either calculated or extracted from the publications. Vaccine efficacy and vaccine effectiveness were either extracted from the publications or calculated as [1-(risk ratio or rate ratio comparing vaccine and control recipients)] × 100. Since only one study per outcome and study design was identified in this review, no meta-analyses were performed. According to the review protocol, analyses were performed in two subgroups: (1) all study participants, irrespective of HPV infection at enrolment, and (2) study participants who were seronegative and PCR-negative for the relevant HPV types at enrolment.

Results

We identified a total of 5196 entries in electronic databases. After exclusion of duplicates, 3318 articles remained for title screening. Of these, 3065 papers were judged to be irrelevant according to their titles and were excluded. The abstracts of the remaining 253 publications were subsequently screened, and 167 of them were considered irrelevant and therefore excluded. We then assessed the full text of the remaining 86 articles. Of these, 79 were excluded due to lack of relevant data ($n = 16$), lack of data on men ($n = 14$), being a modelling study ($n = 1$), being a conference abstract of an included study ($n = 3$), lack of comparator ($n = 16$), lack of original data ($n = 22$) or not being a vaccination study ($n = 7$). Thereby, we finally included seven studies in the analysis (for details, see Fig. 1). Bibliographic data of the 79 studies that were excluded after full-text assessment are reported in Additional file 2.

We included four RCTs [26, 31–33] and three non-randomized studies [24, 25, 34]. The studies comprised data of a total of 5294 study participants. One included RCT [33] was a subtrial of another included study [32], but it reported different outcomes. The main study characteristics are shown in Table 1. Three of these trials were international multicentre studies [26, 32, 33], while the remaining four studies were performed solely in the USA or in Turkey. Four of the studies included both heterosexual men and MSM [25, 32–34]. One study included only self-identified heterosexual men [31]. The other two studies recruited male and female participants, but only the results for males are reported here. One of these studies was performed in adolescents and young adults with behaviorally acquired HIV [24], whereas the other one included HIV-positive adults [26]. The age of the participants at study entry ranged from 12 to 76 years. In all studies, the quadrivalent vaccine (Gardasil) was used. Six studies provided information on potential conflicts of interest [24–26, 32–34]. Two studies were registrative studies and reported sponsorship by a pharmaceutical company [32, 33].

Only two of the studies reported data on HPV-naïve participants [32, 33]. These studies were registrative trials and comprised a total of 2032 participants in the vaccinated and 2033 participants in the placebo arm. Of those, 1397 subjects in the vaccinated and 1408 in the

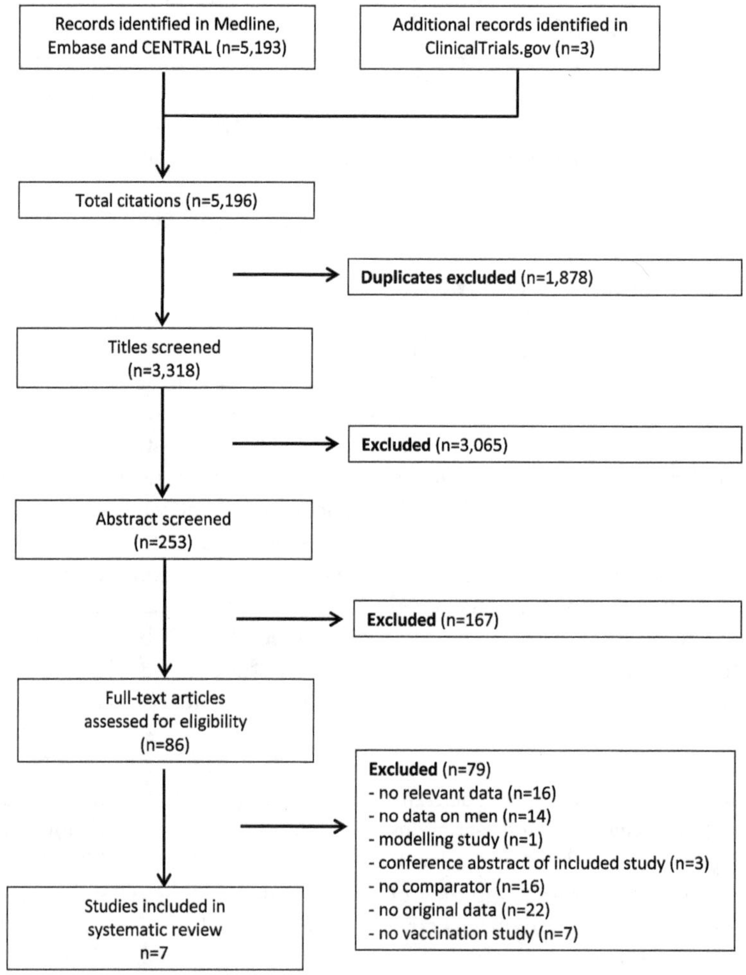

Fig. 1 Flow diagram

placebo group were HPV-naïve men. The mean age in the vaccinated group was 20.6 years (standard deviation (SD) 2.0; range 16–26 years); it was 20.5 years (SD 2.0; range 15–27 years) in the placebo group. The median length of follow-up was 2.9 years for both groups.

Of the 12 outcomes defined a priori in the review protocol, ten were reported in the included studies (Table 2). In two of the RCTs [32, 33], the primary efficacy endpoints defined by the investigators were compound endpoints comprising malignant and benign anal or genital lesions, but only those data that correspond to the outcomes predefined in our protocol were used for the following analyses. We considered the outcome "DNA detection" reported in these two trials [32, 33] as being equivalent to "incident infection". Furthermore, because different sampling techniques were used, we separated "anal infection" from "anogenital infection" in these two studies [32, 33]. A total of four studies reported data on condyloma acuminatum, while two studies reported on the outcomes AIN grade 2, AIN grade 3 and/or severe adverse events. For the remaining outcomes, only one study per outcome was identified. We did not identify any relevant studies investigating the outcomes 10 "squamous cell carcinoma of the head and neck region" or 11 "epithelial dysplasia related to squamous cell carcinoma of the head and neck region".

Risk of bias was low in three of the RCTs (Table 3). In the remaining RCT [31], risk of bias was judged to be high due to the lack of a placebo-controlled study arm (controls were unvaccinated). The three non-randomized studies were judged to have a serious (two studies) or critical risk of bias (one study) due to residual confounding, risk of selection bias and missing data (Table 4).

Table 5 shows vaccine efficacy and effectiveness against infection with HR HPV types (HPV 16 or HPV 18), irrespective of HPV infection status at enrolment. Vaccine efficacy was low against incident anogenital infections caused by HPV 16 (28%) and HPV 18 (33.9%), but was higher against incident anal infections (45.1%

Table 1 Characteristics of included studies

Study	Location	Design	Study period	Inclusion criteria	Exclusion criteria	Age at enrolment (median (range))	Duration of follow-up (median)	Vaccine/ comparator	Study sponsorship	Conflict of interest	Number of participants	Outcomes
Giuliano et al. 2011 [32]	Multicentre (18 countries)	RCT	2004–ongoing (enrolled until 08/2008)	Heterosexual men 16–23 years of age who had 1–5 life-time sex partners or MSM 16–26 years. of age who had 1–5 male or female life-time sex partners	Men with clinically detectable anogenital warts or genital lesions or history of such findings	20 years. (16–26 years)	2.9 yrs	Gardasil/placebo	Merck; National Institutes of Health	Merck, GlaxoSmith-Kline (GSK), Qiagen, AstraZeneca	Vaccinated: 2032; placebo: 2033	PIN grade 2 or 3; penile, perineal or perianal cancer; persistent anogenital infection; incident anogenital infection; genital condyloma acuminatum; severe adverse events
Palefsky et al. 2011 [33]	Multicentre (7 countries)	RCT (substudy of Giuliano et al. 2011 [32])	2004– ongoing (enrolled until 08/2008)	MSM 16–26 years. of age who had 1–5 male or female life-time sex partners and were engaged in insertive or receptive anal intercourse with another man in the past year	Men with history or presence of clinically detectable anogenital warts or genital lesions or intra-anal lesion on anoscopy consistent with AIN or condyloma	22 years. (16–26 years)	2.2 years	Gardasil/placebo	Merck; National Institutes of Health	Merck, GSK, Qiagen, Pharmajet, Aura Biosciences, Roche, GenProbe	Vaccinated: 301; placebo: 301	AIN grade 2; AIN grade 3; anal cancer; persistent anal infection; incident anal infection; anal condyloma accuminatum; severe adverse events
Swedish et al. 2012 [25]	USA	Cohort study	2007–2011	MSM 18 years. or older with a history of biopsy-proven and treated high-grade AIN	Less than three vaccine doses; high-grade AIN at study start	40.4 years. (20.3–72.3 years)	Vaccinated: 489 days; unvaccinated: 722 days	Gardasil/ unvaccinated	NR	Merck, Qiagen, Asha	Vaccinated: 88; unvaccin-ated: 114	Recurrent high-grade AIN (AIN grade 2 or 3)
Coskuner et al. 2014 [31]	Turkey	RCT (not placebo-controlled)	2009–2013	Men with new onset genital warts living in the same area for at least 1 year	Previous treatment for preexisting warts; medical disorders that needed chronic treatment; immune suppression (incl. HIV)	Mean: 34 years. (+/− 7.6)	4 years after first dose	Gardasil/ unvaccinated	NR	NR	Vaccinated: 91; unvaccinated: 80	Recurrent condyloma acuminatum
Swedish and Goldstone 2014 [34]	USA	Cohort study	2007–2013 (vaccinated until 2010)	Self-identified MSM, HIV-negative, no prior history of anal condyloma or previously treated anal condyloma but recurrence-free for at least 12 months prior to study entry	Men with anal or penile condyloma at study start	42.2 years. (range 26.1–76 years)	Up to 4 years. (vacc: median 880 days; unvacc: median 1039 days)	Gardasil/ unvaccinated	None	Merck	Vaccinated: 116; unvaccinated: 197	Anal condyloma

Table 1 Characteristics of included studies *(Continued)*

Study	Location	Design	Study period	Inclusion criteria	Exclusion criteria	Age at enrolment (median (range))	Duration of follow-up (median)	Vaccine/ comparator	Study sponsorship	Conflict of interest	Number of participants	Outcomes
Kahn et al. 2015 [24]	USA (5 centres)	Cross-sectional study	2011–2012	Youth with behaviorally acquired HIV	Serious psychiatric illness, intoxication with alcohol or drugs	21.5 years. (range 12–24 years)	NA	Gardasil/ unvaccinated	National Institutes of Health	Merck	Vaccinated: 23; unvaccinated: 48	(Incident) oral infection (HPV 16 and/ or HPV 18)
NCT01461096 [26, 47]	USA, Brazil	RCT	2012–2015 (stopped due to futility)	HIV-infected adults	History of cancer, history of AIN, previous HPV vaccination, anticoagulation, allergies, drug/ alcohol dependence, serious illness, immunomodulatory treatment; hepatitis B/C treatment	47 years (intraquartile range: 41–53)	2.1 years. (median)	Gardasil/placebo	National Institute of Allergy and Infectious Diseases	Gilead, Bristol Meyer Squibb, GSK	Vaccinated: 236; placebo: 236	Persisting oral infection[a]

AIN anal intraepithelial neoplasia, *MSM* men who have sex with men, *NA* not applicable, *NR* not reported, *PIN* penile, perineal or perianal neoplasia, *RCT* randomized controlled trial

[a]Data on other outcomes available for combined analysis of males and females

Table 2 Overview of outcomes reported in the studies

Study	Incident oral infection	Persisting oral infection	Incident anogenital infection		Persisting anogenital infection		Condyloma acuminatum		AIN grade 2	AIN grade 3 or carcinoma	PIN grade 2	PIN grade 3 or carcinoma	Severe adverse events
			Anogenital	Anal	Anogenital	Anal	Genital	Anal					
Randomized trials													
Giuliano et al. 2011 [32]			x		x		x				x[a]	x[a]	x
Palefsky et al. 2011 [33]				x		x		x	x	x			x[b]
Coskuner et al. 2014 [31]							x						
NCT01461096 [26]		x											
Non-randomized studies													
Swedish et al. 2012 [25]									x[c]	x[c]			
Swedish and Goldstone 2014 [34]								x					
Kahn et al. 2015 [24]	x												

[a]PIN 2 and PIN 3 analysed together
[b]Subgroup of Giuliano et al. [32]; therefore, all severe adverse events already reported there
[c]defined as "high-grade anal intraepithelial neoplasia", comprising AIN 2 and AIN 3 (Goldstone, personal communication). Applying a conservative approach, results are reported here as AIN 2

Table 3 Risk of bias in randomized controlled trials

Study	Random sequence generation	Allocation concealment	Blinding of participants and personnel	Blinding of outcome assessment	Incomplete outcome data	Selective reporting	Other bias
Giuliano et al. 2011 [32]	+	+	+	+	+	+	+
Palefsky et al. 2011 [33]	+	+	+	+	+	+	+
Coskuner et al. 2014 [31][a]	+	+	–	–	+	+	+
NCT01461096 [26]	+	+	+	+	+	+	+

+ low risk of bias, – high risk of bias
[a]Controls received no vaccination, yet blinding was not possible

against HPV 16; 49.5% against HPV 18), although the 95% CIs were overlapping. Vaccine efficacy estimates for preventing persisting (defined as ≥ 6 months) anogenital and anal infections were higher than those for incident infections (46.9–73.6%). Two of the RCTs also reported vaccine efficacy in participants who were seronegative and PCR-negative for the respectively studied HPV types at enrolment. As shown in Table 6, vaccine efficacy estimates were higher for all outcomes compared with those in the analyses performed irrespective of HPV status, ranging from 41.1% (incident anogenital infection with HPV 16) to 100% (incident and persisting anal infection with HPV 18), with wide confidence intervals.

Incident oral infections with HR HPV types were investigated in only one study, which used a non-randomized design. Here, a vaccine effectiveness of 91% was observed; however, the 95% CI was very wide and no confounder-adjusted estimate was reported. For persistent oral HPV infections, an efficacy of 88% was reported in one RCT (Table 5).

Estimates of vaccine efficacy and effectiveness against anogenital lesions are shown in Tables 7 and 8. Efficacy against genital condyloma acuminatum was investigated in two of the RCTs: one RCT reported a vaccine efficacy of 67.2%, whereas the other one did not show a protective effect (– 26%). However, the latter RCT included only participants with a history of condyloma and had a high risk of bias. Efficacy and effectiveness against anal condyloma was assessed in one RCT and in one non-randomized study. Both studies reported very similar results (57.2% and 55%, respectively), but their confidence intervals were wide. Vaccine efficacy against AIN grade 2 was reported to be 61.9% in one RCT, while vaccine effectiveness was slightly lower in a non-randomized study (50%). AIN grade 3 was investigated in only one RCT, which reported a non-significant efficacy of 46.8%. Likewise, PIN grade 2 or 3 was reported in one RCT, but the number of cases was too small in both the vaccinated ($n = 3$) and placebo groups ($n = 2$) to generate a meaningful estimate of vaccine efficacy. Since no cases of anal cancer or penile/perineal/perianal cancer were observed in the included studies, efficacy or effectiveness against these outcomes could not be calculated. Table 8 shows the respective estimates for those RCT participants who were HPV-negative at study entry [32, 33]. In this subgroup, estimates of vaccine efficacy for the prevention of anogenital lesions were higher than among individuals irrespective of HPV status, but the case numbers were small and did not lead to meaningful efficacy estimates against AIN (grade 2: efficacy 75.8%, 11 cases; grade 3: efficacy 63.7%, 8 cases), PIN (grade 2 or 3: efficacy 100%, 1 case) or cancer (no cases).

Severe adverse events following immunization were reported in two of the included RCTs [32, 33]. Because the smaller [33] was composed of a subgroup of participants from the larger RCT [32], all severe adverse events reported in the former had already been included and reported in the latter. Therefore, only data from the larger RCT were considered here. During the entire study period, 8 adverse events were observed in the vaccinated group (2020 participants) and 11 events occurred in the placebo group (2029 participants). This finding corresponds to a risk ratio of 0.73 (95% CI 0.25–1.99) and a risk difference of – 0.2 (95% CI –0.7 to 0.3). According to the trial investigators, none of these adverse events were judged to be vaccine-related.

Table 4 Risk of bias in non-randomized studies

Study	Confounding	Selection bias	Classification of intervention	Deviation from intervention	Missing data	Outcome measurement	Selection of reported results	Overall risk of bias
Swedish et al. 2012 [25][a]	+	–	++	++	–	++	++	–
Swedish and Goldstone 2014 [34][a]	+	–	++	++	–	++	++	–
Kahn et al. [24][b]	– –	–	–	++	–	++	++	– –

++ low risk of bias, + moderate risk of bias, – serious risk of bias, – –- critical risk of bias
[a]Unclear selection into study; differences in follow-up time between groups; loss-to-follow up
[b]Only unadjusted data available; unclear selection into study; loss-to-follow up; possible misclassification of intervention

Table 5 Efficacy or effectiveness of vaccination against human papillomavirus in males: infections in participants irrespective of their HPV status at enrolment

Study	Design	No. of events/no. of participants		Unadjusted estimate (95% CI)	Confounder-adjusted estimate (95% CI)	VE (95% CI)
		Vaccine	Control			
Incident anogenital infection						
HPV 16						
Giuliano et al. 2011 [32][a]	RCT	189/4070.0 pyrs	259/4014.2 pyrs	NR	NA	28.0% (12.9–40.7%)
HPV 18						
Giuliano et al. 2011 [32][a]	RCT	89/4205.4 pyrs	133/4151.5 pyrs	NR	NA	33.9% (13.0–50.1%)
Persisting anogenital infection						
HPV 16						
Giuliano et al. 2011 [32][a]	RCT	71/4199.5 pyrs	131/4112.7 pyrs	NR	NA	46.9% (28.6–60.8%)
HPV 18						
Giuliano et al. 2011 [32][a]	RCT	25/4267.0 pyrs	56/4210.1 pyrs	NR	NA	56.0% (28.8–73.7%)
Incident anal infection						
HPV 16						
Palefsky et al. 2011 [33][a]	RCT	40/615.7 pyrs	71/599.9 pyrs	NR	NA	45.1% (18.0–63.7%)
HPV 18						
Palefsky et al. 2011 [33][a]	RCT	20/651.2 pyrs	39/641.3 pyrs	NR	NA	49.5% (11.3–72.1%)
Persisting anal infection						
HPV 16						
Palefsky et al. 2011 [33][a]	RCT	24/636.6 pyrs	51/622.3 pyrs	NR	NA	54% (23.9–72.9%)
HPV 18						
Palefsky et al. 2011 [33][a]	RCT	7/668.4 pyrs	26/656.3 pyrs	NR	NA	73.6% (37.5–90.3%)
Incident oral infection						
HPV 16 and/or HPV 18						
Kahn et al. 2015 [24][a]	Cross-sectional study	0/23	9/48	NR	NR	91% (−59–99.5%)
Persisting oral infection						
NCT01461096 [26][b]	RCT	1/236	8/236	0.12 (0.02–0.98)[c]	NR	88% (2–98%)

NA not applicable, *NR* not reported, *pyrs* person-years, *VE* vaccine efficacy or effectiveness
[a]VE as reported in the primary study
[b]VE calculated from unadjusted estimate
[c]Hazard ratio (95% CI)

Evidence quality according to GRADE was judged "high" only for the outcome condyloma acuminatum. For five of the included outcomes (incident anogenital infection, persisting oral infection, persisting anogenital infection, AIN grade 2 and severe adverse events following immunization), evidence quality was downgraded to "moderate" due to serious imprecision (wide 95% CIs). The outcome AIN grade 3 was judged to provide "low" quality evidence due to very serious imprecision (very wide 95% CI). Incident oral infection was assessed to provide "very low" quality evidence due to the non-randomized study design and serious imprecision. The evidence quality for PIN grade 2/3 was judged to be "very low" due to serious indirectness (the outcome in the trial comprised penile, perineal and perianal neoplasia) and very serious imprecision (see the GRADE evidence profile in Additional file 3 for details).

Discussion

This systematic review of randomized and non-randomized studies evaluated the efficacy, effectiveness and safety of HPV vaccination in males. When vaccinating individuals irrespective of their HPV status, vaccination is moderately effective against genital HPV infection and high-grade anal intraepithelial lesions. Higher vaccine efficacy was observed in those participants who were naïve for the respective HPV types assessed in the individual studies. No meaningful estimate of vaccine efficacy could be calculated for high-grade penile intraepithelial lesions, and no data were available regarding vaccine efficacy or effectiveness against anal, penile or head and neck squamous cell cancer. Due to their imprecision of estimates, the GRADE evidence quality was moderate to low for the majority of outcomes.

To our knowledge, this is the first systematic review on the efficacy, effectiveness and safety of HPV

Table 6 Efficacy or effectiveness of vaccination against human papillomavirus in males: infections in participants who were seronegative and PCR-negative at enrolment

Study	Design	No. of events/no. of participants		Unadjusted estimate (95% CI)	Confounder-adjusted estimate (95% CI)	VE (95% CI)
		Vaccine	Control			
Incident anogenital infection						
HPV 16						
Giuliano et al. (2011) [32][a]	RCT	62/2337.7 pyrs	103/2287.8 pyrs	NR	NA	41.1% (18.5–57.7%)
HPV 18						
Giuliano et al. (2011) [32][a]	RCT	25/2441.3 pyrs	66/2440.6 pyrs	NR	NA	62.1% (39.2–77.1%)
Persisting anogenital infection						
HPV 16						
Giuliano et al. (2011) [32][a]	RCT	9/2382.4 pyrs	41/2312.9 pyrs	NR	NA	78.7% (55.5–90.9%)
HPV 18						
Giuliano et al. (2011) [32][a]	RCT	1/2461.9 pyrs	25/2453.5 pyrs	NR	NA	96% (75.6–99.9%)
Incident anal infection						
HPV 16						
Palefsky et al. (2011) [33][a]	RCT	6/326 pyrs	25/322.8 pyrs	NR	NA	76.2% (40.7–92%)
HPV 18						
Palefsky et al. (2011) [33][a]	RCT	0/346.3 pyrs	16/375.1 pyrs	NR	NA	100% (71.9–100%)
Persisting anal infection						
HPV 16						
Palefsky et al. (2011) [33][a]	RCT	1/331.5 pyrs	16/329.9 pyrs	NR	NA	93.8% (60.0–99.9%)
HPV 18						
Palefsky et al. (2011) [33][a]	RCT	0/346.3 pyrs	10/376.2 pyrs	NR	NA	100% (51.5–100%)

NA not applicable, *NR* not reported, *pyrs* person-years, *VE* vaccine efficacy or effectiveness
[a]VE as reported in the primary study

vaccination in males. In contrast, at least seven systematic reviews of studies assessing the effects of HPV vaccination in females have been published demonstrating high efficacy and effectiveness of HPV vaccination against infection and dysplasia, particularly in HPV-naïve study participants [35–41]. Considerable differences exist in the body of evidence between male and female HPV vaccination regarding the primary study base. While our current systematic review comprised data from about 5000 participants, randomized trials on HPV vaccination in females included more than 46,000 participants in total [41]. Beyond study size, considerable differences exist between HPV trials in males and females regarding the validity of outcomes and evidence quality. For precancerous lesions of the cervix (cervical intraepithelial neoplasia), robust data from the above-mentioned systematic reviews show that vaccination against HPV prevents high-grade lesions over a time period of more than 6 years. As shown in our systematic review, the evidence base is weaker regarding precancerous lesions in males, particularly for penile lesions. Furthermore, evidence on efficacy, effectiveness and safety of HPV vaccination in males is currently restricted to a period of 4 years after vaccination. Similar to findings from HPV vaccination in females, a considerably higher vaccine efficacy has been found in men who were seronegative and PCR-negative at study entry [41].

Our systematic review has several strengths. It was conducted based on a comprehensive and published review protocol, and internationally accepted tools for the assessment of risk of bias were applied. We performed an outcome-specific assessment of the available data and assessed the quality of the body of evidence for each outcome using the GRADE methodology. We performed a comprehensive review by including different study designs and populations (MSM as well as heterosexual men). The limitations of this review mainly arise from the limitations of the included primary studies. The two major RCTs included here were designed to evaluate compound endpoints comprising malignant and benign lesions. Consequently, neither of these studies had enough power to detect premalignant or malignant lesions as defined in our protocol. Furthermore, the existing non-randomized studies have a high risk of bias. A limitation of our systematic review stems from the restriction of the outcomes to clinical endpoints. For example, we did not

Table 7 Efficacy or effectiveness of vaccination against human papillomavirus in males: anogenital lesions in participants irrespective of their HPV status at enrolment (corresponding to intention-to-treat analysis in RCTs)

Study	Design	No. of events/no. of participants		Unadjusted estimate (95% CI)	Confounder-adjusted estimate (95% CI)	VE (95% CI)
		Vaccine	Control			
Condylomata acuminata						
Genital						
Giuliano et al. 2011 [32][a]	RCT	24/4635.4 pyrs	72/4558.8 pyrs	NR	NA	67.2% (47.3–80.3%)
Coskuner et al. 2014 [31][b]	RCT	45/91	35/80	1.26 (0.69–2.30)	NR	−26% (− 130 to 31%)
Anal						
Palefsky et al. 2011 [33][a]	RCT	13/651.3 pyrs	31/664.2 pyrs	NR	NA	57.2% (15.9–79.5%)
Swedish & Goldstone 2014 [34][d, e]	Cohort study	10/269.3 pyrs	37/604.3 pyrs	0.49 (0.24–0.98)	0.45 (0.22–0.92)	55% (8–78%)
Anal intraepithelial neoplasia grade 2						
Palefsky et al. 2011 [33][a]	RCT	11/668 pyrs	29/671.5 pyrs	NR	NA	61.9% (21.4–82.8%)
Swedish et al. 2012 [25][c, e]	Cohort study	12/117.6 pyrs	35/222.8 pyrs	0.52 (0.27–1.0)	0.50 (0.26–0.98)	50% (2–74%)
Anal intraepithelial neoplasia grade 3						
Palefsky et al. 2011 [33][a]	RCT	10/665.9 pyrs	19/672.8 pyrs	NR	NA	46.8% (−20 to 77.9%)
Anal cancer						
Palefsky et al. 2011 [33]	RCT	0/678.4 pyrs	0/694.8 pyrs	NR	NA	–
Penile, perineal or perianal neoplasia grade 2 or 3						
Giuliano et al. 2011 [32][a]	RCT	3/4663.1 pyrs	2/4628.6 pyrs	NR	NA	−48.9% (− 1682.6 to 82.9%)
Penile, perineal or perianal cancer						
Giuliano et al. 2011 [32]	RCT	0/4670.6 pyrs	0/4630.5 pyrs	NR	NA	–

[a]VE as reported in the primary study
[b]Recurrent lesions
[c]All participants with a history of high-grade AIN (data for 24-month follow-up period); VE calculated from unadjusted estimate
[d]103/313 participants with recurrent lesions
[e]VE calculated from confounder-adjusted estimate
NA not applicable, *NR* not reported, *pyrs* person-years, *VE* vaccine efficacy or effectiveness

search for immunogenicity data and can therefore not draw conclusions from studies that used them as surrogate markers for protection. A further limitation of our systematic review may arise from the decision to focus on all lesions rather than on type-specific lesions. This approach might lead to an underestimation of the efficacy and effectiveness of the vaccine. However, our approach was chosen since it is likely to consider clinical impact and the patient perspective more appropriately than an approach that focusses on type-specific lesions. For future updates of this review, several strategies might be tested in order to improve the specificity of the search results. One could, for instance, use the "NOT" operator to exclude certain types of articles that do not contain data (such as comments or editorials) from the search. Furthermore, it appears possible to focus the search on certain study types (such as RCTs, cohort studies, case-control studies) that are relevant for the PICO (Patient, problem or population; Intervention; Comparison, control or comparator; Outcome) question.When HPV status prior to vaccination is not considered, efficacy of HPV vaccination in males is moderate, particularly regarding incident infections, and the corresponding confidence intervals are wide. In cases where only HPV-naïve participants are vaccinated, the vaccine efficacy estimates are higher, but the corresponding confidence intervals are still wide. These wide confidence intervals might be due at least partly to variations in sampling techniques, because the sampling in men has not been as standardized as it is in women [42], and the main results on genital and anal infections came from multicentre studies [32, 33]. However, the estimates reported here might be conservative, given that data from females suggest that the efficacy of HPV vaccination increases with longer follow-up due to the effect on incident but not prevalent infections [43].

Evidence on efficacy and effectiveness of HPV vaccination in males is particularly scarce regarding oral infections; only one RCT with a small number of events and one small observational study with a high risk of bias reported data on this outcome. However, supporting evidence regarding vaccine effectiveness against oral HPV infections comes from two sources. Using data from the

Table 8 Efficacy or effectiveness of vaccination against human papillomavirus in males: anogenital lesions in participants who were seronegative and PCR-negative at enrolment

Study	Design	No. of events/no. of participants		Unadjusted estimate (95% CI)	Confounder-adjusted estimate (95% CI)	VE (95% CI)
		Vaccine	Control			
Condylomata acuminata						
Genital						
Giuliano et al. (2011) [32][a]	RCT	3/2830.9 pyrs	28/2813.9 pyrs	NR	NA	89.4% (65.5–97.9%)
Anal						
Palefsky et al. (2011) [33][a]	RCT	0/386.8 pyrs	6/418.2 pyrs	NR	NA	100% (8.2–100%)
Anal intraepithelial neoplasia grade 2						
Palefsky et al. (2011) [33][a]	RCT	2/384.5 pyrs	9/418.6 pyrs	NR	NA	75.8% (−16.9 to 97.5%)
Anal intraepithelial neoplasia grade 3						
Palefsky et al. (2011) [33][a]	RCT	2/385.4 pyrs	6/419.7 pyrs	NR	NA	63.7 (−103 to 96.4%)
Anal cancer						
Palefsky et al. (2011) [33]	RCT	0/386.8 pyrs	0/421.1 pyrs	NR	NA	–
Penile, perineal or perianal neoplasia grade 2 or 3						
Giuliano et al. (2011) [32][a]	RCT	0/2833.3 pyrs	1/2824.7 pyrs	NR	NA	100% (− 3788.2 to 100%)
Penile, perineal or perianal cancer						
Giuliano et al. (2011) [32]	RCT	0/2833.3 pyrs	0/2826.2 pyrs	NR	NA	–

NA not applicable, *NR* not reported, *pyrs* person-years, *VE* vaccine efficacy or effectiveness
[a]VE as reported in the primary study

Costa Rica Trial, Herrero et al. performed a post hoc analysis of the impact of female vaccination with the bivalent vaccine on the prevalence of oral infections 4 years after the first vaccine dose. In this study, vaccine effectiveness against oral HPV 16/18 infections was 93.3% (95% CI 63–100%) [44]. Furthermore, vaccinating adult men with the quadrivalent vaccine was shown to induce neutralizing antibodies in the oral cavity in 65.5% (HPV 18) to 93.2% (HPV 16) of participants [45].

In a number of countries, HPV vaccination of girls and women has already been implemented for nearly a decade. If vaccination coverage in girls and women is high enough, indirect (herd) protection of heterosexual men can be achieved [46]. In the presence of herd protection effects, it is not possible to study the effectiveness of HPV vaccination of men in isolation. Therefore, we examined whether the results of the studies included in our systematic review could have been affected by HPV vaccination programs targeting girls and women in the respective study countries. In fact, five of the included studies were conducted in settings where HPV vaccination of females was implemented [24–26, 31, 34]. However, two of those studies included MSM who do not benefit from such herd protection effects [25, 34]. For the remaining three studies one cannot exclude the possibility that herd protection effects might have slightly influenced the respective study estimates.

Conclusions

This systematic review shows that the currently available evidence on the efficacy/effectiveness and safety of HPV vaccination in males is limited due to the small number of relevant studies, imprecise estimates and lack of data for some critical outcomes. Vaccine effectiveness drops markedly in individuals who are already infected with the corresponding HPV type. This supports a recommendation for early vaccination of boys with the goal of establishing optimal vaccine-induced protection before the onset of sexual activity. This might not be a realistic option when implementing a program that intends to target only high-risk males such as MSM or HIV-positives. On the other hand, even if the relative vaccine efficacy in such a population with a high prevalence of infection is low, the impact of the vaccine in MSM may be much higher because of the high absolute risk in this group. While the limitations of the evidence base point to a need for further studies in men, it is important to bear in mind that the results of population-based studies might be difficult to interpret in the presence of the above-mentioned herd protection effects. Furthermore, mathematical modelling studies will still be needed to assess the effects of adding males to existing HPV vaccination programs in more detail. The two available studies with vaccination of HPV-naïve males showed high efficacy for reducing dysplasia.

Additional files

Additional file 1: Search strategy. (DOCX 13 kb)
Additional file 2: List of excluded studies. (DOCX 34 kb)
Additional file 3: GRADE evidence profile. (DOCX 24 kb)

Acknowledgements

The authors would like to thank Dr. Jessica Kahn, Cincinnati, Dr. Stephen Goldstone, New York, and Dr. Timothy Wilkin, New York, for kindly providing additional data and information on their studies. Dr. Martin Terhardt, Berlin, and Dr. Fred Zepp, Mainz, are members of the HPV working group of the German Standing Committee on Vaccination (STIKO) and are kindly acknowledged for comments on the review protocol. We thank Katie Oakley, Ph.D., from Edanz Group (www.edanzediting.com/ac) for editing a draft of this manuscript.

Authors' contributions

All authors were involved in the conception and design of the study and interpretation of the results. MWP and TH performed the search and were responsible for data extraction, data analysis and drafting of the article. OW supervised the extraction and analysis process. SJK and MABVDS critically revised the paper regarding analysis and interpretation of the data. All authors revised the manuscript critically and contributed to the final draft. MWP and TH are guarantors. All authors read and approved the final manuscript.

Competing interests

The authors declare that they have no competing interests.

Author details

[1]Robert Koch Institute, Immunization Unit, Seestrasse 10, 13353 Berlin, Germany. [2]Department of Sport and Health Sciences, Technical University Munich, Chair of Epidemiology, Munich, Germany. [3]Institute of Tropical Medicine, Antwerp, Belgium.

References

1. Ciccarese G, Herzum A, Rebora A, Drago F. Prevalence of genital, oral, and anal HPV infection among STI patients in Italy. J Med Virol. 2017;89:1121–4.
2. Giuliano AR, Harris R, Sedjo RL, Baldwin S, Roe D, Papenfuss MR, Abrahamsen M, Inserra P, Olvera S, Hatch K. Incidence, prevalence, and clearance of type-specific human papillomavirus infections: the Young Women's Health Study. J Infect Dis. 2002;186(4):462–9.
3. Stanley M. Pathology and epidemiology of HPV infection in females. Gynecol Oncol. 2010;117(2 Suppl):S5–10.
4. Jaisamrarn U, Castellsague X, Garland SM, Naud P, Palmroth J, Del Rosario-Raymundo MR, Wheeler CM, Salmeron J, Chow SN, Apter D, et al. Natural history of progression of HPV infection to cervical lesion or clearance: analysis of the control arm of the large, randomised PATRICIA study. PLoS One. 2013;8(11):e79260.
5. Koshiol J, Lindsay L, Pimenta JM, Poole C, Jenkins D, Smith JS. Persistent human papillomavirus infection and cervical neoplasia: a systematic review and meta-analysis. Am J Epidemiol. 2008;168(2):123–37.
6. Schiffman M, Castle PE, Jeronimo J, Rodriguez AC, Wacholder S. Human papillomavirus and cervical cancer. Lancet. 2007;370(9590):890–907.
7. Cogliano V, Baan R, Straif K, Grosse Y, Secretan B, El Ghissassi F, WHO International Agency for Research on Cancer. Carcinogenicity of human papillomaviruses. Lancet Oncol. 2005;6(4):204.
8. de Sanjose S, Alemany L, Ordi J, Tous S, Alejo M, Bigby SM, Joura EA, Maldonado P, Laco J, Bravo IG, et al. Worldwide human papillomavirus genotype attribution in over 2000 cases of intraepithelial and invasive lesions of the vulva. Eur J Cancer. 2013;49(16):3450–61.
9. Walboomers JM, Jacobs MV, Manos MM, Bosch FX, Kummer JA, Shah KV, Snijders PJ, Peto J, Meijer CJ, Munoz N. Human papillomavirus is a necessary cause of invasive cervical cancer worldwide. J Pathol. 1999; 189(1):12–9.
10. Alemany L, Cubilla A, Halec G, Kasamatsu E, Quiros B, Masferrer E, Tous S, Lloveras B, Hernandez-Suarez G, Lonsdale R, et al. Role of human papillomavirus in penile carcinomas worldwide. Eur Urol. 2016;69(5): 953–61.
11. Steinau M, Unger ER, Hernandez BY, Goodman MT, Copeland G, Hopenhayn C, Cozen W, Saber MS, Huang Y, Peters ES, et al. Human papillomavirus prevalence in invasive anal cancers in the United States before vaccine introduction. J Low Genit Tract Dis. 2013;17(4):397–403.
12. WHO-IARC: List of classifications by cancer sites with sufficient or limited evidence in humans, Volumes 1 to 121. 2018. https://monographs.iarc.fr/ENG/Classification/Table4.pdf.
13. Castellsague X, Alemany L, Quer M, Halec G, Quiros B, Tous S, Clavero O, Alos L, Biegner T, Szafarowski T, et al. HPV involvement in head and neck cancers: comprehensive assessment of biomarkers in 3680 patients. J Natl Cancer Inst. 2016;108(6):djv403.
14. Gargano JW, Unger ER, Liu G, Steinau M, Meites E, Dunne E, Markowitz LE. Prevalence of genital human papillomavirus in males, United States, 2013-2014. J Infect Dis. 2017;215(7):1070–9.
15. van Aar F, Mooij SH, van der Sande MA, Speksnijder AG, Stolte IG, Meijer CJ, Verhagen DW, King AJ, de Vries HJ, Schim van der Loeff MF. Anal and penile high-risk human papillomavirus prevalence in HIV-negative and HIV-infected MSM. AIDS. 2013;27(18):2921–31.
16. Kreimer AR, Bhatia RK, Messeguer AL, Gonzalez P, Herrero R, Giuliano AR. Oral human papillomavirus in healthy individuals: a systematic review of the literature. Sex Transm Dis. 2010;37(6):386–91.
17. Buttmann-Schweiger N, Delere Y, Klug SJ, Kraywinkel K. Cancer incidence in Germany attributable to human papillomavirus in 2013. BMC Cancer. 2017; 17(1):682.
18. Kraut AA, Schink T, Schulze-Rath R, Mikolajczyk RT, Garbe E. Incidence of anogenital warts in Germany: a population-based cohort study. BMC Infect Dis. 2010;10:360.
19. Joura EA, Pils S. Vaccines against human papillomavirus infections: protection against cancer, genital warts or both? Clin Microbiol Infect. 2016;22(Suppl 5):S125–7.
20. Serrano B, Alemany L, Ruiz PA, Tous S, Lima MA, Bruni L, Jain A, Clifford GM, Qiao YL, Weiss T, et al. Potential impact of a 9-valent HPV vaccine in HPV-related cervical disease in 4 emerging countries (Brazil, Mexico, India and China). Cancer Epidemiol. 2014;38(6):748–56.
21. Schmeler KM, Sturgis EM. Expanding the benefits of HPV vaccination to boys and men. Lancet. 2016;387(10030):1798–9.
22. Guardian T. Give HPV vaccine to boys to protect against cancers, experts say. 2016. https://www.theguardian.com/science/2016/jul/09/vaccine-boys-cancer-men-hpv.
23. Moher D, Liberati A, Tetzlaff J, Altman DG, Group P. Preferred reporting items for systematic reviews and meta-analyses: the PRISMA statement. Ann Intern Med. 2009;151(4):264–9. W264
24. Kahn JA, Rudy BJ, Xu J, Secord EA, Kapogiannis BG, Thornton S, Gillison ML. Behavioral, immunologic, and virologic correlates of oral human papillomavirus infection in HIV-infected youth. Sex Transm Dis. 2015; 42(5):246–52.
25. Swedish KA, Factor SH, Goldstone SE. Prevention of recurrent high-grade anal neoplasia with quadrivalent human papillomavirus vaccination of men who have sex with men: a nonconcurrent cohort study. Clin Infect Dis. 2012;54(7):891–8.
26. NCT01461096: Evaluating the effectiveness of the quadrivalent human papillomavirus (HPV) vaccine at preventing anal HPV infection in HIV-infected men and women. www.clinicaltrials.gov. Accessed 18 Apr 2017.
27. Higgins JP, Altman DG, Gotzsche PC, Juni P, Moher D, Oxman AD, Savovic J, Schulz KF, Weeks L, Sterne JA, et al. The Cochrane Collaboration's tool for assessing risk of bias in randomised trials. BMJ. 2011;343:d5928.
28. Sterne JA, Hernan MA, Reeves BC, Savovic J, Berkman ND, Viswanathan M, Henry D, Altman DG, Ansari MT, Boutron I, et al. ROBINS-I: a tool for assessing risk of bias in non-randomised studies of interventions. BMJ. 2016;355:i4919.
29. Guyatt GH, Oxman AD, Schunemann HJ, Tugwell P, Knottnerus A. GRADE guidelines: a new series of articles in the Journal of Clinical Epidemiology. J Clin Epidemiol. 2011;64(4):380–2.
30. Guyatt GH, Oxman AD, Vist GE, Kunz R, Falck-Ytter Y, Alonso-Coello P, Schunemann HJ, Group GW. GRADE: an emerging consensus on rating quality of evidence and strength of recommendations. BMJ. 2008;336(7650):924–6.
31. Coskuner ER, Ozkan TA, Karakose A, Dillioglugil O, Cevik I. Impact of the quadrivalent HPV vaccine on disease recurrence in men exposed to HPV infection: a randomized study. J Sex Med. 2014;11(11):2785–91.

32. Giuliano AR, Palefsky JM, Goldstone S, Moreira ED Jr, Penny ME, Aranda C, Vardas E, Moi H, Jessen H, Hillman R, et al. Efficacy of quadrivalent HPV vaccine against HPV infection and disease in males. N Engl J Med. 2011; 364(5):401–11.
33. Palefsky JM, Giuliano AR, Goldstone S, Moreira ED Jr, Aranda C, Jessen H, Hillman R, Ferris D, Coutlee F, Stoler MH, et al. HPV vaccine against anal HPV infection and anal intraepithelial neoplasia. N Engl J Med. 2011;365(17): 1576–85.
34. Swedish KA, Goldstone SE. Prevention of anal condyloma with quadrivalent human papillomavirus vaccination of older men who have sex with men. PLoS One. 2014;9(4):e93393.
35. Rambout L, Hopkins L, Hutton B, Fergusson D. Prophylactic vaccination against human papillomavirus infection and disease in women: a systematic review of randomized controlled trials. CMAJ. 2007;177(5):469–79.
36. La Torre G, de Waure C, Chiaradia G, Mannocci A, Ricciardi W. HPV vaccine efficacy in preventing persistent cervical HPV infection: a systematic review and meta-analysis. Vaccine. 2007;25(50):8352–8.
37. Medeiros LR, Rosa DD, da Rosa MI, Bozzetti MC, Zanini RR. Efficacy of human papillomavirus vaccines: a systematic quantitative review. Int J Gynecol Cancer. 2009;19(7):1166–76.
38. Lu B, Kumar A, Castellsague X, Giuliano AR. Efficacy and safety of prophylactic vaccines against cervical HPV infection and diseases among women: a systematic review & meta-analysis. BMC Infect Dis. 2011;11:13.
39. Rey-Ares L, Ciapponi A, Pichon-Riviere A. Efficacy and safety of human papilloma virus vaccine in cervical cancer prevention: systematic review and meta-analysis. Arch Argent Pediatr. 2012;110(6):483–9.
40. Malagon T, Drolet M, Boily MC, Franco EL, Jit M, Brisson J, Brisson M. Cross-protective efficacy of two human papillomavirus vaccines: a systematic review and meta-analysis. Lancet Infect Dis. 2012;12(10):781–9.
41. Delere Y, Wichmann O, Klug SJ, van der Sande M, Terhardt M, Zepp F, Harder T. The efficacy and duration of vaccine protection against human papillomavirus: a systematic review and meta-analysis. Dtsch Arztebl Int. 2014;111(35–36):584–91.
42. Capra G, Nyitray AG, Lu B, Perino A, Marci R, Schillaci R, Matranga D, Firenze A, Caleca M, Bellavia C, et al. Analysis of persistence of human papillomavirus infection in men evaluated by sampling multiple genital sites. Eur Rev Med Pharmacol Sci. 2015;19(21):4153–63.
43. Lehtinen M, Lagheden C, Luostarinen T, Eriksson T, Apter D, Harjula K, Kuortti M, Natunen K, Palmroth J, Petaja T, et al. Ten-year follow-up of human papillomavirus vaccine efficacy against the most stringent cervical neoplasia end-point-registry-based follow-up of three cohorts from randomized trials. BMJ Open. 2017;7(8):e015867.
44. Herrero R, Quint W, Hildesheim A, Gonzalez P, Struijk L, Katki HA, Porras C, Schiffman M, Rodriguez AC, Solomon D, et al. Reduced prevalence of oral human papillomavirus (HPV) 4 years after bivalent HPV vaccination in a randomized clinical trial in Costa Rica. PLoS One. 2013;8(7):e68329.
45. Pinto LA, Kemp TJ, Torres BN, Isaacs-Soriano K, Ingles D, Abrahamsen M, Pan Y, Lazcano-Ponce E, Salmeron J, Giuliano AR. Quadrivalent human papillomavirus (HPV) vaccine induces HPV-specific antibodies in the oral cavity: results from the mid-adult male vaccine trial. J Infect Dis. 2016;214(8):1276–83.
46. Drolet M, Benard E, Boily MC, Ali H, Baandrup L, Bauer H, Beddows S, Brisson J, Brotherton JM, Cummings T, et al. Population-level impact and herd effects following human papillomavirus vaccination programmes: a systematic review and meta-analysis. Lancet Infect Dis. 2015;15(5):565–80.
47. Wilkin TJ, Chen H, Cespedes M, Paczuski P, Godfrey C, Chiao E, Luque A, Webster-Cyriaque JY, Bastow B, Cranston R, et al. ACTG A5298: a phase 3 trial of the quadrivalent HPV vaccine in older HIV+ adults. In: Conference on Retroviruses and Opportunistic Infections. Session O-14. Boston: Conference on Retroviruses and Opportunistic Infections Foundation; 2016.

16

Perinatal health outcomes and care among asylum seekers and refugees

Nicola Heslehurst*, Heather Brown, Augustina Pemu, Hayley Coleman and Judith Rankin

Abstract

Background: Global migration is at an all-time high with implications for perinatal health. Migrant women, especially asylum seekers and refugees, represent a particularly vulnerable group. Understanding the impact on the perinatal health of women and offspring is an important prerequisite to improving care and outcomes. The aim of this systematic review was to summarise the current evidence base on perinatal health outcomes and care among women with asylum seeker or refugee status.

Methods: Twelve electronic database, reference list and citation searches (1 January 2007–July 2017) were carried out between June and July 2017. Quantitative and qualitative systematic reviews, published in the English language, were included if they reported perinatal health outcomes or care and clearly stated that they included asylum seekers or refugees. Screening for eligibility, data extraction, quality appraisal and evidence synthesis were carried out in duplicate. The results were summarised narratively.

Results: Among 3415 records screened, 29 systematic reviews met the inclusion criteria. Only one exclusively focussed on asylum seekers; the remaining reviews grouped asylum seekers and refugees with wider migrant populations. Perinatal outcomes were predominantly worse among migrant women, particularly mental health, maternal mortality, preterm birth and congenital anomalies. Access and use of care was obstructed by structural, organisational, social, personal and cultural barriers. Migrant women's experiences of care included negative communication, discrimination, poor relationships with health professionals, cultural clashes and negative experiences of clinical intervention. Additional data for asylum seekers and refugees demonstrated complex obstetric issues, sexual assault, offspring mortality, unwanted pregnancy, poverty, social isolation and experiences of racism, prejudice and stereotyping within perinatal healthcare.

Conclusions: This review identified adverse pregnancy outcomes among asylum seeker and refugee women, representing a double burden of inequality for one of the most globally vulnerable groups of women. Improvements in the provision of perinatal healthcare could reduce inequalities in adverse outcomes and improve women's experiences of care. Strategies to overcome barriers to accessing care require immediate attention. The systematic review evidence base is limited by combining heterogeneous migrant, asylum seeker and refugee populations, inconsistent use of definitions and limited data on some perinatal outcomes and risk factors. Future research needs to overcome these limitations to improve data quality and address inequalities.

Systematic registration: Systematic review registration number: PROSPERO CRD42017073315.

Keywords: Migrant health, Asylum seeker, Refugee, Perinatal health, Pregnancy, Access to care, Systematic review

* Correspondence: Nicola.heslehurst@ncl.ac.uk
Institute of Health & Society, Newcastle University, Baddiley-Clark Building, Richardson Road, Newcastle upon Tyne NE2 4AX, UK

Background

Gobalisation, poor living conditions, war and conflict are major factors contributing to forced migration. In 2016, the number of people displaced by conflict and persecution worldwide was estimated to be 65.6 million. Of these 2.8 million were estimated to be asylum seekers and 22.5 million refugees, which the United Nations High Commissioner for Refugees (UNHCR) suggests is the highest level ever recorded [1]. Among this population, 49% of refugees were women, a similar proportion as reported annually since 2003 [1]. The impact of migration on health is far-reaching, making migrant populations particularly vulnerable, fuelling health inequalities and resulting in serious implications for global health.

Research on migrant populations is challenged by the diverse terminology and definitions used. For the purposes of this systematic review, we use the following UNHCR definitions [1]:

- *Asylum seekers* are individuals who have sought international protection and whose claims for refugee status have not yet been determined, irrespective of when they may have been lodged. An *asylum seeker* has applied for asylum on the grounds of persecution in their home country relating to their race, religion, nationality, political belief or membership of a particular social group. This population remains classified as asylum seeker for as long as the application is pending.
- *Refugees* have been forced to leave their country in order to escape war, persecution or natural disaster. The 1951 Convention relating to the Status of Refugees describes a refugee as "a person who owing to a well-founded fear of being persecuted for reasons of race, religion, nationality, membership of a particular social group, or political opinion, is outside the country of this nationality and is unable to or, owing to such fear, is unwilling to avail himself of the protection of that country". A *refugee* is an asylum seeker whose application has been successful.
- *Migrants* include those who move, either temporarily or permanently from one place, area or country of residence to another for reasons such as work or seeking a better life (i.e. economic migrants), for family reasons or to study. People also migrate to flee conflict or persecution, which is where the definition converges with the terms refugee and asylum seeker.

Timely access to perinatal healthcare is an effective method to optimise pregnancy outcomes and the lifelong health of women and their offspring. Late access to maternity care can result in adverse perinatal outcomes. Vulnerable pregnant women, including women with asylum seeker and refugee status, face barriers to accessing healthcare [2] including maternity care [3]. A recent report of vulnerable women in social crisis in Europe included pregnant women seeking or having been refused asylum and found that 65% had no access to antenatal care, 42% accessed care after 12 weeks of pregnancy and two thirds were classified as being 'at risk' requiring urgent or semi-urgent care [4]. This disparity in access to, and use of, perinatal healthcare can lead to significant health inequalities. Failure to effectively reach and provide optimal perinatal care for women with asylum seeker and refugee status will result in failure to reduce health inequalities for this vulnerable group of women and their babies.

There has been a recent escalation of systematic reviews investigating different aspects of perinatal health in women who have migrated, which includes asylum seeker and refugee populations. For example, multiple systematic reviews were published in 2016 and 2017 on topics including perinatal health outcomes [5–8] and experiences of antenatal care [9–11]. However, there is a lack of published systematic reviews that explicitly address pregnancy among asylum seeker and refugee populations, and there is a tendency to group all migrant populations together in syntheses. Given this, we have chosen to undertake a systematic review of systematic reviews to assess the research gaps and provide direction to future research specifically relating to women with asylum seeker and refugee status. The aim of this systematic review was to provide an overview of the existing evidence base drawn from systematic reviews that have examined perinatal healthcare and outcomes among women with asylum seeker or refugee status.

Methods

The Joanna Briggs Institute (JBI) methodology for umbrella reviews was used to guide this systematic review of systematic reviews [12]. The Preferred Reporting Items for Systematic Reviews and Meta-Analyses (PRISMA) reporting guidelines and checklist (Additional file 1) have been used to report each stage of the systematic review methods and findings [13]. The protocol for this systematic review has been registered in the PROSPERO database (CRD42017073315).

Identification of studies

Electronic bibliographic databases were searched using PICOS criteria: Population (asylum seekers or refugees); Intervention (pregnancy); Comparator (non-asylum seekers or refugees for quantitative reviews only, no comparator group required for qualitative reviews); Outcome (defined as selected perinatal health outcomes or care); Study design (quantitative, qualitative or mixed methods systematic reviews). A search strategy for database-specific search terms and subject headings was developed with the support of an information scientist for the databases MEDLINE, Embase, Scopus, Cumulative Index to Nursing and Allied Health Literature, JBI database, PROSPERO, Cochrane Database of Systematic Reviews, Google Scholar, Science Direct, Web of Science, PubMed and ProQuest (see Additional file 2 for database search terms).

Database searches were supplemented with hand searching of the reference lists of all included systematic reviews to identify any further relevant reviews. All included systematic reviews were also subjected to citation searches using all citations produced by Google Scholar. Any systematic reviews identified by the supplementary searches which met the inclusion criteria were also subject to reference list and citation searches until no further eligible reviews were identified. The detailed search strategy was carried out between June and July 2017 and restricted to systematic reviews published within the past 10 years (since January 2007) as per the JBI recommendation [12]. No restrictions were placed on country or region of study or on low-, middle- or high-income status of the host countries. Inclusion criteria were as follows:

- Systematic reviews with a quantitative, qualitative or mixed methods evidence synthesis
- Published in the English language
- Included any perinatal health outcomes (e.g. postnatal depression, low birth weight) or perinatal care (e.g. access to maternity services, experiences of care) during the preconception, antenatal and postnatal periods
- Clearly stated that women with asylum seeker or refugee status were populations within the included studies. This included reviews of migrant women where asylum seekers and refugees were part of the included population

Reviews were excluded if they were:

- Scoping reviews which aimed to identify the extent and nature of the evidence base without a formal evidence synthesis
- Published abstracts without full texts and protocols of systematic reviews. We searched for any subsequent full text publications of these works
- Reviews that focussed on refugees living in camps

Two authors independently screened titles, abstracts and full texts for inclusion in the review. Disagreements regarding eligibility for inclusion were resolved through discussion; a third independent reviewer was available where no agreement could be reached (not required). References were managed and recorded in EndNote version X7. The flow of reviews through each stage of the searches and screening and the reasons for exclusions are presented using a PRISMA diagram (Fig. 1). Data extraction and quality assessments were carried out in duplicate for all included systematic reviews. Independent data extractions and quality assessments were combined by two authors and agreed with recourse to a third reviewer if no agreement could be reached (not required).

Quality assessment

The JBI Critical Appraisal Checklist for Systematic Reviews and Research Syntheses [12] was used for quality assessment. The checklist comprises 11 questions relating to methodological rigor, transparency of reporting and appropriateness of conclusions and recommendations, with options of 'yes' if the review clearly meets the checklist criteria and 'no', 'unclear' or 'not applicable' if the review does not clearly meet the criteria (see Additional file 3). The reviews were awarded a score of 1 for each checklist criterion clearly met, with a maximum possible score of 11. The reviews were considered to be of high quality if they scored 8–11, moderate quality for scores of 4–7 and low quality for scores of 0–3. No reviews were excluded based on quality score. The percentage of included reviews meeting the criteria was calculated for each of the 11 checklist questions.

Data extraction

The JBI umbrella review data extraction form was adapted to meet the needs of this mixed methods systematic review of systematic reviews (see Additional file 3). The following data were extracted for each included systematic review: aim, objectives and focus of the review including review type, aims, objectives, type/definition of included population, inclusion and exclusion criteria and outcomes included in search strategy; search details including date range of the search, search strategy and restrictions to the search; appraisal rating including whether the quality appraisal was reported, what method/tool was used and summary of quality of included studies; key results including the number of included studies, publication date range, sample size, host countries, description of included population, summary results and conclusions for the overall population and also detailed results and conclusions explicitly relating to asylum seekers and refugee populations.

We implemented a process of systematically extracting data which was directly relevant to women with asylum seeker and refugee status for all of the systematic reviews which combined data from multiple populations in their syntheses (e.g. migrants including asylum seekers and refugees). This involved two stages of searching for relevant data in the tables, figures and

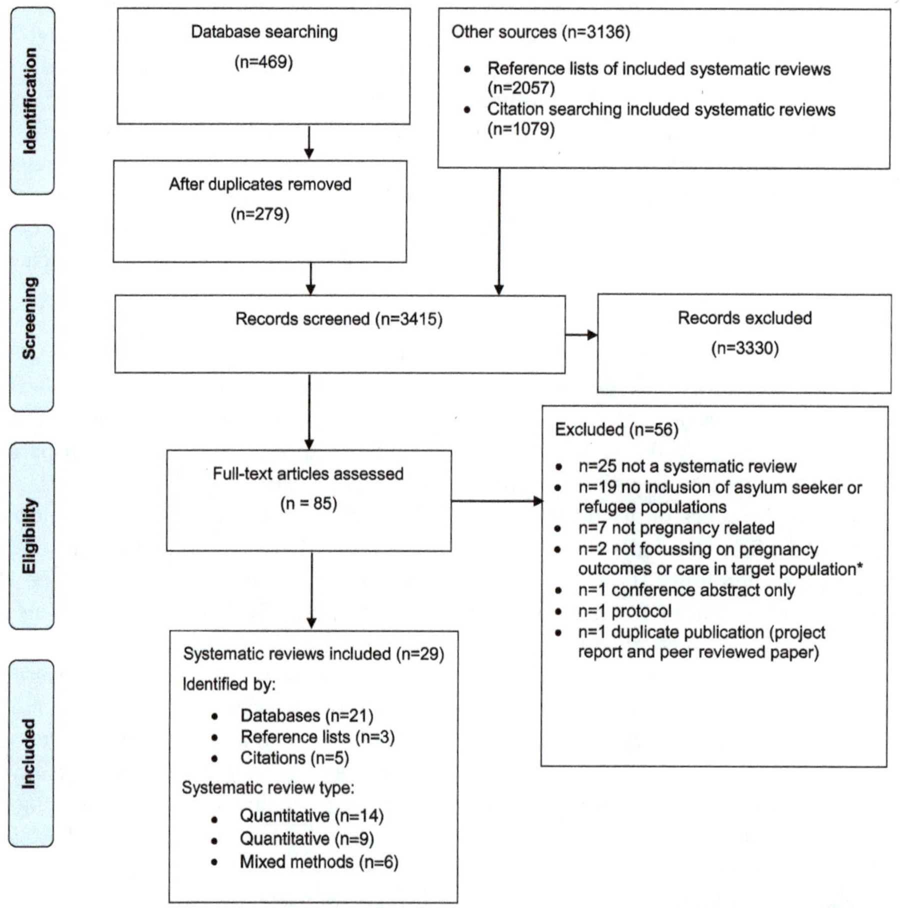

* one review explored interventions to reduce adverse pregnancy outcomes in socially disadvantaged and vulnerable women, including asylum seekers and refugees, but did not specifically relate to pregnancy outcomes or care in this population; one was a review of methodological issues in studies on reproductive health of migrants to Western countries.

Fig. 1 PRISMA flowchart of searches, screening, and inclusion and exclusion of studies

narrative in the results, discussion and conclusions sections of the included systematic reviews. First, the relevant sections of the reviews were searched for data that the authors had explicitly described as being relevant to asylum seeker or refugee populations, and these data were extracted. The second stage involved identifying whether any of the included studies in the systematic reviews were exclusively among asylum seeker or refugee populations. When studies which were exclusively among these populations were identified, data were extracted for any results which had cited these studies as part of the evidence base which informed that specific result. This second stage was only carried out if we were confident that the population of the included study were exclusively asylum seekers and/or refugees; for example, data were not extracted for studies which included migrants and refugees, as we could not be confident that the data that had informed the result originated from women who were migrants or refugees.

Evidence synthesis

Evidence synthesis in systematic reviews of systematic reviews should provide a summary of existing research syntheses in tabular format with a more detailed narrative description of the systematic review characteristics and relevant quantitative and qualitative results [12]. The results have therefore been summarised in tables to describe the characteristics of the included systematic reviews, results for overall populations included in the systematic reviews and also results explicitly relevant to women with asylum seeker and refugee status. Tables are supplemented with a narrative discussion of the included systematic reviews grouped by the review themes of perinatal health outcomes and perinatal healthcare access and experiences for women who are migrants and for asylum seekers and refugees. Each theme has several data-driven sub-themes. As per reporting recommendations [12], any overlap in original research studies in the included systematic reviews is reported in the results table and narrative for the asylum seeker- and refugee-specific data. Evidence synthesis was carried out in duplicate. The first stage of synthesis was performed by JR, HB and AP to group the systematic review data into the review themes and to provide a descriptive summary of the topic-specific data. The second stage involved NH validating the review themes and performing a detailed synthesis of sub-theme data reported in the systematic reviews.

Results

Included systematic reviews

A total of 3415 records were identified by searches, of which 29 were systematic reviews which met the inclusion criteria (Fig. 1). Twenty-one systematic reviews were identified through the database searches, three from reference list and five from citation searching. Fourteen of the included reviews were quantitative, eight of which included a meta-analysis, nine were qualitative and six involved mixed methods (Table 1). The systematic reviews were published between 2009 and 2017; the fewest reviews were published in 2011 and 2012 ($n = 1$ per year), and most were published in 2017 ($n = 7$ published between January and the date of the searches in July and August). The number of studies included in the reviews ranged from eight to 133, and the publication years of the included studies were from 1956 to 2016. Only one systematic review identified was exclusively focussed on women with asylum seeker status [14]. The populations included in the remaining systematic reviews were migrant populations including women with asylum seeker and/or refugee status ($n = 27$) and marginalised women ($n = 1$), which included those with asylum seeker and/or refugee status along with women who had experienced domestic violence, minority ethnic groups, travelling communities, women of low income, those with substance abuse problems, teenagers and women who were homeless. There was no consistent definition in the use of terminology to describe women, and many reviews did not adequately define their populations. We use the terms asylum seeker, refugee and migrant as previously defined, and the term 'women in the host country' to collectively describe comparison groups that have been reported in the systematic reviews which include a range of definitions including non-migrant, native-born, etc. (see Additional file 4 for a detailed description of the study populations).

Quality of evidence

The quality scores ranged from six to 11 ($n = 10$ categorised as moderate quality, $n = 19$ high quality, Additional file 5). Of the 11 questions in the JBI Critical Appraisal Checklist for Systematic Reviews and Research Syntheses, all of the included reviews scored 'yes' in four questions (is the review question clearly stated; were the methods used to combine the studies appropriate; were recommendations for policy and/or practice supported by the reported data; and were the specific directives for new research appropriate?), while only six reviews scored 'yes' for the question 'was the likelihood of publication bias assessed?' (see Additional file 5). Additionally, only 14 reviews used methods to minimise data extraction errors (e.g. duplicate data extraction), 18 carried out quality appraisal and only 21 used adequate sources and resources to search for studies (e.g. database searches supplemented with additional search methods) as recommended in guidelines for systematic reviews of observational studies [15].

Perinatal health outcomes amongst women who are migrants (including asylum seekers and refugees)

Nineteen systematic reviews reported perinatal health outcomes including perinatal mental health, mortality (maternal and offspring), mode of delivery, birth weight, preterm birth, congenital anomalies and additional morbidities. The results are summarised in Table 2, and a narrative summary is presented for each outcome.

Perinatal mental health

Mental health, which included postnatal depression, antenatal depression, anxiety and post-traumatic stress disorder, was the most frequently reported outcome and was included in eleven systematic reviews; six were quantitative [5, 6, 16–19], three were qualitative [8, 20, 21] and two mixed methods [22, 23]. The reviews reported prevalence and risk factors for mental health disorders.

Prevalence of perinatal mental health disorders All systematic reviews reporting prevalence data concluded that perinatal mental health disorders were more frequent in migrant women than in women from the host countries [5, 6, 16–19, 22]. Postnatal depression was the most frequently reported perinatal mental health outcome in the systematic reviews. Prevalence of postnatal depression amongst migrant women was reported as 11.2–60% [16], < 1–59% [5], 24–42% [18], 2.9–52% [22] and 20% (95% confidence interval (CI) 17–23%) [17]. Prevalence of antenatal depression amongst migrant women was reported to be 12–45% [5], and prevalence of any depressive disorder was 31% (95% CI 23.2–40%) [6]. There were also significantly increased associations with mental health disorders amongst migrant women compared with women from the host countries. Anderson et al. [5] reported that anxiety was increased in migrant women with non-English-speaking backgrounds, and post-traumatic stress disorder was 15% compared with 0% amongst non-migrant women. Nilaweera et al. [22] reported that odds ratios (ORs) for postnatal depression in their included studies ranged

Table 1 Summary of included systematic reviews

Author, year	Aim of the systematic review	Methods	Population included	Search strategy (years, databases and supplementary searches)
Alhasanat and Fry-McComish 2015 [16]	To identify the prevalence and risk factors for postnatal depression amongst immigrant women in industrialised countries and compare it with prevalence and risk factors amongst Arab women in their home countries	Quantitative with narrative	Migrant including asylum seekers and/or refugees	1990–2013 Four databases searched No supplementary searches
Anderson et al. 2017 [5]	To evaluate the prevalence and risk factors of mental disorders in the perinatal period amongst migrant women	Quantitative with meta-analysis	Migrant including asylum seekers and/or refugees	From inception of database to Oct 2015 Six databases searched No supplementary searches
Aubrey et al. 2017 [9]	To broadly explore and synthesise current evidence surrounding women's preference for female physicians in obstetrics and gynaecology	Mixed methods	Migrant including asylum seekers and/or refugees	From inception of database Five databases searched Supplementary searches: reference list, citations
Balaam et al. 2013 [30]	To explore migrant women's perceptions of their needs and experiences related to pregnancy and childbirth	Qualitative	Migrant including asylum seekers and/or refugees	1996–2010 Seven databases searched No supplementary searches
Bollini et al. 2009 [26]	To explore whether differences in pregnancy outcomes observed across receiving countries in Europe are associated with varying degrees of implementation of integration policies	Quantitative with meta-analysis	Migrant including asylum seekers and/or refugees	1966–2004 One database searched No supplementary searches
Collins et al. 2011 [18]	To review the rates and risk factors associated with postnatal depression in refugees, asylum seekers and migrant women	Quantitative with narrative	Migrant including asylum seekers and/or refugees	1990–2009 Ten databases searched No supplementary searches
De Maio 2010 [19]	This review investigates the health of immigrants to Canada by critically examining differences in health status between immigrants and the native-born population and by tracing how the health of immigrants changes after settling in the country	Quantitative with narrative	Migrant including asylum seekers and/or refugees	1990–2010 Four databases searched Supplementary searches: reference list
Downe et al. 2009 [31]	To locate and synthesise qualitative accounts of barriers to antenatal care as reported by high-risk, marginalised, pregnant women in the UK	Qualitative	Marginalised populations including asylum seekers and/or refugees	1980–2007 Seven databases searched Supplementary searches: reference list
Falah-Hassani et al. 2015 [17]	Estimate the prevalence of postpartum depressive systems in immigrant women. Compare this prevalence to non-immigrant women. Determine risk factors for postpartum depressive systems in immigrant women	Quantitative with meta-analysis	Migrant including asylum seekers and/or refugees	1950–2014 Seven databases searched Supplementary searches: reference list
Fellmeth et al. 2017 [6]	Summarise and synthesise evidence on prevalence, associated factors and effectiveness of interventions for any perinatal mental disorder in migrant women	Quantitative with meta-analysis	Migrant including asylum seekers and/or refugees	No specific start date until January 2015 Eight databases searched Supplementary searches: hand searching journals, reference list
Gagnon et al. 2009 [25]	To assess whether migrants in western industrialised countries have consistently poorer perinatal health than receiving-country women	Quantitative with meta-analysis	Migrant including asylum seekers and/or refugees	1995–2008 Four databases searched Supplementary searches: reference list, citations
Gissler et al. 2009 [27]	To determine if migrants in western industrialised countries have consistently higher risks of stillbirth, neonatal mortality or infant mortality; if there are migrant sub-groups at potentially higher risk; and what might be the explanations for any risk differences found	Quantitative with meta-analysis	Migrant including asylum seekers and/or refugees	1995–2006 Four databases searched Supplementary searches: reference list
Hadgkiss and Renzaho 2014 [14]	To document physical health problems that asylum seekers experience on settlement in the community and to assess their utilisation of healthcare services and barriers to care, in an international context	Mixed methods	Asylum seekers	2002–2012 Four databases searched Supplementary searches: reference list

Table 1 Summary of included systematic reviews *(Continued)*

Author, year	Aim of the systematic review	Methods	Population included	Search strategy (years, databases and supplementary searches)
Heaman et al. 2013 [35]	Do migrant women in Western industrialised countries have higher odds of inadequate prenatal care compared to receiving-country women, and what factors are associated with inadequate prenatal care amongst migrant women in Western industrialised countries?	Quantitative with narrative	Migrant including asylum seekers and/or refugees	1995–2010 Three databases searched Supplementary searches: reference list
Higginbottom et al. 2015 [36]	What are the experiences of immigrant women in Canada in accessing and navigating maternity and healthcare services from conception to 6 months postpartum?	Mixed methods	Migrant including asylum seekers and/or refugees	Inception to 2013 Ten databases searched Supplementary searches: hand searches within journal websites
Higginbottom et al. 2014 [32]	To synthesise qualitative literature to describe how immigrant women experience maternity services in Canada	Qualitative	Migrant including asylum seekers and/or refugees	Inception to March 2012 Eight databases searched Supplementary searches: contacting authors, reference list
Higginbottom et al. 2012 [23]	To identify and descriptively synthesise current empirical literature on immigrants' experiences of maternity healthcare services in Canada, to outline practice implications and/or to offer recommendations for future research	Mixed methods	Migrant including asylum seekers and/or refugees	2000–2010 Five databases searched Supplementary searches: reference list, citations
Mengesha et al. 2016 [10]	To identify studies that focussed on the views and experiences of culturally and linguistically diverse women in accessing sexual and reproductive health care in Australia	Mixed methods	Migrant including asylum seekers and/or refugees	April 1990–May 2015 Seven databases searched Supplementary searches: reference list
Merry et al. 2013 [28]	To determine if migrants in Western industrialised countries consistently have different rates of caesarean than receiving-country-born women and to identify the reasons that explain these differences	Quantitative with meta-analysis	Migrant including asylum seekers and/or refugees	Inception to Jan 2012 Eleven databases searched Supplementary searches: reference list
Merry et al. 2016 [7]	To provide a synthesis to what is known regarding caesarean births amongst migrants living in high-income countries	Quantitative with narrative	Migrant including asylum seekers and/or refugees	2012–2015 Thirteen databases searched No supplementary searches
Nilaweera et al. 2014 [22]	To summarise the available evidence about the prevalence, nature and determinants of postpartum mental health problems amongst women born in South Asian countries who had migrated to high-income countries, and identify barriers and enablers to seeking health care for these difficulties	Mixed methods	Migrant including asylum seekers and/or refugees	Inception to February 2013 Four databases searched No supplementary searches
Pedersen et al. 2014 [24]	A meta-analysis of all published observational studies from Western European countries comparing the risk of maternal mortality between the receiving-country women and a defined migrant population	Quantitative with meta-analysis	Migrant including asylum seekers and/or refugees	1970–2013 Four databases searched Supplementary searches: reference list
Schmied et al. 2017 [8]	To report the findings of a meta-ethnographic study of the experiences, meanings and ways of 'dealing with' symptoms or a diagnosis of postnatal depression amongst migrant women living in high-income countries with a view to informing culturally appropriate health service design and delivery	Qualitative	Migrant including asylum seekers and/or refugees	1999–2016 Five databases searched Supplementary searches: reference list, citations
Small et al. 2014 [33]	There were two review questions: 1. What do immigrant and non-immigrant women want from their maternity care? 2. How do immigrant and non-immigrant women's experiences and ratings of care compare, both within and across included countries?	Qualitative	Migrant including asylum seekers and/or refugees	1989–2011 Five databases searched No supplementary searches
Tobin et al. 2017 [20]	To synthesise qualitative research on refugee and immigrant women's experiences of postpartum depression to gain insight into the unique needs of this group of women	Qualitative	Migrant including asylum seekers and/or refugees	2004–2014 Five databases searched Supplementary searches: reference list

Table 1 Summary of included systematic reviews *(Continued)*

Author, year	Aim of the systematic review	Methods	Population included	Search strategy (years, databases and supplementary searches)
Villalonga-Olives et al. 2016 [29]	To discuss differences between the USA and Europe regarding reproductive health outcomes of immigrants and to elucidate why these differences occur	Quantitative with narrative	Migrant including asylum seekers and/or refugees	Dates not clear Two databases searched No supplementary searches
Wikberg and Bondas 2010 [34]	To explore and describe a patient perspective in research on intercultural caring in maternity care	Qualitative	Migrant including asylum seekers and/or refugees	1995–2009 Twelve databases searched Supplementary searches: reference list
Winn et al. 2017 [11]	To understand the experiences of pregnant immigrant women accessing perinatal care in North America	Qualitative	Migrant including asylum seekers and/or refugees	Inception to July 2016 Five databases searched Supplementary searches: reference list
Wittkowski et al. 2017 [21]	To appraise and assimilate qualitative findings of postnatal depression in immigrant mothers	Qualitative	Migrant including asylum seekers and/or refugees	1990–2014 Six databases searched Supplementary searches: reference list

from 1.8–2.5 for migrant populations. Meta-analyses performed by Anderson et al. [5] and Falah Hassani et al. [17] also showed a higher odds of suffering from postnatal depression for migrant women compared to those from the host country (OR 1.56 (95% CI 1.31–1.86) and an adjusted OR (aOR) of 2.17 (95% CI 1.54–3.06 respectively)). When Falah Hassani et al. [17] adjusted for publication bias, the association decreased but remained significant (OR 1.67, 95% CI 1.12–2.30). Anderson et al. [5] also reported that associations differed for both antenatal and postnatal depression when stratifying the meta-analyses by country of study: antenatal depression USA (OR 0.71, 95% CI 0.51–0.99) and Canada (OR 1.86, 95% CI 1.32–2.62); postnatal depression USA (OR 0.87, 95% CI 0.59–1.28), Australia (OR 1.115, 95% CI 0.96–1.38) and Canada (OR 1.98, 95% CI 1.57–2.49).

Risk factors for the development of perinatal mental health disorders Seven systematic reviews reported quantitative and qualitative evidence of factors associated with increased risk, or having a protective effect on perinatal mental health disorders [5, 6, 16–19, 22]. There were similarities between the systematic reviews, and results are reported under the themes of stress and support, adjustments to host country, pregnancy care and infant feeding, health status and history and socio-demographics.

- *Stress and support.* This was the most frequently and consistently reported risk factor for the development of mental health disorders amongst migrant women. Examples provided included emotional stress, a history of violence or abuse, having witnessed or experienced stressful life events and their premigration experience such as having migrated for political reasons or problems with the police or army in their home country [5, 6, 16–18]. Lack of social support and lack of family support were also reported to be important risk factors. There was a consistent pattern of low social support increasing the risk and good social support being protective against perinatal mental health disorders [5, 6, 17–19, 22]. Having no relatives or friends, a lack of emotional support from their spouse, being unmarried, having no partner, having migrated for marriage, marital adjustment problems and a lack of domestic decision-making power in relation to the child were all risk factors for perinatal mental health disorders amongst migrant women, whereas having a close relationship with their partner was reported to be protective [5, 6, 16, 17, 22].
- *Adjustment to host country.* The most commonly reported risk factors for perinatal mental health disorders were difficulties with the host country language [5, 6, 17, 19, 22] and being unfamiliar with local life [19]. Anderson et al. [5] reported inconsistent evidence in their included studies relating to the length of time resident in the host country, whereas other reviews reported that shorter duration of residence was a risk factor for perinatal mental health disorders [6, 17]. Fellmeth et al. [6] reported that adherence to traditional postpartum practices was protective against postnatal depression in migrant populations.
- *Pregnancy care and infant feeding.* Experience of perinatal healthcare including operative caesarean and instrumental delivery and poor satisfaction with support [6, 18] and also infant feeding experience including formula feeding and feeding problems [6, 17, 22] were risk factors for the development of perinatal mental health disorders reported by four systematic reviews [7, 17, 18, 22].

Table 2 Summary of results for all included study populations (migrant including asylum seeker and refugee women)

Author, year	Number of studies	Publication date range	Sample size[1]	Topic area of results	Summary of author conclusions
Alhasanat and Fry-McComish 2015 [16]	26	1998–2013 (date range of migrant studies)	9089	Perinatal health outcomes (mental health); access, utilisation and experience of perinatal healthcare	Some similarities in the risk factors for postnatal depression amongst migrant women and Arabic women in their country of birth: lack of social support, stressful life events, lack of emotional support from the partner, history of antenatal depression and marital dissatisfaction. Immigration stress and lack of access to health care services were found amongst migrant women. Lack of social support was more predominant in studies on migrant women
Anderson et al. 2017 [5]	53	1986–2015	119,076 (for the 52 studies which reported sample size)	Perinatal health outcomes (mental health)	Depression is common amongst pregnant and postpartum migrant women, although there is no evidence for an overall increased risk of depression amongst migrant women when compared to non-migrant women
Aubrey et al. 2017 [9]	54	2002–2016 (data for only 10 included studies reported)	Not reported	Access to and utilisation of perinatal healthcare	A key finding of both qualitative and quantitative studies was a preference for female providers because of religious reasons and comfort with a female provider. Provider competence was prioritised over gender
Balaam et al. 2013 [30]	16	2000–2010	393 (excluding men and health professionals)	Access, utilisation and experience of perinatal healthcare	Migrant women's vulnerable situation when pregnant and giving birth must be improved
Bollini et al. 2009 [26]	65	1966–2004	18,322,978 women including 1,632,401 migrant women	Perinatal health outcomes (neonatal intensive care, offspring mortality, preterm birth, low birth weight, congenital anomalies, postpartum haemorrhage)	Risk ratios for low birth weight, preterm delivery, perinatal mortality and congenital anomalies between immigrant and native-born women were more similar in countries with strong integration policies. There was a migrant penalty for those European countries with weak integration policies
Collins et al. 2011 [18]	8	1998–2008	4574 (for the 7 studies which reported sample size)	Perinatal health outcomes (mental health)	Nearly all studies found rates of probable postnatal depression were higher in migrant women than native-born women
De Maio 2010 [19]	51	2006–2010	Not reported	Perinatal health outcomes (mental health, low birth weight, preterm birth, placental dysfunction); access to and utilisation of perinatal healthcare	Mental health issues are less prevalent amongst migrants than the Canadian-born population. However, this advantage diminishes as length of residence in Canada increases. Living in areas with a high density of migrants may help immigrants to retain this advantage
Downe et al. 2009 [31]	8	1998–2006	569 (excluding men and health professionals)	Perinatal healthcare access and experiences	A non-threatening, non-judgemental antenatal service run by culturally sensitive staff may increase access to antenatal care for marginalised women. Multiagency initiatives aimed at raising awareness of, and providing access to, antenatal care may also increase uptake
Falah-Hassani et al. 2015 [17]	24	1995–2013	63,926	Perinatal health outcomes (mental health)	The prevalence of depressive symptoms is 1.5–2.0 higher in migrant women compared with non-migrant women. Migrant women were more likely to develop depressive symptoms if they had shorter residency in the destination country, lower levels of social support, poorer marital adjustment and insufficient household income

Table 2 Summary of results for all included study populations (migrant including asylum seeker and refugee women) *(Continued)*

Author, year	Number of studies	Publication date range	Sample size[1]	Topic area of results	Summary of author conclusions
Fellmeth et al. 2017 [6]	45	1986–2013	19,439 (including 7985 migrant)	Perinatal health outcomes (mental health)	Higher prevalence of postnatal depression in migrant women. Local language ability, length of residency and adhering to traditional birth practices were protective factors
Gagnon et al. 2009 [25]	133	1968–2005	20,152,134	Perinatal health outcomes (maternal and offspring mortality, mode of delivery, low birth weight, preterm birth, maternal health, congenital anomalies, maternal and infant infections, infant morbidities); access to and utilisation of perinatal healthcare	Of 9 outcome categories, 2 appear to be better amongst migrant women (health-promoting behaviour and birth weight), 6 appear worse (infection, congenital anomalies and infant morbidity, prenatal care, maternal health, feto-infant mortality and mode of delivery) and 1 did not differ in most studies (preterm birth)
Gissler et al. 2009 [27]	34	1980–2002	Not reported	Perinatal health outcomes (offspring mortality)	In the European studies, all non-refugee migrants had higher crude stillbirth rates, perinatal mortality rates, neonatal mortality rates and infant mortality rates
Hadgkiss and Renzaho 2014 [14]	32	2002–2012	Not reported	Perinatal health outcomes (offspring mortality, mode of delivery, birth weight, preterm birth, complex obstetric issues)	This study highlights the health inequities faced by asylum seekers residing in the communities of host countries, internationally
Heaman et al. 2013 [35]	29	1996–2007	24,362,611	Access to and utilisation of perinatal healthcare	Migrant women were more likely to receive inadequate prenatal care than receiving-country women. Inadequate prenatal care varied widely by country of birth, indicating that this is not a homogeneous group
Higginbottom, et al. 2012 [23]	30	Not reported	Not reported	Perinatal health outcomes (mental health); access to and utilisation of perinatal healthcare	New migrants are ten times more likely than Canadian-born women to experience personal barriers when accessing healthcare. Language is a particular problem, and current interpreting services are either underutilised or unavailable
Higginbottom et al. 2014 [32]	22	1990–2011	510 (for 21 studies that reported data, excluding 2 studies exclusively with health professionals)	Access, utilisation and experience of perinatal healthcare	Experiences in maternity healthcare for migrant women are deeply embedded in the social position of the women which influences the availability of social supports, communication possibilities with health professionals and socio-economic status, all of which relate to the organisational environment. Furthermore, migrants and healthcare staff have different beliefs and values which form their perceptions on how maternity healthcare should be provided. Cultural knowledge, beliefs, religious and traditional customs were most relevant for migrants, whereas healthcare staff emphasise biomedical needs
Higginbottom et al. 2015 [36]	24	1995–2011	10,339	Access, utilisation and experience of perinatal healthcare	Analysis of these 24 studies led to the development of five interrelated themes: utilisation of prenatal care and educational classes; adequacy of perinatal care; barriers to maternity care in the pre- and postnatal periods; isolation and limited social support; and outcomes related to the access to and the use of services

Table 2 Summary of results for all included study populations (migrant including asylum seeker and refugee women) *(Continued)*

Author, year	Number of studies	Publication date range	Sample size[1]	Topic area of results	Summary of author conclusions
Mengesha et al. 2016 [10]	22	1998–2014	1943	Access, utilisation and experience of perinatal healthcare	Although culturally and linguistically diverse women in Australia have the opportunity to obtain necessary health services, they experience numerous barriers in accessing and utilising sexual and reproductive healthcare
Merry et al. 2013 [28]	76	1956–2010	1,029,454	Perinatal health outcomes (mode of delivery)	Sub-Saharan African, Somali and South Asian migrants consistently have higher caesarean rates while Eastern-European and Vietnamese migrants have lower overall caesarean rates compared to receiving-country-born women. North African, West Asian and Latin American migrant women have higher emergency caesarean rates
Merry et al. 2016 [7]	33	2012–2015	Not reported	Perinatal health outcomes (mode of delivery)	Women from sub-Saharan Africa and South Asia consistently show overall higher rates of caesarean compared with non-migrant women. Women from Latin America, North Africa and Middle East consistently show higher rates of emergency caesarean. Higher rates are more common with emergency caesareans than with planned caesareans
Nilaweera et al. 2014 [22]	15	2003–2012	102,427 (quantitative studies), 84 (qualitative studies)	Perinatal health outcomes (mental health); access, utilisation and experience of perinatal healthcare	The prevalence of clinically significant symptoms of postnatal depression and diagnosed postnatal depression for South Asian women who migrate to high-income countries is between 5 and 20%. This rate is likely to be under-reported because of a lack of specific sub-group analyses and studies on South Asian countries. Barriers to accessing healthcare need to be addressed including proficiency in English language, unfamiliarity with local services and lack of attention to mental health by healthcare providers
Pedersen et al. 2014 [24]	13	1969–2008	42,290,654 women including 6,102,663 migrant	Perinatal health outcomes (maternal mortality)	Migrant women in Western European countries have a doubled risk of dying during or after pregnancy when compared with indigenous-born women. A higher risk of death from direct causes suggests sub-standard obstetric care may be responsible for the majority of the excess deaths amongst migrant women
Schmied et al. 2017 [8]	15	1999–2015	256	Perinatal health outcomes (mental health); access, utilisation and experience of perinatal healthcare	Women who are migrants report higher levels of depressive symptoms, which can severely compromise mother-baby interaction and subsequent attachment relationships
Small et al. 2014 [33]	22	1990–2012	Sample sizes ranged from 6 to 432, with a total of 2498 migrant women	Access, utilisation and experience of perinatal healthcare	What migrant and non-migrant women want from maternity care is similar: safe, high-quality, attentive and individualised care, with adequate information and support. Migrant women were less positive about their care than non-migrant women. Communication problems and lack of familiarity with care systems negatively affected migrant women's experiences, as did perceptions of discrimination and care which was not kind or respectful

Table 2 Summary of results for all included study populations (migrant including asylum seeker and refugee women) *(Continued)*

Author, year	Number of studies	Publication date range	Sample size[1]	Topic area of results	Summary of author conclusions
Tobin et al. 2017 [20]	13	2004–2013	139	Perinatal health outcomes (mental health); access, utilisation and experience of perinatal healthcare	Migrant women with postnatal depression may lack understanding of their condition, are often isolated, alone, fear stigmatisation and risk being considered an unfit mother. Raising awareness with healthcare providers of the meaning of postnatal depression for migrant women is key to the provision of effective care
Villalonga-Olives et al. 2016 [29]	68	1994–2013	80,572,311 (6 studies no data reported)	Perinatal health outcomes (low birth weight)	The prevalence of low birth weight amongst migrants varies by the host country characteristics as well as the composition of migrants to different regions. The primary driver of migrant health is the migrant 'regime' in different countries at specific periods of time. The 'healthy migrant effect' in the USA is largely missing from Europe
Wikberg and Bondas 2010 [34]	40	1988–2008	More than 1160 women from more than 50 cultures	Experience of perinatal healthcare	*Alice in Wonderland* emerged as an overarching metaphor to describe intercultural caring in maternity care. There are specific cultural and maternity care features in intercultural caring: an inner core of caring consisting of respect, presence and listening, as well as external factors such as economy and organisation that affect intercultural caring. Legal status, power relationships and racism influence intercultural caring
Winn et al. 2017 [11]	19	1995–2015	Not reported	Access, utilisation and experience of perinatal healthcare	Three main meta-themes were developed: (1) Expectations Of Pregnancy As Derived From Home, (2) Reality Of Pregnancy In The Host Health Care System. These two themes were connected by our third meta-theme: Support
Wittkowski et al. 2017 [21]	16	1996–2011	337	Perinatal health outcomes (mental health); access, utilisation and experience of perinatal healthcare	Migrant mothers living in Western countries are subject to multifaceted and multifactorial stressors following the birth of their child, possibly making them more susceptible to developing postnatal depression and influencing their subsequent healthcare behaviour. These stressors are related to migration or being a migrant in a Western society as well as cultural influences which are harder to comply with as a migrant living in a different country, removed from their socio-cultural context. Social support appears to play an integral and mediating role for migrant mothers living in Western countries

[1.] If the total sample size was not explicitly reported by the authors of the systematic review, then it was calculated from the table of included studies where possible

- *Health status and history.* The risk of perinatal mental health disorders was increased when migrant women perceived their overall health to be low [17, 19] or had a history of mental health disorders [6, 22]. Fellmeth et al. [6] reported ORs for postnatal depression to be between 24.9 and 29.7 when there was a personal or family history of depression.
- *Socio-demographics.* Risk factors included low income or socio-economic status, unemployment [5, 16, 17], low education [17], having a visible minority status [19] and primiparity [6]. Fellmeth et al. [6] also reported that maternal age > 30 years and < 25 years were risk factors for increased postnatal depression.

Mortality

Two systematic reviews reported data on maternal mortality (death of a woman during pregnancy, childbirth or in the first 42 days after delivery) [24, 25]. Pedersen et al. [24] reported the relative risk (RR) to be twofold amongst migrant women in Western European countries compared with women from the host countries (RR 2.00, 95% CI 1.72–2.33) and the absolute risk difference to be 9 additional maternal deaths per 100,000 deliveries per year for migrant women (95% CI 5.9–15.2). The strongest association was observed for direct causes of death amongst this population including hypertensive disorders (primarily preeclampsia and eclampsia), deep vein thrombosis and pulmonary embolism (RR 2.65, 95% CI 1.88–3.74) rather than indirect causes (unspecified) (RR 1.83, 95% CI 1.37–2.45) [24]. Gagnon et al. [25] included maternal mortality in a composite outcome for maternal health, although this article did not report the results for this outcome exclusively.

Three systematic reviews, all published in 2009, included offspring mortality [25–27]. Gissler et al. reported increased risks of stillbirth (RR 1.40, 95% CI 1.22–1.58), perinatal mortality (RR 1.35, 95% CI 1.26–1.45), neonatal mortality (RR 1.34, 95% CI 1.30–1.38) and infant mortality (RR 1.33, 95% CI 1.30–1.36) amongst migrant women in European countries compared with women from the host countries [27]. When the meta-analyses were restricted to migrants from non-European countries, the risk increased for stillbirths (RR 1.88, 95% CI 1.58–2.23) and slightly increased for perinatal, neonatal and infant mortality (RR 1.54, 95% CI 1.39–1.69; RR 1.40, 95% CI 1.36–1.44; RR 1.37, 95% CI 1.34–1.40 respectively). Conversely, migrant women in the USA had better outcomes than USA-born ethnic minorities (RR 0.77, 95% CI 0.63–0.65), demonstrating a healthy migrant effect. Adjustments for risk factors in the meta-analyses only accounted for a small proportion of the excess mortality risk [27]. Gagnon et al. [25] reported meta-analyses for feto-infant mortality (neonatal, infant mortality and spontaneous abortion). They found that Asian and North African migrant women had a significantly increased association with feto-infant mortality than women in the host country (aOR 1.29, 95% CI 1.02–1.63; aOR 1.25, 95% CI 1.10–1.41 respectively). There was no significant difference between majority-receiving-country women and European-born migrants (aOR 1.14, 95% CI 0.75–1.72) or Latin American-born migrants (aOR 1.02, 95% CI 0.76–1.39) [25]. The meta-analysis for African women showed the largest effect size, but this was not significant (OR 2.43, 95% CI 0.99–5.96) [25]. Note that these meta-analyses only included two or three studies for each country of origin and had high levels of heterogeneity. Bollini et al. [26] found an increased association between offspring mortality (including stillbirth, perinatal, neonatal, postnatal and infant mortality) and migrant women compared to women from the European host countries (OR 1.50, 95% CI 1.47–1.53). The authors hypothesised that pregnancy outcomes amongst migrant women were influenced by the degree of implementation of integration policies in the host countries, where a strong integration policy would be demonstrated by countries which had entrenched equality and social cohesion in their societies [26]. They carried out further meta-analyses adjusting for maternal age, parity and national level of implementation of integration policies and found the associations to be attenuated when there were strong implementation policies (aOR 1.25, 95% CI 1.17–1.34) compared with weak implementation policies (aOR 1.45, 95% CI 1.13–1.86); although the implementation of strong integration policies attenuated the association with offspring mortality, the difference in effect did not reach significance ($p = 0.241$) [26].

Mode of delivery

Three quantitative systematic reviews investigated mode of delivery amongst migrant women compared to women from host countries [7, 25, 28]. Gagnon et al. [25] reported that 40% of the 25 studies included in their review found operative modes of delivery (caesarean and operative vaginal) to be higher amongst migrant women; the remaining studies reported reduced operative mode of delivery outcomes for migrant women (20%), mixed results (12%) or no difference between migrant women and women from the host country (28%). Merry et al. also reported mixed results for caesarean delivery in their 2013 review [28]; associations between migrant women and caesarean varied by country of origin and by receiving country. The authors reported a significantly increased odds of caesarean amongst women migrating from former colonised Caribbean states (OR 1.91, 95% CI 1.37–2.66), South Asia (OR 1.28, 95% CI 1.22–1.35), the Philippines (OR 1.19, 95% CI 1.1–1.29) and Somalia (OR 1.13, 95% CI 1.02–1.26). Women migrating from Africa had increased odds of caesarean which differed according to receiving country: France (OR 2.22, 95% CI 1.92–2.58), Australia (OR 1.17, 95% CI 1.11–1.24), Canada (OR 1.34, 95% CI 1.08–1.67) and North/West Europe (OR 1.43, 95% CI 1.16, 1.77). However, these increased odds were not observed amongst women migrating from North Africa to Canada (OR 0.81, 95% CI 0.74–0.90) or France (OR 1.09, 95% CI 0.95–1.26). Similarly, women migrating from Latin America had significantly increased odds for caesarean in Norway (OR 2.41, 95% CI 1.79–3.23) and Canada (OR 1.43, 95% CI 1.29–1.59), but not in Southern Europe (OR 1.03, 95% CI 0.94–1.12). Odds for caesarean were significantly reduced or no different from those of women from receiving countries when women migrated from Vietnam (OR 0.68, 95% CI 0.66–0.71), Kosovo (OR 0.49, 95% CI 0.36–0.67), Russia/Baltic States (OR 0.75, 95% CI 0.66–0.85) and East Asia (receiving countries: Southern Europe (OR 0.59, 95% CI 0.47–0.73), USA (OR 0.73, 95% CI 0.71–0.75), and Australia, UK, Canada or Finland (OR 0.99, 95% CI 0.95–1.03)) [28]. The 2016 review of Merry et al. [7] was an update of the 2013 review and identified that migrant women from sub-Saharan Africa had higher caesarean section rates, whereas migrant women from Eastern Europe had lower rates than women in the host countries. Higher emergency caesarean deliveries were also reported for women migrating from Latin America, North Africa and the Middle East compared with women in the host countries [7].

Birth weight

Low birth weight (LBW) or small for gestational age (SGA) outcomes were reported by four reviews [19, 25, 26, 29] with contradictory results. A meta-analysis of LBW (< 2500 g) amongst migrant women residing in European countries showed significantly increased association compared with women in the European host countries (OR 1.42, 95% CI 1.42–1.44) [26]. There was a significant attenuation of LBW when analyses adjusted for age, parity and level of implementation of integration policies ($p < 0.001$); weak implementation resulted in an increased association (aOR 1.77, 95% CI 1.63–1.92) and strong implementation reduced the association (aOR 1.08, 95% CI 1.03–1.13), although the association remained significantly increased compared with results for non-migrant women [26]. Conversely, a meta-analysis of international data not restricted to women residing in Europe showed a reduced aOR for LBW and SGA amongst migrant women with borderline significance (aOR 0.92, 95% CI 0.85–1.00) [25]. Meta-analysis by migrant origin showed increased odds amongst women born in African and Asian countries and reduced odds amongst European, Latin American and North African-born women, although no sub-group meta-analysis reached statistical significance [25].

The paradoxical healthy migrant effect in relation to reduced risk of LBW and SGA was discussed by De Maio [19] and Villalonga-Olives et al. [29], although there were some reported inconsistent findings. The systematic review by De Maio [19] discusses how the patterns of reduced risk amongst migrants compared with women in the host countries are influenced by maternal socio-economic status, country of origin and maternal education, where migrant women with low levels of education have better outcomes and there is an increased risk of SGA and LBW amongst migrant women with higher education [19]. Villalonga-Olives et al. [29] discuss how the apparent healthy migrant effect in the USA (where migrant populations often have improved outcomes compared with non-migrant populations) is contrasted by the health inequalities in Europe, where the associations are reversed. The US studies show a reduced risk of LBW and SGA amongst Latina migrants, although this does not extend to Black and Puerto Rican migrants—who have increased risks—and Asian women show no difference in risk compared to women from the host country [29]. In contrast, there is a lack of a healthy migrant effect in Europe with the exception of studies from two countries, Spain and Belgium. However, data from these countries are also conflicting, showing that outcomes differ by migrant origins (e.g. increased risk amongst migrants from Morocco and Turkey) and also by the severity of outcome (e.g. women in host countries have a higher risk of moderate LBW, whereas migrant women have an increased risk of very LBW) [29].

Preterm birth

Three reviews reported preterm birth outcomes [19, 25, 26]. A meta-analysis by Bollini et al. [26] identified a higher odds of preterm birth (< 37 weeks gestation) amongst migrant women in Europe (OR 1.24, 95% CI 1.22–1.26). There was a significant attenuation when analyses adjusted for age, parity and level of implementation of integration policies ($p < 0.001$); weak implementation resulted in increased odds of preterm birth (aOR 2.88, 95% CI 2.50–3.32) and strong implementation policy decreased the odds (aOR 1.18, 95% CI 1.14–1.22) [26]. A meta-analysis reported by Gagnon et al. [25] found differences in risk of preterm birth by migrant origin. Compared with women in the host countries, there was a higher odds for migrant women from Asia (aOR 1.14, 95% CI 1.06–1.21) and Africa (aOR 1.29, 95% CI 1.04–1.60); a lower odds for Latina migrant women (aOR 0.83, 95% CI 0.72–0.95); and no difference for migrant women from Europe and North Africa [25]. De Maio [19] discusses the healthy migrant effect for preterm birth outcomes being influenced by maternal education and length of residence in the receiving country. Migrants with < 5 years residence had a lower prevalence of preterm birth compared with women in the host countries (4.7% vs 6.2%), and those residing > 15 years had the highest prevalence (7.4%) [19]. Further, a 5-year increase in length of residence significantly increased the odds of preterm birth amongst migrant women (aOR 1.14, 95% CI 1.10–1.19), which was potentially influenced by maternal stress and discrimination [19].

Congenital anomaly

Two reviews reported on congenital anomalies [25, 26]. Migrant women had a significantly increased risk of a pregnancy affected by a congenital anomaly compared to women in the host countries (OR 1.61, 95% CI 1.57–1.65). There was a significant attenuation of congenital anomalies when analyses adjusted for age, parity and level of implementation of integration policies ($p < 0.001$); when there was weak implementation, a significant increased association remained (aOR 1.20, 95% CI 0.95–1.52), whereas having a strong implement policy resulted in a significantly lower odds of congenital anomalies amongst migrant women (aOR 0.87, 95% CI 0.78–0.95) [26]. Gagnon et al. [25] combined congenital anomalies with other infant morbidity (such as neonatal intensive care unit (NICU) admission and low Apgar score) and found that 62.5% of the 16 studies included in their review reported worse outcomes for migrant women compared with women from the host country; no studies found this outcome to be better for migrant women.

Additional morbidities

Three reviews reported additional maternal or infant morbidities [19, 26]. Bollini et al. [26] investigated maternal postpartum haemorrhage, but no summary data were reported. De Maio [19] identified a healthy migrant effect for risk of placental dysfunction amongst women residing in Ontario, Canada, for < 5 years which was influenced by length of residence: the lowest odds were for women residing < 3 months (OR 0.53, 95% CI 0.47–0.61), which increased the longer the duration of residence (residing 48–59 months OR 0.82, 95% CI 0.77–0.87); however, the OR remained lower than that for women in the host country for all durations of residency. Gagnon et al. [25] had a composite outcome for maternal health (including but not limited to mortality, pregnancy-related morbidity, extended length of labour, episiotomy) and reported that 50% of their 32 included studies showed worse outcomes for migrant women, 21.9% showed better outcomes and the remaining studies were mixed or reported no difference. The authors also reported maternal and infant infections (including HIV, toxoplasmosis, sexually transmitted infections and rubella seronegativity) to be worse amongst migrant women in 63.6% of included studies and better in 9.1%; the remaining studies showed mixed results [25]. Bollini et al. [26] and Gagnon et al. [25] reported that admission to a NICU or special care was higher amongst offspring of migrant women (Gagnon et al. included NICU admission in their composite outcome for infant morbidities).

Perinatal healthcare access and experiences amongst women who are migrants (including asylum seekers and refugees)

Twenty systematic reviews reported access to, and experience of, perinatal healthcare amongst migrant women; 11 were qualitative [8, 9, 11, 16, 20, 21, 30–34], 5 were quantitative [6, 18, 19, 25, 35] and 4 were mixed methods systematic reviews [10, 22, 23, 36]. Results are summarised in Table 2, and a narrative summary is presented of the themes and sub-themes relating to: (1) access to and utilisation of perinatal healthcare and (2) experience of perinatal healthcare.

1. Access to and utilisation of perinatal healthcare
   Sixteen systematic reviews reported data relating to access or utilisation of perinatal healthcare [8–11, 16, 19–23, 25, 30, 32, 33, 35, 36]. All systematic reviews reported that access to perinatal care, including routine care and specialist care such as mental health support for postnatal depression, was worse amongst migrant women. Heaman et al. [35] reported that 86% of the 29 studies included in their review showed inadequate prenatal care for migrant women compared with women in the host countries, with 15 studies reporting large effect sizes (aORs > 2.0). Gagnon et al. [25] reported that prenatal care was worse amongst migrant women compared with women in the host countries in 58.3% of their 12 included studies, and no studies reported care to be better amongst migrant women. Barriers to accessing care were consistent across all systematic reviews and are summarised here under the themes of structural and organisational barriers, social barriers and personal and cultural barriers.
   a. Structural and organisational barriers
      Ten systematic reviews reported unfamiliarity with local healthcare provision, culture and systems as a barrier [8, 10, 19–22, 30, 32, 33, 36]. Issues included a lack of knowledge and awareness of services and support on offer, a lack of information provision about how to get support, difficulties with navigating healthcare systems, managing bureaucracy and a lack of information about regular appointments and check-ups which resulted in missed appointments. Ten systematic reviews reported language barriers to accessing perinatal healthcare [10, 11, 19–23, 32, 35, 36] including proficiency in being able to verbally communicate with health professionals, access to translators and understanding written communication. Physician availability, long waiting lists for services, especially those specialising in migrant care, a lack of postnatal follow-up and perceptions that health services did not want to take migrant women were additional structural and organisational barriers reported in three systematic reviews [20, 23, 36].
   b. Social barriers
      Nine systematic reviews reported social barriers to accessing care which centred on the competing priorities of *real life worries* [21] that migrant women faced such as poverty, safe housing, employment and caring for their other children [8, 10, 11, 20, 21, 31, 32, 35, 36]. Financial constraints were frequently reported including a lack of health insurance, cost of care and wider poverty issues such as having no phone, childcare or transport [8, 10, 11, 20, 21, 32, 35, 36]. Further social barriers included

having an unplanned pregnancy, being single and maternal education level [31, 35].

c. Personal and cultural barriers
Six systematic reviews reported personal and cultural barriers to accessing services [8, 9, 20, 21, 23, 36]. Three reviews focussed on accessing perinatal mental health services [8, 20, 21] and reported a reluctance amongst migrant women to talk about mental health, a lack of cultural acceptability to seek help, beliefs about women's strength and self-coping, the fear of labelling, stigma and alienation in some cultures, beliefs that depression was not a real health condition, that health professionals and services were for physical health, a lack of understanding of the condition and associated terminology and fears of having their child removed. Additional barriers reported were a lack of culturally appropriate therapists and services available [20, 36] and a preference for female health professionals due to religious reasons and the intimacy of body areas during pregnancy [9, 23]. However, the preference for female providers was negated in emergency situations, and the competency of the health professional was considered more important than gender [9].

2. Experience of perinatal healthcare
Twelve systematic reviews reported data relating to migrant women's experiences of perinatal healthcare [8, 10, 11, 16, 20–22, 30, 32–34, 36]. There were some consistent experiences reported in the systematic reviews, and these are summarised under the themes of negative communication and discrimination, relationships with health professionals, cultural clashes and the receipt of clinical perinatal healthcare.

a. Negative communication and discrimination
Language barriers and having to rely on translators had an impact on communication experiences [8, 10, 11, 30, 32–34]. Systematic reviews also reported themes of insensitive and hurtful communication, perceptions of racism, cultural stereotyping and discriminatory interactions between migrant women and health professionals [10, 33, 34, 36]. Small et al. [33] reported that the migrant women felt that care was not kind or respectful and that they were less likely to be spoken to with respect, understanding and in a way they could comprehend.

b. Relationship with health professionals
The interpersonal relationship between migrant women and health professionals was reported to be an important influence on experience of perinatal care. A positive experience resulted from health professionals who were kind and friendly and who listened to the woman's concerns [10, 32]. However, the majority of data related to struggles with relationships and a lack of connection; migrant women were less likely to describe health professionals positively than women in the host countries [20, 30, 32, 33]. There was a common theme of migrant women feeling rushed during interactions with health professionals [8, 10, 32, 36], misunderstandings with health professionals and a lack of confidence to express concerns or ask questions [11, 30].

c. Cultural clashes
Ten systematic reviews reported a lack of cultural knowledge and sensitivity in their experiences of perinatal healthcare [8, 10, 11, 20, 21, 30, 32–34, 36]. The majority of these clashes stemmed from differences between cultural, religious and traditional beliefs and practices and Western biomedical approaches to perinatal healthcare. The systematic reviews reported that migrant women lacked understanding about Western medicine and care, felt pressure to adapt and were labelled as non-compliant if they resisted Western approaches in favour of traditional practices [11, 20, 21, 30, 32, 34, 36].

d. Clinical perinatal healthcare
Nine systematic reviews reported migrant women's experiences of clinical perinatal healthcare including breastfeeding support, decision making about care and Western approaches to medicine and technology [10, 16, 20–22, 30, 32, 33, 36]. Higginbottom et al. [36] reported some positive experiences amongst migrant women relating to provision of breastfeeding support in hospital; however, the remaining data relate to negative experiences of care. The reviews reported that migrant women were less positive about the care they received and reported that health professionals discussed their care with them less frequently than with women in the host countries, especially relating to mental healthcare needs [16, 22, 33, 36]. The reviews also reported that migrant women did not feel involved in decision making about their care or did not feel they had options [10, 33, 36]. There were reports of poor experiences of care and pain management amongst migrant women who had female genital mutilation (FGM) [30, 33, 36], too much focus on technological and procedural approaches to care and childbirth [30, 32] and an over-reliance on

prescription of medications which were culturally or religiously inappropriate rather than access to supportive care (e.g. counselling for depression) [20, 21, 30, 32].

Results specific to women with asylum seeker or refugee status

Twenty-two of the included systematic reviews either explicitly reported results relevant to women with asylum seeker or refugee status, or they cited studies where the participants were exclusively women with asylum seeker or refugee status [5–11, 14, 16, 18–20, 23, 27–34, 36]. In total, the reviews cited 54 studies, although there was some overlap in the original studies relevant to asylum seekers and refugees included in the systematic reviews and used to inform the analyses (Additional file 5); data from 43 unique studies were cited by these 22 systematic reviews. Eight systematic reviews use primary data that view asylum seekers and refugees as separate sub-groups [5, 6, 16, 18, 19, 23, 30, 36]. Five systematic reviews [7, 9–11, 34, 36] combine asylum seekers and refugees as a sub-group of the migrant population. Seven systematic reviews [8, 20, 27–29, 32, 33] use primary data solely involving refugees. Two systematic reviews [14, 31] use primary data looking at asylum seekers only. Seven systematic reviews [17, 21, 22, 24–26, 35] do not distinguish asylum seekers and refugees from other types of immigrants in their analysis.

The data reported for asylum seekers and refugees were limited, and the majority of detailed data came from qualitative studies on women's access to and experiences of perinatal healthcare. The results table is summarised in Additional file 6, and a narrative summary is presented for perinatal health outcomes and healthcare access and experiences amongst women with asylum seeker or refugee status.

Perinatal health outcomes amongst women with asylum seeker and refugee status

Fourteen systematic reviews reported perinatal health outcomes for asylum seeker and refugee populations [5–7, 14, 16, 18–20, 23, 27–30, 36]. Perinatal health results are presented for perinatal mental health, offspring mortality, mode of delivery, birth weight, preterm birth and additional morbidities. Perinatal mental health was reported most frequently by the systematic reviews. No data specific to asylum seekers or refugees were reported for maternal mortality or congenital anomaly outcomes.

Perinatal mental health amongst women with asylum seeker or refugee status Nine systematic reviews reported data for asylum seekers and refugees [5, 6, 16, 18–20, 23, 30, 36] citing 11 original studies [37–47].

Prevalence of perinatal mental health disorders Five reviews cited data from Stewart et al. [37] which found that rates of postnatal depression were significantly higher amongst women with refugee and asylum seeker status (25.7% and 31.1% respectively) compared with women in the host country of Canada (8.1%, $p = 0.008$). They also found a significantly increased odds of scoring 10 or more on the Edinburgh Postnatal Depression Scale for refugees (OR 4.80, 95% CI, 1.57–14.69) and asylum seekers (OR 3.06, 95% CI, 1.06–8.82) [5, 16, 18, 19, 23]. Similar rates were reported in a systematic review by Fellmeth et al. [6]; 37.3% of refugees and 41.8% of asylum seekers living in Canada experienced symptoms of depression, somatisation or anxiety and significantly increased odds for the prevalence of any depressive order (OR prevalence 0.25, 95% CI 0.21–0.29) (data from Gagnon et al. [48]). Increased prevalence for post-traumatic stress disorder were reported, where asylum-seeking women had the highest prevalence (48.2% above the cut-off), followed by refugees (33.8%) and migrants (15%) [5, 6] (data from Gagnon et al. [48]). Higginbottom et al. [36] reported that of 50 refugee mothers who received a home visit at 4 months postpartum, 26 were found to have symptoms of postpartum depression (data from Merry et al. [39]). Data from original studies exclusively on women with asylum seeker or refugee status [40–44, 47] were used in a meta-synthesis by Balaam et al. [30] and contributed to the findings that stress and low self-esteem were common, and that women had mental health problems such as depression, feelings of loneliness and isolation and expressed sadness, vulnerability and anxiety together with severe nausea.

Risk factors for the development of perinatal mental health disorders Three systematic reviews reported risk factors for the development of perinatal mental health disorders specifically relevant to asylum seekers and refugees [6, 18, 19]. Fellmeth et al. [6] reported data from Matthey et al. [45] which showed statistically significant associations between anxiety and the number of premigration traumatic events experienced or witnessed, but no association with anxiety or post-traumatic stress disorder and history of living in a refugee camp prior to resettlement. Collins et al. [18] and De Maio [19] presented data from Stewart et al. [37] which found that refugees and asylum seekers had significantly lower social support than women in the host country of Canada ($p < 0.001$), including support from family, friends, groups and systems, as well as personal, emotional and instrumental social support. Tobin et al. [20] also reported that women who were refugees attributed their depression to social factors such as family problems or economic hardship rather than biological factors (data from Edge [46]).

Offspring mortality amongst women with asylum seeker and refugee status Two systematic reviews [14, 27] reported offspring mortality amongst women who were refugees using data from nine original studies [40, 49–56]. Gissler et al. [27] reported that in European studies women who were registered refugees or originated from refugee source countries at the time of arrival (including Africa, sub-Saharan Africa, Romania, Kosovo and Russia) had a significantly increased risk of stillbirth (RR 2.01, 95% CI 1.41–2.06), early neonatal mortality (RR 2.77, 95% CI 1.85–4.13) and perinatal mortality (RR 1.71, 95% CI 1.41–2.06) compared to women in the host countries of Norway, Sweden, Ireland and the Netherlands. However, women from Vietnamese backgrounds had lower mortality than women in the host country of Norway [27]. Evidence from the former Yugoslavia showed that women who were refugees had increased risk of early neonatal mortality (RR 3.66, 95% CI 1.92–6.99) and perinatal mortality (RR 3.07, 95% CI 2.05–4.62) but no difference in risk of stillbirth (RR 1.19, 95% CI 0.56–2.50). Deaths attributed to congenital anomalies, pregnancy complications or intrauterine growth restriction were similarly distributed amongst refugees and women in the host country.

Live birth and abortion There were additional data relevant to offspring mortality for women with asylum seeker and refugee status that were not reported in the data for migrant women. Hadgkiss and Renzaho [14] reported that asylum seekers had a higher incidence of sexual assault, unwanted pregnancies and induced abortion-to-live birth ratio compared with women in the host countries (1:2.5 vs 1:7.5) (data from Goosen et al. [55], Kurth et al. [40] and Rogstad and Dale [56]). Asylum seekers with longer duration of stay (compared with those arriving in the previous 6 months) had a lower live birth and abortion rate [14] (data from Goosen et al. [55]).

Mode of Delivery amongst women with asylum seeker and refugee status Three systematic reviews [7, 14, 28] reported caesarean delivery for refugee and asylum seeker women using data from four original studies [38, 40, 57, 58] with conflicting results. Merry et al. [28] and Hadgkiss and Renzaho [14] reported data from two studies [40, 57] which found no significant difference in caesarean delivery rates amongst asylum seekers compared to native-born women (OR 0.93, 95% CI 0.74–1.17) (data from Gagnon et al. [57]). However, Merry et al. [7] reported that refugees and asylum seekers were at a reduced risk of an emergency caesarean compared with economic and student migrants (data from Gagnon et al. [38]) but an increased risk compared with women in the host country of Canada (data from Kandasamy et al. [58]).

Birth weight amongst women with asylum seeker and refugee status Two systematic reviews [14, 29] reported data for low birth weight (LBW) and intrauterine growth retardation using data from five original studies [40, 49, 59–61]. Villalonga-Olives et al. [29] reported no difference in LBW between refugee populations in Ireland or undocumented Latina migrants in the USA and women in the host countries (data from Kelaher and Jessop [61] and Lalchandani et al. [49]). However, Somali refugees in Belgium, Canada, Finland, Norway and Sweden had lower rates of LBW compared with women in the host countries (data from Small et al. [59]). Hadgkiss and Renzaho [14] reported prevalence of intrauterine growth restriction to be one of the most prevalent outcomes amongst women who were seeking asylum, 7% of the population (data from Kurth et al. [40]; no comparison data were reported for women in the host countries).

Preterm birth amongst women with asylum seeker and refugee status Two systematic reviews [14, 27] reported preterm birth amongst women who were refugees using data from two original studies [40, 54]. Hadgkiss and Renzaho [14] reported premature labour to be one of the most prevalent outcomes in women seeking asylum at 15% of the population (data from Kurth et al. [40]), and Gissler et al. [27] reported that women who were displaced from the former Yugoslavia had higher preterm rates than women in the host country (data from Nedic et al. [54]).

Additional morbidities amongst women with asylum seeker and refugee status Two systematic reviews [14, 30] reported additional maternal morbidities and data from six original studies [40–42, 55, 56, 62]. The additional morbidity outcomes reported for women with asylum seeker and refugee status (eclampsia, obstetric haemorrhage and maternal infections) are similar to those reported for migrant women (placental dysfunction, postpartum haemorrhage and maternal infection). There were additional data reported explicitly for women with asylum seeker and refugee status that were not reported for migrant women (including asylum seekers and refugees) showing increased risk of severe acute maternal morbidity (SAMM), gestational diabetes, anaemia and uterine rupture. There was a lack of data explicitly for women with asylum seeker and refugee status and offspring infection and admission to special care units. Hadgkiss and Renzaho [14] reported that asylum seekers faced a range of complex obstetric issues including bleeding, gestational diabetes, anaemia, 4.5 times higher incidence of SAMM than the general obstetric population (31.0 vs 6.8 per 1000 births), uterine rupture (15 vs 8.4%) and eclampsia (27.5 vs 9.1%); but lower incidence of obstetric haemorrhage (42.5 vs 63. 3%) (data from Kurth et al. [40], Goosen et al. [55], Rogstad and Dale [56], Van Hanegem et al. [62]). Baalam et al. [30] reported poor health amongst women with asylum seeker and refugee status which caused complications for the women and the newborn babies, including infected wounds, HIV and hepatitis (data from Kennedy and Murphy-Lawless [41] and McLeish [42]).

Healthcare access and experiences amongst women with asylum seeker and refugee status

Twelve systematic reviews reported access to or experience of perinatal healthcare amongst women with asylum seeker and refugee status [8–11, 20, 23, 30–34, 36]. The sub-themes presented are the same as the results for migrant women. However, there are additional results within the sub-themes for asylum seekers and refugees that were not present, or not as detailed, for migrant women.

Access to perinatal healthcare amongst women with asylum seeker and refugee status The barriers to accessing care are summarised here under the themes of structural and organisational barriers, social barriers and personal and cultural barriers.

1. Structural and organisational barriers
   Seven systematic reviews reported structural or organisational barriers for women with asylum seeker and refugee status to access perinatal healthcare [10, 11, 23, 30, 31, 33, 36] including data from 15 original studies [39–44, 47, 57, 63–69]. Results relating to limited ability to speak the language of the host country or understand the verbal or written information provided [10, 23, 30, 33] were similar to the results for the overall migrant population, as were challenges navigating, and a lack of familiarity with, the healthcare systems and inadequate information about what support services exist [10, 11, 30, 31, 33, 36]. Additional data relevant to asylum seekers and refugees included a lack of knowledge about availability of support services which led to feelings of social isolation [36]. There were assumptions amongst asylum seekers and refugees that they would have to pay for perinatal healthcare when they were entitled to free care [10, 31] and mistrust of healthcare professionals who were perceived to be a threat to the emotional and physical safety of asylum seekers who did not engage with antenatal care [31]. Higginbottom et al. [23] also reported that learning the host country language was not a priority for women, and that the men in the household attended language classes while the women stayed at home.
2. Social barriers
   Six systematic reviews reported social barriers to accessing perinatal healthcare [8, 10, 11, 30, 32, 36] including data from 12 original studies [39–44, 64, 66, 70–73]. Many of the social barriers to accessing or continuing with perinatal healthcare were similar to those for migrant populations such as a lack of finances, transport, issues with housing and a lack of family and friend networks [8, 10, 11, 30, 32, 36]. However, these difficulties were described in the systematic reviews to be particularly challenging for women with asylum seeker or refugee status due to temporary and uncertain status, not being permitted to work in their host countries and the impact of these factors on available resources and having a 'normal life' [8, 36]. For example, Higginbottom et al. [36] describes postnatal refugees skipping meals because of a lack of resources, and Balaam et al. [30] reported that some types of accommodation for refugees and asylum seekers are restricted by fixed mealtimes which imposed practical challenges with flexibility to attend appointments. Mengesha et al. [10] reported that home visits by refugee health nurses were positively received, and Balaam et al. [30] reported that childbirth was a critical milestone towards a better social status, and that the baby represented a new beginning and a health resource.
3. Personal and cultural barriers
   Five systematic reviews reported personal and cultural barriers to accessing perinatal healthcare [9, 20, 23, 30, 32] including data from 11 original studies [40–44, 67, 71, 74–77]. The systematic reviews reported similar results to those for migrants in relation to a lack of cultural understanding of postnatal depression and a preference for female health professionals. Further context was provided on gender preference for asylum seekers and refugees. Aubrey et al. [9] reported that higher rates of caesarean deliveries amongst Syrian refugee women resulted from avoidance in seeking antenatal care due to the lack of female health professionals and the fact that only 5 out of 18 African refugee women in the USA would accept care from a male health professional. However, these findings were in conflict with other studies in their review which reported that African refugee women accessing obstetric care in Australia,

and Somali women in the USA, would accept care from a male health professional in an emergency [9].

Experience of perinatal healthcare amongst asylum seekers and refugees The themes identified in the systematic reviews around experience of care related to negative communication and discrmination, relationship with health professionals, cultural clashes, and clinical perinatal care are summarised below.

1. Negative communication and discrimination
   Seven systematic reviews reported negative communication and discrimination data for asylum seeker and refugee women [10, 11, 23, 30, 33, 34, 36] reporting data from 12 original studies [39–44, 63, 64, 66–68, 73]. There were similar negative communication experiences to the results for migrant women, including reliance on interpreters and experience of discrimination. However, these negative experiences were more widely represented in the data specific to women with asylum seeker and refugee status than for general migrant populations. Balaam et al. [30] reported that refugee and asylum-seeking women were less willing to state their needs and wishes. Data relating to reliance on interpreters represented an inadequacy of service provision leading to delayed care, women's reliance on body language and facial expressions to communicate, their needs not being met and the women being unable to express their concerns. There was a reported need for more consistent professional interpreting support for women with asylum seeker or refugee status including integrated services, continuity of competent interpreters and improving of health professionals' knowledge of when interpreting services are required [10, 23, 30, 33, 36].
   The systematic reviews reported that the most vulnerable women with asylum-seeking or refugee status had the most difficult situation and negative encounters with health professionals including openly racist and discriminatory care, cultural stigma, disrespect, hostility, stereotyping and being treated as 'primitive people' [10, 30, 33, 34]. These experiences are demonstrated in a quote from an included study reported in the systematic review by Wikberg and Bondas [34]: "An African woman asked for help when she got an infection but was not met with respect: She looked at me like this and said,'You are OK'.. . She said to another midwife,'These Africans. .. they come here, they eat nice food, sleep in a nice bed, so now she doesn't want to move from here!' . .. When she said this I didn't say anything, I just cried... she doesn't know me, who I am in my country. And the other midwife said 'What's wrong with them, these Africans?' and some of them they laughed" (data from McLeish [42]). Women reported that these interactions were influenced by skin colour, their language ability and communication problems, and that they wanted supportive, non-discriminatory care [30, 33].
2. Relationship with health professionals
   Four systematic reviews reported data on the relationships between health professionals and women with asylum seeker and refugee status [10, 11, 30, 33] from 10 original studies [40–44, 47, 63, 64, 68, 70]. There were similar findings to the results for overall migrant populations in relation to the importance of a supportive relationship with health professionals, negative experiences such as feeling health professionals were too busy and a lack of confidence to discuss their issues with health professionals [10, 30, 33]. Positive interactions were experienced when health professionals had respect for practices from the country of origin or were of the same ethnicity or religion, and positive support increased confidence in asking questions and acceptance of the new healthcare system and practices [11, 30].
3. Cultural clashes
   Five systematic reviews reported cultural clashes in perinatal healthcare experience amongst women with asylum seeker and refugee status [10, 11, 30, 32, 33], reporting data from five original studies [63, 64, 66, 70, 71]. All data specific to women with asylum seeker and refugee status duplicate the findings of the overall migrant women, such as tensions between feeling the need to adapt to host country medical practices and women's preferences for traditional cultural or religious practices. No new findings were identified in the data specific to women with asylum seeker and refugee status.
4. Clinical perinatal healthcare
   Six systematic reviews reported issues with the clinical perinatal healthcare amongst women with asylum seeker and refugee status [10, 20, 30, 32, 33, 36] reporting data from 15 original studies [39–44, 47, 57, 63, 64, 66, 68, 71, 73, 78]. There were some similarities with the results for migrant women relating to negative experiences amongst women with asylum seeker and refugee status, health professionals showing a lack of knowledge and sensitivity relating to FGM, women receiving poor explanations of care and lack of discussion of options, a lack of assessment and referrals for postnatal depression, an over-reliance on technology and Western practices which lacked cultural

sensitivity [10, 30, 32, 33, 36]. Additional findings in the data for women with asylum seeker and refugee status include the following: outcomes being better amongst women who were able to exhibit resilience and adjust and change their cultural beliefs; disappointment and lack of preparation for the lack of practical postnatal help and support; recommendations for advocacy or link-worker schemes; and the need for culturally appropriate health education materials on labour and delivery and health professional training on Somali refugee women's culture, traditions, values and expectations [30, 33]. The systematic review by Tobin et al. [20] reported discrepancies on the topic of support groups for postnatal depression in their included studies; one study reported limited use for refugee women who preferred individual therapy due to privacy, confidentiality and a cultural stigma related to the condition, whereas another study found that social networking and support groups were important in facilitating help seeking and the healing process.

Discussion

This systematic review of systematic reviews aimed to summarise the existing evidence base of perinatal health outcomes and perinatal healthcare amongst women with the status of asylum seeker and refugee. Although all included reviews incorporated data for women with asylum seeker or refugee status in order to be eligible for inclusion, the data reported specific to this population were limited. Only one included systematic review was exclusively focussed on asylum seekers, and the remaining data for asylum seeker and refugee women were grouped with those for heterogeneous migrant populations or other vulnerable women in the evidence syntheses. We found that a number of perinatal health outcomes were worse for migrant women than women in the host country, including mental health disorders, maternal mortality, preterm birth and congenital anomalies. The qualitative and quantitative evidence specifically relevant to women with asylum seeker and refugee status suggests that they have worse outcomes and experiences compared to the evidence from wider migrant populations (including asylum seekers and refugees) and to women in the host country, particularly relating to complex obstetric issues (e.g. SAMM, uterine rupture, eclampsia), mental health, offspring mortality, sexual assault and unwanted pregnancy, FGM, infectious disease and anaemia. However, similarities in population risk between asylum seekers, refugees and wider migrant populations were observed for some perinatal health outcomes, such as caesarean deliveries. The healthy migrant effect was reported in some of the systematic reviews, particularly relating to LBW where the risk was similar to or better than that for women in the host countries. This was reported by some authors as being an explanation for better outcomes. The evidence suggests that the healthy migrant effect is context-specific and does not translate across all migrants from all countries of origin or receiving countries. Systematic reviews reported a healthy migrant effect amongst specific populations (primarily Latina migrants in the USA) where outcomes tended to be improved compared with women in the host country, either native-born or other migrant groups. However, health inequalities were reported amongst migrant populations from other origin and/or host countries and amongst refugee and asylum seekers who, for certain outcomes, fared worse than either other migrant women or women from the host country. The heterogeneity between migrant, asylum seeker and refugee population leads us to further question the appropriateness of grouping migrant populations in research, practice and policy. Combining populations may mask the true differences in perinatal health outcomes and care requirements, and without these data the development of targeted interventions to prevent adverse outcomes is hindered.

Despite the lack of systematic reviews exclusively focussing on women with asylum seeker and refugee status, there were some data on these populations available to explore perinatal health issues amongst these groups of women. The majority of the literature which specifically focussed on women with refugee and asylum seeker status explored access to and experience of perinatal healthcare. These data showed similar barriers to access and use of perinatal healthcare as for wider migrant populations. However, additional depth of data relevant to asylum seeker and refugee women included social isolation resulting from barriers to care, mistrust of health professionals and financial concerns and poverty; the latter barriers were particularly challenging due to the inability to work and temporary and uncertain status of residency. Women's experiences of care also showed similarities to those for wider migrant populations but with apparently increased challenges with language and communication barriers and more widespread experience of racism, discrimination, stigma and stereotyping in encounters with perinatal healthcare services and professionals.

This systematic review has several strengths, particularly the comprehensive search strategy. We searched 12 databases, using a search strategy developed with an information scientist with expertise in database searching. The search strategy was developed and pre-tested using MEDLINE, then refined and retested until we were confident that it was both sensitive and specific. We also searched the reference lists of all of the included systematic reviews and implemented citation searching. These supplementary searches identified a further eight systematic reviews, which demonstrates the importance of supplementing rigorous database searches with additional search strategies. This is particularly important when searching for qualitative or observational evidence, which can be limited when using databases alone, and is a recommended approach to search strategies in the Meta-analysis Of Observational Studies in Epidemiology (MOOSE) guidelines [15]. The quality of the included reviews was judged to be either moderate or high; no review was considered to be of poor quality. However, supplementing electronic database search strategies was only carried out by authors of 20 included systematic reviews, which suggests that there may be some element of publication bias in the existing evidence syntheses. Only 21% of studies explored publication bias, which may compound bias from combining heterogeneous migrant population definitions in the analysis. A further strength includes screening and data extraction carried out independently by two researchers. We used a validated quality assessment tool to assess the quality of each included review. However, despite our use of a comprehensive search strategy, we cannot be certain that we have retrieved all relevant reviews, as our searches were restricted to English language reviews.

The main limitation of this systematic review of systematic reviews relates to data availability in the existing reviews. We had set out to consider selected pregnancy care and perinatal health outcomes specifically for women who were asylum seekers or refugees, but this couldn't be undertaken in depth as the existing evidence identified often did not allow for these sub-groups to be analysed separately. Despite the large number of studies of migration and perinatal health, there was limited evidence available for a number of pregnancy outcomes including pregnancy complications such as obstetric haemorrhage, maternal infections, maternal mortality and congenital anomalies, and although all reviews included data for women with asylum seeker and refugee status, there were limited results specific to this population. This highlights that although studies on migrant health have increased in recent years, certain maternal and offspring health outcomes remain under-researched, which limits the conclusions that can be drawn. There were also limited data exploring the risk factors for developing adverse outcomes between different migrant populations. The majority of risk factor data related to the development of mental health disorders, although these data were not stratified by the specific migrant population in question, which challenges the interpretation and application into routine care.

A review of systematic reviews will naturally result in overlapping data from multiple reviews incorporating the same original study data. We have addressed this in our review relating to the analysis of data specific to asylum seekers and refugees, detailing the number of unique studies that contributed to the results and listing these studies in Additional file 6: Asylum and Refugee Data, and by reporting the data explicitly for women with asylum seeker and refugee status separately from the results for migrant women including asylum seekers and refugees. Due to the primary focus of this review being on asylum seekers and refugees, and the volume of data relating to migrant populations (which included asylum seekers and refugees), it was not feasible to go into this level of detail for overlapping studies for this population; this is a limitation. However, we do not believe that the identification of overlapping studies included in the systematic reviews that were not explicitly related to asylum seeker and refugee populations would have added to the interpretation of results, given that the major challenge to interpretation was in the grouping of these heterogeneous populations.

Our systematic review of systematic reviews suggests a number of areas that warrant further research. There is limited evidence for women with asylum seeker and refugee status on particular perinatal outcomes such as maternal mortality, obstetric complications such as haemorrhage and infections and congenital anomalies. There is also a paucity of research into the potential causal pathways between migrant statuses and adverse health outcomes. Migrants, asylum seekers and refugees are specific populations; investigating health outcomes for these groups when they are combined presents challenges for furthering research as well as for policy and practice. When it was possible to compare migrant populations including asylum seekers and refugees with asylum seekers and refugees in this review, we were able to demonstrate some similar findings for particular health outcomes but also different and worse outcomes which are masked when groups are combined. We were unable to analyse data specific to asylum seekers and specific to refugees. We only identified one systematic review specific to asylum seekers, which suggests that further research is needed. Our systematic review specifically searched for systematic reviews on asylum seekers and refugees, but studies on other groups of vulnerable women, e.g. undocumented and migrant workers, are also needed. The development of effective interventions to support these women will not be possible if heterogeneous groups continue to be combined for research.

Our findings on the healthcare experiences of women with asylum seeker and refugee status have implications for practice. Interactions with healthcare professionals were far from optimum, with communication, discrimination and stereotyping reported. Current UK [79] and Australian [80]) guidelines share the common recommendations of health professionals needing to understand the specific needs of these groups of women; that a variety of means should be used to support women; and that there is a need to inform women of antenatal services and how to use them. Given the findings of this review on risks of maternal mental health and obstetric complications, the provision of mental health services and facilitation of timely access to antenatal care is essential for this population of women. Healthcare commissioners should also have a clear understanding of local needs so that appropriate services can be planned [79]. Implementing these recommendations into practice and providing culturally specific training for health professionals have the potential to reduce some of these negative experiences for women and also for health professionals.

Conclusions

This systematic review of systematic reviews demonstrates that women with asylum seeker and refugee status have worse perinatal health outcomes, including mental health, offspring mortality and preterm birth, compared to women from other migrant groups. Further research is warranted on particular perinatal health outcomes, e.g. maternal mortality, as well as on understanding potential causal pathways. Access, use and experience of perinatal healthcare were also reported to be far from optimal. This represents inequalities for migrant women, especially those with asylum seeker or refugee status. Improvements in care are urgently needed to increase access and enhance the experience amongst these vulnerable populations. There is an urgent need for the inclusion of unambiguous definitions of migrant groups to be used in research and for analysis to be stratified by migrant status and other migration indicators, e.g. country of origin and length of time spent in the host country. The results of this review support the need for future research on perinatal health which can make specific recommendations for policy and practice.

Additional files

Additional file 1: PRISMA checklist. Completed PRISMA reporting checklist. (DOC 58 kb)

Additional file 2: Database searches. A summary of the database search terms used in the search strategy. (DOCX 17 kb)

Additional file 3: Sample data extraction and quality appraisal. A completed example of the data extraction and quality assessment templates used in the systematic review. (DOCX 89 kb)

Additional file 4: Description of included systematic review populations. Table providing a description of the populations included in the systematic reviews that were included in this systematic review of systematic reviews. (DOCX 25 kb)

Additional file 5: Quality assessment of included systematic reviews. Table of scoring for each included systematic review against quality assessment criteria. (DOCX 17 kb)

Additional file 6: Summary of results and data sources relevant to women with asylum seeker or refugee status directly referred to by the included systematic reviews. Table providing an overview of data relating to asylum seekers and refugee women in the included systematic reviews. (DOCX 35 kb)

Abbreviations

aOR: Adjusted odds ratio; CI: Confidence interval; FGM: Female genital mutilation; JBI: Joanna Briggs Institute; LBW: Low birth weight; NICU: Neonatal intensive care unit; OR: Odds ratio; PICOS: Population Intervention Comparator Outcome Study design; RR: Relative risk; SAMM: Severe acute maternal morbidity; SGA: Small for gestational age; UK: United Kingdom; UNCHR: United Nations High Commissioner for Refugees; USA: United States of America

Acknowledgements

The authors would like to thank Alex Inskip, Librarian, Newcastle University, for his support with the development of the search strategy.

Funding

AP is funded by a UK Economic and Social Research Council North East Doctoral Training Centre Award (Ref: 160149300).

Authors' contributions

NH coordinated the project. AP, NH and JR designed the data extraction form, which was piloted by NH. AP organised the references. AP, HC and NH carried out the searches and screening. All authors performed data extraction. NH and JR drafted the paper. NH, AP and HB organised the tables for inclusion in the paper and the additional files. All authors commented and agreed on the final draft of the manuscript.

Competing interests

The authors declare that they have no competing interests.

References

1. United Nations High Commission for Refugees. Global trends: forced displacement in 2016. Geneva: United Nations High Commissioner for Refugees; 2017.
2. Cheng IH, Drillich A, Schattner P. Refugee experiences of general practice in countries of resettlement: a literature review. Br J Gen Pract. 2015;65(632): e171–6.
3. Khanlou N, Haque N, Skinner A, Mantini A, Kurtz Landy C: Scoping review on maternal health among immigrant and refugee women in Canada: prenatal, intrapartum, and postnatal care. J Pregnancy 2017, Article ID 8783294. https://doi.org/10.1155/2017/8783294.
4. Chauvin P, Simonnot N, Douay C, Vanbiervliet F: Access to healthcare for the most vulnerable in a Europe in social crisis. Doctors of the World/ Médecins du Monde International Network Position Paper; 2015.
5. Anderson FM, Hatch SL, Comacchio C, Howard LM. Prevalence and risk of mental disorders in the perinatal period among migrant women: a systematic review and meta-analysis. Archives Women's Mental Health. 2017;20(3):449–62.
6. Fellmeth G, Fazel M, Plugge E. Migration and perinatal mental health in women from low-and middle-income countries: a systematic review and meta-analysis. BJOG Int J Obstet Gynaecol. 2017;124(5):742–52.
7. Merry L, Vangen S, Small R. Caesarean births among migrant women in high-income countries. Best Practice Res Clin Obstet Gynaecol. 2016;32:88–99.
8. Schmied V, Black E, Naidoo N, Dahlen HG, Liamputtong P. Migrant women's experiences, meanings and ways of dealing with postnatal depression: a meta-ethnographic study. PLoS One. 2017;12(3):e0172385.
9. Aubrey C, Chari R, Mitchell BFP, Mumtaz Z. Gender of provider—barrier to immigrant women's obstetrical care: a narrative review. J Obstet Gynaecol Can. 2017;39(7):567–77.
10. Mengesha ZB, Dune T, Perz J. Culturally and linguistically diverse women's views and experiences of accessing sexual and reproductive health care in Australia: a systematic review. Sex Health. 2016;13(4):299–310.
11. Winn A, Hetherington E, Tough S. Systematic review of immigrant women's experiences with perinatal care in North America. JOGNN. 2017;46(5):764–75.
12. The Joanna Briggs Institute. The Joanna Briggs Institute reviewers' manual 2014: methodology for JBI umbrella reviews. Adelaide: The Joanna Briggs Institute; 2014.

13. Moher D, Liberati A, Tetzlaff J, Altman DG, PRISMA Group. Preferred reporting items for systematic reviews and meta-analyses: the PRISMA statement. PLoS Med. 2009;6(7):e1000097.
14. Hadgkiss EJ, Renzaho AMN. The physical health status, service utilisation and barriers to accessing care for asylum seekers residing in the community: a systematic review of the literature. Aust Health Rev. 2014; 38(2):142–59.
15. Stroup DF, Berlin JA, Morton SC, Olkin I, Williamson GD, Rennie D, Moher D, Becker BJ, Sipe TA, Thacker SB. Meta-analysis of observational studies in epidemiology: a proposal for reporting. Meta-analysis Of Observational Studies in Epidemiology (MOOSE) group. JAMA. 2000;283(15):2008–12.
16. Alhasanat D, Fry-McComish J. Postpartum depression among immigrant and Arabic women: literature review. J Immigr Minor Health. 2015;17(6):1882–94.
17. Falah-Hassani K, Shiri R, Vigod S, Dennis C-L. Prevalence of postpartum depression among immigrant women: a systematic review and meta-analysis. J Psychiatr Res. 2015;70:67–82.
18. Collins CH, Zimmerman C, Howard LM. Refugee, asylum seeker, immigrant women and postnatal depression: rates and risk factors. Archives Women's Mental Health. 2011;14(1):3–11.
19. De Maio FG. Immigration as pathogenic: a systematic review of the health of immigrants to Canada. Int J Equity Health. 2010;9(1):27.
20. Tobin CL, Di Napoli P, Beck CT. Refugee and immigrant women's experience of postpartum depression: a meta-synthesis. J Transcult Nurs. 2018;1:84–100.
21. Wittkowski A, Patel S, Fox JR. The experience of postnatal depression in immigrant mothers living in Western countries: a meta-synthesis. Clin Psychology Psychotherapy. 2017;24(2):411–27.
22. Nilaweera I, Doran F, Fisher J. Prevalence, nature and determinants of postpartum mental health problems among women who have migrated from South Asian to high-income countries: a systematic review of the evidence. J Affect Disord. 2014;166:213–26.
23. Higginbottom G, Bell AS, Arsenault J, Pillay J. An integrative review of experiences of maternity services for immigrant women in Canada. Diversity Equality Health Care. 2012;9:253–66
24. Pedersen GS, Grøntved A, Mortensen LH, Andersen A-MN, Rich-Edwards J. Maternal mortality among migrants in Western Europe: a meta-analysis. Matern Child Health J. 2014;18(7):1628–38.
25. Gagnon AJ, Zimbeck M, Zeitlin J. Migration to western industrialised countries and perinatal health: a systematic review. Soc Sci Med. 2009;69(6):934–46.
26. Bollini P, Pampallona S, Wanner P, Kupelnick B. Pregnancy outcome of migrant women and integration policy: a systematic review of the international literature. Soc Sci Med. 2009;68(3):452–61.
27. Gissler M, Alexander S, Macfarlane A, Small R, Stray-Pedersen B, Zeitlin J, Zimbeck M, Gagnon A. Stillbirths and infant deaths among migrants in industrialized countries. Acta Obstet Gynecol Scand. 2009;88(2):134–48.
28. Merry L, Small R, Blondel B, Gagnon AJ. International migration and caesarean birth: a systematic review and meta-analysis. BMC Pregnancy Childbirth. 2013;13:27.
29. Villalonga-Olives E, Kawachi I, von Steinbüchel N. Pregnancy and birth outcomes among immigrant women in the US and Europe: a systematic review. J Immigr Minor Health. 2017;6:1469–87.
30. Balaam MC, Akerjordet K, Lyberg A, Kaiser B, Schoening E, Fredriksen AM, Ensel A, Gouni O, Severinsson E. A qualitative review of migrant women's perceptions of their needs and experiences related to pregnancy and childbirth. J Adv Nurs. 2013;69(9):1919–30.
31. Downe S, Finlayson K, Walsh D, Lavender T. 'Weighing up and balancing out': a meta-synthesis of barriers to antenatal care for marginalised women in high-income countries. BJOG Int J Obstet Gynaecol. 2009;116(4):518–29.
32. Higginbottom GMA, Hadziabdic E, Yohani S, Paton P. Immigrant women's experience of maternity services in Canada: a meta-ethnography. Midwifery. 2014;30(5):544–59.
33. Small R, Roth C, Raval M, Shafiei T, Korfker D, Heaman M, McCourt C, Gagnon A. Immigrant and non-immigrant women's experiences of maternity care: a systematic and comparative review of studies in five countries. BMC Pregnancy Childbirth. 2014;14:152.
34. Wikberg A, Bondas T. A patient perspective in research on intercultural caring in maternity care: a meta-ethnography. Int J Qual Stud Health Well-being. 2010;5(1):4648.
35. Heaman M, Bayrampour H, Kingston D, Blondel B, Gissler M, Roth C, Alexander S, Gagnon A. Migrant women's utilization of prenatal care: a systematic review. Matern Child Health J. 2013;17(5):816–36.
36. Higginbottom GMA, Morgan M, Alexandre M, Chiu Y, Forgeron J, Kocay D, Barolia R. Immigrant women's experiences of maternity-care services in Canada: a systematic review using a narrative synthesis. Systematic Reviews. 2015;4(1):13.
37. Stewart DE, Gagnon A, Saucier J-F, Wahoush O, Dougherty G. Postpartum depression symptoms in newcomers. Can J Psychiatry. 2008;53(2):121–4.
38. Gagnon AJ, Merry L, Haase K. Predictors of emergency cesarean delivery among international migrant women in Canada. Int J Gynecol Obstet. 2013; 121(3):270–4.
39. Merry LA, Gagnon AJ, Kalim N, Bouris SS. Refugee claimant women and barriers to health and social services post-birth. Can J Public Health. 2011;4: 286–90.
40. Kurth E, Jaeger FN, Zemp E, Tschudin S, Bischoff A. Reproductive health care for asylum-seeking women—a challenge for health professionals. BMC Public Health. 2010;10(1):659.
41. Kennedy P, Murphy-Lawless J. The maternity care needs of refugee and asylum seeking women in Ireland. Fem Rev. 2003;73(1):39–53.
42. McLeish J: Maternity experiences of asylum seekers in England. Br J Midwifery 2005, 13(12):782–785.
43. Briscoe L, Lavender T: Exploring maternity care for asylum seekers and refugees. Br J Midwifery 2009, 17(1):17–23.
44. Iliadi P. Refugee women in Greece: a qualitative study of their attitudes and experience in antenatal care. Health Sci J. 2008;2(3):173–180
45. Matthey S, Silove D, Barnett B, Fitzgerald MH, Mitchell P. Correlates of depression and PTSD in Cambodian women with young children: a pilot study. Stress Health. 1999;15(2):103–7.
46. Edge D: Perinatal depression: its absence among Black Caribbean women. Br JMidwifery 2006, 14(11):646–652.
47. Reynolds B, White J. Seeking asylum and motherhood: health and wellbeing needs. Community Practitioner. 2010;830(20):3.
48. Gagnon AJ, Dougherty G, Wahoush O, Saucier J-F, Dennis C-L, Stanger E, Palmer B, Merry L, Stewart DE. International migration to Canada: the post-birth health of mothers and infants by immigration class. Soc Sci Med. 2013;76:197–207.
49. Lalchandani S, MacQuillan K, Sheil O. Obstetric profiles and pregnancy outcomes of immigrant women with refugee status. Ir Med J. 2001;94(3):79–80.
50. Essén B, Hanson BS, ÖStergren PO, Lindquist PG, Gudmundsson S. Increased perinatal mortality among sub-Saharan immigrants in a city-population in Sweden. Acta Obstet Gynecol Scand. 2000;79(9):737–43.
51. Schulpen TWJ, Van Steenbergen JE, Van Driel HF. Influences of ethnicity on perinatal and child mortality in the Netherlands. Arch Dis Child. 2001;84(3):222–6.
52. Vangen S, Stoltenberg C, Johansen REB, Sundby J, Stray-Pedersen B. Perinatal complications among ethnic Somalis in Norway. Acta Obstet Gynecol Scand. 2002;81(4):317–22.
53. Kuvacic I, Skrablin S, Hodzic D, Milkovic G. Possible influence of expatriation on perinatal outcome. Acta Obstet Gynecol Scand. 1996;75(4):367–71.
54. Nedić B, Loncar S, Ravić J, Komazec J. Deliveries in the outpatient birthing facility in Ruma during 1989 and between 1992 and 1995. Med Pregl. 1999; 52(1–2):53–6.
55. Goosen S, Uitenbroek D, Wijsen C, Stronks K. Induced abortions and teenage births among asylum seekers in The Netherlands: analysis of national surveillance data. J Epidemiology Community Health. 2009;7: 528–33.
56. Rogstad KE, Dale H. What are the needs of asylum seekers attending an STI clinic and are they significantly different from those of British patients? Int J STD AIDS. 2004;15(8):515–8.
57. Gagnon AJ, Stanger E, Dougherty G, Oxman-Martinez J, Platt RW, Saucier J-F, Wahoush O, Merry L, George A, Stewart DE. Refugee and refugee-claimant women and infants post-birth: migration histories as a predictor of Canadian health system response to needs. Can J Public Health. 2007;4:287–91.
58. Kandasamy T, Cherniak R, Shah R, Yudin MH, Spitzer R. Obstetric risks and outcomes of refugee women at a single centre in Toronto. J Obstet Gynaecol Can. 2014;36(4):296–302.
59. Small R, Gagnon A, Gissler M, Zeitlin J, Bennis M, Glazier RH, Haelterman E, Martens G, McDermott S, Urquia M. Somali women and their pregnancy outcomes postmigration: data from six receiving countries. BJOG Int J Obstet Gynaecol. 2008;115(13):1630–40.
60. Reed MM, Westfall JM, Bublitz C, Battaglia C, Fickenscher A. Birth outcomes in Colorado's undocumented immigrant population. BMC Public Health. 2005;5(1):100.

61. Kelaher M, Jessop DJ. Differences in low-birthweight among documented and undocumented foreign-born and US-born Latinas. Soc Sci Med. 2002; 55(12):2171–5.
62. Van Hanegem N, Miltenburg AS, Zwart JJ, Bloemenkamp KWM, Van Roosmalen JOS. Severe acute maternal morbidity in asylum seekers: a two-year nationwide cohort study in the Netherlands. Acta Obstet Gynecol Scand. 2011;90(9):1010–6.
63. Harper Bulman K, McCourt C. Somali refugee women's experiences of maternity care in west London: a case study. Critical Public Health. 2002; 12(4):365–80.
64. Herrel N, Olevitch L, DuBois DK, Terry P, Thorp D, Kind E, Said A. Somali refugee women speak out about their needs for care during pregnancy and delivery. J Midwifery Women's Health. 2004;49(4):345–9.
65. Dartnall L, Ganguly N, Batterham J. Access to Maternity Services Research Report. London: COI and Department of Health; 2005.
66. Riggs E, Davis E, Gibbs L, Block K, Szwarc J, Casey S, Duell-Piening P, Waters E. Accessing maternal and child health services in Melbourne, Australia: reflections from refugee families and service providers. BMC Health Serv Res. 2012;12:117
67. Redwood-Campbell L, Thind H, Howard M, Koteles J, Fowler N, Kaczorowski J. Understanding the health of refugee women in host countries: lessons from the Kosovar re-settlement in Canada. Prehospital and Disaster Medicine. 2008;23(4):322–7.
68. Carolan M, Cassar L. Pregnancy care for African refugee women in Australia: attendance at antenatal appointments. Evidence-Based Midwifery. 2007;5(2):54–9.
69. Carolan M, Cassar L. Antenatal care perceptions of pregnant African women attending maternity services in Melbourne, Australia. Midwifery. 2010;26(2): 189–201.
70. Hill N, Hunt E, Hyrkäs K. Somali immigrant women's health care experiences and beliefs regarding pregnancy and birth in the United States. J Transcult Nurs. 2012;23(1):72–81.
71. Kulig JC. Childbearing beliefs among Cambodian refugee women. West J Nurs Res. 1990;12(1):108–18.
72. O'Mahony JM, Donnelly TT, Bouchal SR, Este D. Cultural background and socioeconomic influence of immigrant and refugee women coping with postpartum depression. J Immigr Minor Health. 2013;15(2):300–14.
73. Allotey P, Manderson L, Baho S, Demian L. Reproductive health for resettling refugee and migrant women. Health issues. 2004;78:12–7.
74. Carroll J, Epstein R, Fiscella K, Gipson T, Volpe E, Jean-Pierre P. Caring for Somali women: implications for clinician–patient communication. Patient Educ Couns. 2007;66(3):337–45.
75. Murray L, Windsor C, Parker E, Tewfik O. The experiences of African women giving birth in Brisbane, Australia. Health Care Women Int. 2010;31(5):458–72.
76. Beine K, Fullerton J, Palinkas L, Anders B. Conceptions of prenatal care among Somali women in San Diego. J Nurse Midwifery. 1995;40(4):376–81.
77. Huster KMJ, Patterson N, Schilperoord M, Spiegel P. Cesarean sections among Syrian refugees in Lebanon from December 2012/January 2013 to June 2013: probable causes and recommendations. Yale J Biology Medicine. 2014;87(3):269.
78. O'Mahony JM, Donnelly TT, Bouchal SR, Este D. Barriers and facilitators of social supports for immigrant and refugee women coping with postpartum depression. Adv Nurs Sci. 2012;35(3):E42–56.
79. National Institute of Health and Care Excellence (NICE) CG110 Pregnancy and complex social factors: a model for service provision for pregnant women with complex social factors 2010. https://www.nice.org.uk/guidance/cg110. Accessed 25 Jan 2018.
80. Department of Health. Clinical Practice Guidelines: Pregnancy Care. Canberra: Australian Government Department of Health; 2018.

Baseline exposure, antibody subclass, and hepatitis B response differentially affect malaria protective immunity following RTS,S/AS01E vaccination in African children

Itziar Ubillos[1], Aintzane Ayestaran[1], Augusto J Nhabomba[2], David Dosoo[3], Marta Vidal[1], Alfons Jiménez[1,4], Chenjerai Jairoce[2], Hèctor Sanz[1], Ruth Aguilar[1], Nana Aba Williams[1], Núria Díez-Padrisa[1], Maximilian Mpina[5], Hermann Sorgho[6], Selidji Todagbe Agnandji[7,8], Simon Kariuki[9], Benjamin Mordmüller[10], Claudia Daubenberger[5,10], Kwaku Poku Asante[3], Seth Owusu-Agyei[3], Jahit Sacarlal[2,11], Pedro Aide[2], John J Aponte[1,2], Sheetij Dutta[12], Ben Gyan[3,13], Joseph J Campo[1,2], Clarissa Valim[14,15], Gemma Moncunill[1,2] and Carlota Dobaño[1,2*]

Abstract

Background: The RTS,S/AS01E vaccine provides partial protection against malaria in African children, but immune responses have only been partially characterized and do not reliably predict protective efficacy. We aimed to evaluate comprehensively the immunogenicity of the vaccine at peak response, the factors affecting it, and the antibodies associated with protection against clinical malaria in young African children participating in the multicenter phase 3 trial for licensure.

Methods: We measured total IgM, IgG, and IgG_{1-4} subclass antibodies to three constructs of the *Plasmodium falciparum* circumsporozoite protein (CSP) and hepatitis B surface antigen (HBsAg) that are part of the RTS,S vaccine, by quantitative suspension array technology. Plasma and serum samples were analyzed in 195 infants and children from two sites in Ghana (Kintampo) and Mozambique (Manhiça) with different transmission intensities using a case-control study design. We applied regression models and machine learning techniques to analyze immunogenicity, correlates of protection, and factors affecting them.

Results: RTS,S/AS01E induced IgM and IgG, predominantly IgG1 and IgG3, but also IgG2 and IgG4, subclass responses. Age, site, previous malaria episodes, and baseline characteristics including antibodies to CSP and other antigens reflecting malaria exposure and maternal IgGs, nutritional status, and hemoglobin concentration, significantly affected vaccine immunogenicity. We identified distinct signatures of malaria protection and risk in RTS,S/AS01E but not in comparator vaccinees. IgG2 and IgG4 responses to RTS,S antigens post-vaccination, and anti-CSP and anti-*P. falciparum* antibody levels pre-vaccination, were associated with malaria risk over 1-year follow-up. In contrast, antibody responses to HBsAg (all isotypes, subclasses, and timepoints) and post-vaccination IgG1 and IgG3 to CSP C-terminus and NANP were associated with protection. Age and site affected the relative contribution of responses in the correlates identified.

(Continued on next page)

* Correspondence: carlota.dobano@isglobal.org
[1]ISGlobal, Hospital Clínic, Universitat de Barcelona, Carrer Rosselló 153 CEK building, E-08036 Barcelona, Catalonia, Spain
[2]Centro de Investigação em Saúde de Manhiça (CISM), Rua 12, Cambeve, Vila de Manhiça, CP 1929 Maputo, Mozambique
Full list of author information is available at the end of the article

(Continued from previous page)

Conclusions: Cytophilic IgG responses to the C-terminal and NANP repeat regions of CSP and anti-HBsAg antibodies induced by RTS,S/AS01E vaccination were associated with malaria protection. In contrast, higher malaria exposure at baseline and non-cytophilic IgG responses to CSP were associated with disease risk. Data provide new correlates of vaccine success and failure in African children and reveal key insights into the mode of action that can guide development of more efficacious next-generation vaccines.

Keywords: Malaria, Vaccine, Antibody, RTS,S, *Plasmodium falciparum*, Immunogenicity, Correlate protection, African children, Hepatitis B

Background

Malaria was estimated to cause 445,000 deaths globally in 2016, mostly attributable to *Plasmodium falciparum* in African children [1]. A reduction in malaria-associated deaths and morbidity has been attained in the last years by combining malaria control interventions, such as vector-targeted measures including distribution of long-lasting insecticide-treated bednets and indoor residual spraying, as well as mass drug administration [2]. However, emerging mosquito resistance to insecticides [3], parasite resistance to drugs [4–7], and non-sustained surveillance strategies [8] can jeopardize malaria elimination strategies. Furthermore, there is a potential for a rebound of malaria illness if immunity is lost as a result of sustained elimination campaigns, in case *P. falciparum* transmission is later reintroduced [9]. In this scenario, an effective malaria vaccine remains an essential tool to reduce and sustain malaria burden at low levels and facilitate elimination [10].

RTS,S/AS01E (Mosquirix™) has consistently provided partial protection against malaria in African children, as demonstrated in phase 3 clinical trial [11–15]. RTS,S/AS01E is based on virus-like particles with the hepatitis B surface antigen (HBsAg) and a fragment of the *P. falciparum* circumsporozoite protein (CSP), which comprises the central repeat region $(NANP)_n$ and the C-terminus (C-term) [16], formulated with GlaxoSmithKline's proprietary adjuvant AS01. RTS,S/AS01E generates high IgG titers to the CSP NANP immunodominant B cell epitope that remains above naturally acquired titers for years [17]. However, such antibodies have not consistently correlated with protection across all ages and malaria endpoints [14, 18]. Since only total IgG responses to NANP have been measured in field trials thus far, it is possible that (i) other CSP antigenic epitopes are targets of vaccine-induced protective immunity and (ii) the isotype/subclass balance, important for effector function of antibodies, is more relevant in protection against malaria than the magnitude of the IgG response. Binding kinetics of anti-NANP antibodies has been analyzed in pilot experiments and showed no strong association with protection in African children, although longitudinal analyses indicated an effect of previous exposure to vaccine or natural infection [19, 20] that can be mimicked by fractional last doses [21]. This shows that it is crucial to understand how RTS,S immunogenicity and vaccine efficacy are affected by baseline factors like age at first vaccination, sex, maternal antibodies, and malaria transmission intensity (MTI) [22]. Efforts to improve RTS,S efficacy to rationally develop and deploy second-generation vaccines should rely on a better understanding of its mode of action, currently unknown, to unravel why RTS,S does not prevent a higher proportion of malaria episodes in African children and what are the factors affecting this.

In this study, we set out to characterize in detail the immunogenicity of the RTS,S/AS01E vaccine in the African pediatric multicenter phase 3 clinical trial and assess the association between the fine epitope specificity and isotype/subclass of the antibody response and protection against clinical malaria. We measured total IgG and, for the first time, IgM as well as IgG1, IgG2, IgG3, and IgG4 responses to the HBsAg and to three CSP constructs: a full-length (FL) and two truncated proteins, one with the central $NANP_{16}$ repeat region and the other with the C-term region [16]. In addition, we investigated the effect of baseline variables including age, malaria exposure, maternal antibodies, sex, and nutritional status on immunogenicity and protection. By applying regression models and machine learning techniques, we identified novel antibody signatures at baseline and induced by RTS,S/AS01E vaccination that correlated with protection and risk from clinical malaria, defined their antigen targets and Ig isotypes/subclasses, and assessed their determinants.

Methods

Design

This study was carried out in two of the seven sites included in the multicenter immunology study MAL067, ancillary to the phase 3 randomized clinical trial MAL055 (NCT00866619)—Kintampo in Ghana (representative of moderate-high MTI) and Manhiça in Mozambique (representative of low MTI) [18], to be able to assess the effect of MTI on vaccine responses. These two sites were prioritized due to higher availability of sufficient numbers and volumes of samples from both study visits and age cohorts. Subjects were followed up by passive case detection (PCD) starting 14 days after sample collection at month (M) 3, approximately 44 days after the third dose (M2), for the subsequent 12 months, when they were censored.

Children age 5–17 months and infants age 6–12 weeks with ≥ 150 μL plasma/serum samples available at M0 (baseline) and M3 were selected. We included 129 RTS,S/AS01E-vaccinated and 66 comparator-vaccinated children and infants from both sites (Fig. 1, Additional file 1: Table S1). For the correlates of malaria disease protection and risk analysis, 78 children and infants were randomly selected from Kintampo, 117 participants were selected from Manhiça according to a prior case-control study of cellular markers [23], and all were analyzed in a case-control design.

Antibody assays

Quantitative suspension array technology (qSAT) [24, 25] was used to measure antibody responses to three CSP constructs (FL, NANP repeat, and C-term [residues 274 to 387: KNNQG...SSIGL] recombinant proteins from WRAIR) and HBsAg (Abcam). The qSAT assays applied the xMAP™ technology (Luminex Corp., TX) and were previously standardized and optimized to control for sources of variability [26, 27]. The multiplex antigen panel also included 32 *P. falciparum* proteins [26, 27] analyzed as markers of malaria exposure and maternally transferred antibodies (see below). Briefly, antigen-coupled multiplex beads were mixed with 50 μL of test sample, negative or positive control [28, 29] at multiple dilutions (see Additional file 1: Supplementary methods). After incubation and washing, biotinylated secondary antibodies were added. Following streptavidin-R-phycoerythrin incubations, samples were acquired with a Luminex 100/200 analyzer and antibody levels measured as median fluorescence intensity (MFI). Data pre-processing is detailed in Additional file 1: Supplementary methods.

Statistical analysis

RTS,S/AS01E immunogenicity was evaluated for all antigens/Ig using basic descriptive methods (see Additional file 1: Supplementary methods) and longitudinal linear mixed effects models [30] including vaccination, visit (M0, M3) and the interaction between them, and adjusting by site. The effect of the vaccine on Ig responses at M3, and on change on Ig levels from M0 to M3, was assessed through tests of the corresponding fixed effects. All models included a random intercept for the individual and a random slope for changes over time among predictors (see Additional file 1: Supplementary methods). To evaluate more thoroughly the impact of age on post-vaccination levels and association between pre- and post-vaccination in RTS,S vaccinees, mixed effects models adjusted by site were also estimated across age cohorts (children and infants).

To understand the effect of the remaining study covariates on M3 Ig levels to all antigens, we fitted first univariate and next multivariable linear regression models (coefficient, 95% confidence intervals (CI), adjusted p values) including only RTS,S vaccinees, with the following predictors: sex, malaria transmission season at M3, having clinical malaria episodes between M0 and M3, and baseline variables like

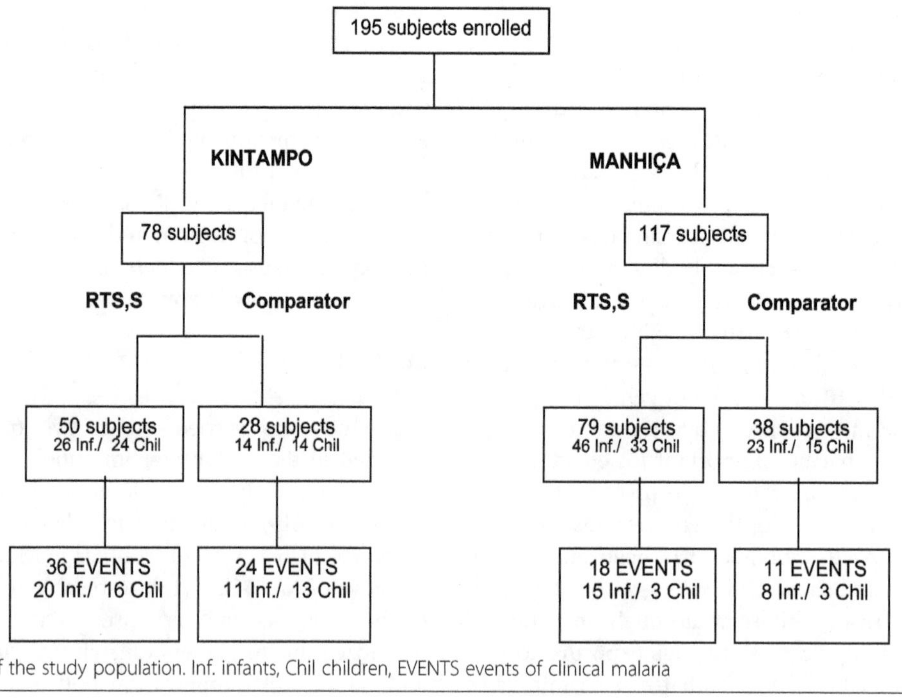

Fig. 1 Flowchart of the study population. Inf. infants, Chil children, EVENTS events of clinical malaria

age (in weeks), antibody levels, hemoglobin (Hb) concentrations, weight-for-age Z score (WAZ), and height-for-age Z score (HAZ). For comparison purposes, models were also fitted at pre-vaccination and on comparator vaccinees at M3. Malaria transmission season was defined as high between April–October for Kintampo and November–April for Manhiça; the remaining months were defined as low transmission. The effect of baseline antibody levels was evaluated in three different ways. First, using the same antigen/Ig as the outcome variable at M3. Second, a *P. falciparum* exposure index was defined as follows [27, 31]. Upon examination of antibody responses to the 32 antigen panel [26, 27], we selected 28 markers in which IgM responses were M3 > M0 and thus acquired with age (e.g., children > infants) and exposure (e.g., Kintampo > Manhiça). Principal component analysis (PCA) of IgM responses to these antigens was performed to construct the corresponding variables, and the first component (PC1) that explained 63% of the variability was selected. Third, a *P. falciparum* maternal antibody index was defined in subjects < 10 months of age [27, 31]. For this, 17 antigens including two VAR2CSA pregnancy-specific antigen constructs were selected which IgG responses were M0 > M3 and thus declined with age (e.g., infants > children) and were higher in infants from the high MTI site (e.g., Kintampo > Manhiça). The construction of the maternal score was done in the same way as the exposure score. We selected the first component that explained 54% of the variability. Linearity of the associations with continuous covariates was evaluated through penalized splines in generalized additive models (GAM); variables were modeled as linear. A stepwise algorithm was used in multivariable models.

Analysis of correlates of protection was based on the case-control design. The outcome was clinical malaria detected by PCD defined by fever > 37.5 °C with any parasitemia in the 12 months after the start of follow-up (M3 plus 14 days). Logistic regression models (odds ratio (OR), 95% CI, adjusted p values) were fitted first univariate and next multivariable to obtain the effect of different predictors in the odds of having malaria. Main predictors included levels ($\log_{10}$MFI) of antibodies at M3, increment of antibody levels between M0 and M3, and ratios (IgG1 + IgG2)/(IgG2 + IgG4) at M3, in RTS,S vaccinees (comparators modeled separately for comparison purposes). The impact of the other covariates (same as above) on the association between antibody responses and clinical malaria risk/protection was also assessed. The linearity of the $\log_{10}$-transformed antibody levels was evaluated when the outcome was case-control. Univariate models were adjusted by site.

Next, multivariable models were obtained in RTS,S-vaccinated subjects through the stepwise algorithm, R package *MASS*, and function *stepAIC*. Both backwards and forward methods were combined to obtain the model with the minimum Akaike information criterion (AIC). All potential single variables were proposed in the first step of the model, not only the significant ones. For the assessment of the maternal index, only subjects < 10 months were taken into account. Correction for multiple testing was done by Holm [32] when analyzing IgG and IgM (with the following predictors: M3 antibody levels and M0–M3 change in antibodies) and IgG subclass ratios. Benjamini-Hochberg [33] was used when IgG_{1-4} subclass levels were the predictors. Holm was used to control for family wise error when there were few tests, whereas Benjamini-Hochberg was used to control for the false discovery rate when there were more tests (e.g., IgG_{1-4}). HBsAg was analyzed separately from CSP constructs.

Finally, to identify the most relevant antibody variables associated with clinical malaria in multi-marker analysis, three machine learning algorithms were computed: (i) elastic net, which is a shrinkage regression that simultaneously does automatic variable selection and continuous shrinkage and can select groups of correlated variables; (ii) recursive feature elimination algorithm using support vector machines (SVM) [34] with linear kernel, which recursively removes features of low importance (computed using the weights of the linear SVM); and (iii) random forest, which constructs a multitude of uncorrelated decision trees and defines the importance of each variable by applying the permutation of the variable's values approach [35]. The optimal tuning parameter values for each machine learning method, i.e., α and λ penalty parameters of elastic net, cost parameter of linear SVM, and number of trees and number of variables to be included in each iteration of random forest, were computed using a 5-fold cross-validation approach [36].

Results

RTS,S/AS01E vaccine immunogenicity

Three doses of RTS,S/AS01E vaccination at 1-month intervals induced a highly statistically significant increase in antibody levels ($\log_{10}$MFI) to CSP FL, NANP repeat, and C-term antigens and to HBsAg, from baseline (M0) to 1 month after the third dose (M3) for all Ig isotypes and subclasses ($p < 0.001$) (Fig. 2). Comparisons of the magnitude of antibody responses to the RTS,S antigens between the various isotypes/subclasses, and the correlations among them, are shown in Additional file 1: Supplementary results Table S2. Fold changes in RTS,S-specific antibody levels at post-vaccination compared to baseline were evaluated with mixed models (Additional file 1: Table S3). Overall differences between pre- and post-vaccination conferred by RTS,S were significant; for IgG, IgG1, and IgG3, they were substantially higher than for IgG2 and IgG4; changes for HBsAg were lesser than those for CSP. Comparator vaccinees had no or negligible increases in responses

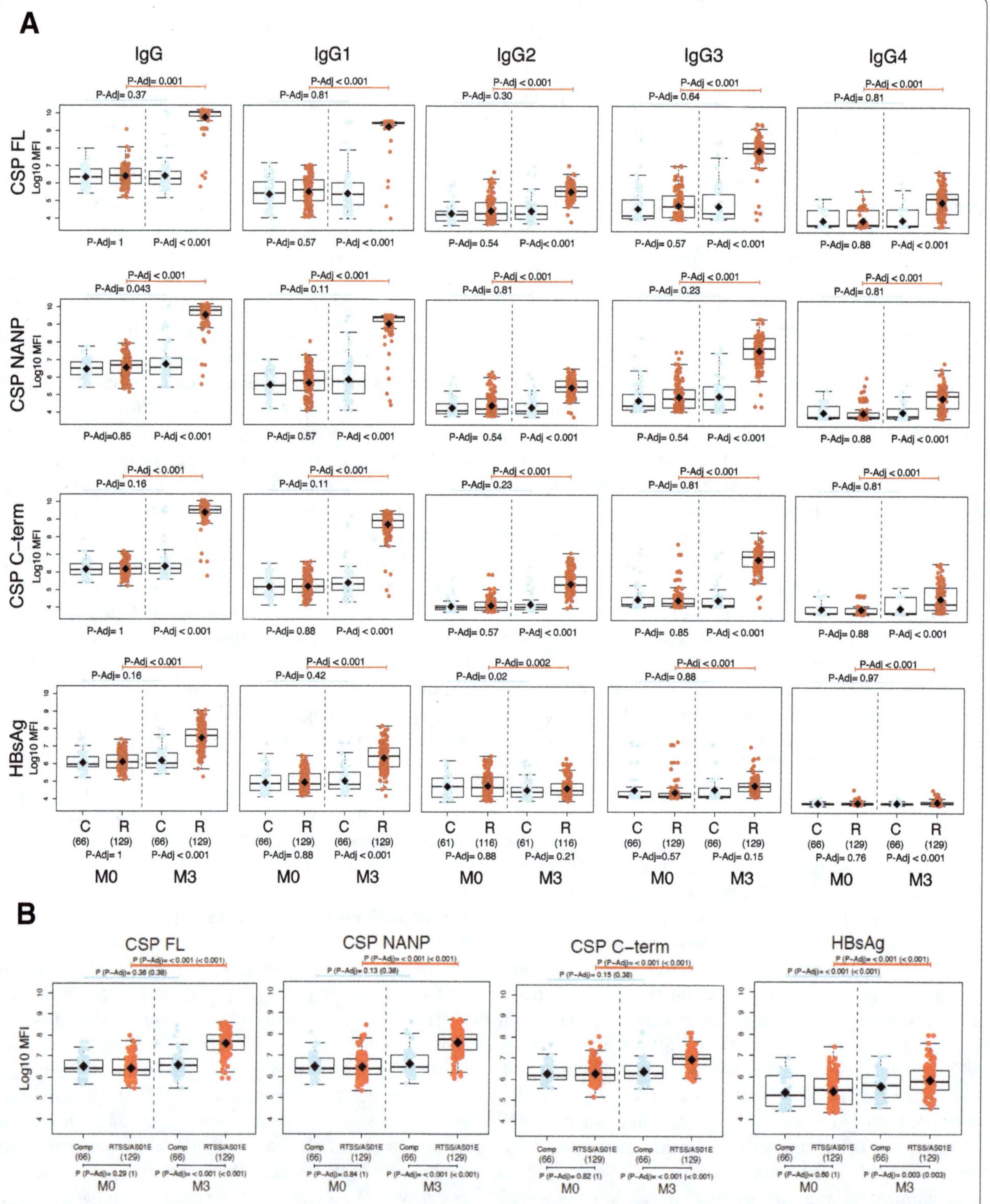

Fig. 2 RTS,S/AS01E vaccine immunogenicity: CSP and HBsAg antibody responses in RTS,S and comparator vaccinees comparing pre- and post-vaccination. **a** IgG antibody levels (*R* = RTS,S; *C* = comparators). **b** IgM antibody levels. Groups were compared through *t* tests and *p* values adjusted by Holm for IgG and IgM and by Benjamini-Hochberg for IgG_{1-4}, as explained in the "Methods" section

from pre- to post-vaccination. When contrasting RTS,S vs comparators at post-vaccination, the highest ratios were again recorded for IgG and IgG1 and the lowest for IgM, followed by IgG4 and IgG2 (Additional file 1: Figure S4).

Effect of age

Children vaccinated with RTS,S/AS01E had significantly higher levels of IgG to all CSP constructs, and of IgG1 and IgG3 (but not other isotypes/subclasses) to NANP and C-term, than infants at M3 (Additional file 1: Figure S5). Levels of antibodies to HBsAg at M3 were also higher in RTS,S-vaccinated children than infants, except for IgG2. Regarding changes in antibody levels from pre- to post-vaccination, children had a greater increase to all RTS,S antigens than infants, particularly for CSP FL (all isotypes and subclasses) (Additional file 1: Table S3 and Figure S6). Statistically significant or marginally significant differences between infants and children were recorded in IgG (CSP FL, C-term, and NANP), IgG1 (CSP FL), IgG2 (CSP FL and NANP), and IgG3 (CSP FL, C-term, and NANP). For HBsAg, RTS,S-vaccinated children had significantly higher pre- to post-vaccination changes for IgG, IgM, and IgG1 than infants. Ratios of antibody levels in RTS,S to comparators at post-vaccination in infants and children are reported in Additional file 1: Figure S7. Using univariate linear models adjusted by site, we evaluated whether Ig levels induced by RTS,S vaccination changed with age when computed as a continuous variable within infant and children cohorts (Additional file 1: Table S4). We found that for HBsAg (but not CSP), $\log_{10}$MFIs for most antibodies significantly increased for every 1-week increase in age at baseline in infants and children. Antibody seropositivity was consistent between age groups except for HBsAg (Additional file 1: Table S5).

Effect of site

Levels of IgG, IgG1, and IgG3 to CSP or HBsAg in RTS,S vaccinees at M3 were not different in the two sites (Additional file 1: Figures S8 and S9 stratified also by age), whereas levels of IgG2 to all CSP constructs and IgG4 to CSP FL were significantly higher in Kintampo (high MTI) than Manhiça (low MTI). Levels of anti-CSP IgM at M3 did not differ by site, but anti-HBsAg IgMs and IgG4 were higher in Manhiça than Kintampo (Additional file 1: Table S6). Some associations between prior clinical malaria episodes or between malaria transmission season at M3 and antibody responses in univariate analysis were lost when adjusted by site (data not shown).

Effect of baseline CSP and HBsAg antibodies

Anti-CSP IgG levels at M0 were usually higher in infants than children but not statistically significant with this limited sample size (Additional file 1: Figure S6). Significantly higher IgM and lower IgG2 to HBsAg were detected in children, who had been previously vaccinated with the pentavalent DTwP-HBV-Hib vaccine (as part of the routine expanded program of immunization (EPI)) compared to infants ($p < 0.001$). Consistent with higher MTI, levels of IgG, IgG1, IgG2, and IgG3 to CSP constructs (and of IgM in children) were higher in Kintampo than Manhiça at baseline, but this did not happen for antibodies against HBsAg (Additional file 1: Table S7). In fact, pre-vaccination levels of anti-HBsAg IgG2, and of IgG4 in children, were significantly higher in Manhiça than in Kintampo.

We tested whether pre-vaccination levels had an impact on post-RTS,S vaccination responses by fitting regression models in each age group [18] and found no consistent associations with anti-CSP antibodies. Correlation coefficients were low and with varying direction, although a trend ($p = 0.05$) was observed for CSP NANP whereby infants with higher M0 had lower M3 IgG and IgG1 levels (Additional file 1: Figure S6, Fig. 3), but no effect was detected in children, except for CSP FL IgG2. However, there was a significant effect for HBsAg whereby children with higher M0 IgG, IgM, and IgG2 (also for infants) had higher M3 levels. There was no significant correlation between baseline HBsAg antibodies and CSP responses at M3, or the opposite (data not shown).

Effect of baseline maternal P. falciparum antibodies

Summary scores based on IgGs to malarial antigens at baseline in subjects younger than 10 months are shown on Additional file 1: Table S8 and Figure S10. At M0, there was a significant positive association between the maternal malaria antibody index and anti-CSP IgGs, but this was not the case for CSP IgM or for anti-HBsAg antibodies, except IgG2 (Additional file 1: Table S9). In fact, there was a significant negative association with anti-HBsAg IgM (also in comparator vaccines at M3) and IgG3 levels at baseline and a positive association for IgG2. Regarding the impact on M3 RTS,S responses, maternal antibodies were significantly negatively associated with IgG and IgG1 HBsAg levels (borderline associations to some CSP constructs) (Additional file 1: Table S9).

Effect of baseline P. falciparum exposure antibodies

Summary scores based on naturally acquired antimalarial IgM (to distinguish from maternally derived IgG) are shown in Additional file 1: Table S8 and Figure S10. At M0, there was a significant positive association between malaria exposure and IgMs to all CSPs and HBsAg (Additional file 1: Table S10). When stratifying by age, the association with HBsAg IgM was only significant in infants (data not shown). Regarding the impact on M3 responses to RTS,S, the malaria exposure index was significantly and positively associated with IgG, IgG1, and

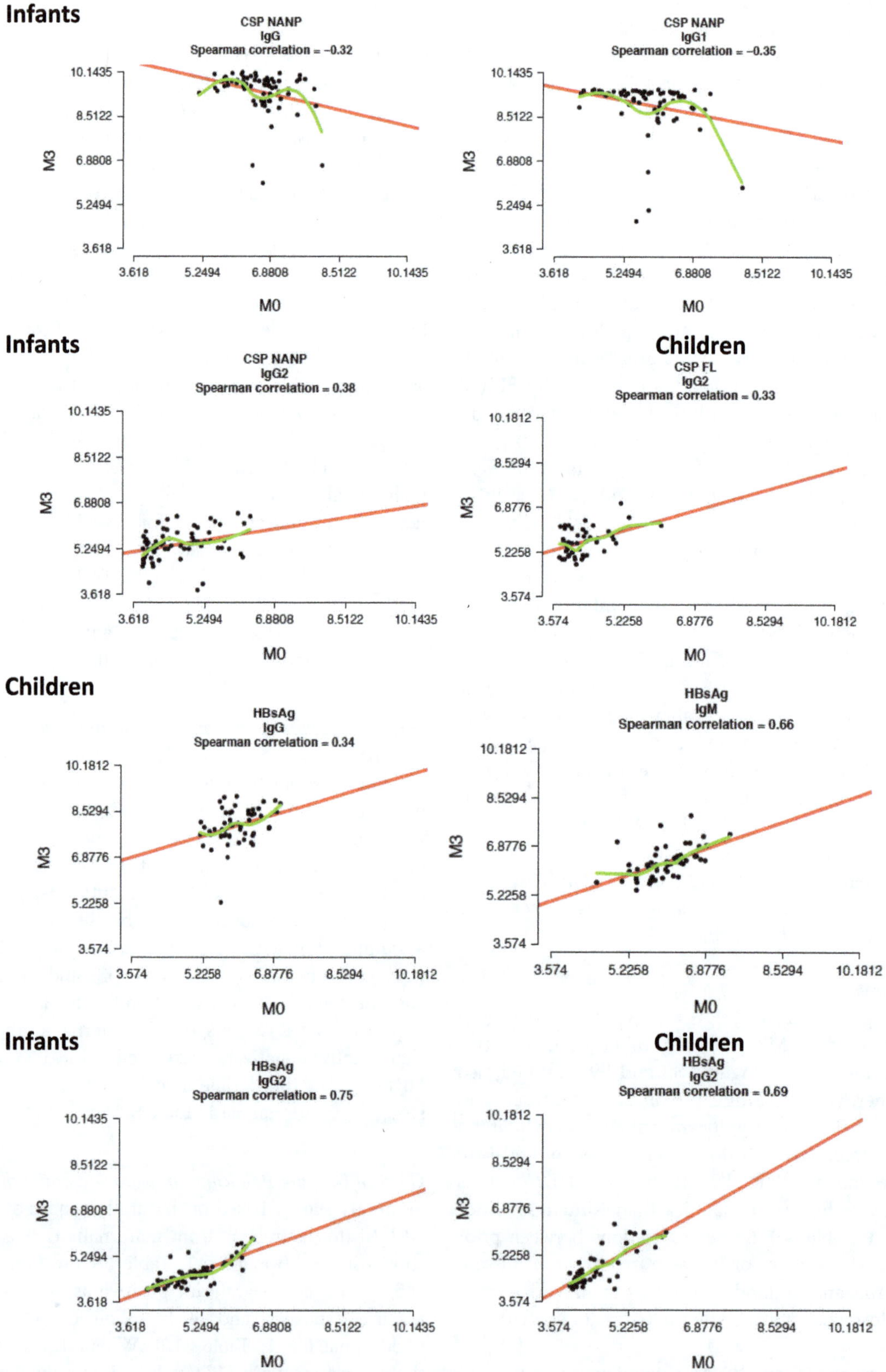

Fig. 3 Effect of pre-vaccination (M0) antibody levels on post-vaccination (M3) RTS,S immunogenicity. Some representative examples of antibody isotypes/subclasses and antigens are shown. Spearman correlation coefficients are included as well as linear regression and non-parametric LOESS estimations, as red and green lines, respectively. See Additional file 1: Figure S6 for further details

IgM (borderline for IgG3) HBsAg levels, also in comparator vaccinees for IgM (Additional file 1: Table S10).

Multivariable linear regression analysis of immunogenicity

Factors significantly affecting the magnitude of RTS,S antibody responses at M3 depending on the antigen/Ig are shown in Table 1. Whilst all Ig tended to increase with age, C-term and FL (but not NANP) CSP IgG2 levels decreased in subjects younger than 10 months (Additional file 1: Table S11). Site strongly affected HBsAg antibody levels, not only for IgM but also for IgGs (Table 1), particularly in subjects of age < 10 months (Additional file 1: Table S11), which were higher in Manhiça than Kintampo, as well as IgG2 and IgG4 to CSPs, which were higher in Kintampo than Manhiça. Here, prior malaria episodes (rather than exposure index) were significantly associated with higher HBsAg IgG, IgG1, and IgM, and CSP (NANP and C-term) IgG4, M3 levels. Furthermore, a statistically significant negative impact of high baseline NANP (borderline for C-term) CSP IgG on M3 responses emerged, and the positive effect of baseline HBsAg IgG2 and IgM remained. Higher anti-*P. falciparum* maternal IgG at M0 was also inversely associated with CSP (not HBsAg) IgG levels at M3 in subjects age < 10-month old (Additional file 1: Table S11).

RTS,S/AS01E-induced antibody correlates of malaria disease protection

Crude $\log_{10}$MFI levels of IgG, IgG1, and IgG3 to CSP constructs at M3 in RTS,S vaccinees were higher but not significantly in those who did not present with clinical malaria vs those who did over the 12-month follow-up period. In contrast, levels of IgG2 to all CSP constructs and of IgG4 to CSP FL were significantly lower in non-malaria controls than in malaria cases (Additional file 1: Figures S10–S13). A combined analysis of all IgG subclasses showed that the ratio of cytophilic (IgG1 + IgG3) to non-cytophilic (IgG2 + IgG4) antibodies to all CSP constructs was significantly higher among controls than cases in RTS,S vaccinees but not in comparator vaccinees (Fig. 5). Stratified by age, this difference occurred in children but not in infants (Additional file 1: Figure S14). Stratified by site, this was only seen for Kintampo but not for Manhiça (Additional file 1: Figures S15 and S16).

Baseline levels of CSP IgG were generally higher in subjects who developed clinical malaria than in those who did not (Additional file 1: Table S12). An analysis of the change in antibody responses between M0 and M3 in RTS,S vaccinees revealed significantly higher increase of Ig CSP levels in those who were protected than in those who subsequently suffered clinical malaria (Fig. 4). Stratified by age, this difference was significant in children but not in infants (Additional file 1: Figure S14). Stratified by site, this was more apparent for Kintampo than Manhiça (Additional file 1: Figure S15).

Regarding responses to the HBsAg component of the RTS,S vaccine, levels of IgG, IgG1, IgG3, and IgM at M3 in RTS,S vaccinees but not in comparators were lower in those who had clinical malaria over the 12-month follow-up period vs those who did not (Additional file 1: Figures S11–S13).

The covariates significantly associated with clinical malaria risk in univariate logistic regression models (including all vaccinees) were site, previous malaria episodes, WAZ, HAZ, baseline CSP IgG (and IgG1), *P. falciparum* maternal and exposure antibodies (Additional file 1: Tables S13–S14). When adjusted by site (Kintampo had higher odds of malaria than Manhiça), only age cohort and baseline *P. falciparum* maternal and exposure antibodies were statistically significant. Within RTS,S vaccinees, age cohort and baseline *P. falciparum* maternal antibodies remained significant. We next assessed if these covariates affected the associations between CSP and HBsAg Ig responses (M3 levels, M3-M0 changes, and M3 IgG subclass ratios) and clinical malaria in RTS,S vaccines. In multivariable regression models, the associations between antibody responses and clinical malaria remained statistically significant after correction for multiple comparisons for anti-C-term CSP IgG2 levels, M3–M0 changes in IgG and IgG1, and cytophilic to non-cytophilic IgG subclass ratio, as well as anti-HBsAg levels (IgG, IgG1, IgG3) and subclass ratio (Table 2). In these models, age and site significantly affected clinical malaria and, in some cases, also baseline antibodies. Sex was not significantly associated with clinical malaria, but there were some significant interactions with antibody responses to RTS,S vaccination; and antibodies appeared more strongly associated with malaria disease protection in males rather than females (data not shown). In addition, sex ($p = 0.1$) was retained in all models including C-term CSP IgG2 responses (Table 2).

Machine learning multi-marker analyses (Fig. 5) revealed a signature of protection against clinical malaria in RTS,S vaccinees composed of antibodies to HBsAg (IgG3, IgG4, IgM, and IgG1 at M3 and M0, and IgG2 at M0), to CSP NANP (IgG3 at M3), and C-term (IgG1 and IgG at M3). In analysis stratified by age and site, IgG3 NANP was more prominent in infants in Manhiça, and IgG1 C-term in children in Kintampo (Additional file 1: Table S14). Moreover, a signature of malaria disease risk was also identified composed of IgG2 responses to CSP C-term, NANP, and HBsAg at M3; baseline responses to CSP C-term, NANP (IgG1, IgG, IgG3, and IgM), and *P. falciparum* antigens (exposure and maternal indices); and IgG4 responses to CSP NANP and C-term at M3 (Fig. 5). In addition, IgG3 and IgM to CSP C-term at M3 (in detriment of IgG1), and IgG1 and IgM to CSP NANP at M3 (in detriment of IgG3), were also associated with increased risk. In stratified analysis, M0

Table 1 Factors affecting the immunogenicity of RTS,S/AS01E. Multivariable linear models including RTS,S/AS01E vaccinees at month 3

Isotype	Antigen	Age*	Site	Prior episode†	Season	Baseline Ig	Exposure index	Sex	Hb	WAZ	HAZ
IgG	CSP FL	1.21 (0;2.43), *0.05*									
	CSP C-term	1.1 (0.01;2.2), *0.048*		99.08 (− 16.6;375.18), 0.12		− 43.99 (− 69.72;3.61), 0.06			− 13.8 (− 28.2;3.5), 0.11		
	CSP NANP	1.55 (0.3;2.82), *0.02*				− 46.15 (− 65.99;-14.73), *0.009*			− 14.99 (− 30.87;4.5), 0.12		
	HBsAg	3.97 (2.83;5.12), *< 0.001*	93.14 (9.18;241.67), *0.02*	238.29 (29.17;785.95), *0.01*					− 18.02 (− 32.07;− 1.06), *0.04*		
IgG1	CSP FL									− 21.26 (− 41.39;5.8), 0.11	
	CSP C-term	1.54 (0.17;2.94), *0.03*	91.17 (− 7.67;295.82), 0.08	166.93 (− 18.55;774.83), 0.1						− 21.42 (− 42.4;7.22), 0.13	
	CSP NANP					− 44.3 (− 63.7;-14.7), 0.08	8.62 (0.4;17.5), *0.04*				
	HBsAg	4.28 (3.09;5.49), *< 0.001*	90.61 (4.9;246.35), *0.03*	161.88 (− 4.42;617.53), *0.06*					− 17.52 (− 32.3;0.43), *0.005*		
IgG2	CSP FL		− 69.3 (− 78.86;-55.43), *< 0.001*				3.28 (− 7.2;0.8), 0.11				
	CSP C-term		− 74.77 (− 84.4;-59.2), *< 0.001*								
	CSP NANP	1.2 (0.25;2.16), *0.01*	− 45.45 (− 66.66;− 10.72), *0.02*			30.86 (− 8.56;87.27), 0.14	− 5.93 (− 10.55;-1.07), *0.02*	25.18 (− 6.89;68.29), 0.14		− 24.23 (− 37.63;− 7.94), *0.006*	
	HBsAg	2.45 (1.75;3.15), *< 0.001*				318.44 (234.5;423), *< 0.001*					
IgG3	CSP FL			144.38 (− 20.29;649.19), 0.12						− 22.63 (− 43.2;5.31), 0.1	
	CSP C-term	1.05 (− 0.17;2.29), 0.09					5.84 (− 0.92;13.06), 0.09				
	CSP NANP	1.38 (− 0.13;2.91), 0.07		197.82 (− 8.62;870.67),					− 23.08 (− 40.14;− 1.15),		

Table 1 Factors affecting the immunogenicity of RTS,S/AS01E. Multivariable linear models including RTS,S/AS01E vaccinees at month 3 *(Continued)*

Isotype	Antigen	Age*	Site	Prior episode†	Season	Baseline Ig	Exposure index	Sex	Hb	WAZ	HAZ
				0.07					*0.041*		
	HBsAg	1.96 (1.23;2.71), *< 0.001*									20.89 (3.3;41.43), *0.002*
IgG4	CSP FL		− 52.07 (− 75.66;− 5.61), *0.03*	123.51 (− 21.64;537.55), 0.13			8.6 (1.45;16.2), *0.02*				− 22.32 (− 40.8;2.03), 0.07
	CSP C-term	0.93 (− 0.38;2.25), 0.16	72.93 (− 13.56;245.99), 0.12	215.08 (0.49;887.87), *0.049*		− 49.59 (− 76.34;7.39), 0.08				− 26.52 (− 45.39;− 1.14), *0.042*	
	CSP NANP			304.28 (72.25;848.85), *0.002*							
	HBsAg	0.57 (0.33;0.82), *< 0.001*	18.49 (4.39;34.49), *0.009*	19.24 (− 2.74;46.19), 0.09		55.36 (− 6.46;158.1), 0.09			− 4 (− 7.75;− 0.1), *0.045*	8.14 (1.42;15.3), *0.02*	− 5.15 (− 11.05;1.14), 0.11
IgM	CSP FL				− 76.82 (− 96.23;42.51), 0.11				− 14.68 (− 27.4;0.32), 0.055		
	CSP C-term		62.15 (6.71;146.4), *0.02*	95.03 (− 0.67;282.94), 0.052					− 18.52 (− 28.3;− 7.4), *0.002*		− 12.64 (− 26.4;3.73), 0.12
	CSP NANP	1.07 (0.05;2.09), *0.04*									
	HBsAg	2.17 (0.87;3.48), *0.001*	212.61 (97.4;395.11), *< 0.001*	190.2 (38.4;508.6), *0.005*		120.31 (49.19;225), *< 0.001*			− 15.86 (− 27.03;− 2.99), *0.02*		− 15.53 (− 30.01;1.95), 0.08

The coefficients indicate the percent change for a unit change in the predictor (95% confidence intervals), the *p* values indicated are for statistically significant covariates (in italics) and for those that improved the model. Malaria transmission season at month 3 sample collection (low vs high). Baseline antibodies to the same Ig/antigen. Baseline anti-*P. falciparum* exposure IgM levels (exposure PC1 index).
Sex male vs female, *Hb,g/dL* baseline hemoglobin, *WAZ* weight-for-age Z scores, *HAZ* height-for-age Z scores

*Continuous age at weeks. Site (Manhiça vs Kintampo)

†Malaria episode between month 0 and month 3 (yes vs no)

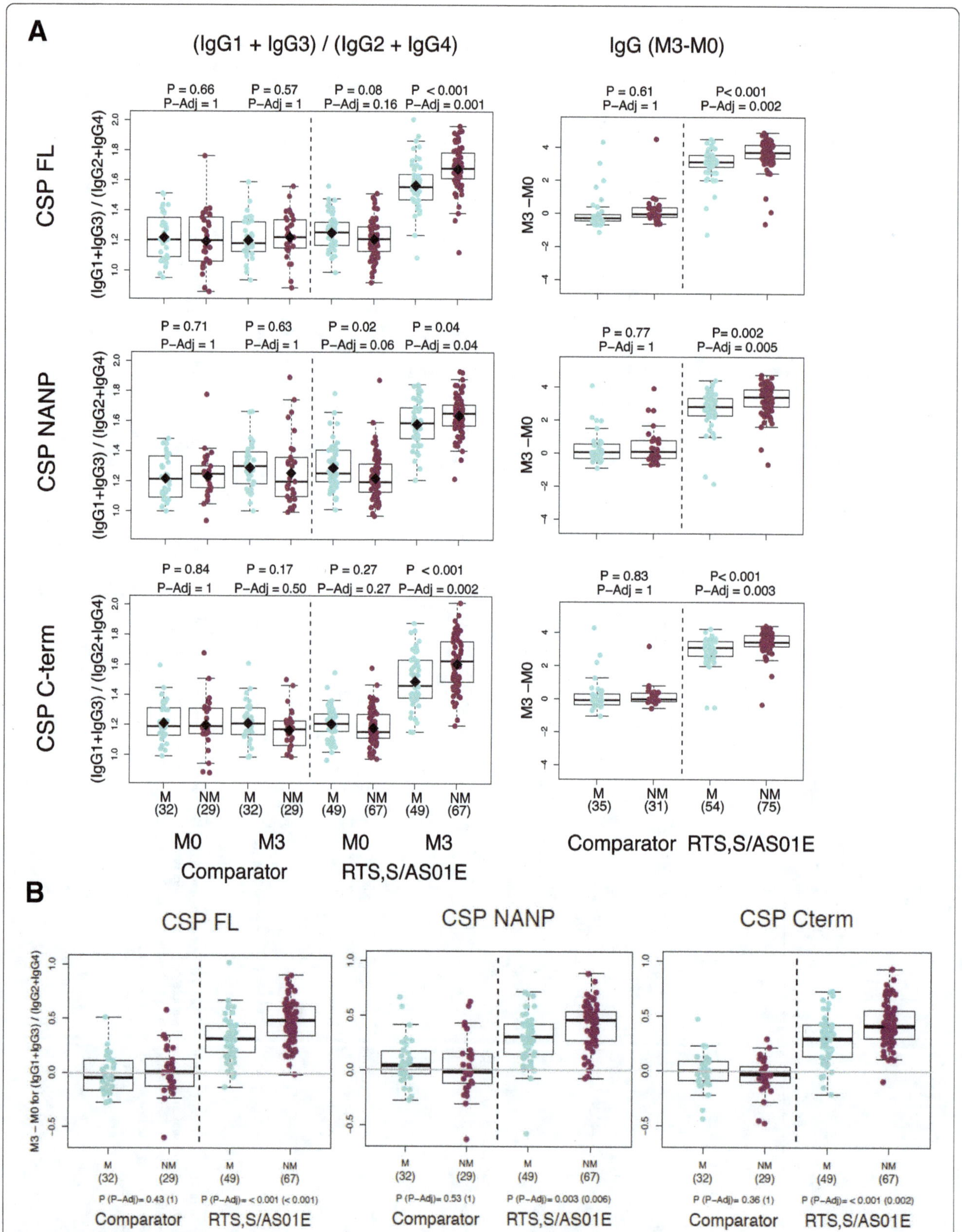

Fig. 4 (See legend on next page.)

(See figure on previous page.)
Fig. 4 Association between CSP Ig responses after vaccination and RTS,S-induced protection. **a** Ratio of cytophilic IgG1 and IgG3 vs non-cytophilic IgG2 and IgG4 antibodies, and increment of IgG levels between month 0 and month 3 in protected (NM = no clinical malaria) and non-protected (M = clinical malaria). **b** Difference between month 3 and month 0 (M3–M0) cytophilic/non-cytophilic ratios. Groups were compared through *t* tests and *p* values adjusted by Holm

IgG2 to CSP NANP and M0 IgG4 to CSP C-term were also associated with risk in infants. These protective signatures were not found in comparator vaccinees, in whom malaria exposure index was the strongest risk variable.

Discussion

Our study confirms prior knowledge on RTS,S/AS01E immunogenicity and goes a significant step beyond in understanding its determinants and mode of action. The data corroborate that vaccination induces a substantial increase in anti-CSP and HBsAg IgG responses, higher in children than in infants, which contributes to protection against clinical malaria [18]. In addition, a set of novel findings expand the breadth of knowledge about RTS,S immunogenicity and potential correlates of protection.

First, we showed that antibodies to other CSP epitopes in its C-terminal region are also elicited by RTS,S/AS01E in African children (although seemingly at lower levels compared to NANP repeat) and are the only ones associated with clinical malaria protection in multivariable analysis in our study population. Inclusion of a CSP FL construct allowed detecting responses of lower magnitude possibly due to the additive response to multiple B cell epitopes.

Second, we characterized Ig responses not previously assessed, including IgM and IgG subclasses for all antigens. We found that IgG1 predominates upon RTS,S vaccination, followed by IgG3, with lower production of IgG2 and IgG4. Furthermore, our data support that the balance of anti-CSP IgG subclasses more than the total IgG levels is important for protection against clinical malaria, as a higher ratio of cytophilic IgG1 and IgG3 to non-cytophilic IgG2 and IgG4 antibodies was associated with antimalarial immunity. Thus, children who predominantly produced anti-CSP (particularly C-term) IgG2 and IgG4 in detriment of IgG1 and IgG3 as a response to vaccination were at higher risk of suffering malaria disease. This is consistent with the notion that acquired immunity is attributed to cytophilic rather than non-cytophilic IgGs [37] due to their functional capacity to fix complement and opsonize parasites for Fc binding and phagocytosis [38, 39]; these mechanisms could also be acting in CSP-mediated sporozoite immunity. Antibodies to C-term CSP seem not important in blocking hepatocyte invasion by sporozoites but could mediate these other protective mechanisms. Recent studies have shown that acquired human antibodies, and antibodies to CSP, can fix and activate complement on the sporozoite surface, leading to inhibition of motility [40]. This potential antibody-mediated mechanism of action of RTS,S needs to be confirmed in future functional studies. Our findings are, however, not in line with observations by Chaudhury et al. [41], where IgG4 was associated with protection against sporozoite challenge in RTS,S-vaccinated naïve adults and IgG4 inhibited phagocytosis mediated by IgG1 and IgG3 when using the THP1 pro-monocytic cell line. That study also found that phagocytic activity using THP1 cells was not associated with vaccine efficacy. It is possible that the mechanisms of immunity differ between vaccinated malaria-naive adults and children resident in a malaria-endemic region. Furthermore, using THP-1 cells may not represent all Fc-receptor interactions that occur with phagocytes in vivo due to differences in Fc-receptor expression and function between THP1 cells, monocytes, neutrophils, and other cells. Recent studies have also highlighted differences in opsonic phagocytosis activity when using purified monocytes versus whole-blood assays [42].

Third, we characterized the effect of baseline status, including variables related to malaria exposure, on RTS,S immunogenicity and efficacy. At the individual level, the presence of antibodies at the time of vaccination due to maternal transfer and/or to past/present infections or to other vaccinations [43, 44] likely varies in infants and children and may differentially affect RTS,S outcomes. As expected, Kintampo had higher M0 levels of CSP antibodies than Manhiça. The site did not seem to have a major role in CSP antibody levels at M3, but because of the different baselines, it had a significant effect on change from M0 to M3 CSP responses. Thus, individuals exposed to higher MTI had higher M0 Ig levels and lower change in antibodies from M0 to M3. This was manifested differently depending on age group: (i) higher M0 IgG levels in infants than children presumably represented passively transferred maternal antibodies that, in the absence of vaccination (comparators), decayed from M0 to M3, and these were generally higher in Kintampo than Manhiça due to higher malaria exposure in the mothers; (ii) higher M0 IgG and IgM levels in children represented those acquired upon infection and were also higher in Kintampo than Manhiça. Season did not impact the outcomes (consistent with a recent report [45]) as the majority of volunteers were vaccinated within restricted time periods.

A prior analysis of the effect of baseline anti-NANP CSP IgGs within the phase 3 trial [18] reported that

Table 2 Association between RTS,S-induced antibody responses and protection against clinical malaria

		Univariate All subjects			Multivariable All subjects				Multivariable Subjects age < 10 months			
Antibody	Antigen	OR	95%CI	*p*	OR	95%CI	*p*	Covariates*	OR	95%CI	*P*	Covariates**
IgG M3	CSP FL	0.74	0.41; 1.23	0.25				*Age*, *site*, exposure				*Age*, *site*, exposure
	CSP C-term	0.58	0.28; 1.05	0.21	0.6	0.26; 1.18	0.17	Age, *site*, M0, exposure				*Age*, *site*, M0, exposure
	CSP NANP	0.67	0.37; 1.08	0.21				Age, *site*, M0				*Age*, *site*
	HBsAg	0.50	0.29; 0.82	*0.02*	0.38	0.2; 0.7	*0.002*	*Site*, exposure	0.42	0.18; 0.9	*0.03*	*Site*, *M0*, exposure, maternal
IgM M3	CSP FL	0.94	0.5; 1.75	1				*Age*, *site*, exposure				*Age*, *site*, M0
	CSP C-term	1.09	0.49; 2.44	1				*Age*, *site*, exposure				*Age*, *site*, M0
	CSP NANP	0.79	0.43; 1.44	1				*Age*, *site*, exposure				*Age*, *site*, M0
	HBsAg	0.46	0.25; 0.82	*0.03*				*Site*, *M0*, exposure				*Site*, *M0*, exposure
IgG1 M3	CSP FL	0.86	0.52; 1.36	0.54				*Age*, *site*, exposure				*Age*, *site*, exposure
	CSP C-term	0.60	0.34; 0.97	0.09	0.64	0.36; 1.06	0.1	Age, *site*, exposure				*Age*, *site*, M0, exposure
	CSP NANP	0.83	0.53; 1.25	0.48				*Age*, *site*, *M0*, exposure				*Age*, *site*, *M0*, exposure
	HBsAg	0.58	0.35; 0.92	*0.057*	0.49	0.27; 0.85	*0.01*	*Site*, exposure				*Age*, *site*, exposure
IgG2 M3	CSP FL	4.38	1.75; 12.29	*0.006*				Age, *site*				*Site*, *maternal*
	CSP C-term	4.08	2.07; 8.79	< *0.001*	2.62	1.18; 6.11	*0.02*	*Site*, sex	2.69	1.09; 7.32	*0.04*	*Maternal*, site, sex
	CSP NANP	2.63	1.2; 6.25	*0.049*				Age, *site*				*Maternal*, *site*
	HBsAg	0.76	0.37; 1.49	0.49				Age, *site*				*Maternal*, *site*
IgG3 M3	CSP FL	0.88	0.56; 1.35	0.54				*Age*, *site*, exposure				*Age*, *site*, exposure
	CSP C-term	0.75	0.44; 1.26	0.46				*Age*, *site*, exposure				*Age*, *site*, exposure
	CSP NANP	0.81	0.53; 1.21	0.46	0.63	0.38; 1.02	0.07	Age, *site*, exposure				*Age*, *site*, exposure
	HBsAg	0.19	0.06; 0.51	*0.004*	0.1	0.02; 0.34	< *0.001*	*Site*, exposure	0.26	0.06; 0.92	*0.05*	*Site*, maternal, exposure
IgG4 M3	CSP FL	2.15	1.31; 3.66	*0.009*				*Age*, *site*, exposure				*Age*, *site*, exposure
	CSP C-term	1.27	0.79; 2.04	0.46	1.63	0.92; 3	0.1	*Age*, *site*				*Age*, *site*, exposure
	CSP NANP	1.27	0.74; 2.24	0.48				*Age*, *site*, M0, exposure				*Age*, *site*, exposure
	HBsAg	0.11	0.01; 1.51	0.20				*Age*, *site*, exposure				*Age*, *site*, exposure
IgG M3–M0	CSP FL	0.47	0.27; 0.73	*0.001*				*Age*, *site*, exposure				*Age*, *site*, exposure
	CSP C-term	0.36	0.18; 0.65	*0.001*	0.51	0.26; 0.88	*0.03*	Age, *site*, exposure				*Age*, *site*, exposure
	CSP NANP	0.55	0.35; 0.8	*0.003*	0.72	0.46; 1.06	0.11	Age, *site*, exposure				*Age*, *site*, exposure
	HBsAg	0.73	0.49; 1.07	0.11				*Age*, *site*, exposure				*Age*, *site*, exposure
IgM M3–M0	CSP FL	0.72	0.43; 1.18	0.38				*Age*, *site*, exposure				*Age*, *site*, exposure
	CSP C-term	0.64	0.36; 1.11	0.35				*Age*, *site*, exposure				*Site*, *maternal*
	CSP NANP	0.62	0.38; 0.97	0.14				*Age*, *site*, exposure				*Age*, *site*, exposure

Table 2 Association between RTS,S-induced antibody responses and protection against clinical malaria *(Continued)*

		Univariate All subjects			Multivariable All subjects				Multivariable Subjects age < 10 months			
Antibody	Antigen	OR	95%CI	*p*	OR	95%CI	*p*	Covariates*	OR	95%CI	*P*	Covariates**
	HBsAg	0.79	0.42; 1.41	0.42				*Age*, *site*, exposure				*Age*, *site*, exposure
IgG1 M3–M0	CSP FL	0.52	0.33; 0.76	*0.007*				*Age*, *site*, exposure				*Age*, *site*, exposure
	CSP C-term	0.54	0.33; 0.81	*0.01*	0.63	0.39; 0.96	*0.04*	Age, *site*, exposure	0.66	0.4; 1.02	0.07	*Age*, *site*, exposure
	CSP NANP	0.63	0.44; 0.86	*0.01*	0.75	0.52; 1.03	0.08	Age, *site*, exposure	0.78	0.54; 1.08	0.14	*Age*, *site*, exposure
	HBsAg	0.73	0.51; 1.05	0.19				*Age*, *site*, exposure				*Age*, *site*, exposure
IgG2 M3–M0	CSP FL	0.72	0.41; 1.21	0.34				Age, *site*				*Site*, *maternal*
	CSP C-term	2.30	1.29; 4.33	*0.02*	1.86	0.95; 3.81	0.08	*Site*, sex	2.46	1.1; 6.13	*0.04*	*Site*, *maternal*, sex
	CSP NANP	0.86	0.52; 1.43	0.60				Age, *site*				*Site*, *maternal*
	HBsAg	1.32	0.65; 2.73	0.56				Age, *site*				*Site*, *maternal*
IgG3 M3–M0	CSP FL	0.65	0.45; 0.91	*0.03*	0.77	0.52; 1.11	0.16	Age, *site*, exposure				*Age*, *site*, exposure
	CSP C-term	0.79	0.53; 1.17	0.35				*Age*, *site*, exposure				*Age*, *site*, exposure
	CSP NANP	0.72	0.53; 0.97	0.07	0.73	0.52; 1.02	0.07	Age, *site*, exposure				*Age*, *site*, exposure
	HBsAg	0.76	0.48; 1.16	0.34				*Age*, *site*, exposure				*Age*, *site*, exposure
IgG4 M3–M0	CSP FL	1.67	1.08; 2.66	*0.053*				*Age*, *site*, exposure				*Age*, *site*, exposure
	CSP C-term	1.15	0.78; 1.71	0.56	1.44	0.9; 2.37	0.14	Age, *site*				*Age*, *site*, exposure
	CSP NANP	1.19	0.75; 1.9	0.56				*Age*, *site*, exposure				*Age*, *site*, exposure
	HBsAg	0.78	0.08; 7.09	0.82				*Age*, *site*, exposure	18.1	0.57;967	0.11	*Age*, *site*, exposure
IgG1 + IgG3/IgG2 + IgG4 M3	CSP FL	0.01	0; 0.12	*< 0.001*	0.11	0.01; 1.9	0.13	Age, *site*				*Site*, *maternal*
	CSP C-term	0.03	0; 0.22	*0.002*	0.03	0; 0.35	*0.007*	*Site*, sex	0.04	0; 0.79	*0.04*	*Site*, *maternal*, sex
	CSP NANP	0.06	0; 0.82	*0.07*	0.06	0; 1.26	0.07	Age, *site*, exposure				*Site*, *maternal*
	HBsAg	0.07	0; 1.14	*0.07*	*0*	0; 0.15	*0.004*	*Site*, exposure				*Site*, *maternal*

Logistic regression models of the association between (i) levels of antibodies (log_{10}MFI) at month (M) 3, (ii) increments from M0 to M3 antibodies (iii), ratio of cytophilic to non-cytophilic antibodies at M3, and clinical malaria (yes/no), in RTS,S/AS01E vaccinees, expressed as odds ratio (OR), 95% confidence interval (CI), and *p* values (corrected for multiple comparisons, see the "Methods" section). The associations between predictors and outcome shown here were not found in comparator vaccines at month 3 (data not shown). Multivariable analysis models were done with the minimum Akaike information criterion (AIC); statistically significant variables are marked in italics. A combination of backward and forward stepwise algorithms was used to obtain the model with the minimum AIC.

*Variables that were statistically significant (italics) or improved the multivariable model. Exposure = malaria exposure antibody index, age in weeks; M0 = baseline antibody levels to the respective antigen/Ig

**Analyses included also antimalarial maternal antibody index (maternal)

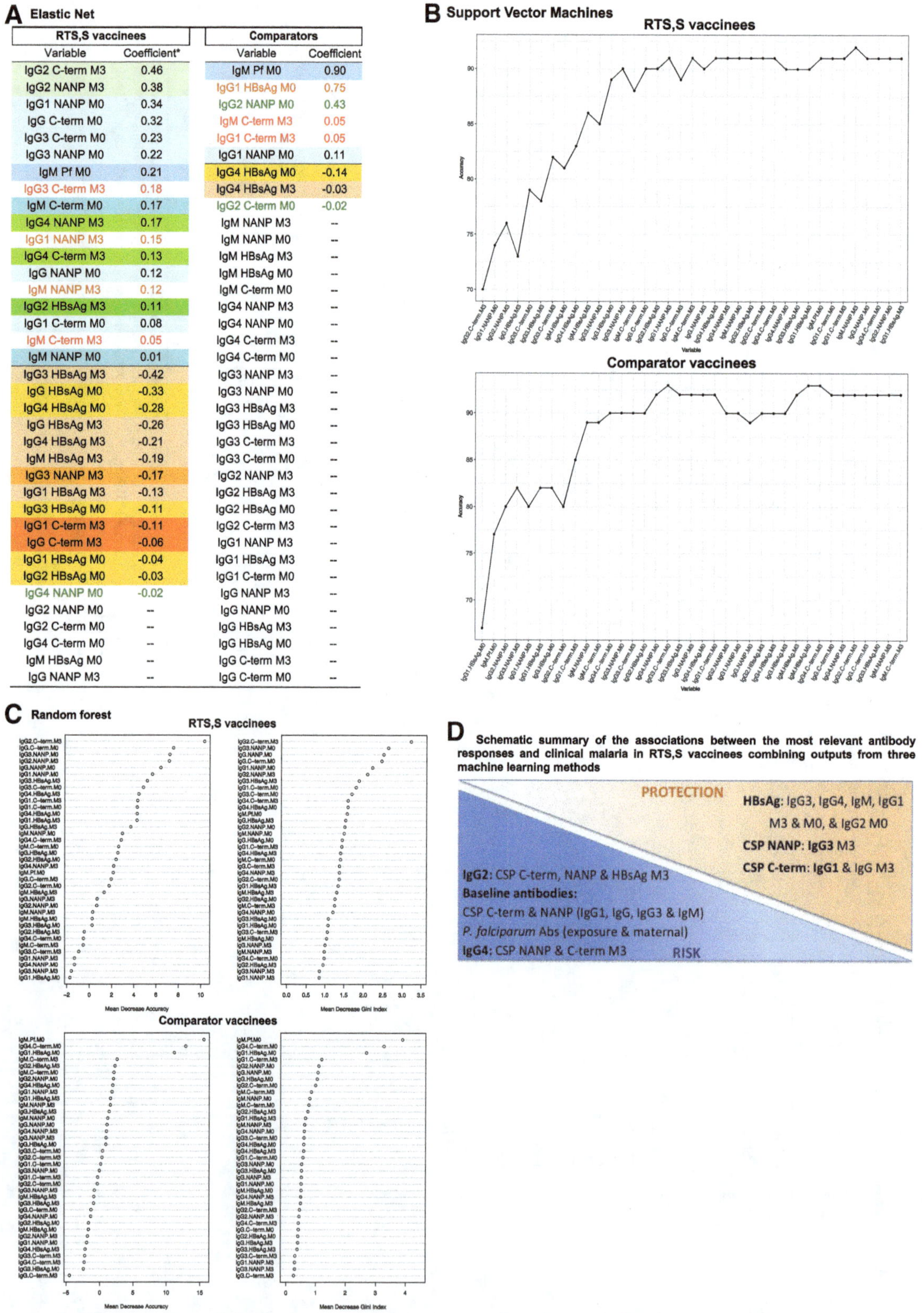

A Elastic Net

RTS,S vaccinees		Comparators	
Variable	Coefficient*	Variable	Coefficient
IgG2 C-term M3	0.46	IgM Pf M0	0.90
IgG2 NANP M3	0.38	IgG1 HBsAg M0	0.75
IgG1 NANP M0	0.34	IgG2 NANP M0	0.43
IgG C-term M0	0.32	IgM C-term M3	0.05
IgG3 C-term M0	0.23	IgG1 C-term M3	0.05
IgG3 NANP M0	0.22	IgG1 NANP M0	0.11
IgM Pf M0	0.21	IgG4 HBsAg M0	-0.14
IgG3 C-term M3	0.18	IgG4 HBsAg M3	-0.03
IgM C-term M0	0.17	IgG2 C-term M0	-0.02
IgG4 NANP M3	0.17	IgM NANP M3	--
IgG1 NANP M3	0.15	IgM NANP M0	--
IgG4 C-term M3	0.13	IgM HBsAg M3	--
IgG NANP M0	0.12	IgM HBsAg M0	--
IgM NANP M3	0.12	IgM C-term M0	--
IgG2 HBsAg M3	0.11	IgG4 NANP M3	--
IgG1 C-term M0	0.08	IgG4 NANP M0	--
IgM C-term M3	0.05	IgG4 C-term M3	--
IgM NANP M0	0.01	IgG4 C-term M0	--
IgG3 HBsAg M3	-0.42	IgG3 NANP M3	--
IgG HBsAg M0	-0.33	IgG3 NANP M0	--
IgG4 HBsAg M0	-0.28	IgG3 HBsAg M3	--
IgG HBsAg M3	-0.26	IgG3 HBsAg M0	--
IgG4 HBsAg M3	-0.21	IgG3 C-term M3	--
IgM HBsAg M3	-0.19	IgG3 C-term M0	--
IgG3 NANP M3	-0.17	IgG2 NANP M3	--
IgG1 HBsAg M3	-0.13	IgG2 HBsAg M3	--
IgG3 HBsAg M0	-0.11	IgG2 HBsAg M0	--
IgG1 C-term M3	-0.11	IgG2 C-term M3	--
IgG C-term M3	-0.06	IgG1 NANP M3	--
IgG1 HBsAg M0	-0.04	IgG1 HBsAg M3	--
IgG2 HBsAg M0	-0.03	IgG1 C-term M0	--
IgG4 NANP M0	-0.02	IgG NANP M3	--
IgG2 NANP M0	--	IgG NANP M0	--
IgG2 C-term M0	--	IgG HBsAg M3	--
IgG4 C-term M0	--	IgG HBsAg M0	--
IgM HBsAg M0	--	IgG C-term M3	--
IgG NANP M3	--	IgG C-term M0	--

Fig. 5 Multi-marker correlates analyses by machine learning techniques. Results from three complementary methods are shown stratified by vaccination group. **a** Elastic Net. **b** Support vector machines. **c** Random forest. **d** Schematic summary of the associations between the most relevant antibody responses and clinical malaria in RTS,S vaccinees combining outputs from three machine learning methods

pre-vaccination titers were associated with lower RTS,S immunogenicity in infants and higher immunogenicity in children. We also found a significant negative association between anti-NANP CSP pre-vaccination levels and post-vaccination IgG and IgG1 responses, particularly in younger children. At baseline, anti-CSP IgGs in infants < 10 months correlated with IgG to *P. falciparum* antigens used as markers of maternal antibodies, and anti-CSP IgGs in children correlated with IgM to *P. falciparum* antigens that are markers of current/recent exposure. These maternal and exposure indices, obtained using an unprecedented breadth of pre-erythrocytic and erythrocytic stage proteins, were significantly associated to some CSP and HBsAg Ig responses at M3. Overall, the data show that high concentrations of maternal CSP IgG at baseline could interfere with RTS,S immunization by binding the vaccine proteins and impeding antigen presentation and subsequent response, resulting in lower immunogenicity in newborns.

More importantly, higher malaria exposure prior to M0 positively predicted the occurrence of malaria cases over the 12-month follow-up period after M3, while lower levels of antibodies to CSP or *P. falciparum* antigens at M0 predicted lower risk of clinical malaria during the post-vaccination follow-up; this also applied for comparator vaccinees at M3. Here, naturally acquired CSP antibody levels also indicated malaria exposure. In this line, it is well established that the strongest risk factor for future malaria disease is having had malaria episodes in the past [37]. In fact, malaria events prior to M3 rendered participants more susceptible to future malaria episodes, but this was largely explained by site, with higher baseline MTI and malaria incidence in Kintampo than Manhiça. As RTS,S vaccination induced a potent increase in anti-CSP antibodies at M3, individuals protected against clinical malaria had a significantly higher increase in M0 to M3 Ig levels than the non-protected, more remarkably for C-term Ig. The associations were significant mostly for Kintampo (where the effect of malaria exposure was heavier) and children (in whom there were little maternal antibodies and RTS,S elicited higher M3 Ig levels). Thus, it appears that RTS,S exerts a larger benefit (vaccine efficacy) when vaccinees have had less malaria exposure before M0, thus that they are able to mount a higher (on average) CSP IgG response at M3 upon vaccination, and this contributes more efficiently to controlling *P. falciparum* infection. This is in line with the results from the main MAL055 trial with regard to the significant interaction between vaccine efficacy and site in children (not infants) whereby lower efficacy was generally estimated in sites of higher MTI [14].

We and others have shown that malaria exposure alters the phenotype and functional characteristics of memory B lymphocytes [46, 47] and other cells, e.g., T helper [48], that are responsible for antibody production. Individuals under higher MTI may have an immune system that is suppressed, de-regulated, or primed by natural exposure to produce a different immune response that upon RTS,S vaccination could deviate CSP response to predominantly non-cytophilic antibodies and/or overall lower IgG levels. Elicitation of IgE rather than IgG CSP responses [49] and of T_H2 rather than T_H1 [23] may also be associated with lower RTS,S efficacy. Induction of greater IgG1 and IgG3 relative to lower IgG2 and IgG4 in individuals under lower MTI would lead to a better quality and more balanced immune response associated with functional CSP antibody-mediated vaccine protection. Our data strongly support this assertion. Levels of IgG2 to all CSP constructs and IgG4 to CSP FL (but not of IgG1 or IgG3) induced by RTS,S vaccination were significantly higher with heavier MTI. Other baseline variables not previously assessed in RTS,S studies could influence the immune balance, and particularly, the role of sex deserves more investigation because of the increased overall mortality in girls than boys found in a secondary analysis [50]. Baseline Hb, WAZ, and HAZ were associated with antibody levels at M3, suggesting that the health status of the child might also affect the initial response to the vaccine, but this was not significant after adjustment. Due to sample sizes, these observations should be interpreted with caution but merit further assessment. Thus, determinants of IgG2, IgG4, or IgE CSP responses and exhausted T_H and B cells associated with malaria infections need to be disentangled as they appear relevant for vaccine success.

Remarkably, higher HBsAg antibody levels were associated with less malaria disease risk in RTS,S vaccinees, and this was consistent across Ig isotypes, ages, and sites and confirmed in machine learning analysis. This unforeseen result could be an indirect association related to a better general immune status in the volunteers protected against clinical malaria, who may respond more potently to non-malarial antigen epitopes upon vaccination, or a surrogate of other protective mechanisms. Alternatively, there may be a direct immunological mediation whereby HBsAg-specific T cells might provide help to B cells to produce CSP antibodies by virtue of being presented together (hapten-carrier hypothesis). The complex relationship between malaria exposure, HBsAg antibodies, and clinical malaria risk will be the subject of future investigations.

Our study design had some limitations that can be mitigated in follow-up studies. In Kintampo, all children who fulfilled the inclusion criteria, most of whom had malaria, were analyzed. Whereas in Manhiça, a case-control design was needed because there were fewer cases; a cohort design would have required to increase the number of samples substantially to have power to detect association with protection. In Manhiça, there was also an age imbalance, as most cases were in infants. Despite this and having many markers and multiple comparisons, the results were coherent and biologically plausible. Thus, the impacts of CSP IgG subclasses, baseline malaria exposure, and of HBsAg Ig levels, on clinical malaria risk, were consistent.

Conclusions

Our characterization of an expanded breadth of antigen epitopes and Ig isotypes/subclasses induced by RTS,S, including non-CSP *P. falciparum* antigens as markers of maternal antibodies and malaria exposure, led to a better understanding of baseline determinants of vaccine take and protection against clinical malaria. We identified new potential correlates of malaria disease risk and protection, including IgG subclasses, baseline antibody levels, and HBsAg antibodies. These data shed new light into the mode of action of RTS,S, further evidencing that it is more complex and multifactorial than previously thought. Future studies should assess the function of the antibodies, their correlation with cellular immune responses associated with clinical malaria protection and risk, and the kinetics of peak and post-booster CSP and HBsAg responses over time. Elucidating mechanisms of RTS,S immunity and correlates will be translated into a more rational development, testing, and deployment of next-generation vaccines. Protective responses identified could be favored with appropriate adjuvants, delivery systems, and/or vaccination schedules, including combination with antimalarial drugs.

Acknowledgements
We are grateful to the volunteers and their families; the clinical, field, and lab teams at the research institutions; the MAL067 Vaccine Immunology Consortium investigators and Working Groups; the hyper-immune plasma suppliers (NIBSC, UK); David Lanar, Virander Chauhan, Chetan Chitnis, Deepak Gaur, Ross Coppel, David Cavanagh, Benoit Gamain, Evelina Angov, and James Beeson for *P. falciparum* antigen supply; and Claudia Hernández for project assistance. We thank GlaxoSmithKline Biologicals S.A. for their support in the conduct of the MAL067 study.

Funding
Funding was obtained from the NIH-NIAID (R01AI095789), PATH Malaria Vaccine Initiative (MVI), Ministerio de Economía y Competitividad (Instituto de Salud Carlos III, PI11/00423), and EVIMalaR and AGAUR-Catalonia (2014 SGR991). ISGlobal is a member of the CERCA Program, Generalitat de Catalunya.

Authors' contributions
CD and IU wrote the first draft of the manuscript. CD, JJA, JJC, and GM conceived the study. AA, HS, IU, JJA, and CV performed the database management, statistical analysis, and experimental design of the manuscript. AJN, DD, CJ, JJC, GM, CD, and SO collected the samples and data and participated in the clinical trial. MV, AJ, and IU performed the experiments. NAW, NDP, and CD coordinated the study. MM, HS, STA, SK, BM, and CDa participated in the conception and implementation of the multicenter immunology study. JJA, IU, CD, JJC, GM, and CV participated in the design of the analysis. SD provided the antigens. GM, JJC, BM, HS, AA, RA, and CV contributed to the write up of the manuscript. All reviewed and approved the manuscript.

Competing interests
The authors declare that they have no competing interests.

Author details
[1]ISGlobal, Hospital Clínic, Universitat de Barcelona, Carrer Rosselló 153 CEK building, E-08036 Barcelona, Catalonia, Spain. [2]Centro de Investigação em Saúde de Manhiça (CISM), Rua 12, Cambeve, Vila de Manhiça, CP 1929 Maputo, Mozambique. [3]Kintampo Health Research Centre, Kintampo, Ghana. [4]Spanish Consortium for Research in Epidemiology and Public Health (CIBERESP), Barcelona, Spain. [5]Ifakara Health Institute, Bagamoyo Research and Training Center, P.O. Box 74, Bagamoyo, Tanzania. [6]Institut de Recherche en Sciences de la Santé, Nanoro, Burkina Faso. [7]Centre de Recherches Médicales de Lambaréné (CERMEL), BP 242, Lambaréné, Gabon. [8]Institute of Tropical Medicine and German Center for Infection Research, University of Tübingen, Wilhelmstraße 27, 72074 Tübingen, Germany. [9]Kenya Medical Research Institute (KEMRI)/Centre for Global Health Research, Kisumu, Kenya. [10]Swiss Tropical and Public Health Institute, Socinstrasse 57, 4002 Basel, Switzerland. [11]Facultade de Medicina, Universidade Eduardo Mondlane, Maputo, Mozambique. [12]Walter Reed Army Institute of Research (WRAIR), Silver Spring, MD, USA. [13]Noguchi Memorial Institute for Medical Research, University of Ghana, Accra, Ghana. [14]Department of Osteopathic Medical Specialties, Michigan State University, 909 Fee Road, Room B 309 West Fee Hall, East Lansing, MI 48824, USA. [15]Department of Immunology and Infectious Diseases, Harvard T.H. Chen School of Public Health, 675 Huntington Ave., Boston, MA 02115, USA.

References

1. WHO. World Malaria Report 2017. 2017. Available from: http://www.who.int/malaria/publications/world-malaria-report-2017/en/.
2. WHO. A framework for malaria elimination. 2017. Available from: http://www.who.int/malaria/publications/atoz/9789241511988/en/.
3. Benelli G, Beier JC. Current vector control challenges in the fight against malaria. Acta Trop. 2017;174:91–6.
4. von Seidlein L, Dondorp A. Fighting fire with fire: mass antimalarial drug administrations in an era of antimalarial resistance. Expert Rev Anti-Infect Ther. 2015;13(6):715–30.
5. White NJ, Pongtavornpinyo W, Maude RJ, Saralamba S, Aguas R, Stepniewska K, Lee SJ, Dondorp AM, White LJ, Day NP. Hyperparasitaemia and low dosing are an important source of anti-malarial drug resistance. Malar J. 2009;8:253.
6. Brady OJ, Slater HC, Pemberton-Ross P, Wenger E, Maude RJ, Ghani AC, Penny MA, Gerardin J, White LJ, Chitnis N, et al. Role of mass drug administration in elimination of Plasmodium falciparum malaria: a consensus modelling study. Lancet Glob Health. 2017;5(7):e680–7.
7. Poirot E, Skarbinski J, Sinclair D, Kachur SP, Slutsker L, Hwang J. Mass drug administration for malaria. Cochrane Database Syst Rev. 2013;12:CD008846.
8. Bridges DJ, Winters AM, Hamer DH. Malaria elimination: surveillance and response. Pathog Glob Health. 2012;106(4):224–31.
9. Cheah PY, White NJ. Antimalarial mass drug administration: ethical considerations. Int Health. 2016;8(4):235–8.
10. Healer J, Cowman AF, Kaslow DC, Birkett AJ. Vaccines to accelerate malaria elimination and eventual eradication. Cold Spring Harb Perspect Med. 2017;7(9).
11. Agnandji ST, Lell B, Soulanoudjingar SS, Fernandes JF, Abossolo BP, Conzelmann C, Methogo BG, Doucka Y, Flamen A, Mordmuller B, et al. First results of phase 3 trial of RTS,S/AS01 malaria vaccine in African children. N Engl J Med. 2011;365(20):1863–75.
12. Agnandji ST, Lell B, Fernandes JF, Abossolo BP, Methogo BG, Kabwende AL, Adegnika AA, Mordmuller B, Issifou S, Kremsner PG, et al. A phase 3 trial of RTS,S/AS01 malaria vaccine in African infants. N Engl J Med. 2012;367(24):2284–95.
13. Olotu A, Fegan G, Wambua J, Nyangweso G, Leach A, Lievens M, Kaslow DC, Njuguna P, Marsh K, Bejon P. Seven-year efficacy of RTS,S/AS01 malaria vaccine among young African children. N Engl J Med. 2016;374(26):2519–29.
14. RTS SCTP. Efficacy and safety of RTS,S/AS01 malaria vaccine with or without a booster dose in infants and children in Africa: final results of a phase 3, individually randomised, controlled trial. Lancet. 2015;386(9988):31–45.
15. RTS SCTP: Efficacy and safety of the RTS,S/AS01 malaria vaccine during 18 months after vaccination: a phase 3 randomized, controlled trial in children and young infants at 11 African sites. PLoS Med 2014;11(7):e1001685.
16. Chaudhury S, Ockenhouse CF, Regules JA, Dutta S, Wallqvist A, Jongert E, Waters NC, Lemiale F, Bergmann-Leitner E. The biological function of

antibodies induced by the RTS,S/AS01 malaria vaccine candidate is determined by their fine specificity. Malar J. 2016;15:301.

17. Campo JJ, Sacarlal J, Aponte JJ, Aide P, Nhabomba AJ, Dobano C, Alonso PL. Duration of vaccine efficacy against malaria: 5th year of follow-up in children vaccinated with RTS,S/AS02 in Mozambique. Vaccine. 2014;32(19):2209–16.
18. White MT, Verity R, Griffin JT, Asante KP, Owusu-Agyei S, Greenwood B, Drakeley C, Gesase S, Lusingu J, Ansong D, et al. Immunogenicity of the RTS,S/AS01 malaria vaccine and implications for duration of vaccine efficacy: secondary analysis of data from a phase 3 randomised controlled trial. Lancet Infect Dis. 2015;15(12):1450–8.
19. Olotu A, Clement F, Jongert E, Vekemans J, Njuguna P, Ndungu FM, Marsh K, Leroux-Roels G, Bejon P. Avidity of anti-circumsporozoite antibodies following vaccination with RTS,S/AS01E in young children. PLoS One. 2014;9(12):e115126.
20. Ajua A, Lell B, Agnandji ST, Asante KP, Owusu-Agyei S, Mwangoka G, Mpina M, Salim N, Tanner M, Abdulla S, et al. The effect of immunization schedule with the malaria vaccine candidate RTS,S/AS01E on protective efficacy and anti-circumsporozoite protein antibody avidity in African infants. Malar J. 2015;14:72.
21. Regules JA, Cicatelli SB, Bennett JW, Paolino KM, Twomey PS, Moon JE, Kathcart AK, Hauns KD, Komisar JL, Qabar AN, et al. Fractional third and fourth dose of RTS,S/AS01 malaria candidate vaccine: a phase 2a controlled human malaria parasite infection and immunogenicity study. J Infect Dis. 2016;214(5):762–71.
22. Olotu A, Fegan G, Wambua J, Nyangweso G, Awuondo KO, Leach A, Lievens M, Leboulleux D, Njuguna P, Peshu N, et al. Four-year efficacy of RTS,S/AS01E and its interaction with malaria exposure. N Engl J Med. 2013;368(12):1111–20.
23. Moncunill G, Mpina M, Nhabomba AJ, Aguilar R, Ayestaran A, Sanz H, Campo JJ, Jairoce C, Barrios D, Dong Y, et al. Distinct TH1 and TH2 cellular responses associated with malaria protection and risk in RTS,S/AS01E vaccinees. Clin Infect Dis. 2017;65(5):746–55.
24. Ubillos I, Campo JJ, Jimenez A, Dobano C. Development of a high-throughput flexible quantitative suspension array assay for IgG against multiple Plasmodium falciparum antigens. Malar J. 2018;17(1):216.
25. Vidal M, Aguilar R, Campo JJ, Dobano C. Development of quantitative suspension array assays for six immunoglobulin isotypes and subclasses to multiple Plasmodium falciparum antigens. J Immunol Methods. 2018;455:41–54.
26. Ubillos I, Aguilar R, Sanz H, Jimenez A, Vidal M, Valmaseda A, Dong Y, Gaur D, Chitnis CE, Dutta S, et al. Analysis of factors affecting the variability of a quantitative suspension bead array assay measuring IgG to multiple Plasmodium antigens. PLoS One. 2018;13(7):e0199278.
27. Ubillos I, Jimenez A, Vidal M, Bowyer PW, Gaur D, Dutta S, Gamain B, Coppel R, Chauhan V, Lanar D, et al. Optimization of incubation conditions of Plasmodium falciparum antibody multiplex assays to measure IgG, IgG1-4, IgM and IgE using standard and customized reference pools for sero-epidemiological and vaccine studies. Malar J. 2018;17(1):219.
28. Bryan D, Silva N, Rigsby P, Dougall T, Corran P, Bowyer PW, Ho MM. The establishment of a WHO reference reagent for anti-malaria (Plasmodium falciparum) human serum. Malar J. 2017;16(1):314.
29. Alonso PL, Sacarlal J, Aponte JJ, Leach A, Macete E, Milman J, Mandomando I, Spiessens B, Guinovart C, Espasa M, et al. Efficacy of the RTS,S/AS02A vaccine against *Plasmodium falciparum* infection and disease in young African children: randomised controlled trial. Lancet. 2004;364(9443):1411–20.
30. Fitzmaurice GM, Laird NW, Ware JH. Applied longitudinal analysis. Hoboken: Wiley; 2011.
31. Aguilar R, Unbillos I, Vidal M, Balanza N, Crespo N, Jiménez A, Nhabomba A, Jairoce C, Dosoo D, Gyan B, et al. Antibody responses to α-Gal in African children vary with age and site and are associated with malaria protection. Sci Rep. 2018;8:9999.
32. Holm S. A simple sequentially rejective multiple test procedure. Scand J Stat. 1979;6:65–70.
33. Benjamini Y, Hochberg Y. Controlling the false discovery rate: a practical and powerful approach to multiple testing. J R Stat Soc. 1995;B57:289–300.
34. Guyon I, Weston J, Barnhill S, Vapnik V. Gene selection for cancer classification using support vector machines. Mach Learn. 2002;46(1–2):389–42.
35. Breiman L. Random forests. Mach Learn. 2001;45(1):5–32.
36. Hastie T, Tibshirani R, Friedman J. The elements of statistical learning. New York: Springer New York Inc; 2001. p. 241–9.
37. Dobano C, Quelhas D, Quinto L, Puyol L, Serra-Casas E, Mayor A, Nhampossa T, Macete E, Aide P, Mandomando I, et al. Age-dependent IgG subclass responses to Plasmodium falciparum EBA-175 are differentially associated with incidence of malaria in Mozambican children. Clin Vaccine Immunol. 2012; 19(2):157–66.
38. Boyle MJ, Reiling L, Feng G, Langer C, Osier FH, Aspeling-Jones H, Cheng YS, Stubbs J, Tetteh KK, Conway DJ, et al. Human antibodies fix complement to inhibit Plasmodium falciparum invasion of erythrocytes and are associated with protection against malaria. Immunity. 2015;42(3):580–90.
39. Osier FH, Feng G, Boyle MJ, Langer C, Zhou J, Richards JS, McCallum FJ, Reiling L, Jaworowski A, Anders RF, et al. Opsonic phagocytosis of Plasmodium falciparum merozoites: mechanism in human immunity and a correlate of protection against malaria. BMC Med. 2014;12:108.
40. Kurtovic L, Behet M, Feng G, Reiling L, Fowkes F, Kazura J, Chelimo K, A.D, Sauerwein R, Beeson J: Antibodies promote complement activation against *Plasmodium falciparum* sporozoites, providing a novel mechanism of anti-malarial immunity. ASTMH Annual Meeting 2017.
41. Chaudhury S, Regules JA, Darko CA, Dutta S, Wallqvist A, Waters NC, Jongert E, Lemiale F, Bergmann-Leitner ES. Delayed fractional dose regimen of the RTS,S/AS01 malaria vaccine candidate enhances an IgG4 response that inhibits serum opsonophagocytosis. Sci Rep. 2017;7(1):7998.
42. Zhou J, Feng G, Beeson J, Hogarth PM, Rogerson SJ, Yan Y, Jaworowski A. CD14(hi)CD16+ monocytes phagocytose antibody-opsonised Plasmodium falciparum infected erythrocytes more efficiently than other monocyte subsets, and require CD16 and complement to do so. BMC Med. 2015;13:154.
43. Aponte JJ, Aide P, Renom M, Mandomando I, Bassat Q, Sacarlal J, Manaca MN, Lafuente S, Barbosa A, Leach A, et al. Safety of the RTS,S/AS02D candidate malaria vaccine in infants living in a highly endemic area of Mozambique: a double blind randomised controlled phase I/IIb trial. Lancet. 2007;370(9598):1543–51.
44. Abdulla S, Oberholzer R, Juma O, Kubhoja S, Machera F, Membi C, Omari S, Urassa A, Mshinda H, Jumanne A, et al. Safety and immunogenicity of RTS,S/AS02D malaria vaccine in infants. N Engl J Med. 2008;359(24):2533–44.
45. Han L, Hudgens MG, Emch ME, Juliano JJ, Keeler C, Martinson F, Kamthunzi P, Tegha G, Lievens M, Hoffman IF. RTS,S/AS01 malaria vaccine efficacy is not modified by seasonal precipitation: results from a phase 3 randomized controlled trial in Malawi. Sci Rep. 2017;7(1):7200.
46. Requena P, Campo JJ, Umbers AJ, Ome M, Wangnapi R, Barrios D, Robinson LJ, Samol P, Rosanas-Urgell A, Ubillos I, et al. Pregnancy and malaria exposure are associated with changes in the B cell pool and in plasma eotaxin levels. J Immunol. 2014;193(6):2971–83.
47. Ubillos I, Campo JJ, Requena P, Ome-Kaius M, Hanieh S, Rose H, Samol P, Barrios D, Jimenez A, Bardaji A, et al. Chronic exposure to malaria is associated with inhibitory and activation markers on atypical memory B cells and marginal zone-like B cells. Front Immunol. 2017;8:966.
48. Illingworth J, Butler NS, Roetynck S, Mwacharo J, Pierce SK, Bejon P, Crompton PD, Marsh K, Ndungu FM. Chronic exposure to Plasmodium falciparum is associated with phenotypic evidence of B and T cell exhaustion. J Immunol. 2013;190(3):1038–47.
49. Rinchai D, Presnell S, Chaussabel D. Blood interferon signatures putatively link lack of protection conferred by the RTS,S recombinant malaria vaccine to an antigen-specific IgE response. F1000Research. 2015;4(919).
50. Klein SL, Shann F, Moss WJ, Benn CS, Aaby P. RTS,S malaria vaccine and increased mortality in girls. MBio. 2016;7(2):e00514–6.

18

Offspring outcomes after prenatal interventions for common mental disorders

Marlies E. Brouwer[1,2], Alishia D. Williams[1,6], Sam E. van Grinsven[1], Pim Cuijpers[3], Mijke P. Lambregtse-van den Berg[4], Huibert Burger[5] and Claudi L. H. Bockting[2*]

Abstract

Background: It is presumed that pharmacological and non-pharmacological treatment of prenatal common mental disorders can mitigate associated adverse effects in offspring, yet strong evidence for the prophylactic benefits of treatment is lacking. We therefore examined the effect of prenatal treatments for common mental disorders on offspring outcomes.

Methods: For this meta-analysis, articles published up to August 31, 2017, were obtained from PubMed, PsycInfo, Embase, and Cochrane databases. Included studies needed to be randomized controlled trials (RCTs) on the effect of treatment of prenatal common mental disorders comparing an intervention to a control condition, including offspring outcome(s). Random effects models were used to calculate Hedges' g in the program Comprehensive Meta-Analysis© (version 3.0).

Results: Sixteen randomized controlled trials among 2778 pregnant women compared offspring outcomes between prenatal interventions and control groups. There were zero pharmacological, 13 psychological, and three other interventions (homeopathy, relaxation interventions, and short psycho-education). Birth weight (mean difference 42.88 g, $g = 0.08$, 95% CI −0.06 to 0.22, $p = 0.27$, $n = 11$), Apgar scores ($g = 0.13$, 95% CI −0.28 to 0.54, $p = 0.53$, $n = 4$), and gestational age ($g = 0.03$, 95% CI −0.06 to 0.54, $p = 0.49$, $n = 10$) were not significantly affected. Other offspring outcomes could not be meta-analyzed due to the inconsistent reporting of offspring outcomes and an insufficient number of studies.

Conclusions: Non-pharmacological interventions had no significant effect on birth outcomes, although this outcome should be considered with caution due to the risk of biases. No randomized controlled trial examined the effects of prenatal pharmacological treatments as compared to treatment as usual for common mental disorders on offspring outcomes. Present clinical guidelines may require more research evidence on offspring outcomes, including child development, in order to warrant the current recommendation to routinely screen and subsequently treat prenatal common mental disorders.

Trial registration: PROSPERO CRD42016047190

Keywords: Common mental disorders, Prenatal interventions, Offspring, Child, Pregnancy, Antidepressant, Psychotherapy, Depression, Anxiety

* Correspondence: c.l.bockting@amc.uva.nl

[2]Department of Psychiatry, Amsterdam University Medical Centres, location AMC, University of Amsterdam, Meibergdreef 9, 1105 AZ Amsterdam, the Netherlands

Full list of author information is available at the end of the article

Background

Leading clinical guidelines advise to screen and treat common mental disorders and symptoms among all pregnant women [1, 2]. Common mental disorders and symptoms generally refer to mood and anxiety disorders, including depression, phobias (including extreme fear of childbirth 'tokophobia'), generalized anxiety disorder, post-traumatic stress disorder, and obsessive-compulsive disorders [2]. Prevalence rates of mental disorders during pregnancy are estimated as high as 12.4% for mood disorders and 15.2% for anxiety disorders [3, 4]. Next to the burden of these common mental disorders for the pregnant women, these disorders may be harmful for the offspring [5]. Adverse effects on the offspring include almost 20% increased odds of low birth weight as compared to offspring from mothers without mental problems [6]. Low birth weight in turn has repeatedly been linked to negative (long term) somatic outcomes such as all-cause mortality, stunted growth, respiratory problems, and obesity [7]. In addition, low birth weight is associated with an increased risk for the development of mental problems [8]. Other adverse effects of prenatal mental disorders on the (unborn) child include a 13% increased risk of premature birth [6] and lower Apgar scores [5]. Similar to the effects of low birth weight, children from women who had a mental disorder during pregnancy have a two to three times increased risk for the development of psychopathology [9]. This includes an increased risk of symptoms of depression in (late) adolescence [10], an increased risk of anxiety in the ages 6 to 9 years old, and internalizing and externalizing (psychiatric) problems at the ages 2 to 6 [2, 11, 12]. Other risks for the offspring of pregnant women with common mental disorders include behavioral, motor, developmental, and cognitive problems such as attention-deficit hyperactivity disorder and an atypical (functional and structural) brain development [2, 9, 13, 14]. Theoretical accounts of the associations between prenatal mental health and offspring outcomes focus on a cascade of processes, such as activation of the stress-response (hypothalamic-pituitary-adrenal [HPA] axis), (epi)genetics, e.g., methylation of "stress" genes, elevated levels of intrauterine cytokines or glucocorticoids, and poor self-care during pregnancy (e.g., smoking, disturbed appetite) or poor mother-child attachment in the postpartum period due to the disabling nature of mental health problems [10, 14–18].

Effective treatments for prenatal common mental disorders are therefore of paramount importance given the recurrent and life-long course of most mental disorders and their association with (chronic) somatic conditions [19]. Although the exact mechanisms through which prenatal mental disorders exert an effect on offspring are currently unknown, the adverse outcomes themselves are clear. Current evidence-based treatments for mental disorders during pregnancy, i.e., medication and/or psychological interventions, are (implicitly) presumed to not only address mental needs of pregnant women, but also to confer prophylactic mental and physical benefits for offspring [20, 21]. As implied in the NICE guidelines, "The impact of any mental health problem may often require more urgent intervention than would usually be the case because of its potential effect on the foetus/baby (..)" [2]. The most used treatment for these disorders during pregnancy is antidepressant medication (AD; 3.7% of all pregnant women in the UK up to 6.2% in the USA [22, 23]), followed by psychological therapies including cognitive behavioral therapy (CBT) [24]. Supporting evidence for the benefits of these treatments is however limited, and the impact is typically restricted to the pregnant woman [1, 2, 24, 25]. Previous meta-analyses indicate that the evidence is restricted to psychological interventions for prenatal depression, for which CBT and interpersonal psychotherapy were shown to be most effective [24].

Given that the recommended treatments for prenatal common mental disorders might paradoxically have an adverse effect on the offspring intrauterine, it is crucial to examine the effects of prenatal maternal treatments on offspring. To our knowledge, no meta-analyses of randomized controlled trials (RCTs) have examined the effect of various treatments on common mental disorders during pregnancy on offspring [1, 2, 24, 25]. One meta-analysis indicated a positive, but small effect of prenatal preventive and acute treatments for depression on child functioning only [26]. Nonetheless, no conclusions regarding the effect of acute treatment for prenatal common mental disorders on offspring could be made, given that the majority of the studies that were included in this review included healthy pregnant women without (a history of) MDD or depressive symptoms (not acute treatment). Moreover, in the review, the authors did not assess the effects of acute treatment alone on child functioning. The last is the main aim of this meta-analysis, i.e., to examine the effect of prenatal treatments for common mental disorders on offspring outcomes. Some studies furthermore report adverse effects of prenatal antidepressants use on preterm birth, birth weight, and Apgar scores [27], persistent pulmonary hypertension (PPHN) [28, 29], development [30, 31], and cardiovascular malformations [32] in offspring. However, these reports are derived from non-randomized studies that do not permit conclusions of causality. The beneficial or possibly iatrogenic effects of psychological interventions on offspring are however less clear, despite the beneficial effects of psychotherapies for perinatal major depressive disorders as reported in previous meta-analyses [24, 25]. A review of the evidence from RCTs is timely and warranted. The primary aim of the current study was to conduct a meta-analysis to examine whether treatments for pregnant women with common mental disorders, as recommended in leading clinical guidelines (including antidepressants and psychotherapy) [1, 2], prevent adverse effects in offspring, both in terms of somatic and mental outcomes.

Method

Search strategy and selection criteria

This meta-analysis was conducted in accordance with the PRISMA guidelines and registered on PROSPERO [33]. A search in PubMed, PsycInfo, Embase, and the Cochrane database of randomized trials was performed on articles published from their origin through April 2016 and updated up to August 31, 2017. Five search strings were composed using standardized vocabulary (e.g., MeSH terms and text words), terms for searching title and abstract, and Boolean operators. The full search string is presented in Additional file 1. The five key strings targeted pregnancy, common mental disorders, interventions, offspring outcomes, and study design.

Included studies needed to (1) be a (cluster) randomized controlled trial; (2) treat (3) one or more prenatal common mental disorders or high levels of symptoms; (4) compare an intervention to a control condition; (5) include at least one offspring outcome; and (6) report sufficient information to calculate effect sizes (or provide this information available upon request). Included common mental disorders and symptoms were mood disorders and anxiety disorders according to the definition of DSM-IV axis I and older [34]. These included obsessive-compulsive disorders and trauma- and stress-related disorders/symptoms. Severe mental illnesses like bipolar disorder, psychosis, schizophrenia, or substance abuse were excluded due to the low prevalence rates [2]. The common mental disorder or symptoms could be assessed by self-report measures or clinical interviews, provided that the participants were primarily selected based upon the presence of mental disorders or high symptom levels. The control condition was defined as care or treatment as usual, wait-list control, or placebo medication. Language was restricted to English and Dutch due to the language proficiency of the authors. Two authors (MEB and SG) independently screened and selected the articles and assessed the risk of bias using the seven criteria as proposed by the Cochrane Handbook for Systematic Reviews of Interventions. Disagreement was solved by consultation of a third rater (CLB) and reaching consensus. The Grading of Recommendations Assessment, Development and Evaluation (GRADE) framework [35] was used to assess the overall level of certainty and strength of evidence for each of the main offspring outcomes. The evidence for each of the main offspring outcomes was potentially downgraded based upon risk of bias, inconsistency, indirectness, imprecision, number of participants, and pooled effect sizes.

Offspring outcome measures

The primary outcomes included all offspring variables collected in the neonatal period, during infancy and early childhood. They included Apgar scores, birth weight, gestational age, and measures of cognitive, motor, and emotional development. Examples of these variables are offspring depressive and anxiety symptoms (e.g., as assessed by the strengths and difficulties questionnaire [36]), general development (e.g., Bayley scales of infant development [37]), child behavior (e.g., child behavior checklist [38]), neurodevelopmental problems (e.g., Brazelton neonatal behaviour assessment scale [39]), and biological measures (e.g., cortisol levels, height, weight). No restrictions were made on the assessment instruments (self-report, reports, observations). Offspring outcomes needed to be reported as continuous outcomes in order to be able to calculate Hedges' g effect sizes. Where applicable, these outcomes were converted to the international system of units (SI), or to equal units (e.g., months to weeks, days to weeks, kilograms to grams). Data was extracted by one author (SG) using a standardized form and fully checked by a second author (MEB). Offspring measures that were reported in less than three studies were excluded from analyses.

Data analysis

The effect sizes for all child outcomes were calculated using Hedges' g and 95% confidence intervals (CI) to correct for small sample bias. Each effect size thus indicates a standardized comparison between the intervention group and control group. To calculate the pooled effect sizes, we extracted the reported mean scores, standard deviations, and number of participants for each group (intervention and control groups separately) for each offspring measurement. The software program Comprehensive Meta-Analysis© (version 3.0) was used to calculate pooled effect sizes, mean differences, forest plots, heterogeneity, and funnel plots. The effect sizes were interpreted according to Cohen's rule of thumb (small = 0.20–0.49; medium = 0.50–0.79; large = 0.80 and higher). As an indicator of heterogeneity among the effect sizes, we used the I^2 statistics (0% = no heterogeneity to 75% = high heterogeneity). We calculated 95% confidence intervals [40] around I^2, using the non-central χ^2-based approach within the heterogi module for Stata [41]. Funnel plots were used to visually inspect for publication bias, which was statistically checked with Egger's test of the intercept and Duval and Tweedie's trim and fill procedure [42].

A priori, we expected substantial heterogeneity between studies and therefore used a random effects model [43] in which a pooled effect size was calculated for each offspring outcome, and one random effects model for the overall pooled effect size. Secondly, several post hoc subgroup analyses were performed, in which pooled effect sizes were calculated for the main DSM disorders or symptoms, DSM disorders or symptoms and the offspring outcomes, type of intervention (psychotherapy, supplements or medication, and other), diagnostic status (through clinical interview or self-reported symptoms), risk of bias (high, low), and whether the author indicated a significant and positive effect of the intervention on maternal main DSM disorders or symptoms (yes, no). A mixed effects model was used in the subgroup analyses, where the pooled effect sizes within subgroups were calculated with the random effects model, and the fixed effects model was used to test the difference between subgroups.

Results

The search yielded 10,160 results up to April 2016. Citations and references of included articles and 207 reviews resulted in 129 additional articles. The search was updated up to August 2017, which resulted in 968 additional articles. A total of 9770 articles were screened after removal of duplicates. The systematic search resulted in 18 eligible articles (0.18%; see Fig. 1 for full details) reporting results of 16 RCTs, which are reported in Table 1. In total, 2778 pregnant women were randomized over 11 different treatment types. Treatment types included (variations of) CBT, massage therapy, psychoeducation, relaxation treatments, and couples therapy. Intensity of the interventions ranged from two psychoeducation phone sessions up to 16 CBT-based home visits. Details of treatment type, intensity, and the effects on maternal psychopathology are reported in Table 1. Seven studies focused on depression only [44–50], two on both depression and anxiety [51, 52], three on anxiety only [53–55], two on fear of childbirth [56, 57], one on posttraumatic stress disorder (PTSD) [58], one on stress in general [59], and one on various common mental disorders [60]. The risk of bias in the included studies was in general high, as reported in Table 1.

The included studies reported 28 different offspring outcome measures. Most outcomes were reported in a single study only. Analyses were restricted to the outcomes that were reported in at least three studies, which resulted in three eligible outcomes: birth weight, Apgar (1, 5, and 10 min combined), and gestational age (Fig. 2). For five studies, it was therefore not possible to aggregate any of the reported offspring outcomes in the meta-analysis, both in terms of target outcome (e.g., cognitive vs. emotional development) and measurement instrument. Effect sizes of the removed outcomes for each study are reported in Fig. 3. The mean values for each included study, and the overall highest and lowest values on the three offspring outcomes are displayed in Table 2.

Since there were no RCTs of pharmacological interventions during pregnancy reporting offspring outcomes, data from 11 non-pharmacological RCTs (reported in 13 articles) were analyzed. First, pooled effect sizes for each selected outcome were calculated. Outcomes of the meta-analysis are reported in Table 3 and displayed in Fig. 2. Birth weight was not significantly affected by interventions as compared to control conditions, corresponding to a mean difference of 42.88 g (95% CI −33.06 to 118.83, $N = 11$, $n = 1583$, $I^2 = 39\%$ [45, 47, 49, 50, 52–55, 57, 59, 60]) between the intervention and control groups. Gestational age and Apgar scores did not significantly improve or worsen by prenatal interventions (gestational age mean difference = 0.08 weeks [95% CI −0.09 to 0.24], $N = 10$, $n = 1669$, $I^2 = 0\%$ [49, 50, 52, 53, 55–57, 59, 60]; Apgar mean difference = 0.21 [95% CI −0.28 to 0.71], $N = 4$, $n = 663$, $I^2 = 68\%$ [51, 52, 55, 57]). The pooled effect size indicated an overall non-significant effect on Apgar scores, birth weight, and gestational age together. Since these three offspring outcomes are heterogeneous in interpretation, this overall result is not further discussed. Heterogeneity across the outcomes was low, $I^2 = 23\%$ (95% CI 0–60%). There was some indication of publication bias, as indicated by Duval and Tweedie's trim and fill procedure (studies trimmed = 2, adjusted $g = 0.05$, 95% CI −0.05 to 0.15). Visual inspection of the funnel plot and the Egger's test ($p = 0.16$) did not indicate publication bias. The evidence for each of the three pooled effect sizes was downgraded using the GRADE assessment to very low certainty of evidence. For each of the outcomes, there was a serious risk of bias, consistency in measures, serious indirectness, and serious imprecision. Birth weight and gestational age were rated as important outcomes, and Apgar scores were rated as not important.

Table 3 displays several subgroup analyses. Studies targeting depression and anxiety, or with a focus on other disorders, did not show a significant pooled effect size, hence did not improve offspring outcomes based on the three selected outcomes. According to the mixed effects analysis, the subgroups did not differ significantly. When investigating the separate offspring outcomes for each disorder (depression, anxiety, and other), it appeared that there was no significant effect of intervention on offspring outcomes within each disorder. The overall effect size in the risk of bias subgroup analysis was not significant. Although studies with a high risk of bias were significantly related to positive birth outcomes ($g = 0.21$, 95% CI 0.00 to 0.42, $p = 0.05$, $N = 7$, $n = 786$, $I^2 = 31\%$ [45, 47, 51, 53, 55, 57, 59]), the mixed effects analysis indicated no significant difference between high and low risk of bias studies ($p = 0.09$). The method

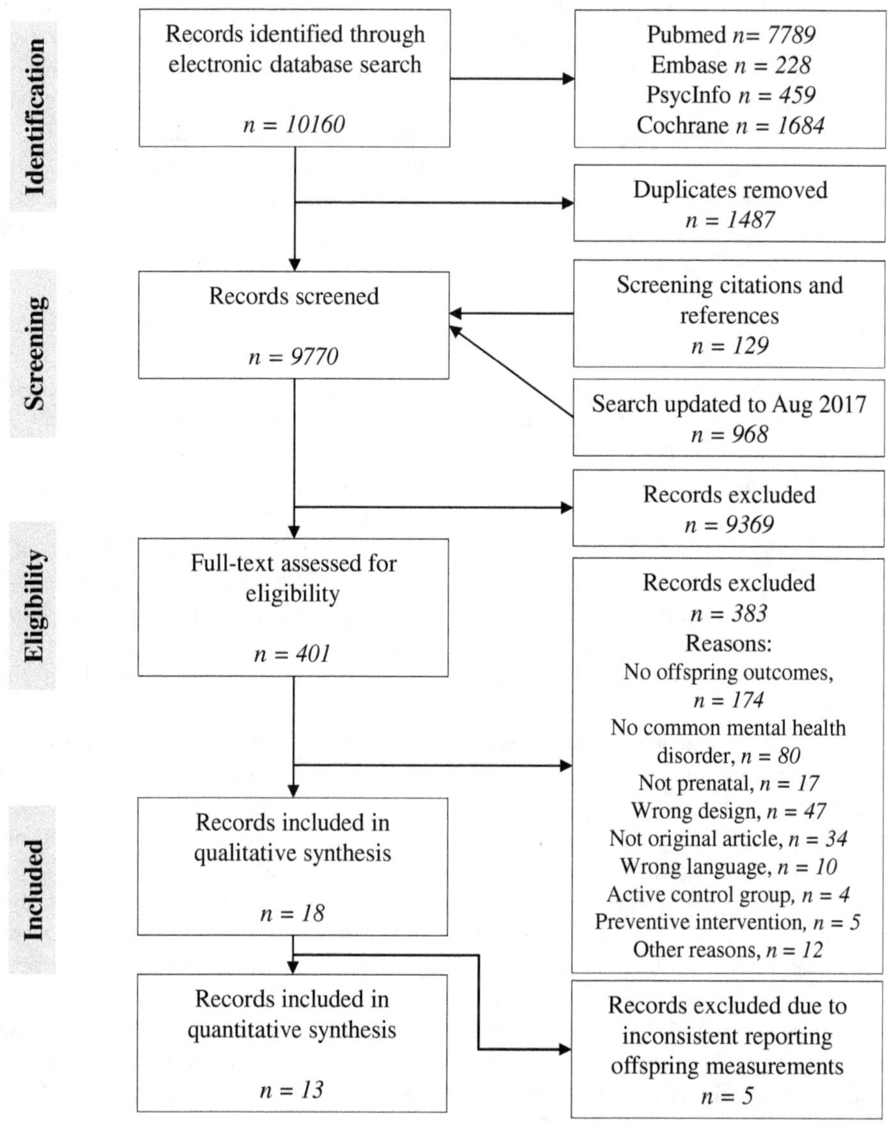

Fig. 1 Flowchart of included studies

through which the (possible) diagnosis was established, i.e., through clinical interview or self-report, whether the authors reported that the intervention had a significant effect on treating maternal common mental disorder (symptoms) compared to the control group, and the type of intervention (psychotherapy versus other types), did not significantly affect offspring outcomes, nor did the mixed effects analyses show differences between the subgroups (Table 3).

Discussion

Leading international clinical guidelines [1, 2] recommend screening and treatment of pregnant women for mental disorders and symptoms, with the clinical view to additionally prevent adverse effects on the offspring. The systematic search identified 16 non-pharmacological RCTs, including 14 psychological interventions that reported offspring outcomes. The results from the current meta-analysis indicate that non-pharmacological interventions do not have a significant effect on improving birth outcomes, and their effects could not be meta-analyzed for (developmental) offspring outcomes. Therefore, based on the current evidence, there is no strong indication of prophylactic effects. Although no statistically significant result was obtained for birth weight, all effect sizes within the 95% confidence interval around the pooled effect estimate were small, indicating that the true effect of prenatal interventions on birth weight is most likely small. Furthermore, the quality of most studies was low and the studies were relatively heterogeneous. An explanation for the non-significant effect size may be a ceiling effect since offspring in the control

Table 1 Overview of included studies

Author, year	Study focus	Selection criteria	Conditions and timing of intervention	No. of participants	Authors conclude sign. Effect of intervention on mother?	Offspring measures	Country	Risk of bias S	C	B	A	I	R	O	T
Bastani, 2006 [53]	Anxiety	STAI > 30	IG: Applied relaxation training, 7 wk. group sessions CG: TAU Prenatal	IG, 52; CG, 52; Total, 104	Yes, on anxiety symptoms	*Medical records:* BW & GA	Iran	?	?	?	?	+	–	?	H
Cappon, 2015 [54] [x]	Anxiety	BAI ≥ 21	IG: Listening to music, 20 to 296 times individually CG: TAU Prenatal	IG, 36; CG, 37; Total, 73	Yes, on anxiety symptoms	*Questionnaire:* BW & GA. *IBQ-r* at age 2 to 3 months	USA	?	?	+	+	–	+	+	L
Chambers, 2009 [55] [x]	Anxiety	STAI; State or trait subscale ≥ 40	IG: 6 wk. individual relaxation training CG: List of tips for reducing stress Prenatal	IG, 10; CG, 12; Total, 22	No	*Medical records:* BW & GA & Apgar scores	USA	+	?	–	+	–	+	–	H
Fenwick, 2015 [56]	Fear of childbirth	W-DEQ ≥ 66	IG: Telephone psycho-education, 2 sessions CG: TAU Prenatal	IG, 91; CG, 93; Total, 184	Yes, on flashbacks	*Medical records:* GA. Hospitalization up to 6 weeks	Australia	+	–	–	+	+	+	+	L
Field, 2009 [45]	Depression	SCID diagnosis MDD	IG: Massage therapy, 12 wk. sessions CG: TAU Prenatal	IG, 88; CG, 61; Total, 149	Yes, on depressive symptoms	*Medical records:* BW & GA. *Saliva* (cortisol) & *BNBAS* at age 2 days	USA	+	?	–	+	–	–	–	H
Karamoozian, 2015 [51]	Depression & Anxiety	EPDS > 9 & PRAQ high score	IG: 12 wk. group CBSM CG: TAU Prenatal	IG, 14; CG, 15; Total, 29	Yes, on anxiety and depressive symptoms	*Apgar scale:* Apgar scores	Iran	?	?	?	?	+	+	–	H
Madigan, 2015 [58]	PTSD in adolescents	CPTSDI PTSD diagnosis *or* AAI unresolved state of mind	IG: 12 wk. trauma focused CBT plus 12 sessions parenting course CG: Parenting course (TAU) Prenatal	IG, 12; CG, 14; Total, 26	No	*ASSP* at age 12 months	Canada	?	?	?	+	+	+	–	L
Maselko, 2015 [46] [a*]	Depression	SCID diagnosis MDD	IG: Thinking healthy programme (CBT based), 7 wk. visits and 9 monthly visits CG: Enhanced routine care Prenatal and postpartum	IG, 289; CG, 295; Total, 584	Yes, less MDD diagnoses in IG	*SDQ, SCAS*, weight, height, and BMI at age 7 years	Pakistan	+	+	+	+	+	–	–	L
Milgrom, 2015 [50]	Depression	SCID diagnosis MDD *and* EPDS ≥ 13	IG: Beating blues before birth (CBT based), 8 sessions CG: TAU Prenatal	IG, 16; CG, 13; Total, 29	Yes, on depressive and anxiety symptoms	*Medical records:* BW & GA. *IBQ-R, ASQ-3, and ASQ-SE* at age 9 months	Australia	+	+	?	+	+	–	–	M
Netsi, 2015 [47]	Depression	CIS diagnosis MDD	IG: 12 sessions individual CBT CG: TAU	IG, 14; CG, 11; Total, 25	Yes, on depressive symptoms	*Medical records:* BW. *ICQ and BISQ* at age 2 months	UK	+	+	–	+	–	+	–	H

Table 1 Overview of included studies *(Continued)*

Author, year	Study focus	Selection criteria	Conditions and timing of intervention	No. of participants	Authors conclude sign. Effect of intervention on mother?	Offspring measures	Country	Risk of bias							
								S	C	B	A	I	R	O	T
			Prenatal												
Rahman, 2008 [44]*	Depression	SCID diagnosis MDD	IG: Thinking healthy programme (CBT based), 7 wk. visits and 9 monthly visits CG: Enhanced routine care Prenatal and postpartum	IG, 440; CG, 463; Total, 903	Yes, on MDD diagnoses	*Records*: Weight, height, health at ages 6 and 12 months	Pakistan	+	+	+	+	+	+	+	L
Rothberg, 1991 [59]	Stress	SRRS ≥ 39	IG: Psychosocial support during each antenatal clinic visit CG: TAU Prenatal	IG, 43; CG, 43; Total, 86	No	*Medical records & Ballard score:* BW & GA. *Height, hospitalization* at birth	South Africa	+	?	?	+	−	+	−	H
Rouhe, 2013 [57]	Fear of childbirth	W-DEQ ≥ 100	IG: 6 sessions psycho-educative group therapy CG: TAU Prenatal and postpartum	IG, 131; CG, 240; Total: 371	Yes, on fear symptoms	*Medical records:* BW & GA & Apgar scores. Arterial Ph. at birth	Finland	+	+	−	−	−	+	−	H
Urizar, 2011 [48]	Depression	CES-D ≥ 16 *or* past history of MDD	IG: 12 wk. group CBSM CG: TAU Prenatal	IG, 24; CG, 29; Total, 53	No	*Saliva* (cortisol) at ages 6 and 18 months	USA	?	?	?	?	+	+	−	H
Verbeek, 2016[52][x]	Depression & Anxiety	EPDS ≥ 12 *or* STAI ≥ 42	IG: 10 to 12 sessions individual CBT CG: TAU Prenatal and postpartum	IG, 121; CG, 120; Total, 241	No	*Medical records:* BW & GA & Apgar scores	NL	+	+	−	+	+	+	+	L
Verbeek, 2016b [52] [b x]	Depression & Anxiety	EPDS ≥ 12 *or* STAI ≥ 42	IG: 10 to 12 sessions individual CBT CG: TAU Prenatal and postpartum	IG, 97; CG, 99; Total, 196	No	*CBCL and BSID* at age 18 months	NL	+	+	−	+	+	+	+	L
Vilhena, 2017 [60]	Common mental disorder in obese women	SRQ-20 ≥ 8	IG: Homeopathy, 2 times a day, 4 days a week CG: Placebo Prenatal	IG, 62; CG, 72; Total, 134	No	*Records:* GA, BW, Apgar of 10 at 5 min after birth	Brazil	+	+	+	?	?	+	−	L
Zhao, 2017 [49]	Depression	EPDS ≥ 9 or PDSS ≥ 20	IG: 6 sessions couple-separated psycho-educational program for first time parents CG: TAU Prenatal	IG, 175; CG, 174; Total, 349	Yes, on depressive status	*Medical records:* GA, BW	China	+	?	?	?	+	+	?	L

All presented studies were randomized controlled trials (RCT), except for *cluster RCT. [x]Doctoral dissertation. [a]Follow-up for Rahman 2008. [b]Follow-up for Verbeek 2016. *IG* intervention group, *CG* control group, *TAU* treatment as usual, *wk* weekly, *MDD* major depressive disorder, *CBSM* cognitive-behavioral stress management, *CBT* cognitive behavioral therapy, *BW* birth weight, *GA* gestational age, *USA* United States of America, *UK* United Kingdom, *NL* the Netherlands, *BAI* Beck anxiety inventory, *STAI* state trait anxiety inventory, *W-DEQ* Wijma delivery expectancy/experience questionnaire, *SCID* structured clinical interview for DSM disorders, *EPDS* Edinburgh postnatal depression scale, *PRAQ* pregnancy-related anxiety questionnaire, *CPTSDI* children's PTSD inventory, *PTSD* posttraumatic stress disorder, *AAI* adult attachment interview, *MDD* major depressive disorder, *CIS* clinical interview schedule, *SRRS* social readjustment rating scale, *CES-D* Centre for Epidemiological Studies depression Scale, *SRQ-20* self-report questionnaire, *IBQ-R* infant behaviour questionnaire revised, *ASQ-3* ages and stages questionnaire, *ASQ-SE* ages and stages questionnaire social emotional, *SDQ* strengths and difficulties questionnaire, *SCAS* Spence children's anxiety scale, *ASSP* Ainsworth strange situation procedure, *BNBAS* Brazelton neonatal behaviour assessment scale, *ICQ* infant characteristic questionnaire, *BISQ* brief infant sleep questionnaire, *BSID* Bayley scales of infant development, *CBCL* child behaviour checklist. Risk of bias criteria are represented as *S* = sequence generation, C = allocation concealment, B = blinding of participants and personnel, A = blinding of outcome assessors, I = incomplete outcome data, R = selective reporting, O = other sources of bias, and are coded as + = low risk of bias (0 points), − = high risk of bias (2 points),? = unclear risk of bias (1 point). T = total risk of bias, in which H = high risk of bias, L = low risk of bias. Total risk of bias is scored as < 6 = low risk, > 6 high risk

Author, year	Study focus	g	95% CI Lower - Upper		p-value
Chambers, 2009	Anxiety	-0.64	-1.48	0.20	0.14
Karamoozian, 2015	Mixed	1.04	0.28	1.80	0.01
Rouhe, 2013	Fear of childbirth	0.15	-0.19	0.49	0.37
Verbeek, 2016	Mixed	0.00	-0.25	0.25	1.00
	Apgar, pooled	**0.13**	**-0.28**	**0.54**	**0.53**
Bastani, 2006	Anxiety	0.52	0.13	0.91	0.01
Cappon, 2015	Anxiety	0.04	-0.42	0.49	0.87
Chambers, 2009	Anxiety	-0.52	-1.34	0.30	0.21
Field, 2009	Depression	0.22	-0.11	0.54	0.19
Milgrom, 2015	Depression	0.07	-0.57	0.71	0.83
Netsi, 2015	Depression	0.34	-0.43	1.11	0.39
Rothberg, 1991	Stress	0.15	-0.27	0.57	0.49
Rouhe, 2013	Fear of childbirth	0.09	-0.13	0.30	0.42
Verbeek, 2016	Mixed	-0.09	-0.34	0.16	0.48
Vilhena, 2017	Common mental health	0.23	-0.10	0.57	0.17
Zhao, 2017	Depression	-0.18	-0.39	0.03	0.10
	BW, pooled	**0.08**	**-0.06**	**0.22**	**0.27**
Bastani, 2006	Anxiety	0.00	-0.38	0.38	1.00
Chambers, 2009	Anxiety	-0.54	-1.36	0.29	0.20
Fenwick, 2015	Fear of childbirth	0.03	-0.26	0.32	0.85
Field, 2009	Depression	0.22	-0.11	0.54	0.19
Milgrom, 2015	Depression	0.00	-0.68	0.68	1.00
Rothberg, 1991	Stress	0.14	-0.28	0.56	0.52
Rouhe, 2013	Fear of childbirth	0.06	-0.15	0.28	0.56
Verbeek, 2016	Mixed	-0.12	-0.38	0.13	0.33
Vilhena, 2017	Common mental health	0.27	-0.07	0.61	0.11
Zhao, 2017	Depression	-0.02	-0.23	0.19	0.82
	GA, pooled	**0.03**	**-0.06**	**0.13**	**0.49**

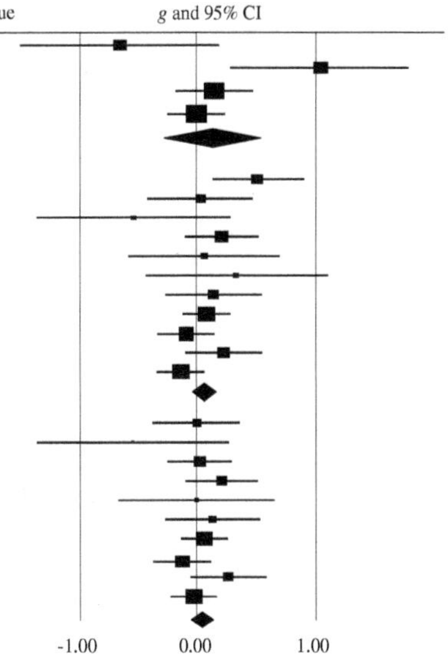

Fig. 2 Forest plots for Apgar scores, birth weight, and gestational age. BW = birth weight, GA = gestational age, *g* = Hedges' *g*, mixed = combination of multiple common mental disorders and/or symptoms

and intervention groups had a birth weight within the normal range. The birth weight in the trials ranged from 2883 to 3626 g, indicating there was no low birth weight according to the worldwide standards for low birth weight, that is less than 2500 g [61].

Secondly, the meta-analysis did not show that the somatic outcomes indexed by Apgar scores and gestational age were significantly associated with the non-pharmacological interventions. As for birth weight, the confidence intervals around the pooled effect estimates for Apgar scores and gestational age indicate that a true effect is most likely small. It was furthermore not possible to investigate the impact of prenatal interventions on preventing preterm birth, since the included studies had different definitions of preterm birth (different gestational age), or did not report enough information to calculate effect sizes. Additionally, five out of 16 studies reported different measures of (long term) offspring outcomes. It was therefore not possible to investigate the effects of interventions on non-somatic outcomes, such as psychopathology or developmental problems. Although previous research and clinical

Author, year	Study focus	Outcome measure	Timing	g	95% CI Lower - Upper		p-value
Behavioral outcomes							
Milgrom, 2015	Depression	Combined	9 months	0.42	-0.30	1.15	0.25
Field, 2009	Depression	Combined	1 day	0.41	0.09	0.74	0.01
Netsi, 2015	Depression	Combined	2 months	-0.57	-1.35	0.21	0.15
Verbeek, 2016b	Mixed	Combined	18 months	-0.05	-0.35	0.24	0.71
Cappon, 2015	Anxiety	Combined	2-3 months	1.49	0.97	2.01	0.00
Biological outcomes							
Field, 2009	Depression	Cortisol levels	0	1.04	0.69	1.39	0.00
Maselko, 2015	Depression	Combined	7 years	-0.07	-0.23	0.09	0.41
Rahman, 2008	Depression	Combined	Combined	0.14	-0.01	0.28	0.06
Rothberg, 1991	Stress	Length	0	-0.28	-0.70	0.14	0.19
Rouhe, 2013	Fear of childbirth	Combined	0	-0.04	-0.34	0.26	0.79
Urizar, 2011	Risk of PPD	Combined	Combined	0.19	-0.36	0.74	0.50
Social/ developmental / emotional outcomes							
Madigan, 2015	PTSD	ASSP Disorg.	12 months	-0.07	-0.82	0.67	0.85
Maselko, 2015	Depression	Combined	7 years	-0.06	-0.22	0.10	0.45
Milgrom, 2015	Depression	Combined	9 months	0.58	-0.14	1.31	0.12
Netsi, 2015	Depression	Difficult temp.	2 months	0.08	-0.68	0.84	0.83
Urizar, 2011	Risk of PPD	Combined	18 months	-0.21	-0.78	0.36	0.48
Verbeek, 2016b	Mixed	Combined	18 months	-0.10	-0.40	0.20	0.51
Cognitive outcomes							
Verbeek, 2016b	Mixed	BSID Cognitive	18 months	-0.14	-0.43	0.15	0.35

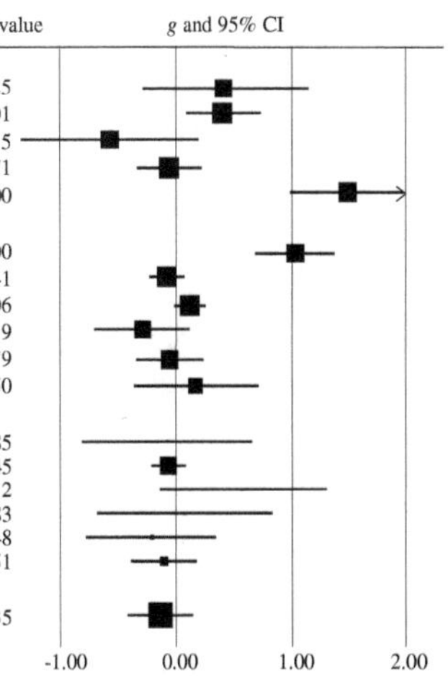

Fig. 3 Forest plots of excluded offspring outcomes. *g* = Hedges' *g*, mixed = combination of multiple common mental disorders and/or symptoms, combined = combination of multiple offspring outcomes and/or timing of offspring outcomes, PPD = peripartum depression, ASSP Disorg = Ainsworth stranger situation disorganized attachment measure, BSID Cognitive = Bayley scales of infant development-cognitive subscale, difficult temp = difficult temperament

Table 2 Study offspring outcomes

Author, year	Mean birth weight (Sd.) in grams	Mean Apgar score (Sd.)	Mean gestational age (Sd.) in weeks
Bastani, 2006 [53]	IG, 3168 (420) CG, 2883 (640)	n/a	IG, 38 (5.9) CG, 38 (4.4)
Cappon, 2015 [54]	IG, 3366 (523) CG, 3344 (773)	n/a	n/a
Chambers, 2009 [55]	IG, 3232 (695) CG, 3562 (529)	IG, Apgar 1 min: 7.8 (1.3) CG, Apgar 1 min: 8 (1.1) IG, Apgar 5 min: 8.5 (0.7) CG, Apgar 5 min: 9.1 (0.3)	IG, 38.4 (2.5) CG, 39.5 (1.4)
Fenwick, 2015 [56]	n/a	n/a	IG, 39.2 (1.6) CG, 39.1 (2.0)
Field, 2009 [45]	IG, 3318 (360) CG, 3226 (492)	n/a	IG, 39 (1.2) CG, 38.7 (1.6)
Karamoozian, 2015 [51]	n/a	IG, Apgar 1 min: 8.9 (0.3) CG, Apgar 1 min: 8.1 (0.8) IG, Apgar 5 min: 9.7 (0.5) CG, Apgar 5 min: 9.3 (0.7)	n/a
Milgrom, 2015 [50]	IG, 3626 (786) CG, 3575 (595)	n/a	IG, 40 (1) CG, 40 (2)
Netsi, 2015 [47]	IG, 3423 (503) CG, 3180 (871)	n/a	n/a
Rothberg, 1991 [59]	IG, 3214 (649) CG, 3113 (690)	n/a	IG, 38.7 (3) CG, 38.3 (2.7)
Rouhe, 2013 [57]	IG, 3532 (550) CG, 3486 (518)	IG, Apgar 1 min: 8.7 (1.1) CG, Apgar 1 min: 8.5 (1.4) IG, Apgar 5 min: 9.3 (1.0) CG, Apgar 5 min: 9.1 (1.2) IG, Apgar 10 min: 9.7 (0.8) CG, Apgar 10 min: 9.5 (0.9)	IG, 39.7 (1.5) CG, 39.6 (1.6)
Verbeek, 2016; Verbeek, 2016b [52]	IG, 3419 (651) CG, 3474 (561)	IG, Apgar 1 min: 8.6 (n/a) CG, Apgar 1 min: 8.6 (n/a) IG, Apgar 5 min: 9.5 (n/a) CG, Apgar 5 min: 9.5 (n/a) IG, Apgar 10 min: 9.8 (n/a) CG, Apgar 10 min: 9.8 (n/a)	IG, 38.9 (2.3) CG, 39.2 (1.8)
Vilhena, 2017 [60]	IG, 3390 (440) CG, 3270 (560)	n/a	IG, 39.4 (1.2) CG, 38.9 (1.9)
Zhao, 2017 [49]	IG, 3256 (522) CG, 3349 (529)	n/a	n/a
Combined range per offspring outcome	Lowest value, 2883 Highest value, 3626	Lowest value, 7.8 Highest value, 9.8	Lowest value, 38 Highest value, 40

IG intervention group, *CG* control group

guidelines [1, 2] report on harmful effects of prenatal mental disorders on offspring, including an increased risk of low birth weight [6], the current meta-analysis could not support the notion that treatment can mitigate this effect. Furthermore, the current results did not indicate that pregnant women in the care as usual or placebo groups had worse or better offspring outcomes. This is to some extent in contrast to a recent meta-analysis, in which it was concluded that prenatal preventive and acute interventions for MDD (symptoms) improved overall child functioning. This effect was however primarily based upon preventive interventions and offspring behaviour [26].

The current meta-analysis found zero RCTs on the effects of antenatal treatment of common mental disorders with medication (i.e., antidepressants) on offspring. This is noteworthy given the fact that antidepressant medication is one of the most used treatments during pregnancy [22]. Furthermore, previous reviews of non-randomized trials indicate an association between prenatal antidepressant use and adverse offspring outcomes, including lower birth weight, preterm birth, lower Apgar scores [27, 62], and cardiovascular malformations [32]. Correspondingly, untreated maternal mental disorders has been associated with similar adverse effects, which in turn are linked to other subsequent

Table 3 Meta-analyses and subgroup analyses results

		N	No. of participants	g	95% CI	p	I^2	95% CI	p^a
Effect of prenatal interventions on offspring outcomes (BW, GA, Apgar)	All studies [45, 47, 49–57, 59, 60]	13	1796	0.09	− 0.03 to 0.21	0.14	23	0–60	
Effect of prenatal interventions for each offspring outcome	BW [45, 47, 49, 50, 52–55, 57, 59]	11	1583	0.08	− 0.06 to 0.22	0.27	39	0–70	
	GA [49, 50, 52, 53, 55–57, 59, 60]	10	1669	0.03	− 0.06 to 0.13	0.49	0	0–53	
	Apgar [51, 52, 55, 57]	4	663	0.13	− 0.28 to 0.54	0.53	68	0–87	
Subgroup analyses									
Type of diagnosis*	Anxiety [52–57]	6	852	− 0.01	− 0.22 to 0.20	0.89	40	0–75	0.41
	BW [52–55, 57]	5	668	0	− 0.33 to 0.32	1	70	22–88	
	GA [52–56]	5	779	− 0.06	− 0.24 to 0.12	0.54	27	0–71	
	Depression [45, 47–50]	5	575	0.02	− 0.15 to 0.18	0.86	0	0–79	
	BW [45, 47–50]	5	575	0.01	− 0.20 to 0.23	0.90	22	0–68	
	GA [45, 48–50]	4	550	0.05	− 0.12 to 0.21	0.58	0	0–85	
	Other [51, 52, 59, 60]	4	283	0.22	− 0.90 to 0.54	0.17	62	0–85	
	BW [52, 59, 60]	3	254	0.06	− 0.15 to 0.27	0.57	22	0–97	
	GA [52, 59, 60]	3	254	0.07	− 0.19 to 0.33	0.60	45	0–84	
Risk of bias	High [45, 47, 51, 53, 55, 57, 59]	7	786	0.21	− 0.00 to 0.42	*0.05*	31	0–70	0.09
	Low [49, 50, 52, 54, 56, 60]	6	1010	− 0.00	− 0.13 to 0.12	0.97	0	0–61	
Diagnosis through clinical interview or self-report	Clinical interview [45, 47, 50]	3	203	0.20	− 0.07 to 0.47	0.15	0	0–90	0.43
	Self-report [49, 51–60]	10	1593	0.08	− 0.06 to 0.22	0.28	36	0–70	
Type of intervention	Psychotherapy [47, 49–52, 57, 59]	7	1130	0.08	− 0.10 to 0.27	0.40	39	0–75	0.67
	Other [45, 53–56, 60]	6	666	0.13	− 0.02 to 0.28	0.09	0	0–74	
Report of sign. Effect of intervention on mother?	No [52, 55, 59, 60]	4	483	0.05	− 0.18 to 0.28	0.68	31	0–75	0.64
	Yes [45, 47, 49–51, 53, 54, 56, 57]	9	1313	0.11	− 0.04 to 0.26	0.14	29	0–67	

[a]The p value indicates whether the subgroups differ from each other. g = Hedges' g, 95% CI = confidence interval 95% of Hedges' g. *In this subgroup analysis, the Verbeek 2016 study subgroups depression, anxiety, and combined (other) were analyzed separately. *BW* birth weight, *GA* gestational age. Superscript numbers refer to included studies in each analysis

offspring problems [7]. Other studies suggest that the effects of antidepressants on offspring might be minimal [63–65]. Due to the nature of the studies (non-randomized cohort trials), there is insufficient evidence of the possible effects of prenatal antidepressant usage. It is therefore not clear what the net effects of antidepressants are for offspring. RCTs and comparative treatment trials are needed to disentangle whether these offspring outcomes are related to antidepressant use or are predominantly the result of the mental disorders of the mother. To estimate the (enduring) relative effects of pharmacological and non-pharmacological interventions on offspring, a RCT comparing the two intervention types may provide more information on the prophylactic effects on offspring. Such design would be more ethical since the pregnant woman receives treatment according to clinical recommendations. Moreover, it would provide more information on the effects of antidepressants.

Collectively, the findings of the meta-analysis indicate that there is insufficient data to support the beneficial effects of prenatal treatments on offspring and that more research on the effects of prenatal treatments on offspring is needed. These results of the meta-analysis must be interpreted in the context of some limitations. In general, the included trials had a high risk of bias and reported different offspring outcomes, and the GRADE assessment indicated very low certainty of evidence, thereby limiting the results. Overall, there is some indication that non-pharmacological interventions may have a positive influence on offspring birth weight; however, the effect was not significant and could be overestimated due to the small samples sizes and high risk of bias. The small sample size of pregnant women, and the small amount of included studies, increases the risk of false-positive and false-negative birth outcomes. Furthermore, other birth outcomes including preterm birth, low birthweight for gestational age, or child development could not be analyzed due to the inconsistent reporting and lack of studies. There is no conclusive evidence that interventions aimed to target prenatal mental disorders are beneficial or iatrogenic for offspring, especially with regard to long-term and psychological impact.

For health care professionals, there is little evidence that prenatal non-pharmacological interventions are beneficial for the offspring with respect to birth weight, gestational age, and Apgar scores. There is not enough support that commonly used treatments for prenatal mental disorders are beneficial to offspring and hence do not provide a scientific foundation to support recommendations of specific treatment options with respect to the benefit for the child. More systematic research with long-term follow-up of the offspring is consequently needed to support (inter)national guidelines for prenatal mental disorders. As a first step, research on prenatal interventions may register birth outcomes from birth reports of (former) participants in RCTs. RCTs focusing on pharmacological interventions as compared to psychotherapy during pregnancy are needed, even though this may be challenging due to ethical considerations and preferences of pregnant women and their health care providers.

Conclusions

The results from the current meta-analysis indicate no significant effects of non-pharmacological interventions on improving birth outcomes. No firm conclusion of prophylactic effects can be drawn due to the reported limitations. Despite the recommendation of leading international clinical guidelines [1, 2] to routinely screen pregnant women for common mental disorders and symptoms, and subsequently treat the mother to reduce perinatal symptomatology and prevent adverse effects on the offspring, there is insufficient data to support the clinical recommendation regarding the safety of prenatal treatments for the offspring. Prior research implies that prenatal interventions improve maternal psychopathology [24, 26], yet more research is warranted to draw stronger conclusions on the impact of prenatal interventions on offspring, especially regarding child development. Potential adverse effects on offspring cannot be ruled out, thereby underscoring the urgent need for properly controlled trials to best inform care approaches for mothers and their offspring.

Abbreviations

AD: Antidepressant medication; CBT: Cognitive behavioral therapy; CI: Confidence intervals; PPHN: Persistent pulmonary hypertension; PTSD: Posttraumatic stress disorder; RCT: Randomized controlled trial

Acknowledgements

Not applicable.

Funding

Not applicable.

Authors' contributions

MEB, SG, and CLB designed the study and study proposal. MEB and SG assessed studies for eligibility, designed data collection tools, and extracted and systematically scored all information from included articles. CLB was the third rated to reach consensus. MEB, SG, and PC analyzed the data, and all authors interpreted the results. MEB, AW, SG, and CLB drafted the article. All authors critically revised the article and approved the final version.

Competing interests

The authors declare that they have no competing interests.

Author details

[1]Department of Clinical Psychology, Utrecht University, Heidelberglaan 1, 3584 CS Utrecht, the Netherlands. [2]Department of Psychiatry, Amsterdam University Medical Centres, location AMC, University of Amsterdam, Meibergdreef 9, 1105 AZ Amsterdam, the Netherlands. [3]Department of Clinical, Neuro and Developmental Psychology, Vrije Universiteit Amsterdam, Van der Boechorststraat 1, 1081 BT Amsterdam, the Netherlands. [4]Department of Psychiatry and Child and Adolescent Psychiatry/Psychology, Erasmus Medical Centre Rotterdam, P.O. Box 2060, 3000 CB Rotterdam, the Netherlands. [5]Department of General Practice, University Medical Centre Groningen, University of Groningen, Antonius Deusinglaan 1, 9713 AV Groningen, the Netherlands. [6]Faculty of Science, School of Psychology, The University of New South Wales, Sydney, NSW 2052, Australia.

References

1. O'Connor E, Rossom RC, Henninger M, Groom HC, Burda BU. Primary care screening for and treatment of depression in pregnant and postpartum women. JAMA. 2016;315:388.
2. National Institute for Health and Clinical Excellence. Antenatal and postnatal mental health: clinical management and service guidance: Updated edition. NICE Clinical Guideline 192. London: NICE; 2014. Available from: https://www.nice.org.uk/guidance/cg192/evidence/full-guideline-pdf-4840896925.
3. Dennis C-L, Falah-Hassani K, Shiri R. Prevalence of antenatal and postnatal anxiety: systematic review and meta-analysis. Br J Psychiatry. 2017;210:315–23.
4. Bennett HA, Einarson A, Taddio A, Koren G, Einarson TRT. Prevalence of depression during pregnancy: systematic review. Obstet Gynecol. 2004;103: 698–709.
5. Alder J, Fink N, Bitzer J, Hösli I, Holzgreve W. Depression and anxiety during pregnancy: a risk factor for obstetric, fetal and neonatal outcome? A critical review of the literature. J Matern Neonatal Med. 2007;20:189–209.
6. Grote NK, Bridge JA, Gavin AR, Melville JL, Iyengar S, Katon WJ. A meta-analysis of depression during pregnancy and the risk of preterm birth, low birth weight, and intrauterine growth restriction. Arch Gen Psychiatry. 2010;67:1012–24.
7. Belbasis L, Savvidou MD, Kanu C, Evangelou E, Tzoulaki I. Birth weight in relation to health and disease in later life: an umbrella review of systematic reviews and meta-analyses. BMC Med. 2016;14:147.
8. Loret de Mola C, Araujo de Franca GV, de Quevedo LA, Horta BL. Low birth weight, preterm birth and small for gestational age association with adult depression: systematic review and meta-analysis. Br J Psychiatry. 2014;205:340–7.
9. O'Donnell KJ, Glover V, Barker ED, O'Connor TG. The persisting effect of maternal mood in pregnancy on childhood psychopathology. Dev Psychopathol. 2014;26: 393–403.
10. Stein A, Pearson RM, Goodman SH, Rapa E, Rahman A, McCallum M, et al. Effects of perinatal mental disorders on the fetus and child. Lancet. 2014; 384:1800–19.
11. Newman L, Judd F, Olsson CA, Castle D, Bousman C, Sheehan P, et al. Early origins of mental disorder - risk factors in the perinatal and infant period. BMC Psychiatry. 2016;16:270.
12. Lahti M, Savolainen K, Tuovinen S, Pesonen A-K, Lahti J, Heinonen K, et al. Maternal depressive symptoms during and after pregnancy and psychiatric problems in children. J Am Acad Child Adolesc Psychiatry. 2017;56:30–39.e7.
13. van den Bergh BRH, Dahnke R, Mennes M. Prenatal stress and the developing brain: risks for neurodevelopmental disorders. Dev Psychopathol. 2018;30:743–62.

14. van den Bergh BRH, van den Heuvel MI, Lahti M, Braeken M, de Rooij SR, Entringer S, et al. Prenatal developmental origins of behavior and mental health: the influence of maternal stress in pregnancy. Neurosci Biobehav Rev. 2017. [Epub ahead of print]
15. Talge NM, Neal C, Glover V. Antenatal maternal stress and long-term effects on child neurodevelopment: how and why? J Child Psychol Psychiatry Allied Discip. 2007;48:245–61.
16. Gluckman PD, Hanson MA, Cooper C, Thornburg KL. Effect of in utero and early-life conditions on adult health and disease. N Engl J Med. 2008;359:61–73.
17. Pearson RM, Evans J, Kounali D, Lewis G, Heron J, Ramchandani PG, et al. Maternal depression during pregnancy and the postnatal period: risks and possible mechanisms for offspring depression at 18 years. JAMA Psychiatry. 2013;70:1312. https://doi.org/10.1001/jamapsychiatry.2013.2163.
18. Barker DJ. The fetal and infant origins of adult disease. BMJ. 1990;301:1111.
19. Bockting CL, Hollon SD, Jarrett RB, Kuyken W, Dobson K. A lifetime approach to major depressive disorder: the contributions of psychological interventions in preventing relapse and recurrence. Clin Psychol Rev. 2015; 41:16–26.
20. Rahman A, Fisher J, Bower P, Luchters S, Tran T, Yasamy MT, et al. Interventions for common perinatal mental disorders in women in low- and middle-income countries: a systematic review and meta-analysis. Bull World Health Organ. 2013;91:593–601I.
21. Lewis AJ, Galbally M, Gannon T, Symeonides C. Early life programming as a target for prevention of child and adolescent mental disorders. BMC Med. 2014;12:33.
22. Charlton RA, Jordan S, Pierini A, Garne E, Neville AJ, Hansen AV, et al. Selective serotonin reuptake inhibitor prescribing before, during and after pregnancy: a population-based study in six European regions. BJOG. 2015; 122:1010–20.
23. Ko JY, Farr SL, Dietz PM, Robbins CL. Depression and treatment among U.S. pregnant and nonpregnant women of reproductive age, 2005–2009. J Womens Heal. 2012;21:830–6.
24. van Ravesteyn LM, Lambregtse-van den Berg MP, WJG H, Kamperman AM. Interventions to treat mental disorders during pregnancy: a systematic review and multiple treatment meta-analysis. PLoS One. 2017;12:e0173397.
25. Cuijpers P, Weitz E, Karyotaki E, Garber J, Andersson G. The effects of psychological treatment of maternal depression on children and parental functioning: a meta-analysis. Eur Child Adolesc Psychiatry. 2014;24:237–45.
26. Goodman SH, Cullum KA, Dimidjian S, River LM, Kim CY. Opening windows of opportunities: evidence for interventions to prevent or treat depression in pregnant women being associated with changes in offspring's developmental trajectories of psychopathology risk. Dev Psychopathol. 2018;30:1179–96.
27. Ross LE, Grigoriadis S, Mamisashvili L, Vonderporten EH, Roerecke M, Rehm J, et al. Selected pregnancy and delivery outcomes after exposure to antidepressant medication: a systematic review and meta-analysis. JAMA Psychiatry. 2013;70:436–43.
28. Huybrechts KF, Bateman BT, Palmsten K, Desai RJ, Patorno E, Gopalakrishnan C, et al. Antidepressant use late in pregnancy and risk of persistent pulmonary hypertension of the newborn. JAMA. 2015;313:2142.
29. Grigoriadis S, Vonderporten EH, Mamisashvili L, Tomlinson G, Dennis C-L, Koren G, et al. Prenatal exposure to antidepressants and persistent pulmonary hypertension of the newborn: systematic review and meta-analysis. BMJ. 2014;348:f6932.
30. Rai D, Lee BK, Dalman C, Newschaffer C, Lewis G, Magnusson C. Antidepressants during pregnancy and autism in offspring: population based cohort study. BMJ. 2017;358:j2811.
31. Man KKC, Chan EW, Ip P, Coghill D, Simonoff E, Chan PKL, et al. Prenatal antidepressant use and risk of attention-deficit/hyperactivity disorder in offspring: population based cohort study. BMJ. 2017;357:j2350.
32. Grigoriadis S, VonderPorten EH, Mamisashvili L, Roerecke M, Rehm J, Dennis C-L, et al. Antidepressant exposure during pregnancy and congenital malformations: is there an association? J Clin Psychiatry. 2013;74:e293–308.
33. van Grinsven S, Brouwer ME, CLH B. Offspring outcomes of prenatal treatment of maternal psychopathology. PROSPERO. 2016; http://www.crd.york.ac.uk/PROSPERO/display_record.asp?ID=CRD42016047190.
34. American Psychiatric Association. Diagnostic and statistical manual of mental disorders (4th ed., text rev.). Washington, DC, US: Author; 2000.
35. Guyatt G, Oxman AD, Akl EA, Kunz R, Vist G, Brozek J, et al. GRADE guidelines: 1. Introduction—GRADE evidence profiles and summary of findings tables. J Clin Epidemiol. 2011;64:383–94.
36. Goodman R. The strengths and difficulties questionnaire: a research note. J Child Psychol Psychiatry. 1997;38:581–6.
37. Bayley N. Bayley scales of infant and toddler development. San Antonio: The Psychological Corporation; 2006.
38. Rescorla LA. Assessment of young children using the Achenbach System of Empirically Based Assessment (ASEBA). Ment Retard Dev Disabil Res Rev. 2005;11:226–37.
39. Brazelton TB. Introduction. Monogr Soc Res Child Dev. 1978;43(5/6):1.
40. Ioannidis JPA, Patsopoulos NA, Evangelou E. Uncertainty in heterogeneity estimates in meta-analyses. Br Med J. 2007;335(7626):914–6.
41. Orsini N, Bottai M, Higgins J, Buchan I. HETEROGI: Stata module to quantify heterogeneity in a meta-analysis. Statistical Software Components S449201, Boston College Department of Economics, revised 25 Jan 2006.
42. Duval S, Tweedie R. Trim and fill: a simple funnel-plot-based method of testing and adjusting for publication bias in meta-analysis. Biometrics. 2000;56:455–63.
43. Borenstein M, Hedges LV, JPT H, Rothstein HR. An introduction to meta-analysis. Chichester: Wiley; 2009.
44. Rahman A, Malik A, Sikander S, Roberts C, Creed F. Cognitive behaviour therapy-based intervention by community health workers for mothers with depression and their infants in rural Pakistan: a cluster-randomised controlled trial. Lancet. 2008;372:902–9.
45. Field T, Diego M, Hernandez-Reif M, Deeds O, Figueiredo B. Pregnancy massage reduces prematurity, low birthweight and postpartum depression. Infant Behav Dev. 2009;32:454–60.
46. Maselko J, Sikander S, Bhalotra S, Bangash O, Ganga N, Mukherjee S, et al. Effect of an early perinatal depression intervention on long-term child development outcomes: follow-up of the Thinking Healthy Programme randomised controlled trial. Lancet Psychiatry. 2015;2:609–17.
47. Netsi E, Evans J, Wulff K, O'Mahen H, Ramchandani PG. Infant outcomes following treatment of antenatal depression: findings from a pilot randomized controlled trial. J Affect Disord. 2015;188:252–6.
48. Urizar GG, Muñoz RF. Impact of a prenatal cognitive-behavioral stress management intervention on salivary cortisol levels in low-income mothers and their infants. Psychoneuroendocrinology. 2011;36:1480–94.
49. Zhao Y, Munro-Kramer ML, Shi S, Wang J, Luo J. A randomized controlled trial: effects of a prenatal depression intervention on perinatal outcomes among Chinese high-risk pregnant women with medically defined complications. Arch Womens Ment Health. 2017;20:333–44.
50. Milgrom J, Holt C, Holt CJ, Ross J, Ericksen J, Gemmill AW. Feasibility study and pilot randomised trial of an antenatal depression treatment with infant follow-up. Arch Womens Ment Health. 2015;18:717–30.
51. Karamoozian M, Askarizadeh G. Impact of prenatal cognitive-behavioral stress management intervention on maternal anxiety and depression and newborns' Apgar scores. Iran J Neonatol. 2015;6:14–23.
52. Verbeek T. Pregnancy and psychopathology. Groningen: University of Groningen; 2016.
53. Bastani F, Hidarnia A, Montgomery KS, Aguilar-Vafaei ME, Kazemnejad A. Does relaxation education in anxious primigravid Iranian women influence adverse pregnancy outcomes? A randomized controlled trial. J Perinat Neonatal Nurs. 2006;20:138–46.
54. Cappon R. Anxious origins: attenuating maternal and fetal anxiety with acoustically modified music. Ann Arbor: ProQuest LLC; 2015.
55. Chambers AS. Relaxation during pregnancy to reduce stress and anxiety and their associated complications. Arizona: The University of Arizona; 2009.
56. Fenwick J, Toohill J, Gamble J, Creedy DK, Buist A, Turkstra E, et al. Effects of a midwife psycho-education intervention to reduce childbirth fear on women's birth outcomes and postpartum psychological wellbeing. BMC Pregnancy Childbirth. 2015;15:284.
57. Rouhe H, Salmela-Aro K, Toivanen R, Tokola M, Halmesmäki E, Saisto T. Obstetric outcome after intervention for severe fear of childbirth in nulliparous women - randomised trial. BJOG An Int J Obstet Gynaecol. 2013; 120:75–84.
58. Madigan S, Vaillancourt K, McKibbon A, Benoit D. Trauma and traumatic loss in pregnant adolescents: the impact of trauma-focused cognitive behavior therapy on maternal unresolved states of mind and posttraumatic stress disorder. Attach Hum Dev. 2015;17:175–98.
59. Rothberg AD, Lits B. Psychosocial support for maternal stress during pregnancy: effect on birth weight. Am J Obstet Gynecol. 1991;165:403–7.
60. de Vilhena EC, de Castilho EA. Homeopathic treatment of overweight and obesity in pregnant women with mental disorders: a double-blind, controlled clinical trial. Altern Ther Health Med. 2016;22:14–22.

61. United Nations Children's Fund and World Health Organization. Low birthweight: country, regional and global estimates. New York: UNICEF; 2004.
62. Grigoriadis S, VonderPorten EH, Mamisashvili L, Eady A, Tomlinson G, Dennis C-L, et al. The effect of prenatal antidepressant exposure on neonatal adaptation. J Clin Psychiatry. 2013;74:e309–20.
63. Huybrechts KF, Palmsten K, Avorn J, Cohen LS, Holmes LB, Franklin JM, et al. Antidepressant use in pregnancy and the risk of cardiac defects. N Engl J Med. 2014;370:2397–407.
64. Brown HK, Ray JG, Wilton AS, Lunsky Y, Gomes T, Vigod SN. Association between serotonergic antidepressant use during pregnancy and autism spectrum disorder in children. JAMA. 2017;317:1544–52.
65. Sujan AC, Rickert ME, Oberg AS, Quinn PD, Hernandez-Diaz S, Almqvist C, et al. Associations of maternal antidepressant use during the first trimester of pregnancy with preterm birth, small for gestational age, autism spectrum disorder, and attention-deficit/hyperactivity disorder in offspring. JAMA. 2017;317:1553–62.

Permissions

All chapters in this book were first published in MEDICINE, by BioMed Central; hereby published with permission under the Creative Commons Attribution License or equivalent. Every chapter published in this book has been scrutinized by our experts. Their significance has been extensively debated. The topics covered herein carry significant findings which will fuel the growth of the discipline. They may even be implemented as practical applications or may be referred to as a beginning point for another development.

The contributors of this book come from diverse backgrounds, making this book a truly international effort. This book will bring forth new frontiers with its revolutionizing research information and detailed analysis of the nascent developments around the world.

We would like to thank all the contributing authors for lending their expertise to make the book truly unique. They have played a crucial role in the development of this book. Without their invaluable contributions this book wouldn't have been possible. They have made vital efforts to compile up to date information on the varied aspects of this subject to make this book a valuable addition to the collection of many professionals and students.

This book was conceptualized with the vision of imparting up-to-date information and advanced data in this field. To ensure the same, a matchless editorial board was set up. Every individual on the board went through rigorous rounds of assessment to prove their worth. After which they invested a large part of their time researching and compiling the most relevant data for our readers.

The editorial board has been involved in producing this book since its inception. They have spent rigorous hours researching and exploring the diverse topics which have resulted in the successful publishing of this book. They have passed on their knowledge of decades through this book. To expedite this challenging task, the publisher supported the team at every step. A small team of assistant editors was also appointed to further simplify the editing procedure and attain best results for the readers.

Apart from the editorial board, the designing team has also invested a significant amount of their time in understanding the subject and creating the most relevant covers. They scrutinized every image to scout for the most suitable representation of the subject and create an appropriate cover for the book.

The publishing team has been an ardent support to the editorial, designing and production team. Their endless efforts to recruit the best for this project, has resulted in the accomplishment of this book. They are a veteran in the field of academics and their pool of knowledge is as vast as their experience in printing. Their expertise and guidance has proved useful at every step. Their uncompromising quality standards have made this book an exceptional effort. Their encouragement from time to time has been an inspiration for everyone.

The publisher and the editorial board hope that this book will prove to be a valuable piece of knowledge for researchers, students, practitioners and scholars across the globe.

List of Contributors

G. Lu
Medical College of Yangzhou University, Yangzhou University, Yangzhou 225001, China
Institute of Public Health, Medical School, Ruprecht-Karls-University Heidelberg, Heidelberg, Germany

M. Nagbanshi, N. Goldau, M. Mendes Jorge, A. Jahn and O. Müller
Institute of Public Health, Medical School, Ruprecht-Karls-University Heidelberg, Heidelberg, Germany

P. Meissner
Department of Paediatric and Adolescent Medicine, Ulm University, Ulm, Germany

F. P. Mockenhaupt
Institute of Tropical Medicine and International Health, Charité-Universitätsmedizin Berlin, Berlin, Germany

Umme Z. Mulla
Centre for Innovative Research Across the Life Course (CIRAL), Faculty of Health and Life Sciences, Coventry University, Coventry CV1 5FB, UK

Petra A. Wark
Centre for Innovative Research Across the Life Course (CIRAL), Faculty of Health and Life Sciences, Coventry University, Coventry CV1 5FB, UK
Global eHealth Unit, Department of Primary Care and Public Health, Imperial College, Imperial College, London SW7 2AZ, UK

Laura J. Hardie, David Murphy and Gregory D. M. Potter
Division of Epidemiology and Biostatistics, Leeds Institute for Cardiovascular and Metabolic Medicine, School of Medicine, University of Leeds, Leeds LS2 9JT, UK

Darren C. Greenwood
Division of Epidemiology and Biostatistics, Leeds Institute for Cardiovascular and Metabolic Medicine, School of Medicine, University of Leeds, Leeds LS2 9JT, UK
Leeds Institute of Data Analytics, University of Leeds, Leeds LS2 9JT, UK

Gary S. Frost, Heather E. Ford and K. Petropoulou
Nutrition and Dietetic Research Group, Division of Diabetes, Endocrinology and Metabolism, Faculty of Medicine, Imperial College London, London W12 ONN, UK

Nisreen A. Alwan
Academic Unit of Primary Care and Population Sciences, Faculty of Medicine, University of Southampton, Southampton SO16 6YD, UK
NIHR Southampton Biomedical Research Centre, University of Southampton and University Hospital Southampton NHS Foundation Trust, Southampton SO166YD, UK

Michelle Carter, Neil Hancock and Janet E. Cade
Nutritional Epidemiology Group, School of Food Science and Nutrition, University of Leeds, Leeds LS2 9JT, UK

Essra A. Noorwali
Nutritional Epidemiology Group, School of Food Science and Nutrition, University of Leeds, Leeds LS2 9JT, UK
Department of Clinical Nutrition, Faculty of Applied Medical Sciences, Umm Al-Qura University, Makkah 21955, Saudi Arabia

Paul Elliott and Elio Riboli
MRC-PHE Centre for Environment and Health, Department of Epidemiology and Biostatistics, School of Public Health, Faculty of Medicine, Imperial College London, London W2 1PG, UK

Michelle A. Morris
Leeds Institute of Data Analytics, University of Leeds, Leeds LS2 9JT, UK

Ushma D. Upadhyay, Nicole E. Johns and Alice F. Cartwright
Department of Obstetrics, Gynecology & Reproductive Sciences, University of California, San Francisco, 1330 Broadway, Suite 1100, Oakland, California 94612, USA

Rebecca Barron, Chantal Tapé, Alyssa Mierjeski and Alyson J. McGregor
Department of Emergency Medicine, Warren Alpert Medical School of Brown University, 593 Eddy Street, Providence, RI 02903, USA

Karen M. Edmond, Khaksar Yousufi and Ariel Higgins-Steele
UNICEF Afghanistan, UNOCA, Jalalabad Road, Kabul, Afghanistan

Zelaikha Anwari
Ministry of Public Health, Reproductive, Maternal, Newborn, Child and Adolescent Directorate, Kabul, Afghanistan

Sayed Masoud Sadat
Ministry of Public Health, Community Based Health Care Department, Kabul, Afghanistan

Shah Mansoor Staniczai
Save The Children, Kabul, Afghanistan

Alexandra L. Bellows and Emily R. Smith
Department of Global Health and Population, Harvard TH Chan School of Public Health, Boston, USA

Kirsten M. Fiest
Departments of Critical Care Medicine and Community Health Sciences, O'Brien Institute for Public Health and Hotchkiss Brain Institute, Cumming School of Medicine, University of Calgary, 2500 University Drive NW, Calgary, AB T2N 1N4, Canada

Christiane Job McIntosh and Danielle Demiantschuk
Department of Critical Care Medicine, Cumming School of Medicine, University of Calgary, 2500 University Drive NW, Calgary, AB T2N 1N4, Canada

Jeanna Parsons Leigh
Department of Critical Care Medicine, O'Brien Institute for Public Health, Cumming School of Medicine, University of Calgary, 2500 University Drive NW, Calgary, AB T2N 1N4, Canada

Henry T. Stelfox
Departments of Critical Care Medicine, Medicine and Community Health Sciences, O'Brien Institute for Public Health, Cumming School of Medicine, University of Calgary, 2500 University Drive NW, Calgary, AB T2N 1N4, Canada

Georgina A. V. Murphy
Centre for Tropical Medicine and Global Health, Nuffield Department of Medicine, University of Oxford, Oxford, UK
Kenya Medical Research Institute - Wellcome Trust Research Programme, Nairobi, Kenya

David Gathara, Jacintah Mwachiro and Jalemba Aluvaala
Kenya Medical Research Institute - Wellcome Trust Research Programme, Nairobi, Kenya

Mike English
Kenya Medical Research Institute - Wellcome Trust Research Programme, Nairobi, Kenya
Centre for Tropical Medicine and Global Health, Nuffield Department of Medicine, University of Oxford, Oxford, UK

Nancy Abuya
Kenya Medical Research Institute - Wellcome Trust Research Programme, Nairobi, Kenya
Nairobi City County Government, Nairobi, Kenya

Masoud Babaei
Division of Clinical Epidemiology and Aging Research, German Cancer Research Center (DKFZ), Im Neuenheimer Feld 581, 69120 Heidelberg, Germany

Lei Huang
Division of Clinical Epidemiology and Aging Research, German Cancer Research Center (DKFZ), Im Neuenheimer Feld 581, 69120 Heidelberg, Germany
Medical Faculty Heidelberg, Heidelberg University, Heidelberg, Germany

Lina Jansen
Division of Clinical Epidemiology and Aging Research, German Cancer Research Center (DKFZ), Im Neuenheimer Feld 581, 69120 Heidelberg, Germany
German Cancer Consortium (DKTK), German Cancer Research Center (DKFZ), Heidelberg, Germany

Hermann Brenner
Division of Clinical Epidemiology and Aging Research, German Cancer Research Center (DKFZ), Im Neuenheimer Feld 581, 69120 Heidelberg, Germany
German Cancer Consortium (DKTK), German Cancer Research Center (DKFZ), Heidelberg, Germany
Division of Preventive Oncology, DKFZ and National Center for Tumor Diseases (NCT), Heidelberg, Germany

Yesilda Balavarca and Petra Schrotz-King
Division of Preventive Oncology, DKFZ and National Center for Tumor Diseases (NCT), Heidelberg, Germany

Lydia van der Geest and Valery Lemmens
The Netherlands Cancer Registry, The Netherlands Comprehensive Cancer Organization (IKNL), Utrecht, the Netherlands

Liesbet Van Eycken and Harlinde De Schutter
Belgian Cancer Registry (BCR), Brussels, Belgium

Tom B. Johannesen
Cancer Registry of Norway (CRN), Oslo, Norway

Maja Primic-Žakelj and Vesna Zadnik
Cancer Registry of Slovenia (CRS), Ljubljana, Slovenia

Marc G. Besselink
Dutch Pancreatic Cancer Group, Amsterdam UMC, University of Amsterdam, Amsterdam, the Netherlands

Alexandra B. Hogan, Peter Winskill, Robert Verity and Azra C. Ghani
Department of Infectious Disease Epidemiology, MRC Centre for Global Infectious Disease Analysis, Imperial College London, School of Public Health, St Mary's Campus, Norfolk Place, London W2 1PG, UK

Jamie T. Griffin
Department of Infectious Disease Epidemiology, MRC Centre for Global Infectious Disease Analysis, Imperial College London, School of Public Health, St Mary's Campus, Norfolk Place, London W2 1PG, UK
School of Mathematical Sciences, Queen Mary University London, Mile End Road, London E1 4NS, UK

Jennifer M. Ross
Division of Allergy and Infectious Diseases, Department of Medicine, University of Washington, Seattle, Washington, USA
Institute for Health Metrics and Evaluation, University of Washington, 2301 5th Ave Suite 600, Seattle, WA 98121, USA

Nathaniel J. Henry, Laura A. Dwyer-Lindgren, Molly H. Biehl, Sarah E. Ray, Robert C. Reiner Jr, Rebecca W. Stubbs, Kirsten E. Wiens, Lucas Earl, Michael J. Kutz, Natalia V. Bhattacharjee, Hmwe H. Kyu, Mohsen Naghavi and Simon I. Hay
Institute for Health Metrics and Evaluation, University of Washington, 2301 5th Ave Suite 600, Seattle, WA 98121, USA

Andrea de Paula Lobo
Department of Public Health, University of Brasilia, Distrito Federal, Brazil
Department of Health Surveillance, Ministry of Health, Brasilia, Brazil

Fatima Marinho de Souza
Department of Health Surveillance, Ministry of Health, Brasilia, Brazil

John Wilding
University of Liverpool, Liverpool, UK

Thomas Godec, Stuart Pocock and Liam Smeeth
London School of Hygiene and Tropical Medicine, London, UK

Kamlesh Khunti
University of Leicester, Leicester, UK

Robin Fox
Bicester Health Centre, Bicester, UK

Per Clauson and Niklas Hammar
AstraZeneca, Gothenburg, Sweden

Peter Fenici
AstraZeneca, Luton, UK

Jesús Medina
AstraZeneca Farmacéutica Spain, Madrid, Spain

Mingwang Shen
Department of Epidemiology and Biostatistics, School of Public Health, Xi'an Jiaotong University Health Science Center, Xi'an, Shaanxi 710061, People's Republic of China
School of Mathematics and Statistics, Xi'an Jiaotong University, Xi'an 710049, People's Republic of China
Department of Integrative Biology, The University of Texas at Austin, Austin, TX 78712, USA

Yanni Xiao
School of Mathematics and Statistics, Xi'an Jiaotong University, Xi'an 710049, People's Republic of China

Lauren Ancel Meyers
Department of Integrative Biology, The University of Texas at Austin, Austin, TX 78712, USA
The Santa Fe Institute, Santa Fe, NM 87501, USA

Libin Rong
Department of Mathematics, University of Florida, Gainesville, FL 32611, USA

Steven E. Bellan
Department of Epidemiology and Biostatistics, College of Public Health, University of Georgia, Athens, GA 30602, USA
Center for Ecology of Infectious Diseases, University of Georgia, Athens, GA 30602, USA

Ludovic Trinquart
Department of Biostatistics, Boston University School of Public Health, Boston, Massachusetts, USA

Adam G. Dunn
Centre for Health Informatics, Australian Institute of Health Innovation, Macquarie University, Sydney, Australia

Florence T. Bourgeois
Department of Pediatrics, Harvard Medical School, Boston, Massachusetts, USA
Center for Pediatric Therapeutics and Regulatory Science, and Computational Health Informatics Program, Boston Children's Hospital, Boston, MA, USA

Sascha Ludwig
Department of Cardiology and Pneumology, Göttingen University Medical Centre, Robert-Koch-Straße 40, D-37075 Göttingen, Germany

Tobias Raupach
Department of Cardiology and Pneumology, Göttingen University Medical Centre, Robert-Koch-Straße 40, D-37075 Göttingen, Germany
Health Behaviour Research Centre, University College London, 1-19 Torrington Place, London WC1E 7HB, UK

Nikolai Schuelper
Department of Haematology and Medical Oncology, Göttingen University Medical Centre, Robert-Koch-Straße 40, D-37075 Göttingen, Germany

Jamie Brown
Health Behaviour Research Centre, University College London, 1-19 Torrington Place, London WC1E 7HB, UK

Sven Anders
Department of Legal Medicine, University Medical Centre Hamburg-Eppendorf, Butenfeld 34, D-22529 Hamburg, Germany

Su Yun Kang, Katherine E. Battle, Harry S. Gibson, Daniel J. Weiss, Ewan Cameron and Peter W. Gething
Malaria Atlas Project, Oxford Big Data Institute, Nuffield Department of Medicine, University of Oxford, Oxford, UK

Rosalind E. Howes
Malaria Atlas Project, Oxford Big Data Institute, Nuffield Department of Medicine, University of Oxford, Oxford, UK
Center for Global Health and Diseases, Case Western Reserve University, Cleveland, OH, USA

Arsène Ratsimbasoa
National Malaria Control Programme, Ministry of Health, Antananarivo, Madagascar
University of Antananarivo, Antananarivo, Madagascar

Stéphanie Ramboarina
National Malaria Control Programme, Ministry of Health, Antananarivo, Madagascar
University of Antananarivo, Antananarivo, Madagascar
Center for Global Health and Diseases, Case Western Reserve University, Cleveland, OH, USA

Milijaona Randrianarivelojosia
Institut Pasteur de Madagascar, Antananarivo, Madagascar
Faculté des Sciences, Université de Toliara, Toliara, Madagascar

Peter A. Zimmerman
Center for Global Health and Diseases, Case Western Reserve University, Cleveland, OH, USA

Thomas Harder, Ole Wichmann and Miriam Wiese-Posselt
Robert Koch Institute, Immunization Unit, Seestrasse 10, 13353 Berlin, Germany

Stefanie J. Klug
Department of Sport and Health Sciences, Technical University Munich, Chair of Epidemiology, Munich, Germany

Marianne A. B. van der Sande
Institute of Tropical Medicine, Antwerp, Belgium

Nicola Heslehurst, Heather Brown, Augustina Pemu, Hayley Coleman and Judith Rankin
Institute of Health & Society, Newcastle University, Baddiley-Clark Building, Richardson Road, Newcastle upon Tyne NE2 4AX, UK

Itziar Ubillos
ISGlobal, Hospital Clínic, Universitat de Barcelona, Carrer Rosselló 153 CEK building, E-08036 Barcelona, Catalonia, Spain

Augusto J Nhabomba
Centro de Investigação em Saúde de Manhiça (CISM), Rua 12, Cambeve, Vila de Manhiça, CP 1929 Maputo, Mozambique

David Dosoo
Kintampo Health Research Centre, Kintampo, Ghana

Maximilian Mpina
Ifakara Health Institute, Bagamoyo Research and Training Center, Bagamoyo, Tanzania

Clarissa Valim
Department of Osteopathic Medical Specialties, Michigan State University, 909 Fee Road, Room B 309 West Fee Hall, East Lansing, MI 48824, USA
Department of Immunology and Infectious Diseases, Harvard T.H. Chen School of Public Health, 675 Huntington Ave., Boston, MA 02115, USA

Sam E. van Grinsven
Department of Clinical Psychology, Utrecht University, Heidelberglaan 1, 3584 CS Utrecht, the Netherlands

Marlies E. Brouwer
Department of Clinical Psychology, Utrecht University, Heidelberglaan 1, 3584 CS Utrecht, the Netherlands
Department of Psychiatry, Amsterdam University Medical Centres, location AMC, University of Amsterdam, Meibergdreef 9, 1105 AZ Amsterdam, the Netherlands

Claudi L. H. Bockting
Department of Psychiatry, Amsterdam University Medical Centres, location AMC, University of Amsterdam, Meibergdreef 9, 1105 AZ Amsterdam, the Netherlands

Alishia D. Williams
Department of Clinical Psychology, Utrecht University, Heidelberglaan 1, 3584 CS Utrecht, the Netherlands
Faculty of Science, School of Psychology, The University of New South Wales, Sydney, NSW 2052, Australia

Pim Cuijpers
Department of Clinical, Neuro and Developmental Psychology, Vrije Universiteit Amsterdam, Van der Boechorststraat 1, 1081 BT Amsterdam, the Netherlands

Mijke P. Lambregtse-van den Berg
Department of Psychiatry and Child and Adolescent Psychiatry/Psychology, Erasmus Medical Centre Rotterdam, 3000 CB Rotterdam, the Netherlands

Huibert Burger
Department of General Practice, University Medical Centre Groningen, University of Groningen, Antonius Deusinglaan 1, 9713 AV Groningen, the Netherlands

Index

www.ingramcontent.com/pod-product-compliance
Lightning Source LLC
LaVergne TN
LVHW061510220926
848485LV00017B/707